MEDICAL MICROBIOLOGY
A Short Course

Ellen Jo Baron
Department of Medicine
UCLA School of Medicine

Robert S. Chang
Department of Medical Microbiology and
    Immunology, School of Medicine
University of California, Davis

Dexter H. Howard
Department of Microbiology and Immunology
UCLA School of Medicine

James N. Miller
Department of Microbiology and Immunology
UCLA School of Medicine

Jerrold A. Turner
Departments of Medicine and Microbiology
    and Immunology
UCLA School of Medicine
Harbor–UCLA Medical Center

Chapter 2. Physiology and Metabolism
Contributed by
Robert P. Gunsalus
Department of Microbiology and Molecular
    Genetics
University of California, Los Angeles

Chapter 3. Genetic Variability of
    Microorganisms
Contributed by
Alexander D. Johnson
Department of Microbiology and Immunology
University of California, San Francisco

MEDICAL MICROBIOLOGY
A Short Course

Ellen Jo Baron
Robert S. Chang
Dexter H. Howard
James N. Miller
Jerrold A. Turner

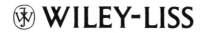

WILEY-LISS

A JOHN WILEY & SONS, INC., PUBLICATION
New York • Chichester • Brisbane • Toronto • Singapore

Address All Inquiries to the Publisher
Wiley-Liss, Inc., 605 Third Avenue
New York, NY 10158-0012

Copyright © 1994 Wiley-Liss, Inc.

Printed in the United States of America

All rights reserved. This book is protected by copyright. No part of it, except brief excerpts for review, may be reproduced, stored in a retrieval system, or transmitted in any form or by any means, electronic, mechanical, photocopying, recording, or otherwise, without permission from the publisher.

Library of Congress Cataloging-in-Publication Data

Medical microbiology : a short course / Ellen Jo Baron . . . [et al.].
        p.   cm.
    Includes bibliographical references and index.
    ISBN 0-471-56728-0
    1. Medical microbiology. I. Baron, Ellen Jo.
    [DNLM: 1. Microbiology. QW 4 M4882 1993]
QR46.M4724   1993
616′.01—dc20
DNLM/DLC
for Library of Congress   93-16481

The text of this book is printed on acid-free paper.

CONTENTS

SECTION II: MYCOLOGY
Dexter H. Howard

SECTION III: VIROLOGY
Robert S. Chang

SECTION IV: PARASITOLOGY
Jerrold A. Turner

FOREWORD

Why was this book written? At a time when so many excellent, extensive, and beautifully illustrated texts flood the bookstores, why offer another one? The reasons are fairly simple and rather unsophisticated. In our collective experience of many years of teaching all kinds of students, we have become convinced that most texts fail their purpose because they overshoot the mark.

Anyone who comes in contact year after year with students, especially medical students in their preclinical years, cannot fail to appreciate the burden under which these students operate. To graduate, they must learn an enormous amount of material on an exceptionally diverse series of subjects, each increasing in scope yearly. As any student can tell you, all lecturers consider their particular topic absolutely "essential." And so, the pile of "essentials" grows and grows. To deal with this difficulty, various curriculum innovations have been proposed and implemented in many schools. Despite such innovations, the basic vocabulary and concepts, and what instructors deem "essential," keep growing.

A second cruel observation arises from long years of teaching and questioning students: many of them are not really interested in one or another of the required disciplines. As excited and all encompassingly passionate about a given discipline that we, the practitioners of that discipline tend to be, the students have many other interests and concerns. High among them is passing many courses, on diverse subjects, all taken simultaneously.

Recognizing these difficulties, a series of *Short Course* texts has been conceived along the lines of the noted architect Mies van der Rohe's dictum ''less is more.'' *Short Course* texts present the bare essentials of the discipline in a palatable form that will enable most students to grasp the vocabulary, essential principles, and important information sufficiently to assimilate the information, pass the course, and develop an adequate foundation for those who want to pursue deeper investigations in the given discipline.

Each book of the *Short Course* series is generally divided into ''bite size'' chapters that mostly approximate the length of an average lecture reading assignment. A short introduction, setting the stage, starts each chapter. The end of each chapter contains a summary and a series of questions designed to evaluate the student's progress and comprehension; the appended answers are meant as a further learning experience. As new terms or concepts are introduced, they are identified in boldface type and defined for easy recognition and recall.

The original book in the series, **Immunology: A Short Course,** continues to enjoy an overwhelming success and popularity among students, validating the *Short Course* teaching and learning approach. The present text, **Medical Microbiology: A Short Course,** has been written with the same pedagogical philosophy in mind. The text presents, in a succinct, yet comprehensive way, background material on various pathogenic organisms, and delineates the epidemiology, transmission, clinical manifestations, diagnosis, and treatment of diseases caused by these organisms. The book is divided into Bacteriology, Mycology, Virology, and Parasitology—the four sections that comprise a course in Medical Microbiology.

The Bacteriology section opens with a chapter written to familiarize students with basic concepts relating to bacterial architecture, pertinent phenotypic characteristics, and general structure-function relationships as they pertain to bacterial pathogenesis. This chapter, together with the chapter on host-parasite relationships, provides the necessary foundation for subsequent chapters designed to convey to the student simplified, clear explanations of mechanisms at play during the inactivation and destruction of microorganisms, bacterial genetics, and bacterial metabolism. A comprehensive survey of significant bacterial diseases is given, including their etiologic agents and mechanisms of pathogenesis.

The section on Mycology presents a succinct summary of the facts about medically important fungi. The areas covered include characteristics of zoopathogenic fungi, epidemiology, pathogenesis, and host responses. A practical summary of the diagnostic approaches available in a clinical laboratory most likely to yield information on the etiology of the infectious process and modality of treatment is also presented. The information in this section, while to some students, only mildly stimulating, is nevertheless useful. More importantly, it may be lifesaving. Care has been taken to present medical mycology in a few well-constructed chapters, thereby covering the subject in a way that allows the reader to prepare for any sort of examination or serving as a guide to the selection of diagnostic approaches in clinical settings.

Medical virology is currently expanding at a phenomenal rate—witness the vast expansion of new knowledge following the emergence of the AIDS epidemic. Nevertheless, the Virology section has been carefully abstracted and is presented in a form that the average student can assimilate in the time allotted for the subject. The first six chapters of the Virology section deal succinctly with basic concepts while the subsequent 11 chapters deal with individual virus families and their medical significance and importance.

In the section on Parasitology, each of the major parasitic diseases of humans is covered. Important features of the organism as well as the epidemiology, transmission, clinical manifestations, and treatment of the disease are included. Less common parasitic diseases are discussed in succinct paragraphs, that nonetheless contain these key elements. Summary tables are provided for most parasites as handy study guides, as are schematic life cycles, in an easily read left to right linear arrangement. A brief chapter describes the role of eosinophils in parasitic infections.

Separately and collectively, the four sections of *Medical Microbiology: A Short Course* present the core material in a form that the average student can easily assimilate. The information provides a more than adequate foundation for the student to comprehend publications in general medical journals dealing with this discipline. This book will also enable students to pass the course and licentiate examinations.

The authors hope that students using this book will avoid the choking sensation so common in many courses, and even conceive a curiosity about the subject that will lead to future study.

Eli Benjamini, Ph.D.
Professor of Immunology (Emeritus)
Department of Medical Microbiology
    and Immunology
School of Medicine
University of California, Davis

BACTERIOLOGY

GENERAL PROPERTIES
OF BACTERIA

The majority of bacteria on this planet are harmless. In fact, many are necessary for the existence of higher orders of life. Certain bacteria mineralize organic
constituents in soil so that plants can utilize them, and others synthesize vitamins
in humans.

Medical bacteriology is the study of the relatively small number of frank
pathogenic and potentially pathogenic bacteria and the interacting bacterial and
host factors that cause and influence infectious processes (pathogenesis). Nonpathogenic bacteria with similar hosts and environmental locations, as well as
structural and antigenic composition, must also be identified and differentiated. It
is essential to present the following general information about bacteria prior to a
detailed consideration of specific bacterial properties, bacterial-host interactions,
and the outcome of their confrontation: riddance vs. infection vs. disease.

VIRULENCE FACTORS

Virulence factors may be defined as substances responsible for the ability of
a bacterium to produce infection or disease. They exist as surface or subsurface
structures or extracellular products produced by the bacterium. Bacterial virulence

is determined by one or more operative factors, including those associated with adherence, invasiveness, antiphagocytic activity, intracellular parasitism, exotoxin production, endotoxin activity, hypersensitivity responsiveness, and/or antigenic variation. Virulence is also influenced by host response and host-parasite relationships that occur following parasite entrance.

CLASSIFICATION OF MICROORGANISMS

With the exception of the viruses, microorganisms are classified as **eukaryotic protists,** which consist of the protozoa, fungi, and algae other than blue-green, and **prokaryotes (Kingdom "Prokaryotae"),** which consist of the bacteria and blue-green algae. The eukaryotic protists can be either unicellular or multicellular, have a true nucleus with a distinct nuclear membrane, undergo typical chromosomal organization during cell division, and may (fungi and algae) or may not (protozoa trophozoites) contain a cell wall. The prokaryotes are unicellular, have neither a well-defined nucleus nor nuclear membrane, undergo amitotic division (binary fission), and (with one exception) contain a cell wall of unique chemical composition.

NOMENCLATURE AND IDENTIFICATION

Genotypic (DNA and RNA homology) and **phenotypic** (e.g., staining and biochemical properties, antigen-antibody reactivity) characteristics are used to name and identify bacteria. As with other living things, bacteria are placed in Orders, Families, Genera, and species. Knowledge of the Genus and species name and their correct written format is a basic requirement for medical and scientific personnel. As an example, the etiologic agent for anthrax is written as *Bacillus anthracis* or as *B. anthracis.*

There are bacteria within a species that exhibit differences in their properties that do not warrant a separate name but are of sufficient importance to be designated in some manner:

1. Based upon a single functional or structural difference, reference may be made to nonmotile strains of *Escherichia coli* or nonpiliated strains of *Neisseria gonorrhoeae.*

2. Based upon phenotypic differences, bacteria in the same Genus and species have been designated as subspecies as a means of differentiation. As an example, despite the almost 100% DNA homology between the etiologic agents of

syphilis and yaws, differences in geographic distribution, transmission, clinical manifestations, and pathogenicity for experimental animals prompted their respective designations as *Treponema pallidum* subsp. *pallidum* and *Treponema pallidum* subsp. *pertenue.*

3. Bacterial species may also be placed in serogroups, serotypes, or serovars based upon the antigenic diversity of their surface or subsurface antigens. To illustrate, most streptococci are grouped on the basis of specific cell wall polysaccharide antigens, *Streptococcus pneumoniae* is serotyped on the basis of its antigenically distinct polysaccharide capsule, and *Leptospira interrogans* species are designated as serovars based upon the antigenic diversity of their outer membrane.

STAINING

Staining of bacteria is necessary to observe them with relative clarity under the ordinary light microscope. A dye or dyes applied to a bacterial preparation may stain uniformly or reveal internal and external structures; these procedures are useful in bacterial classification and identification. A description of the various types of stains follows:

Simple stains refer to the application of a single dye to a bacterial smear (film). Although methylene blue is used as a simple stain to detect the characteristic metachromatic granules of *Corynebacterium diphtheriae* in the diagnosis of diphtheria, simple stains are rarely of value in diagnostic bacteriology.

Differential stains refer to the individual or combined application of two or more dyes to a bacterial smear. The Gram and acid-fast stains are the most important and widely used procedures in the staining of specimens and cultures for microscopic examination.

1. The **Gram stain,** developed by Christian Gram in 1884, permits the separation of bacteria into two broad groups. Bacteria stained with a basic aniline dye (crystal violet) fixed to the organisms with an iodine mordant, may either retain the dye or become decolorized after treatment with alcohol or acetone. Organisms that resist decolorization fail to take up a red basic aniline dye counterstain (safranin), appear purple or violet, and are referred to as **gram-positive.** In contrast, decolorized bacteria take up the counterstain, appear red, and are referred to as **gram-negative.**

The gram reaction is influenced by several factors, such as the age of the bacterial culture, temperature of incubation, constituents and pH of the culture medium, and thickness of the smear. Despite these potential causes for variation, consistently reliable Gram stain results are obtained when the procedure is performed properly. Although the mechanism of the reaction is unclear, it appears to be associated with differences in cell wall structure and permeability. The procedure is useful in the identification of pathogens in and from diagnostic specimens. In addition, architectural and antigenic dissimilarities between the two groups relate to overt differences in their virulence factors, the pathogenesis of the diseases they produce, and their susceptibility to antimicrobial agents.

2. The **acid-fast stain,** first developed by Ehrlich in 1882, is based upon the principle that bacteria belonging to the genera *Mycobacterium* and *Nocardia* are not easily stained with the usual aniline dyes. This is due to their high content of cell wall bound lipids. However, once the organisms belonging to these genera are stained and the dye fixed by a mordant, the dye is retained even when treated with alcohol containing acid. The red dye-phenol mixture first applied to the smear is carbolfuchsin; phenol (carbolic acid) acts as a mordant and fixes the fuchsin dye to the organisms. Methylene blue, added as a counterstain, is taken up only by decolorized organisms. Those organisms resistant to decolorization appear red and are referred to as **acid-fast.** The acid-fast stain is valuable in the diagnosis of nocardiosis and mycobacterial diseases such as tuberculosis, leprosy, and AIDS-associated infection with members of the *Mycobacterium avium-intracellulare* complex (MAC).

STRUCTURE AND STRUCTURE-FUNCTION RELATIONSHIPS

Bacteria range in size from 0.1 to 20 μm in length and from 0.2 to 2 μm in diameter. They are clearly visible under the light microscope at 900–1000× utilizing the oil immersion objective.

Bacteria are found in four forms (Fig. 1.1):

1. **Coccus (spherical).** Cocci may occur in clusters *(Staphylococcus aureus),* pairs *(S. pneumoniae),* or in chains *(Streptococcus pyogenes).*

2. **Bacillus (rod-shaped).** Bacilli may be long with square-cut ends *(B. anthracis)* or short with rounded ends *(Haemophilus influenzae);* if the organisms are so short as to appear as cocci, they are referred to as coccobacillary.

3. **Vibrio (curved).** Curved bacteria have a single turn *(Vibrio cholerae).*

4. **Spirillum, spirochete (spiral).** Spiral organisms have a series of turns or twists *(Borrelia burgdorferi).*

As shown in Figure 1.2, bacteria consist of a cell wall (one exception), cytoplasmic (plasma) membrane enclosing the cytoplasm, mesosomes, a nuclear apparatus, ribosomes, and various cytoplasmic granules. Some bacteria have cap-

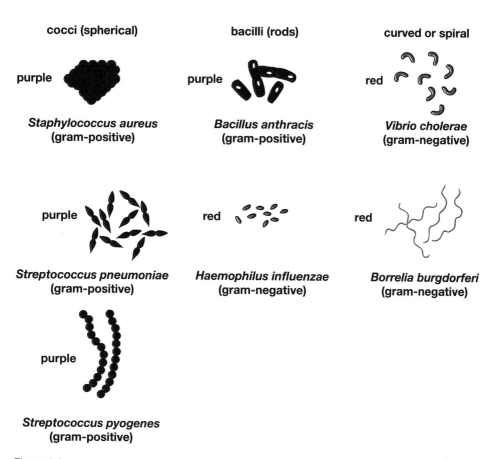

Figure 1.1.

Examples of bacterial shapes. The holes in *B. anthracis* represent unstained spores.

sules, flagella, pili, and/or can produce spores. The cytoplasmic membrane, cell wall, and capsule (if present) are referred to collectively as the **cell envelope.**

The **cytoplasmic (plasma) membrane** is a thin, ductile, elastic, trilaminar structure that encloses the cytoplasm and is composed mostly of proteins and lipoproteins embedded in a phospholipid bilayer (Figs. 1.3 and 1.4). This membrane functions as a significant osmotic barrier to low molecular weight substances, and as a semipermeable membrane controlling the exchange of substances between the cell and surrounding medium. Several enzymatically mediated biosynthetic processes, as well as electron transport and oxidative phosphorylation, take place within the membrane.

Mesosomes are saclike invaginations of the cytoplasmic membrane contain-

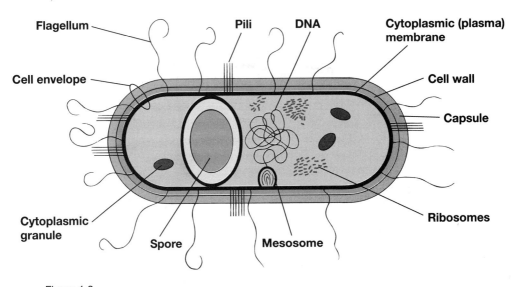

Figure 1.2.

Schematic diagram illustrating bacterial cell structure. The text indicates which of the structures are common to some bacteria and which are common to all bacteria.

ing circular or tubular structures that are attached to DNA chromatin. Mesosomes are thought to be associated in some way with cell division.

The **cell wall** is a constituent of all bacteria, except members of the genus *Mycoplasma* (Figs. 1.3 and 1.4). The cell wall lies in close approximation to the cytoplasmic membrane and has a chemical composition unique to the bacteria. This structure confers rigidity and shape to the bacterial cell and acts as a barrier to low molecular weight substances (<10,000). Inasmuch as mammalian cells lack cell walls, antimicrobial agents that inhibit cell wall synthesis (e.g., penicillin) or trigger cell wall autolysis will have selective activity against bacteria and little or no host toxicity. Bacterial rigidity and shape are attributable to a three-dimensional (3D) latticework layer, which lies closest to the cytoplasmic membrane and is referred to as **peptidoglycan (PG)** (syn: murein, mucopeptide).

As shown in Figure 1.5, PG is a biopolymer consisting of alternating units of *N*-acetyl-D-muramic acid and *N*-acetyl-D-glucosamine with a short peptide linked to the lactyl moiety of the M residues. The sugars are bound by β(1,4) glycosidic linkages, and the general structure of the peptide is as indicated on the diagram. The dibasic amino acid in gram-positive organisms is usually D-lysine and in gram-negative organisms *meso*-diaminopimilic acid (*m*-DAP). Covalent peptide linkages or cross-bridges lead to formation of the 3D, macromolecular "lattice" surrounding the cytoplasmic membrane. The peptide cross-bridges are

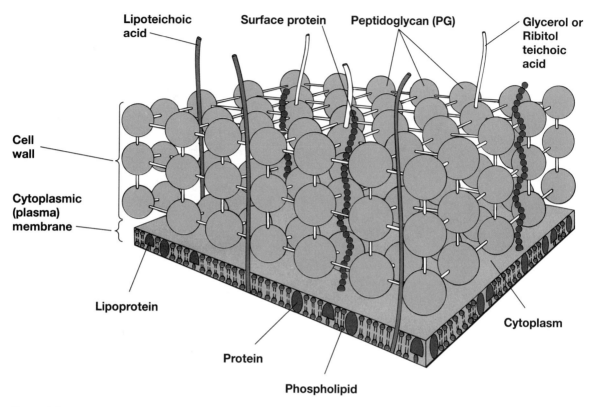

Figure 1.3.

Schematic diagram of the cell wall, cytoplasmic membrane, and cytoplasm of a typical gram-positive bacterium.

synthesized through the enzymatic action of a transpeptidase. The cell walls of gram-positive and gram-negative bacteria differ significantly in several structural aspects as illustrated in Figures 1.3 and 1.4.

The walls of **gram-positive** organisms are thick, compact, and almost exclusively PG (Fig. 1.3). The **teichoic acids**, which are polymers of ribitol or glycerol phosphate, are covalently linked to the PG of many of these organisms and, as major surface antigens, may act as virulence factors. All gram-positive bacteria contain **lipoteichoic acid (LTA)** covalently linked to the cytoplasmic membrane. This surface molecule acts as a virulence factor for *S. pyogenes* by participating in the mediation of attachment to buccal cell epithelium. Several gram-positive bacteria have surface proteins that are anchored or covalently linked to either the cytoplasmic membrane or PG, and may act as virulence factors or serve as the basis for a classification scheme.

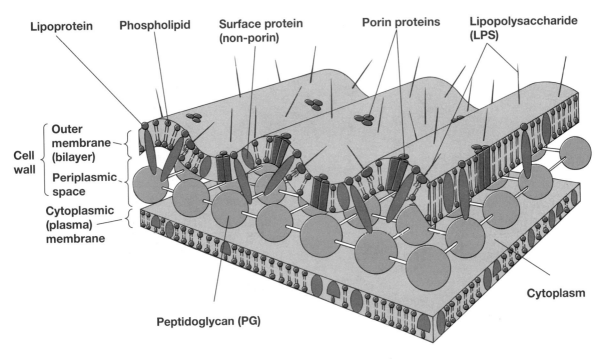

Figure 1.4.

Schematic diagram of the cell wall, cytoplasmic membrane, and cytoplasm of a typical gram-negative bacterium.

In contrast, the walls of **gram-negative** bacteria are thinner, less compact, and more complex in their chemical composition (Fig. 1.4). They are composed of a distinct, convoluted, wrinkled **outer membrane (OM)** bilayer and a distinct, thin PG layer separated from the cytoplasmic membrane by a **periplasmic space** containing binding proteins, which play a role in the specific transport of substances into the cell, and oligosaccharides, which are important in osmotic regulation. The OM is composed essentially of lipoproteins, phospholipids, porins, nonporins, and lipopolysaccharide, the latter making up the outer leaflet of the membrane almost exclusively.

Lipoproteins are the most abundant proteins of gram-negative bacteria; the lipid end is inserted into the OM while the protein end is covalently linked to PG.

Phospholipids form the OM matrix and contribute to OM stabilization.

Porins are OM protein trimers that form channels that permit small molecular weight solutes to diffuse across the OM; because porins are penetrated slowly

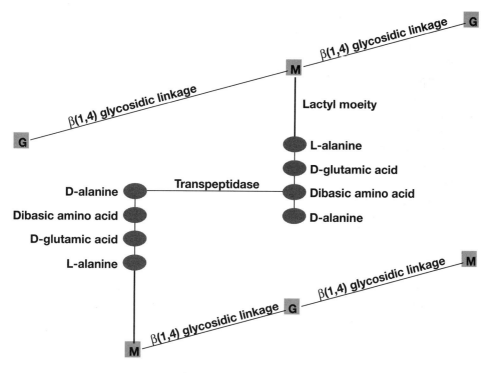

Figure 1.5.

General structure of the peptidoglycan molecule. G, *N*-acetyl-D-glucosamine; M, *N*-acetyl-D-muramic acid.

by large molecules, they may contribute to the relatively high resistance of gram-negative organisms to certain antimicrobial agents.

Nonporin proteins contribute to the anchoring of the OM to PG; certain of these proteins may be responsible for attachment, invasion, and/or iron binding, while the same or others (e.g., OM proteins of *Borrelia* that cause the relapsing fevers) may undergo antigenic variation and thus play a significant role in the pathogenesis and control of disease.

Lipopolysaccharide (LPS) (syn: endotoxin) consists of a glycolipid complex, referred to as lipid A, linked to a polysaccharide made up of a core and a terminal or side chain series of repeating units. LPS is toxic for humans, producing hypotension, fever, shock, intravascular coagulation, and/or tissue necrosis. The **lipid A moiety** is responsible for the **toxicity** of the molecule, the core polysaccharide components constitute the region common to many gram-negative organisms, and the **terminal repeating units or O side chains** consist of major surface antigens with diverse epitopes that confer **specificity** upon the organisms. The immunological specificity may be illustrated by the classification of over 2000 distinct serotypes of *Salmonella* based, in part, on the antigenic diversity among O side chain determinant groups.

Protoplast refers to a shapeless gram-positive bacterium whose cell wall has been removed in an osmotically stabilized medium by lysozyme hydrolysis or by inhibition of cell wall synthesis with an antimicrobial agent such as penicillin. Similar treatment of a gram-negative bacterium results in a nearly cell wall-less organism that has only retained some or all of its OM components and is referred to as a **spheroplast**. Actively growing and multiplying protoplasts and spheroplasts are generally called L forms. Although somewhat controversial, it has been hypothesized that protoplasts, spheroplasts, and L forms may be induced in a host by antimicrobial therapy thus offering a plausible explanation for the persistence or chronicity of infections.

Capsules are well-defined mucoid structures, usually polysaccharide in nature, which closely surround the cell wall of some bacteria. The **antiphagocytic** property of capsules contributes to the virulence of several pathogens, including *S. pneumoniae* and *H. influenzae*. The presence and **antigenic diversity** of capsules within a given bacterial species influence:

1. Pathogenesis. Nonencapsulated *H. influenzae* may produce chronic, noninvasive respiratory disease, but only the encapsulated strain is invasive.

2. Effective vaccine preparation. The immunological specificity of capsular polysaccharides must be considered in the preparation of capsular vaccines directed against diseases due to *S. pneumoniae, Neisseria meningitidis,* and *H. influenzae.*

3. The ability to make a rapid and accurate diagnosis. Antibodies directed against the specific capsular polysaccharides of bacterial pathogens may be utilized in the rapid diagnosis of the diseases they produce.

Flagella are long, slender appendages originating from a basal body and hooklike structure within the cytoplasmic membrane of several bacilli, vibrios, and spirilla. The majority of flagellated pathogens are completely surrounded by numerous flagella and are referred to as peritrichous. All flagella are composed entirely of a single protein subunit called flagellin, which differs in primary structure among different bacterial species. Flagella are responsible for **bacterial motility** that may **enhance bacterial invasion.** The surface of flagella is made up of protein antigens with diverse epitopes useful in the identification and classification of organisms such as those within the genus *Salmonella.* Spirochetes contain a similar motility apparatus, protein in nature, which lies in the periplasmic space between the cytoplasmic and outer membranes; they are referred to as **periplasmic flagella** (syn: endoflagella and axial filaments).

Pili are hairlike, rigid, surface appendages originating in the cytoplasmic membrane and observable by electron microscopy. These appendages are found predominately in gram-negative organisms and are composed of protein subunits called **pilin.** There are two types of pili, referred to as sex (F) pili and common pili (fimbriae).

1. **Sex pili.** Sex pili, of which only 1–4 are found at random bacterial sites, mediate the conjugation of donor and recipient cells and may participate in DNA transfer.

2. **Common pili.** In contrast, as many as 200 common pili may be evenly distributed over the surface of an organism and may act as virulence factors by **mediating adherence to host cell surfaces.** The pili of enterotoxigenic *E. coli* mediate the attachment and colonization of gut mucosal epithelium. The fimbria-like surface M protein of *S. pyogenes,* together with LTA, is responsible for adherence to host buccal epithelial cells. Nonpiliated *N. gonorrhoeae* do not produce disease presumably due to their inability to adhere and colonize. Once piliated bacteria are established within the host, the pili may undergo **antigenic variation** that enables them to **evade the host immune system.**

The bacterial **nuclear apparatus** has no visible nuclear membrane. It is an irregular, thin, fibrillar, single, double-stranded, closed, circular, DNA molecule. During multiplication, DNA never aggregates to form a well-defined chromosome during cell division but rather remains diffuse.

Bacterial ribosomes are located in the cytoplasm and are sites of protein synthesis. These ribosomes are 70S monomers composed of 30S and 50S subunits in contrast to the 80S monomer mammalian ribosomes that are made up of 40S and 60S subunits. The significance of this difference between bacterial and mammalian ribosomes is highlighted by the minimal toxicity of certain antimicrobial agents that act by selectively binding to the bacterial ribosome subunits.

Endospores are refractile bodies produced by vegetative cells after nutritional depletion of the medium in which they are grown. These bodies are highly resistant to heat and chemical agents and are able to survive for years in the environment. Of the bacterial genera that contain pathogens, the only two capable of forming endospores are *Bacillus* and *Clostridium.* Endospores may be oval or round and may be located terminally, subterminally, or centrally within the bacterial cell prior to lysis and release into the environment. A single bacterium produces a single endospore for the purpose of its survival; multiplication does not occur. Under favorable in vitro or in vivo nutritional and environmental conditions, an endospore germinates to produce a single vegetative cell; the significance of this observation is made clear by the fact that only vegetative cells are capable of producing the exotoxins responsible totally or in part for the pathogenesis of disease due to the endospore-forming pathogens.

Cytoplasmic granules are located in the bacterial cytoplasm. These granules represent stored food reserves consisting of protein, polysaccharide, and/or lipid. The presence and location of granules within members of the genus *Corynebacterium* can be accentuated and clearly visualized by growth of the organisms on special media thus serving as an aid in their identification.

SUMMARY

1. Bacterial virulence is determined by one or more operative factors including those associated with adherence, invasiveness, antiphagocytic activity, intracellular parasitism, exotoxin production, hypersensitive responsiveness, and/or antigenic variation.

2. Bacteria are unicellular, have neither a well-defined nucleus nor a nuclear membrane, undergo amitotic division (binary fission), and (with one exception) contain a cell wall of unique chemical composition.

3. The Gram and acid-fast stains are the two most important and widely used procedures in the staining of specimens and cultures for microscopic examination. The Gram stain identifies gram-positive and gram-negative bacteria, which exhibit dissimilarities in their structural and antigenic makeup that relate to overt differences in their virulence factors, in the pathogenesis of the diseases they produce, and in their susceptibility to antimicrobial agents. Inasmuch as only members of the genera *Nocardia* and *Mycobacterium* are acid-fast, this staining procedure is a valuable laboratory adjunct in the diagnosis of nocardiosis and mycobacterial diseases such as tuberculosis, leprosy, and AIDS-associated infection with members of the *Mycobacterium avium-intracellulare* complex (MAC).

4. Bacteria consist of a unique cell wall (with one exception), a cytoplasmic membrane enclosing the cytoplasm, mesosomes, a nuclear apparatus, ribosomes, and various cytoplasmic granules. Some have capsules, flagella, pili, and/or can produce spores.

5. Differences in cell wall structure between gram-positive and gram-

negative bacteria account for differences in their functional properties as well as their susceptibility to antimicrobial agents.

6. Capsules, usually polysaccharide, closely surround the cell wall of some bacteria. These capsules may be antiphagocytic, vaccinogenic, and/or identifiable in rapid diagnostic tests utilizing specific antiserum.

7. Flagella are composed of a single protein subunit called flagellin and are responsible for motility. Flagella may function as virulence factors by enhancing invasion and may be useful in classification and identification because of their unique surface epitopes. Spirochetes contain a similar motility apparatus, protein in nature, which lies in the periplasmic space between the cytoplasmic membrane and the OM.

8. Common and sex (F) pili are hairlike surface protein appendages. Sex pili mediate the conjugation of donor and recipient cells, while common pili (fimbriae) may be associated with virulence by mediating adherence of bacteria to host cell surfaces.

9. Bacterial ribosomes, located in the cytoplasm, are sites of protein synthesis. Endospores are highly resistant refractile bodies produced by the vegetative cells of only the *Bacillus* and *Clostridium* genera of bacteria among pathogens.

REFERENCES

Aronson AI, Fitz-James P (1976): Structure and morphogenesis of the bacterial spore coat. Bacteriol Rev 40:360.

Beveridge TJ (1981): Ultrastructure, chemistry, and function of bacterial wall. Int Rev Cytol 72:229.

Clegg S, Geilach GF (1987): Enterobacterial fimbriae. J Bacteriol 169:939.

Costerton JW, Ingram JM, Cheng KJ (1974): Structure and function of the cell envelope of gram-negative bacteria. Bacteriol Rev 38:87.

MacNab RM (1987): Flagella. In Neidhardt FC (ed): *Escherichia coli* and *Salmonella typhimurium*: Cellular and Molecular Biology. Washington, DC: ASM Press. pp 70–90.

Nikaido H, Vaara M (1985): Molecular basis of outer membrane permeability. Microbiol Rev 49:1.

Ottow JC (1975): Ecology, physiology, and genetics of fimbriae and pili. Annu Rev Microbiol 29:79.

Rietschel ET, Brade H (1992): Bacterial endotoxins. Sci Am 267:54.

Truper HG, Schleifer K-H (1992): Prokaryote characterization and identification. In Balows A, Truper HG, Dworkin M, Harder W, Schleifer K-H (eds): The Prokaryotes. 2nd ed, Vol. I. New York: Springer-Verlag. pp 126–148.

Wheat RW (1992): Bacterial morphology and ultrastructure. In Joklik WK, Willett HP, Amos DB, Wilfert CM (eds): Zinsser Microbiology. 20th ed. Norwalk, CT: Appleton & Lange. pp 18–30.

Widermann BL, Kaplan SL (1992): Microbial virulence factors. In Feigin RD, Cherry JD (eds): Textbook of Pediatric Infectious Diseases. 3rd ed, Vol 1. Philadelphia: W. B. Saunders. pp 119–130.

REVIEW QUESTIONS

For questions 1 to 3, choose the ONE BEST answer or completion.

1. Prokaryotes, which include the bacteria, *differ* from the eukaryotic protists in that the *former*
   a) do not exhibit tissue differentiation
   b) are identified on the basis of phenotypic expression
   c) have neither a distinct nucleus nor a nuclear membrane
   d) are unicellular
   e) contain a cell wall

2. Bacterial virulence factors
   a) always exist as either surface or subsurface structures
   b) are exclusively protein or lipoprotein in nature
   c) may be produced by clostridial spores
   d) exist only among gram-negative organisms
   e) may be single or multiple for a given disease process

3. The Gram stain is a valuable procedure because
   a) it can be used to distinguish members of the genera *Mycobacterium* and *Nocardia* from other bacterial genera containing pathogens
   b) it can be employed to divide bacteria into two broad groups useful as an aid in diagnostic bacteriology
   c) it selectively identifies encapsulated organisms
   d) it utilizes the single application of an aniline dye to a smear followed by acid-alcohol treatment
   e) it differentiates between flagellated and piliated organisms

For questions 4 to 7, ONE or MORE of the completions given is correct. Choose the appropriate answer.

A) if only **1, 2, 3** are correct
B) if only **1 and 3** are correct
C) if only **2 and 4** are correct
D) if only **4** is correct
E) if **all** are correct

4. The cell walls of gram-positive and gram-negative bacteria
   1) are unique in their chemical composition
   2) exhibit significant differences in structure and function
   3) contain peptidoglycan, which is responsible for their shape and rigidity
   4) are composed of an outer membrane bilayer
   5) contain lipopolysaccharide (LPS)

5. The bacterial capsule
   1) may be antiphagocytic and thus contribute to invasiveness
   2) is usually polysaccharide in nature
   3) may be antigenically diverse among the same species of organisms
   4) may stimulate specific protective antibody
   5) may stimulate specific antibody useful as assays for rapid identification and diagnosis

6. Flagella and common pili of bacteria
   1) are found predominantly in gram-negative bacteria
   2) are protein in nature
   3) lie between the cytoplasmic and outer membrane
   4) may function independently as virulence factors
   5) are responsible for motility

7. The bacterial endospore
   1) is produced for the purpose of the organism's survival
   2) is highly resistant to heat, several chemical agents, and environmental conditions
   3) is produced by members of the genera *Bacillus* and *Clostridium,* both of which contain pathogens
   4) germinates under favorable nutritional and environmental conditions to produce a single vegetative cell
   5) of pathogens must germinate if exotoxin is to be produced

ANSWERS TO REVIEW QUESTIONS

1. *c* Only the prokaryotes have neither a distinct nucleus nor nuclear membrane. The other characteristics are exhibited by both prokaryotes and eukaryotic protists..

2. *e* Bacterial virulence is determined by operative single or multiple factors associated with the surface or subsurface structure(s) and/or extracellular products of gram-positive and gram-negative organisms. These virulence factors may be protein, polysaccharide, or lipid in nature and are never produced by spores.

3. *b* The use of the Gram stain to classify the bacteria as gram-positive or gram-negative provides a useful adjunct in diagnostic bacteriology. The Gram and acid-fast stains are differential stains, the latter utilized in the diagnosis of mycobacterial and nocardial disease. Neither staining procedure can be used to selectively identify capsules, flagella, or pili.

4. *A* Only the walls of gram-negative organisms contain an outer membrane bilayer and LPS.

5. **E** All are correct statements.

6. **C** Flagella may be found with equal predominance in both gram-positive and gram-negative bacteria. Only the periplasmic flagella of spirochetes are found between the cytoplasmic and outer membrane. Flagella are the organelles of locomotion while common pili are responsible for adherence.

7. **E** All are correct statements.

PHYSIOLOGY AND METABOLISM

Bacteria compose about one-half of the earth's total biomass and these bacteria recycle much of the organic materials in the biosphere. However, only a relatively small number of the bacterial species affect humans detrimentally. The average healthy human contains numerous species of bacteria on the skin, under nails, in the nose, mouth, vagina and in the intestines and colon, which are either harmless or in some instances highly beneficial. It is estimated that there are more bacterial cells residing in the gut than there are human cells in the entire body.

Of the numerous types of bacteria on earth, each species exhibits a unique set of structural, biochemical, and genetic properties that allows it to be taxonomically identified. If these properties are known, it allows us to relatively easily predict the ability of a species to colonize and multiply in various habitats, including humans. It also allows us to predict the beneficial or deleterious effects on humans. This chapter summarizes the general principles of bacterial growth and nutrition, and the modes of cellular metabolism and energy generation. Bacteria have evolved a variety of strategies to extract useful energy from the available resources in a particular habitat whether it be in the soil, in water, on a plant, or on the inside or outside of a human host. However, these bacteria share very similar properties regarding cell structure, growth, and division.

Growth of the bacterial cell occurs by a vegetative process known as **binary fission,** which is asexual. Binary fission is a rapid process that occurs in a generally predictable manner with time (Fig. 2.1). Upon introduction of a bacterium into a suitable new growth environment, a short **lag phase** occurs while the cell adapts to its new surroundings. During this time, the cell must synthesize any new machinery needed for cellular biosynthesis and energy generation to fuel cell growth. Once optimally adjusted to its new surroundings, the cell initiates a phase of rapid cell growth and division, termed the **exponential** or **log phase.** Bacterial cell numbers increase in an exponential manner until some essential nutrient becomes limiting in the cells environment, or alternatively, a toxic end product of cell metabolism accumulates that is deleterious for the growth process. Cell growth then slows and usually stops within a single cell generation time. The bacteria have entered the **stationary phase** where nearly all cellular biosynthesis have ceased. The cell remains viable but it has readjusted its cellular metabolism to provide for cell maintenance only. If new or alternative nutrients are not encountered, cellular energy supplies are eventually depleted and the cells enter a **death phase.** The population of viable cells decreases until eventually no living cells remain. Cell lysis and the concomitant release of the cell contents reduces the total cell numbers. Depending on the bacterial species, this phase may be relatively short (hours to days) or quite long (months for some soil bacteria). Certain bacterial species can undergo a cellular differentiation process to form cell resting stages known as **spores** and **cysts** that allow survival over long periods of time

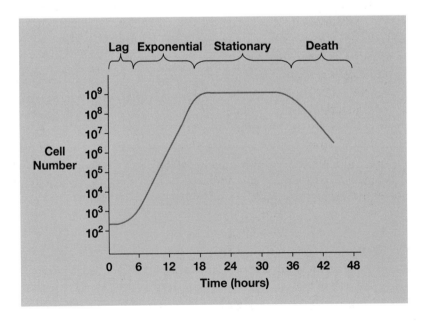

Figure 2.1.

Typical bacterial growth curve.

(i.e., months to years). Spores and cysts show little apparent metabolic activity (described below).

The cell **generation time** or cell **doubling time** refers to the period required to complete one round of cell division (e.g., 1 cell → 2 cells). The length of time is dependent on the bacterial species being considered and the conditions used for cell growth. The latter variables include the composition of the culture medium and environmental conditions, such as temperature, pH, and ionic strength. For the bacterium *Escherichia coli,* the cell doubling time ranges from its fastest time of 20 min during optimal conditions to well over 10 h when nutrients are provided at a highly limited rate of supply. The potential for a rapid increase in bacterial cell populations can be quite impressive (Table 2.1). Over a period of only 5 h, for example, 100 *E. coli* cells can multiply to over 3 million cells at a cell generation time of 20 min. If the cells were able to constantly produce an enterotoxin, it would accumulate and be elevated by four orders of magnitude in concentration!

Cell division by most species of bacteria occurs by a process called **binary fission** (Fig. 2.2A). The cell, whether it be a rod, cocci, vibrio, or spirillum, enlarges by elongation at previously designated growing zones. Virtually every component of the cell is being rapidly synthesized and assembled into a mature cell structure nearly identical to the parent cell except for its relative length. Upon attaining a critical size, the cell begins to divide, a process that upon completion, yields two daughter cells. Each new cell is nearly equal in size and composition: About one half of each cell consists of newly synthesized cell material while the other one half is preexisting material from the parent cell. Each daughter cell receives a newly replicated copy of the bacteria's genome. A physical separation of cells may or may not occur depending on the species.

For some specialized bacterial genera (e.g., *Bacillus, Clostridium, Azotobacter,* or *Chlamydia*) an alternative type of cell developmental process may occur that yields a resting cell form called a **spore** (see Chapter 1) or **cyst,** which in the

TABLE 2.1. Exponential Increase in Bacterial Cell Numbers

Time (h)	Generation times	Number of cells present[a]
0	0	100 (initial cell number)
1	3	800
2	6	6,400
3	9	51,200
4	12	409,600
5	15	3,276,800

[a] Assuming cell doubling every 20 min.

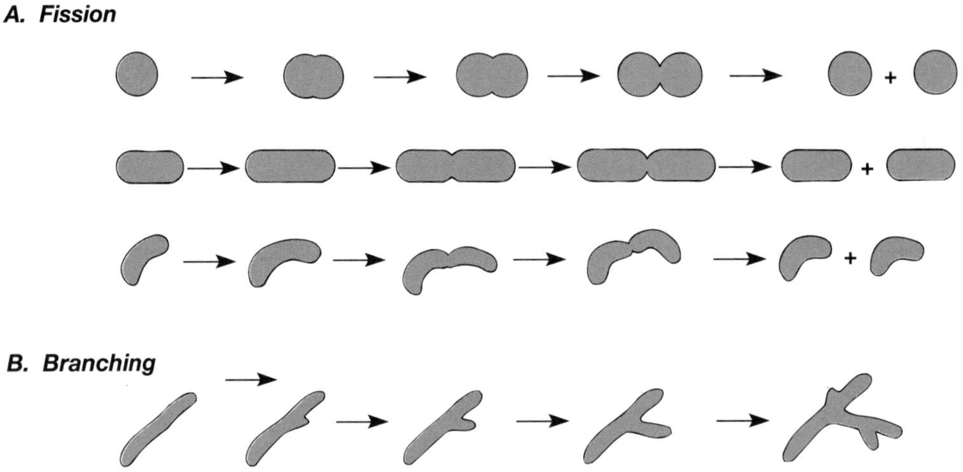

A. Fission

B. Branching

Figure 2.2.
Bacterial cell division occurring by binary fission (**A**) and by branching (**B**).

case of *Chlamydia* is referred to as an **elementary body.** These morphologically distinct cell types have specialized properties that provide advantages in survival and/or dispersal when culture conditions are unfavorable for normal vegetative growth. The morphologies of spores and cysts differ considerably from the vegetative cell as does the capacity to perform biosynthesis and energy generation.

Species of a limited number of bacterial genera exhibit a somewhat variable cell morphology in contrast to the characteristic rod, cocci, vibrio, and spirillum species described above. These species include the mycoplasmas (e.g., *Mycoplasma* or *Ureaplasma*), which do not maintain a uniform cell size or shape due to the lack of a rigid cell wall. Species of certain other bacterial genera may grow in filamentous and cordlike structures (e.g., *Mycobacterium*) or as true filamentous branching mycelia, which eventually may lead to spore formation (e.g., *Nocardia* or streptomycetes). A budding or **branching** process of cell growth occurs for these latter microbes (Fig. 2.2B). New cell growth also initiates at distinct points on existing cells although the locations can appear somewhat variable. Elongation of the new cell may continue for variable lengths of time before new growing points emerge. Distinct cell morphologies result.

BACTERIAL NUTRITION

Nutrients are the various organic and inorganic materials every microbe must acquire from its environment to accomplish cell growth and division. In general, these nutrients include the major and minor elements in proper abundance that constitute a normal healthy cell (Table 2.2). Each nutrient must be available in the immediate vicinity of the bacterium and in the proper form for uptake into the cell and for synthesis of new cell materials.

The number of nutrients the cell requires may differ depending on the bacterial species being considered. Whereas some bacterial species are nutritionally quite demanding, and thus require complex media for their culture, others are nutritionally very simple in their requirements. Bacteria referred to as **nutritionally complex** or **fastidious** require a large array of organic compounds for growth (e.g., some lactobacilli). A **complete medium** may include nearly all of the amino acids, each purine and pyrimidine, all the vitamins, plus the various inorganic cations and anions found within the cell. These molecules are examples of **essential nutrients** in that they are obligatorily for cell growth. Other fastidious organisms may require special types of sugars or lipids in addition to performed enzyme cofactors, such as nicotinamide adenine dinucleotide (NAD^+) or heme. Many bacterial species are considerably less demanding nutritionally and may require only a single organic compound to meet all of their biosynthetic needs (e.g., glucose for *E. coli*) as long as the other essential elements that comprise the cell are provided in proper inorganic forms. These latter nutrients may be provided as a mixture of mineral salts of ammonia or nitrate, sulfate, phosphate, and the less abundant metal ions including iron, magnesium, nickel, copper, etc. (Table 2.2).

Late in the exponential cell growth phase (Fig. 2.1) nutrients are rapidly depleted from the medium. If these cells are not replenished or if alternative nutrients are not present, cell growth slows and usually ceases within one cell generation. For some bacterial species, nutrient depletion may trigger a cellular differentiation process to give rise to spores or cysts that are metabolically inactive or nearly so. Cell survival is thus assured for long periods of time.

EFFECT OF ENVIRONMENTAL FACTORS ON GROWTH

Environmental conditions are also critical for the cells ability to grow and/or survive. The cell must encounter acceptable conditions of temperature, oxygen availability, pH, moisture, and ionic strength. Each species exhibits a characteristic range for each variable that allows growth while the maximum rate of cell growth occurs when all variables are ideal. Some bacteria are **obligate aerobes** (oxygen

TABLE 2.2. **Composition of a Typical Bacterium and Sources of Nutritional Supplements**[a]

Elements	Cell dry weight (%)	May be provided as
Major		
Carbon	50	Sugars, polypeptides, amino acids
Oxygen	20	Organic compounds, water, salts
Nitrogen	14	Amino acids, purines, pyrimidines, ammonia, nitrate, dinitrogen
Hydrogen	8	Water, organic compounds
Phosphorus	3	Phosphate, other phosphorylated compounds
Sulfur	1	Sulfate, sulfide, cysteine, glutathione
Potassium	1	Inorganic salts
Sodium	1	Inorganic salts
Minor (2% in total)		
Ca, Mg, Cl, Fe		Inorganic salts
Zn, Co, Cu, Mo,		Inorganic salts
Mn, Ni, Se		Inorganic salts

[a] The vitamins are not listed in this table but should not be overlooked as essential or nonessential nutrients.

requiring) or **obligate anaerobes** (grow only in the complete absence of molecular oxygen). Adequate provision for this nutrient must be considered for achieving optimal cell culture. Other bacterial species are **facultative** in their need for oxygen and can grow either in the presence or complete absence of oxygen due to their alternative pathways for acquiring energy (e.g., adenosine triphosphate, ATP). **Microaerophilic** bacteria require oxygen for growth but at a reduced level: these bacteria are either unable to grow or grow poorly under either air-saturated or oxygen-free conditions. The **pH** of the culture medium is important as bacterial species grow only over a limited range of hydrogen ion concentrations. The term **acidophile** refers to acid-loving organisms that thrive at low pH, while **alkaliphiles** prefer basic pH growth conditions. Most bacteria of medical significance grow optimally at near-neutral pH values. Finally, some bacterial species require carbon dioxide (CO_2) for growth as it must be incorporated during certain biosynthetic reactions. As the CO_2 level may be low in many environments, additional CO_2 must often be provided to achieve optimal cell growth.

Bacteria often encounter toxic forms of oxygen including hydrogen peroxide (H_2O_2) and superoxide (O_2^-) during the normal course of aerobic growth. The bacteria may also sometimes be exposed to high levels of H_2O_2 generated by eucaryotic cell tissues (e.g., peroxisomes). To minimize cell damage, one or more types of bacterial enzymes may be produced as a detoxification strategy (Table 2.3). The diagnostic oxidase test used for bacterial identification reveals the pres-

TABLE 2.3. Bacterial Response to Oxygen Damage

Enzyme	Substrate	Reaction
Catalase	H_2O_2	$2\ H_2O_2 \rightarrow 2\ H_2O + O_2$
Peroxidase	H_2O_2	$H_2O_2 + NADH \rightarrow 2\ H_2O + NAD$
Superoxide dismutase	O_2^-	$2\ O_2^- + 2\ H^+ \rightarrow H_2O_2 + O_2$

ence of cytochrome c and its ability to oxidize an artificial electron acceptor (e.g., tetramethyl phenylenediamine, TTMP), a process unrelated to oxygen toxicity.

BACTERIAL METABOLISM

Metabolic Pathways of Carbon Flow

To ensure the maintenance of cell functions and to support cell growth energy has to be generated by breaking down nutrients. This process is referred to as **catabolism.** Complex carbohydrates, or disaccharides, like lactose are converted to simple sugars like glucose, which are then **oxidized** to three-carbon (C_3) compounds. **Oxidation** is the withdrawal of electrons from a chemical compound. An oxidation reaction is always coupled to a reduction of a compound. **Reduction** is the transfer reaction of electrons to a chemical substrate.

The oxidation and reduction of chemical compounds is catalyzed by enzymes. **Enzymes** are proteins that recognize and bind specific substrates and exhibit a specific activity to convert the substrate to a product. An important feature of enzymes is that their activity can be regulated by metabolic activators or inhibitors. An activator increases enzyme activity and can be the substrate. An inhibitor decreases the activity and can be the product of the chemical reaction that is catalyzed by the enzyme itself or by a different enzyme. Regulation of enzyme activity ensures that the right amount of substrate is used and a product is made that is important for the coordination of multiple enzyme activities in complex reactions.

Some enzymes require low molecular weight organic compounds to transfer electrons, protons, amino- or methyl groups. These non-polypeptide compounds are referred to as **prosthetic groups** when they are tightly bound to the enzyme. Flavin adenine dinucleotide (FAD) (Fig. 2.3) is one example of a prosthetic group that transfers electrons and protons in oxidation–reduction reactions of certain

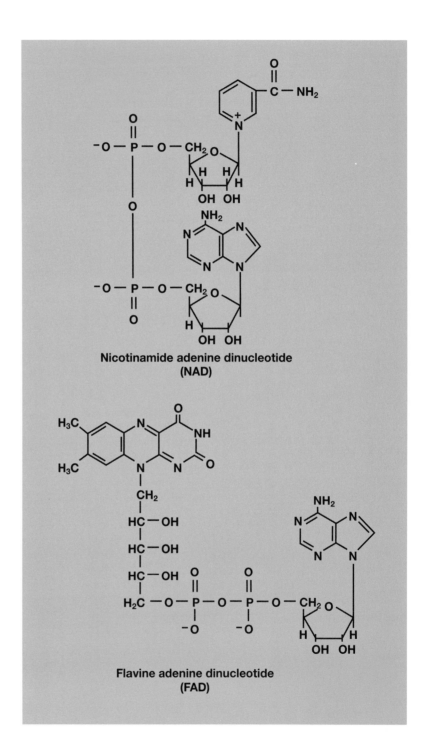

Figure 2.3.
Structure of NAD and FAD. The oxidized forms of nicotinamide adenine dinucleotide (NAD) and flavin dinucleotide (FAD) are shown with the reactive regions indicated in red.

enzymes. **Coenzymes** are small organic compounds that are freely diffusible and bind to enzymes only temporarily. The most important coenzyme in oxidation–reduction reactions is NAD (Fig. 2.3). Since prosthetic groups and coenzymes receive electrons, protons, or chemical groups when reacting with enzymes they must be continually regenerated by interacting with other enzymes of central metabolism.

Metabolic Energy

Catabolic reactions yield energy that is preserved as a metabolic intermediate. The universal form of metabolic energy currency is **ATP** (adenosine triphosphate) (Fig. 2.4). Adenosine triphosphate can be used to fuel energy-requiring processes of cell biosynthesis reactions.

This compound can be generated by two basic processes. First, in **substrate-level phosphorylation** the phosphate group of phosphorylated high-energy intermediates is transferred to ADP by kinase enzymes. Substrate-level phosphorylation occurs in the glycolysis pathway, in the tricarboxylic acid cycle, and in certain fermentation processes. Second, **electron-transport phosphorylation** involves a complex enzyme system to generate an intermediate energy form (e.g., chemiosmotic membrane potential), which is subsequently converted to ATP by the en-

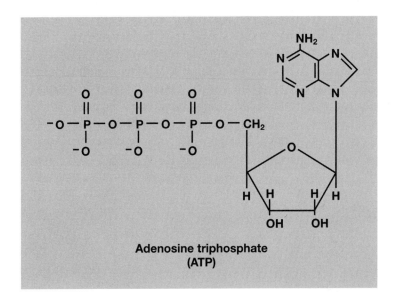

Adenosine triphosphate
(ATP)

Figure 2.4.
Structure of ATP.

zyme ATP synthase (also known as ATPase). Electron-transport phosphorylation is the mode of energy generation during aerobic and anaerobic respiration as well as during photosynthesis. This means of ATP generation is described in more detail below.

Glycolysis

Glycolysis is a sequence of reactions that converts glucose to pyruvate with concomitant production of ATP (Fig. 2.5). Almost all microorganisms, whether aerobic, anaerobic, or microaerophilic, use the glycolysis pathway to oxidize glucose to pyruvate. Glycolysis is also referred to as the Embden–Meyerhof–Parnas pathway or the fructose-1,6-bisphosphate (FBP) pathway. All intermediates between glucose and pyruvate are phosphorylated.

The first of 11 reactions in the glycolysis sequence is the phosphorylation of glucose to glucose 6-phosphate by the enzyme hexokinase. Glucose can also enter the cell via a complex transport system that phosphorylates glucose upon entry. Either PEP or ATP is consumed to form glucose 6-phosphate. The phosphorylation of glucose prevents the substrate from leaving the cell by diffusion. Glucose 6-phosphate is isomerized to fructose 6-phosphate by the enzyme phosphoglucose isomerase. Phosphofructokinase phosphorylates fructose 6-phosphate with ATP to form fructose 1,6-bisphosphate, which is cleaved by the enzyme aldolase to glyceraldehyde 3-phosphate and dihydroxyacetone phosphate. Only glyceraldehyde 3-phosphate is oxidized further in the glycolysis pathway. Dihydroxyacetone phosphate is converted to glyceraldehyde 3-phosphate by the enzyme triose phosphate isomerase. The NAD-dependent enzyme glyceraldehyde 3-phosphate dehydrogenase oxidizes glyceraldehyde 3-phosphate to 1,3-bisphosphoglycerate while generating reduced NAD (NADH). In this reaction inorganic phosphate (P_i) is attached to the substrate to form an energy-rich compound. The enzyme phosphoglycerate kinase then transfers this high-energy phosphate group to ADP, yielding ATP and 3-phosphoglycerate. Phosphoglyceromutase rearranges 3-phosphoglycerate to 2-phosphoglycerate which is then hydrolysed to phosphoenolpyruvate by the enzyme enolase. In the last step of glycolysis the enzyme pyruvate kinase transfers the phosphate group of phosphoenolpyruvate to ADP, generating ATP and pyruvate. Most, but not all, reactions in the glycolytic pathway are reversible.

The net reaction of converting glucose to pyruvate is summarized as follows:

$$\text{Glucose} + 2P_i + 2\text{ ADP} + 2\text{ NAD} \rightarrow 2\text{ pyruvate} + 2\text{ ATP} + 2\text{ NADH} + 2\text{ H}_2\text{O}$$

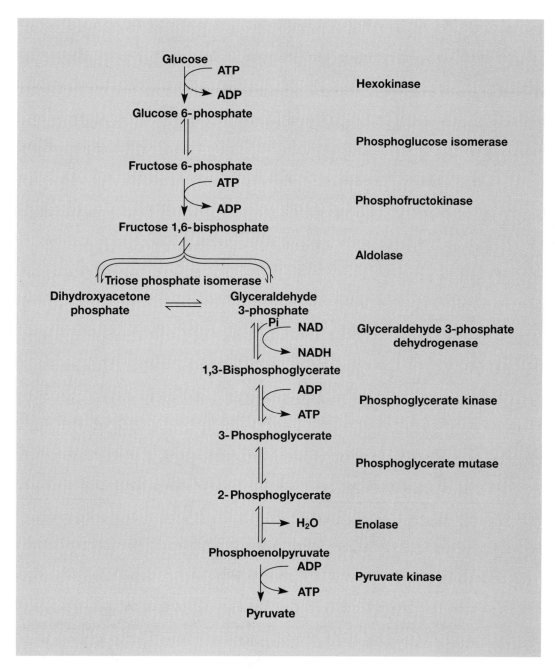

Figure 2.5.

The glycolytic pathway for conversion of glucose to pyruvate.

The two ATP molecules acquired during glycolysis are made by substrate-level phosphorylation. The two newly generated NADH molecules will be reoxidized to NAD in aerobic microorganisms by respiration and in anaerobic microorganisms by fermentation.

Fate of Pyruvate in Aerobic Bacteria

In contrast to glycolysis, which is nearly universal in all organisms, pyruvate can be converted to many different products depending on the particular bacterial species and its growth conditions (e.g., environment).

In **aerobic** microorganisms, pyruvate is converted to **acetyl–coenzyme A (acetyl–CoA)** by the enzyme pyruvate dehydrogenase:

$$\text{Pyruvate} + \text{NAD} + \text{CoA} \rightarrow \text{acetyl–CoA} + \text{NADH}$$

Acetyl–CoA serves as the entry intermediate for the tricarboxylic acid cycle.

Tricarboxylic Acid Cycle

The **tricarboxylic acid (TCA) cycle** describes a sequence of reactions that results in the complete break down of the acetyl group of acetyl–CoA to CO_2. The TCA cycle is also referred to as citric acid or Krebs cycle. This pathway is common to all aerobic and to many but not all anaerobic microorganisms. The cycle also provides intermediates for biosynthesis of amino acids, nucleic acids, and heme.

The first step of the cycle (Fig. 2.6) is the condensation of acetyl–CoA and oxaloacetate to citrate by the enzyme citrate synthase. In this reaction CoA is released. Citrate is rearranged to isocitrate by the enzyme aconitase. Isocitrate is oxidized and decarboxylated by the enzyme isocitrate dehydrogenase to form α-ketoglutarate, CO_2 and NADH. The enzyme α-ketoglutarate dehydrogenase catalyses the subsequent oxidation and decarboxylation of α-ketoglutarate to give succinyl–CoA, CO_2 and NADH. At this point acetyl–CoA has been completely oxidized to two molecules of CO_2. The followings steps of the cycle will regenerate the initial entry intermediate, oxaloacetate. Succinyl–CoA synthetase converts succinyl CoA to succinate by generating a high-energy phosphate intermediate that is used to generate ATP by substrate-level phosphorylation. Succinate is oxidized to fumarate by the enzyme succinate dehydrogenase, which contains as enzyme-bound reduced FAD (FADH) prosthetic group. Fumarase hydroxylates

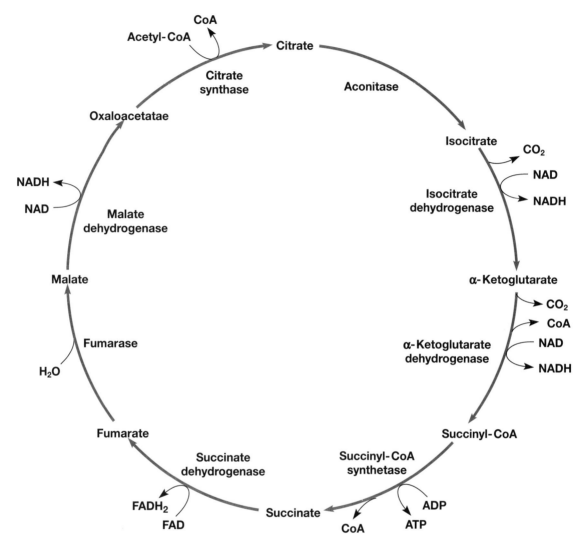

Figure 2.6.
The tricarboxylic acid cycle.

fumarate to malate, which is then oxidized to oxaloacetate by the enzyme malate dehydrogenase, coupled with formation of NADH. All reactions of the TCA cycle with the exception of that catalyzed by citrate synthase are reversible.

The net reaction of converting acetyl–CoA to CO_2 is summarized as follows:

$$\text{Acetyl–CoA} + 3\,\text{NAD} + 1\,\text{FAD} + \text{ADP} + P_i + 2\,\text{H}_2\text{O} \rightarrow 2\,\text{CO}_2 + 3\,\text{NADH} + \text{FADH} + \text{ATP} + \text{CoA}$$

The three molecules of NADH and one molecule of FADH will be regenerated to NAD and FAD by respiration.

Fermentation—Fate of Pyruvate in Anaerobic Bacteria

In **anaerobic** microorganisms pyruvate can be converted by a series of reactions to reduced organic compounds, such as acetate, ethanol, and lactate. All these pathways have in common the ability to consume NADH by regenerating it to NAD. This method is the general strategy of fermentation. **Fermentation** is defined as an ATP generating process in which organic substrates are oxidized incompletely to form acids or alcohols.

Enteric bacteria like *E. coli, Klebsiella pneumoniae,* and *Enterobacter aerogenes* ferment lactose to a variety of organic acids and alcohols. The disaccharide is first cleaved to glucose and galactose, and the latter is converted to glucose. Glucose is then oxidized to pyruvate by the glycolysis pathway. Subsequent reactions convert pyruvate to acetate, lactate, formate, succinate, ethanol, hydrogen, and CO_2. Because of the acidic nature of the majority of the end products this mode of fermentation is referred to as **mixed acid fermentation.** Although *Salmonella, Shigella,* and *Froteus* species cannot utilize lactose, these species do ferment glucose by mixed acid fermentation as described above. The production of acids from either lactose or glucose can be easily diagnosed by incorporation of a pH indicator in the growth medium.

The **lactic acid fermentation** used by the lactic acid bacteria including *Lactobacillus, Staphylococcus,* and *Streptococcus* begins with glucose, which is converted to lactate via pyruvate.

The **alcohol fermentation** performed by yeasts and certain bacteria converts glucose to pyruvate, which is then exclusively converted to ethanol and CO_2.

Clostridium species perform specialized fermentations that are not commonly found in many other microorganisms. *Clostridium perfringens* ferments glucose to butyrate, acetate and lactate, ethanol, CO_2, and H_2. *Clostridium botulinum* ferments proteins and amino acids to mainly acetate and lactate. *Clostridium tetanomorphum* can ferment the amino acids glutamate and histidine to butyrate and acetate.

Gluconeogenesis

Gluconeogenesis refers to the synthesis of glucose from non-carbohydrate compounds, such as the amino acids or lactate. The precursors are first converted to pyruvate, which is then converted to glucose via the gluconeogenesis pathway. The gluconeogenesis pathway shares all but three enzymes with the glycolysis pathway. Three reactions are irreversible in the glycolysis pathway and the gluconeogenesis pathway must employ three distinct enzymes to bypass those irreversible reactions:

1. Phosphoenolpyruvate synthase

   Pyruvate $+$ ATP $+$ H_2O $\rightarrow$ phosphoenolpyruvate $+$ AMP $+$ P_i

2. Fructose 1,6-bisphosphatase

   Fructose 1,6-bisphosphate $+$ H_2O $\rightarrow$ fructose 6-phosphate $+$ P_i

3. Glucose 6-phosphatase

   Glucose 6-phosphate $+$ H_2O $\rightarrow$ glucose $+$ P_i

ENERGY GENERATION BY OXIDATIVE PHOSPHORYLATION

Oxidative phosphorylation is the process in which ATP is formed from ADP and P_i as electrons are transferred from NADH or FADH to O_2. Oxidative phosphorylation reactions generate most of the ATP made in aerobic microorganisms. The associated electron-transport pathway also serves to regenerate NAD and FAD from their reduced forms, which are generated in the glycolysis and TCA pathways. The oxidation of NADH or FADH with concomitant reduction of O_2 to form H_2O is catalyzed by a series of enzymes and coenzymes that are located in the cytoplasmic membrane of the bacterial cell. This membrane bound enzyme system is called the **electron-transport chain** (Fig. 2.7).

The electron-transport chain contains enzymes that "pump" protons across the cytoplasmic membrane from the inside to the outside of the cell. Since the cytoplasmic membrane is impermeable for protons they are "trapped" on the outside of the cell. As a consequence the pH on the outside becomes more acidic, whereas the pH in the interior of the cell is more alkaline. This difference in pH, also referred to as **ΔpH** or pH gradient, can be determined experimentally by use

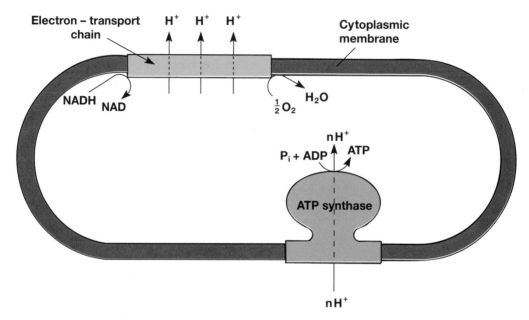

Figure 2.7.

Coupling of electron-transport pathway activity to ATP synthesis.

of a pH electrode. Since protons are positively charged a proton gradient across the cytoplasmic membrane also causes a charge difference (i.e., positive on the outside and negative on the inside of the cell). The difference in charge is referred to as $\Delta\Psi$ or electrical membrane potential, which can be determined using positively charged, radioactive molecules that can freely diffuse into the cell. The combined values of ΔpH and $\Delta\Psi$ are defined as **proton motive force (Δp)** or chemiosmotic membrane potential. The proton motive force can be calculated according to the following equation:

$$\Delta p = \Delta\Psi - Z\,\Delta pH$$

The term Z is a constant that equals 59 mV at 25°C and allows one to convert ΔpH into millivolts (mV). Thus, Δp is expressed in millivolts.

The proton motive force can be considered as a membrane associated energy form that is used by the cell to fuel the energy-requiring processes of ATP synthesis via the membrane-bound ATP synthase (Fig. 2.7). Flagellar movement and transport of nutrients into the cell may also be couple to transfer of protons back into the interior of the cell.

SUMMARY

1. Bacterial species exhibit specific nutritional requirements as well as optimal environmental conditions for their growth.

2. Most types of bacteria reproduce by a process called binary fission. Some species exhibit a branching pattern of cell growth.

3. Under ideal growth conditions, bacterial cell numbers increase exponentially (logarithmically) and continue to do so until some essential nutrient becomes limiting.

4. Most medically related bacteria obtain energy by catabolic reactions and generate ATP by substrate level phosphorylation reactions and/or by oxidative phosphorylation reactions coupled to cellular respiration.

5. Most anaerobic bacteria break down simple sugars to obtain their energy by specific fermentation pathways that yield characteristic end products (alcohols, organic acids, or gases).

6. The toxic forms of oxygen generated by cell metabolism are detoxified by the bacterial enzymes, catalase, peroxidase, and superoxide disumutase.

7. Once nutrients are depleted, cell growth ceases, and the cell remains viable until energy reserves are either used up or the cell suffers some type of irreversible damage. Cell death ensues.

8. Each bacterial species exhibits a characteristic maximal rate of growth but it can also grow at a slower rate depending on the type of the nutrients provided.

9. Glucose is oxidized to pyruvate by the glycolysis pathway by both aerobic and anaerobic microorganisms.

10. Aerobic microbes break down pyruvate to acetyl–CoA, which then is further degraded to CO_2 by enzymes of the TCA pathway.

REFERENCES

Brock TD, Madigan MT (1994): Biology of Microorganisms. Englewood Cliffs, NJ: Prentice Hall.
Gottschalk G (1986) Bacterial Metabolism. NY: Springer-Verlag.
Neidhardt FC, Ingraham JL, Schaechter M (1990): Physiology of the Bacterial Cell. MA: Sinauer Associates.

REVIEW QUESTIONS

> For questions 1 to 4, choose the ONE BEST answer or completion.

1. A bacterial isolate from the skin surface is tested for its ability to grow under different environmental conditions. Given the source of the isolate, which of the following variables are likely to provide unsuitable conditions for its growth?
   a) A complete medium at a pH of 3
   b) Only under anaerobic conditions
   c) A glucose medium at 5° C
   d) A complex medium at 37°C

2. What term refers to a prosthetic group of an enzyme?
   a) An amino acid
   b) FAD
   c) NAD
   d) Magnesium

3. Cell growth is optimized or nearly so during the following phases of a bacterial growth cycle:
   a) Lag phase
   b) Log phase
   c) Stationary phase
   d) Death phase
   e) All of the above

4. The Embden-Meyerhof-Parnas-pathway results in the formation of

   a) acetyl-CoA
   b) ethanol
   c) ATP
   d) NAD
   e) succinate

> For questions 5 and 6, ONE or MORE of the completions given is correct. Choose the appropriate answer.

5. The cell doubling time refers to
   a) the time required for one cell to double in mass
   b) the time required for one cell to form two new cells
   c) the time required for a culture to increase by a factor of two logs
   d) the generation time of a cell
   e) the time to form a spore

6. Different organisms may exhibit different specific nutrient requirements for their growth. Which term represents likely requirements of a fastidious microorganism?
   a) Heme
   b) NAD
   c) Amino acids
   d) Potassium ions
   e) Purines

7. What term refers to a toxic form a oxygen?
   a) O_2
   b) Hydrogen peroxide
   c) Superoxide
   d) H_2O

8. An obligate anaerobe is able to
   a) grow in a complete medium
   b) grow as a micro-aerophile
   c) grow exponentially
   d) obligately form resting stages

For questions 9 and 10, ONE of the completions given is incorrect. Choose the appropriate answer.

9. Anaerobic microorganisms may produce one or more of the following compounds as end products of fermentation:
   a) CO_2
   b) Butyrate
   c) Pyruvate
   d) Ethanol
   e) Lactate

10. The process of oxidative phosphorylation by a cell involves
    a) glucose-l-phosphate
    b) ATP synthase
    c) a proton motive force
    d) generation of a Δ pH gradient
    e) a cell membrane

ANSWERS TO REVIEW QUESTIONS

1. *d* A rich medium at 37°C which mimics the environment of the skin.

2. *b* FAD which is tightly bound to an enzyme.

3. *b* Log phase where the cell is rapidly growing.

4. *c* ATP as an high energy intermediate.

5. *b* and *d* are correct.

6. All answers are correct.

7. *b* and *c* are correct as peroxide and superoxide can give rise to oxidative damage.

8. *a* and *c* are correct; the term obligate limits cell growth to complete absence of oxygen. The ability to form spores is not limited to anaerobes.

9. *c* is incorrect; pyruvate is an intermediate rather than a final product of fermentation.

10. *a* is incorrect.

GENETIC VARIABILITY OF MICROORGANISMS

Bacteria and other microorganisms possess a formidable array of mechanisms that allow for rapid genetic changes. This ability to diversify genetically provides these microorganisms with the means to resist hazards as different as attack by the human immune system or the introduction of a new antibiotic drug. In addition to clinical concerns, the ability of microorganisms (particularly bacteria) to undergo genetic changes has been exploited and studied by scientists interested in basic questions in molecular biology. Indeed, such studies led to the discovery of the tools of recombinant DNA and heralded one of the technological revolutions of the century.

This chapter covers the basic processes that underlie genetic changes observed in microorganisms. The information is arranged according to the molecular mechanism responsible for the change. Where possible, each mechanism is illustrated with an example known to have clinical impact. In several cases, the clinical import is outweighed by the usefulness of the mechanisms to scientists and genetic engineers, and the reader will be alerted to this fact.

SIMPLE MUTATIONS

All organisms replicate their genetic material (almost always DNA) with very high accuracy; however, errors do occur. Such errors produce **mutations,** inheritable changes in the genetic makeup of the organism. For bacteria, it is estimated that the probability of a mistake being passed on to a daughter is about $1/10^9$ per base pair per generation. It is now recognized that this low error rate should not be viewed as the failure rate of an imperfect apparatus; rather, these rare errors provide a continued and important source of genetic variability. This variability is random; that is, the bacterium does not specify when and where in the genome these errors (or more properly, alterations) occur. How, then, is this type of variability useful to the bacterium?

For example, the common bacterium *Escherichia coli,* a natural resident of the human gut, is killed by the antibiotic rifampin, which inhibits the RNA polymerase of bacteria thereby disrupting protein synthesis and DNA replication. However, because of the random errors of replication, a small fraction ($\sim 1/10^7$) of the bacteria in a population is resistant to rifampin. These bacteria contain a particular type of mutation in a gene that codes for a subunit of the RNA polymerase, rendering the polymerase resistant to the drug and enabling the mutant *E. coli* to grow in its presence.

The following simple experiment shows how this process can easily be observed in the laboratory and illustrates the important principle of **genetic selection.** A culture of normal *E. coli* contains a very large number of bacteria ($\sim 10^9$/ml). If a portion of this culture is inoculated into a fresh medium containing rifampin, most of the bacteria fail to grow; however, the small fraction that are resistant to the drug (as a result of random replication errors) will multiply. In a rich medium, *E. coli* divides every 20 min and within a few hours the culture will contain 10^9/ml of rifampin-resistant *E. coli.* In interpreting this experiment, it is important to realize that the drug did not *induce* the mutations; rather, it served to select those rare mutants that previously existed in the culture and allow them to flourish and supplant the original population. These ideas reflect the notions proposed by Darwin (variability coupled with selective pressures) and forms one of the basic concepts of modern biology.

Although mutations in bacteria arise spontaneously as discussed above, certain chemical compounds (e.g., benzpyrenes) and certain types of irradiation (e.g., ultraviolet light) can increase by several hundredfold the frequency of mutations in bacteria. These agents are called **mutagens**; most of them act directly on DNA causing lesions that result in mutations. Since DNA is a universal genetic material, it is not surprising that these same mutagens also damage the DNA of human cells, an event that can lead to many types of cancers. This shared susceptibility has led to the development of very simple and inexpensive tests using bacteria to screen substances in order to predict whether they will be mutagenic (and, therefore, carcinogenic) to humans. For example, this type of bacterial test revealed that certain types of hair dyes marketed in the 1970s were mutagenic; they were replaced by less harmful versions.

PROGRAMMED DNA REARRANGEMENTS

Although the genetic variability produced by simple mutations is a potent means of surviving new environmental challenges, microorganisms also employ several other clever devices apparently designed to evade the immune systems of mammals. The mechanisms underlying these strategies are based on specific types of **DNA rearrangements.** Three of the most important are **translocation, inversion,** and **deletion.**

Translocation

Translocation literally means a change in location. In this case, the locations refer to positions on the genome and the term refers to a specific device possessed by a number of microorganisms. An analogy is sometimes made between this device and a compact disk (CD) player. In Figure 3.1 (top), a segment of a genome is depicted; it contains an expression locus, analogous to the CD player, and a collection of silent genes that would correspond to a library of CDs. In the example shown, gene I resides in the expression locus and is therefore being expressed, that is, transcribed and translated into protein. Figure 3.1 (bottom) depicts the result of a translocation, analogous to the selection of a different CD from the library and its insertion into the player. In the example shown, gene II has replaced gene I at the expression locus causing this second gene to now be expressed in place of the original gene. In this way an organism can maintain a special array of genes (I,II,III, etc.), expressing only one at a time. It should be noted that the CD analogy is not perfect; when a translocation occurs, the selected silent gene is first replicated and the copy is inserted into the expression locus; the copy that previously resided at the expression locus is destroyed in the process. In this way the organism maintains a complete library.

An example of translocation occurs in *Neisseria gonorrhoeae,* the bacterium that causes human gonorrhea. On its surface, this bacteria expresses **pili,** threadlike structures that attach to tissues in the host. These pili, due to their exposed location, are an important attack point for the immune system. However, *N. gonorrhoeae*

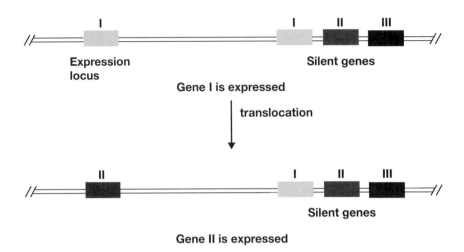

Figure 3.1.

An idealized translocation system showing the relevant portions of a hypothetical genome.

utilizes a translocation system to alter the identity of the pilin, a major structural protein of the pilus. Carried in its genome is a library of at least 12 different types of pilin genes, only one of which is expressed by a bacterium at a given time. Since the organism can switch among different pilins using translocations, it confounds the human immune system by requiring new responses to the different pili. The details of translocation in *N. gonorrhoeae* differ somewhat from the idealized situation of Figure 3.1; in particular, the silent genes are only partial copies of the pilin gene and a translocation event thus replaces only a section of the complete gene located at the expression locus.

Perhaps the most dramatic example of translocation is exhibited not by a bacterium but by a protozoan parasite of the genus *Trypanosoma,* the cause of African sleeping sickness. Here the expression locus reads a gene that encodes a protein, the variable surface glycoprotein (VSG) that resides on the surface of the trypanosome and constitutes a major antigenic feature. A silent library contains as many as 1000 different VSG genes, each encoding a VSG of a different amino acid sequence. Because the parasite can express so many different VSGs (one at a time), an effective immune response is difficult to mount and maintain in the same way that it is difficult to hit a moving target. Again, it should be emphasized that trypanosomes utilize a complex set of reactions that only approximate the idealized translocation situation shown in Figure 3.1.

It is important to note that these translocation systems operate on a probabilistic basis. That is, attack by the immune system does not trigger a change of expression of the surface proteins; rather, the translocations take place spontaneously at a low level, and the immune system exerts a selective pressure, which permits the proliferation of only those organisms expressing a surface protein that has not yet triggered an immune response.

Inversion

This term also applies to a particular type of DNA rearrangement. In this case a mechanism allows a specialized segment of DNA to invert its orientation in the genome. In keeping with the audio-equipment metaphor, inversion would be analogous to flipping over a phonograph record: The inversion has only two states (or sides) and can flip back and forth between them.

How is this inversion device used by microorganisms? Perhaps the best understood example is found in *Salmonella typhimurium,* a bacterium that causes **enterocolitis** in humans. The bacterium propels itself using **flagella,** which extend from the surface of the organism and, therefore, provide a convenient attack point for the immune system. *S. typhimurium* contains two different genes that encode flagellin, which is a major constituent of the flagella. The two types of flagellin (called *H1* and *H2*) have different amino acid sequences. Only one type of flagellin is produced at any one time by a bacterium, but the inversion system allows the bacterium to flip back and forth between the two. A diagram of the complete system in *S. typhimurium* is shown in Figure 3.2. The invertible segment of DNA contains a transcriptional promoter and, in the orientation shown in Figure 3.2 (top), the promoter reads into the *H2* flagellin, allowing its expression. The promoter also expresses transcriptional repressor of the other flagellin gene (*H1*) ensuring that this gene is not expressed. When the segment is inverted (Fig. 3.2, bottom), its promoter points away from the *H2* gene. Since this gene does not contain its own promoter, it is no longer expressed. For the same reason, the repressor is no longer produced, allowing the *H1* gene to be transcribed. In this way the bacterium can switch back and forth between two type of flagella as a means of surviving an immune response.

The switching between the two types of flagella of *S. typhimurium* occurs at a low frequency, approximately $1/10^4$. As for the cases of translocation, the inversion event is not induced by an immune response; rather, the immune response serves as the selective pressure that allows one of the variants to flourish. In the *Salmonella* genome, the invertible segment is flanked by special DNA sequences (indicated by boxes in Fig. 3.2) that specify exactly which part of the genome is to be flipped. The bacteria encode a number of specialized proteins that carry out the inversion process; the most important is encoded on the invertible segment itself.

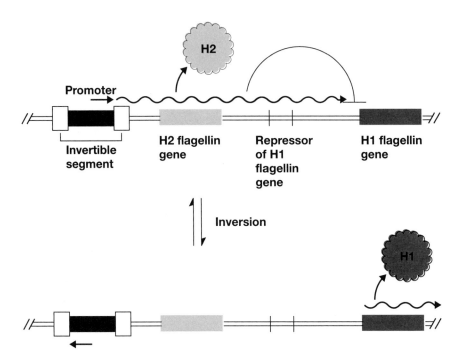

Figure 3.2.

Example of the DNA inversion system found in *S. typhimurium*. It permits the organism to switch back and forth between two flagellar proteins (H1 and H2).

Deletion

As the name implies, this mechanism involves the selective removal of certain parts of the genome. This mechanism has an obvious drawback compared to those discussed above, as the information present on the deleted segment would be lost. Nevertheless, several microorganisms utilize this device as a way of making specialized types of cells that are "dead ends"; that is, they do not reproduce. Despite its limitations, deletion is one of the most important types of DNA rearrangements known in the study of medicine for it is one of the basic mechanisms underlying the remarkable plasticity of the immune system. Although a detailed view is beyond the scope of this chapter, an outline of the basic process is shown in Figure 3.3. As cells of the immune system develop, selective deletions occur that bring variable regions of immunoglobulin genes into proximity with constant region coding sequences. Different cells undergo different deletions resulting in a complex spectrum of immunoglobulin-producing cells. Note that mammals maintain the germ line in a completely different set of cells that do not undergo deletion.

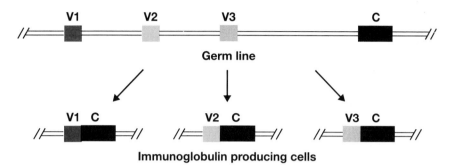

Figure 3.3.
Highly simplified schematic view of the role of deletion in generating the repertoire of immuno-globulin genes in mammals.

The fact that invading microorganisms as well as the human defense system utilize programmed DNA rearrangements to generate diversity is testament to the power of this mechanism; DNA rearrangements are clearly one of the keys to understanding the complex interplay between host and invader.

MOVEMENT OF GENETIC MATERIAL BETWEEN ORGANISMS

Sexual reproduction, which is so common that we take it for granted, must have evolved from the enormous selective advantage offered to organisms that could exchange genetic material. Although most bacteria reproduce asexually, they too have evolved mechanisms that allow them to enjoy the advantages of genetic exchange. In this section, we discuss three of the most important types of genetic exchange.

Transformation

The term **transformation** has a number of distinct meanings in biology. In this chapter, it refers to the ability of bacteria to stably take up DNA from the surroundings. Figure 3.4 depicts a scenario whereby DNA from one bacterium can be transferred to another by this path. How DNA gets across the bacterial membrane is not well understood. It is clear, however, that some bacteria have special receptors for DNA on their membranes, which facilitate the internalization of DNA.

Transformation appears to be a major source of genetic exchange for a num-

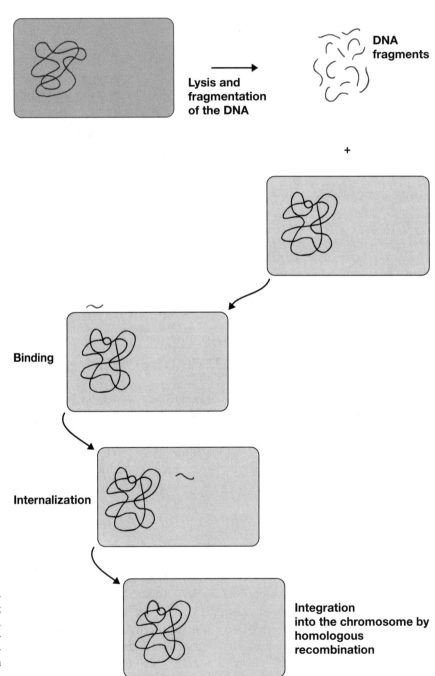

Figure 3.4.

Transformation of one bacterium by a DNA fragment from a second bacterium. The integration of the fragment by homologous recombination is described in Figure 3.10.

ber of bacteria including *N. gonorrhoeae* and *Streptococcus pneumoniae* (a causative agent of pneumonia and other infections). It is difficult to document a particular example of transformation with clinical consequences, but it is easy to imagine the transfer of drug resistance genes by this route.

Perhaps the main impact of transformation lies in the area of recombinant DNA research. Transformation, as a basic tool of recombinant DNA research, is widely exploited by scientists and genetic engineers to introduce DNAs from many different organisms (including humans) into bacteria where they can be easily manipulated experimentally.

Plasmids and Conjugation

The chromosome of the bacterium *E. coli,* to take a typical example, is a single, circular molecule of DNA encoding several thousand genes. In addition to this chromosome, an *E. coli* cell typically contains other, smaller molecules of DNA called **plasmids.** Plasmids are circular DNA molecules that contain their own origins of replication and, therefore, replicate separately from the main chromosome. Many different types of plasmids are found in the bacterial world; they vary in size from two or three genes up to hundreds. One notorious example, the R1 plasmid, is shown in Figure 3.5. This plasmid endows bacteria that carry it with resistance to six different antibiotics, a situation clearly advantageous to the bacteria but problematic in the clinic. In fact, the R1 plasmid was discovered after the widespread use of antibiotics had begun and presumably reflects one of the ways bacteria respond to selective pressures introduced by modern medicine. The R1 plasmid is an example of a **drug resistance** plasmid. Another medically important class of plasmids are the **virulence** plasmids, which carry genes that provide bacteria with pathogenic properties. For example, some virulence plasmids carry genes that enable the bacterium to invade human cells; others are responsible for producing enterotoxins.

A number of plasmids have the ability to move from one bacterium to another by a process called **conjugation.** Conjugation is simply the joining together of two bacteria that results in the exchange of genetic material. Note that the process is distinguished from transformation (above) and transduction (below) in that the donor and recipient bacteria must be physically linked.

A plasmid isolated from *E. coli* called the F (fertility) factor has been intensively studied and serves to illustrate the process of conjugation. It is related to the R1 plasmid and exemplifies the way in which these plasmids move from cell to cell by conjugation. The F plasmid contains approximately 100 genes, some of which are devoted to producing specialized pili (called the F or sex pili) that are

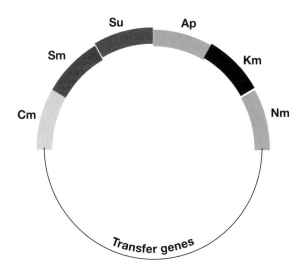

Figure 3.5.

Map (not to scale) of the R1 plasmid. The transfer genes direct the movement of the plasmid from one bacterium to another. Cm, chloramphenicol; Sm, streptomycin; Su, sulfonamide; Ap, ampicillin; Km, kanamycin; Nm, neomycin.

formed on the bacterial surface. Only bacteria that carry the F factor (denoted as F^+) produce these pili, which can attach specifically to a bacterium that does not carry the F factor (denoted as F^-). In a process that is not well understood, the pili bring the cells close together, a bridge is formed between the two cells, and the F factor DNA is copied and transferred from the F^+ to the F^- cell, converting it to an F^+ cell (Fig. 3.6).

The transfer of DNA is also directed by a set of genes carried on the F plasmid. First, the plasmid is cleaved on one strand at a specific site. Next, an end of DNA produced by this cleavage enters the recipient cell and continues to move across until the entire strand is transferred, at which point the ends are joined to form a circular molecule. This single-stranded molecule is then converted to double-stranded DNA by the action of DNA polymerase. During this process, the complementary strand of DNA remains within the donor cell and is also converted to duplex DNA. In this way, the plasmid is transferred to a new cell while the donor cell maintains its copy.

Occasionally, the *E. coli* F factor will integrate itself into the bacterial chromosome by homologous recombination (see below). When this happens, part (and sometimes all) of the *E. coli* chromosome can be transferred to a recipient cell by way of the pathway discussed above. Such *E. coli* strains are denoted Hfr (high frequency of recombination) to indicate that they often transfer chromosomal genes to recipient cells. In the example of Figure 3.7, the rifampin resistance gene was transferred, converting a susceptible bacterium into a resistant one.

Conjugation is a particularly potent device for transferring plasmids (and for Hfr strains, chromosomal genes as well) from one bacterium to another. Several

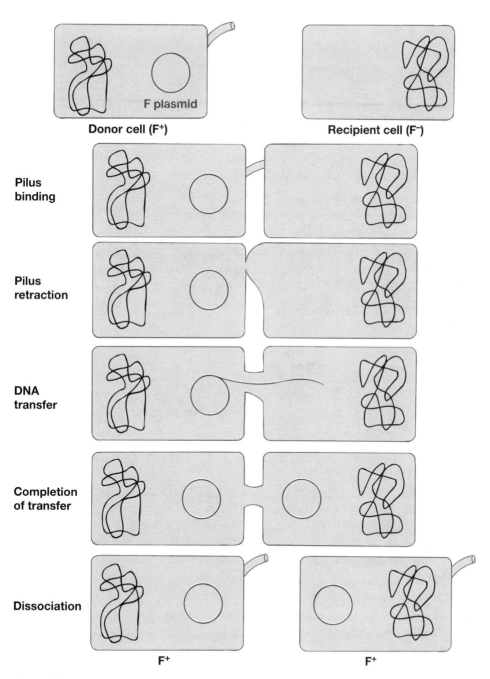

Figure 3.6.

Model for conjugation and DNA transfer directed by the *E. coli* F plasmid.

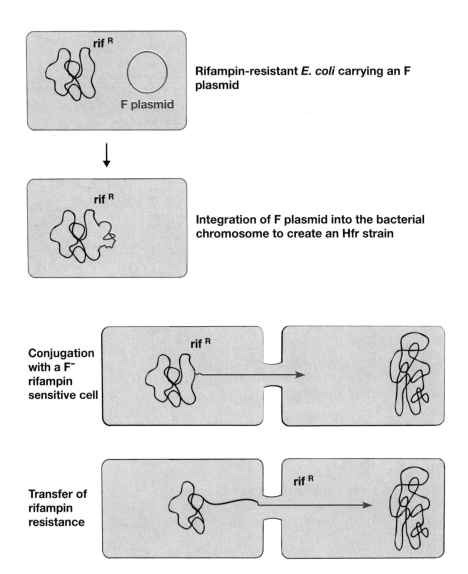

Rifampin-resistant *E. coli* carrying an F plasmid

Integration of F plasmid into the bacterial chromosome to create an Hfr strain

Conjugation with a F⁻ rifampin sensitive cell

Transfer of rifampin resistance

Figure 3.7.

Creation of an Hfr bacterium by integration of the F plasmid into the bacterial chromosome. The lower part of the figure depicts the transfer of rifampin resistance from the Hfr to an F⁻ rifampin-sensitive bacterium.

additional considerations underscore the importance of this process. First, many plasmids are much smaller than R1 or the F factor discussed above and do not carry the array of genes necessary to direct the conjugation process. Nonetheless, in a process called **plasmid mobilization,** these smaller plasmids can be transferred from one bacterium to another using the apparatus provided by a larger, conjugative plasmid. Mobilization does require that the two plasmids both reside in the donor cell. Second, many naturally occurring plasmids enjoy large host ranges; that is, they can exist in and be transferred between different genera of bacteria. This property is presumably an important component in the rapid spread of the drug resistance plasmids that followed the introduction of clinical antibiotics. For example, during an outbreak of dysentery in the late 1950s, the responsible pathogen, *Shigella flexneri,* carried an R plasmid that bore several drug resistance genes. *E. coli* isolated from these patients carried the same plasmid, suggesting that it was exchanged between the two bacterial genera. Finally, certain plasmids can be transferred by conjugation from bacteria (a prokaryote) to fungi and plants (eukaryotes) illustrating that this process can act across one of the major taxonomic divisions in biology.

In addition to their importance to the bacterial world, plasmids are used extensively in recombinant DNA technologies. Foreign DNA (e.g., from humans) can be inserted into bacterial plasmids where it can be easily reproduced and manipulated.

Viruses and Transduction

Transduction is a process by which DNA moves from one bacterium to another by way of a bacterial virus. Bacterial viruses are often called **bacteriophage** (phage for short), a term that distinguishes them from viruses that attack animal or plant cells. An individual phage consists of a genome wrapped in a specialized protective protein coat. In order to reproduce, the phage adsorbs to the surface of a bacterium and injects its genome to the inside of the cell where it directs the synthesis of proteins required to replicate the viral genome and encapsulate it to form new phage. This process is carried out at the expense of the infected cell that typically lyses, releasing hundreds of newly formed phage. Occasionally, segments of the host chromosome are also packaged into phage; upon adsorption of these phage to a naive bacterium, this donor DNA is injected. In this way DNA can be transferred from one bacterium, which is lysed in the process, to another. In a sense, this device resembles that of transformation (above), although in this case, the bacterial DNA is protected in a phage coat and enters a cell using the phage's machinery.

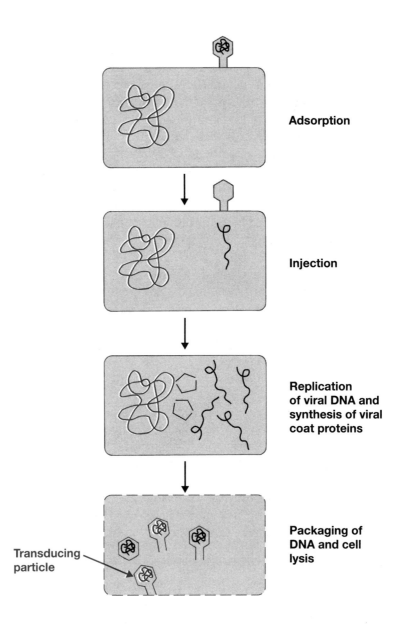

Adsorption

Injection

**Replication
of viral DNA and
synthesis of viral
coat proteins**

**Packaging of
DNA and cell
lysis**

Transducing
particle

Figure 3.8.

Creation of a transducing
phage by generalized transduction.

Transduction falls into two broad classes, **generalized transduction** and **specialized transduction.** In generalized transduction, any of the bacterial genes can be packaged, as shown in Figure 3.8. Each phage coat receives a "headful" of DNA, typically about 20 genes worth. This DNA is usually a phage genome but occasionally a headful of host DNA is received. This DNA can then be passed on to a recipient cell by adsorption and subsequent injection.

Specialized transduction is carried out by a particular class of bacteriophage called **temperate phage.** Upon infection, temperate viruses can reproduce and lyse the host cell as described above. These viruses also have an alternative pathway available to them: they can insert their DNA into the host chromosome and replicate passively as a component of the bacterial chromosome, causing the bacterium no harm (Fig. 3.9A). Such a virus might remain dormant in the bacterium for many generations. However, in response to certain environmental signals, the dormant virus can be induced to grow lytically, killing the host cell and releasing hundreds of progeny phage. This induction begins with the excision of the viral DNA from the host chromosome. This excision (as well as its prior insertion) is carried out by a specialized set of proteins, the most important of which are encoded by the virus. As shown in Figure 3.9B, these proteins occasionally err and excise a piece of DNA that contains both virus genes and host genes. In many cases, these hybrid viral genomes are replicated, packaged, and released as phage particles. On infection of a naive cell, the phage injects this hybrid genome and the infected cell receives bacterial (as well as viral) genes.

In contrast to generalized transduction, specialized transduction has an important limitation: a given temperate virus inserts itself into only one spot on the bacterial chromosome. Therefore, the bacterial genes available for specialized transduction are limited to those lying at or near the site of insertion.

General Recombination

We have seen three ways in which DNA can be transferred from one bacterium to another. These methods of exchange would be relatively useless, however, unless the newly arrived DNA were assimilated into the genetic makeup of the recipient. For plasmids, which can replicate autonomously within a cell, no further step is needed. In contrast, most segments of DNA acquired by transformation or transduction would be rapidly diluted as the bacterium replicates its DNA and divides, unless it was incorporated into the recipient's genome. This incorporation usually occurs by means of **general recombination,** a process that appears so important for maintaining genetic diversity that it is thought to occur in all organisms. (In humans, e.g., the crossing over of chromosomes during egg

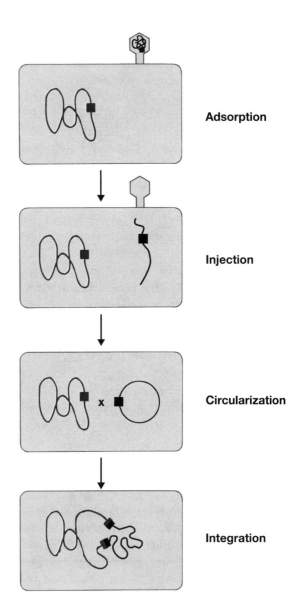

Adsorption

Injection

Circularization

Integration

Figure 3.9A.

Integration of a temperate bacteriophage into a bacterial genome.

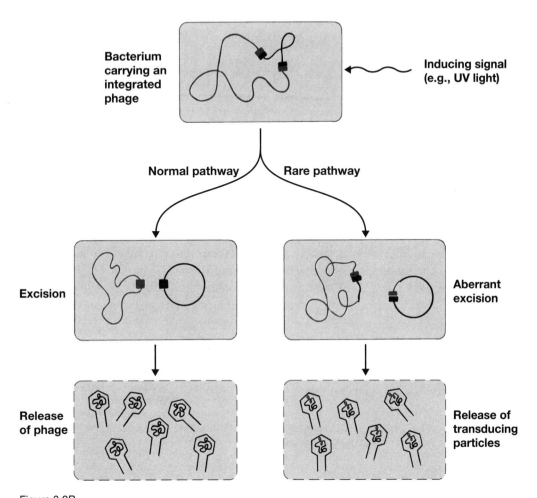

Figure 3.9B.

Creation of transducing phage by specialized transduction. Only temperate phage can participate in specialized transduction.

and sperm cell development utilizes this type of recombination.) Although the precise mechanism is a subject of intense research and a certain amount of controversy, the process involves the breakage and reunion of two double helices. A remarkable feature of this type of exchange is that it occurs only between two DNA duplexes that are homologous, that is, very similar in sequence. This generality arises because the DNA of any sequence can participate in this event, as long as a homolog is available.

As shown in Figure 3.10, DNA transferred into a bacterium by transformation, generalized transduction, or Hfr conjugal transfer can, through a double re-combination event, replace the recipient's copy of the homologous region of the chromosome.

TRANSPOSONS

Some of the rapid evolutionary changes in bacteria can be seen as a conse-quence of **transposons,** which are short segments of DNA that can move around within a cell to many different positions on the bacterial chromosome and plas-mids. Transposition is distinguished from the examples of programmed DNA rearrangements discussed above due to the unpredictability of the movement. Al-though some transposons have highly preferred targets, others can insert them-selves into nearly any location on a bacterial chromosome or plasmid.

The simplest transposons are called **insertion sequences (IS).** These tran-sposons consist of a gene that encodes a **transposase** (the enzyme largely respon-sible for the movement of the transposon) flanked by special DNA sequences that are also required for the movement of the element. The main consequence of the

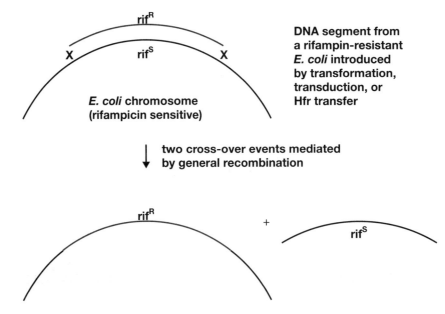

Figure 3.10.

Example showing how two cross-overs can result in the replacement of a section of the *E. coli* chromosome with foreign DNA introduced by transformation, conjugation, or transduction.

movement of IS elements is the inactivation of genes into which they land. At any given time, many copies of IS elements are scattered around the bacterial chromosomes and plasmids and they can serve as portable regions of homology that permit general recombination. For example, the integration of the F plasmid into the bacterial chromosome to form an Hfr strain (above and Fig. 3.7) can occur by recombination between one IS element on the plasmid and a second on the chromosome. Of greater clinical importance is a second class of transposon, the **composite transposons.** These transposons often consist of an antibiotic resistance gene flanked by two insertion sequences (Fig. 3.11). This type of element is thought to have evolved by the fortuitous insertion of IS elements to either side of a drug resistance gene. The composite transposon moves as a unit; that is, the drug resistance gene is carried along with the two IS elements. This design has important consequences for the spread of antibiotic resistance among bacteria. For example, a composite transposon could jump from a bacterial chromosome to a conjugative plasmid present in the same cell. The plasmid could then be transferred to a new cell by conjugation allowing the spread of the transposon. In fact, close inspection of the DNA sequence of the R1 drug resistance plasmid (Fig. 3.5) has suggested that it arose from the insertion in close proximity of several composite transposons, each carrying a different drug resistance gene.

Several additional types of transposons are found in bacteria; some are quite complex, such as the remarkable class present in the genus *Streptococcus.* These transposons, in addition to drug resistance genes, carry genes that encode conjugation systems allowing the transfer of the transposon (along with neighboring DNA) into recipient cells. This appears to be a major pathway for the spread of antibiotic resistance in this genus of bacteria.

Finally, it should be noted that transposons are found in virtually all organ-

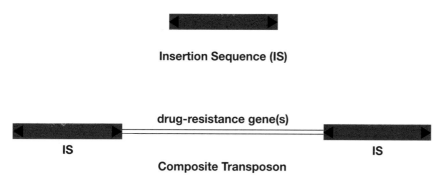

Insertion Sequence (IS)

drug-resistance gene(s)

IS   IS

Composite Transposon

Figure 3.11.

Idealized view of an insertion sequence and a composite transposon.

isms ranging from bacteria to humans. In all cases, they are thought to provide an important and rapid source of genetic diversity on which selective pressure acts to allow the fittest to survive.

SUMMARY

1. The genetic makeup of bacterial cells is continually changing. Selective pressure in the form of antibiotic drugs or the immune system allows rare variants to proliferate and take over a population.

2. Simple mutations, such as those generated by rare errors in DNA replication, are an important source of genetic variability for all organisms.

3. Programmed DNA rearrangements (especially translocations and inversions) constitute one strategy employed by microorganisms to continually change the identity of components on their surfaces.

4. The movement of genetic material between different bacteria (by transformation, conjugation, and transduction) provides yet another source of genetic diversity. The proliferation of drug resistance genes in many different genera of bacteria is testimony to the efficiency of these mechanisms, especially conjugation.

5. Transposons (many of which also carry drug resistance genes) jump to different spots on bacterial chromosomes and plasmids. These transposons can be regarded as drug resistance DNA modules and figure prominently in the dispersion of drug resistance genes among bacteria.

REFERENCES

Alberts B, Bray D, Lewis J, Raff M, Roberts K, Watson JD (1994): Molecular Biology of the Cell. 3rd ed. New York: Garland Publishing.

Berg DE, Howe MM (eds) (1989): Mobile DNA. Washington, DC: American Society for Microbiology.

Jawetz E, Melnick JL, Adelberg EA (1982): Review of Medical Microbiology. 15th ed. Los Altos, NY: Lange Medical Publications.

Kornberg A, Baker TA (1992): DNA Replication, 2nd ed. New York: W.H. Freeman and Co.

Neidhardt FC, Ingraham JL, Low KB, Magasanik B, Schaechter M, Umbarger HE (eds) (1987): *Escherichia coli* and *Salmonella typhimurium* Cellular and Molecular Biology, Vol. 2. 2nd ed. Washington, DC: American Society for Microbiology.

Watson JD, Hopkins NH, Roberts JW, Steitz JA, Weiner AM (1987): Molecular Biology of the Gene, 4th ed. Menlo Park, CA: The Benjamin/Cummings Publishing Co.

REVIEW QUESTIONS

> For questions 1 to 7, choose the ONE
> BEST answer or completion.

1. Which of the following genetic mechanisms
   require that a donor and a recipient bacterium be in physical contact?
   a) Transformation
   b) Conjugation
   c) Transduction
   d) Inversion
   e) All of the above

2. Bacteria can acquire resistance to antibiotics
   by which of the following routes?
   a) Transformation
   b) Simple mutation
   c) Conjugation
   d) Plasmid mobilization
   e) All of the above

3. An Hfr strain of *Escherichia coli* differs from
   an F⁺ strain in which of the following ways:
   a) The flagella of the Hfr strain are shorter.
   b) The Hfr strain has an F factor integrated
      into the bacterial genome.
   c) The Hfr strain is less susceptible to attack
      by antibodies.
   d) The Hfr strain is more susceptible to an-
      tibiotics.
   e) The Hfr strain grows more rapidly.

4. Which of the following statements is NOT
   true for generalized transduction?
   a) The transduction is carried out by bacte-
      riophage.
   b) Any bacterial gene can be transferred.
   c) The donor and recipient bacteria need not
      be in contact.
   d) The transduction is carried out without
      lysis of the donor bacterium.
   e) The transferred genes are packaged into
      a phage.

5. Which of the following mechanisms is responsible for the switching of surface proteins in trypanosomes?
   a) Translocation
   b) Inversion
   c) Conjugation
   d) Transduction
   e) None of the above

6. An F⁺ bacterium differs from an F⁻ bacterium in which of the following ways?
   a) The F⁺ bacterium carries genes respon-
      sible for formation of the sex pilus; the
      F⁻ bacterium cannot make these struc-
      tures.
   b) The F⁺ bacterium can undergo DNA
      transformation, whereas the F⁻ cannot.
   c) The F⁺ bacterium has flagella, whereas
      the F⁻ bacterium does not.

d) During conjugation, the F$^+$ bacteria acts as the recipient and the F$^-$ bacterium acts as the DNA donor.

e) All of the above.

7. Which of the following statements are generally true for plasmids?

a) Plasmids can move from bacterium to bacterium by both conjugation and mobilization.

b) Plasmids can carry more than one drug-resistance gene.

c) Plasmids can be transferred between bacteria of different genera.

d) Plasmids contain their own origins of DNA replication.

e) All of the above.

ANSWERS TO REVIEW QUESTIONS

---

1. *b* During conjugation, the donor and recipient bacteria are joined to allow the passage of DNA.

2. *e* Although conjugation is probably the most common route of drug resistance gene dissemination, drug resistance can be acquired by all four of the mechanisms listed in the question.

3. *b* An F$^+$ strain of *Escherichia coli* becomes an Hfr strain when the F factor integrates into the bacterial genome.

4. *d* In the process of transduction, the recipient bacterium is lysed, releasing transducing particles.

5. *a* Translocation allows trypanosomes to carry many silent copies of VSG genes, any one of which can become active.

6. *a* The F factor carries genes required for formation of the sex pilus, as well as genes required to effect the transfer of DNA from the donor bacterium (the F$^+$) to the recipient bacterium (F$^-$).

7. *e* The answers *a, b,* and *c* are especially important in understanding the rapid spread of R plasmids.

CHAPTER 4

STERILIZATION, DISINFECTION, AND ANTISEPSIS

Sterilization, disinfection, and antisepsis techniques are an inherent part of proper medical and surgical practice. An understanding of the principles and practical applications of these procedures is evident when one considers the many frank and potentially pathogenic organisms that are able to remain viable outside the body for long periods of time, exhibit a high degree of resistance to physical methods and chemical agents, and can be transmitted with relative ease.

DEFINITIONS

Sterilization refers to the destruction or elimination of all microorganisms by physical means, including heat, radiation, and filtration.

Disinfection or germicidal refers to the destruction of pathogenic or potentially pathogenic microorganisms by chemical means. The term usually applies to the treatment of fomites (inanimate objects) but the term ''skin disinfectant'' has been used in medical practice.

Antisepsis refers to the destruction or prevention of growth of pathogenic or potentially pathogenic microorganisms by chemical means. The term usually refers to the external application of a chemical to tissues.

Bacteriostatic agent refers to a chemical or biological agent that prevents the growth and multiplication of but does not destroy pathogenic or potentially pathogenic microorganisms. The term refers to those agents applied to fomites or to external or internal tissues.

Bactericidal agent refers to a chemical or biological agent that destroys pathogenic or potentially pathogenic microorganisms. This term also refers to those agents applied to fomites or to external or internal tissues.

STERILIZATION

Dry Heat

Dry heat destroys microorganisms by lysis or protein denaturation. There are two types of dry heat sterilization: incineration and hot-air ovens.

Incineration is considered the best method to dispose of infected carcasses and organic wastes; sterilization of inoculating loops by passage through a Bunsen burner is another effective form of incineration.

Hot-air ovens produce dry heat by gas or electricity in insulated double-walled metal containers. The temperature and time required for effective sterilization is 180°C for 2 h. Although small hot-air metal ovens are available for physicians' offices, they cannot be used to sterilize rubber or fabrics and are, therefore, of limited value.

Moist Heat

Moist heat is a more efficient and rapid method for denaturating microbial proteins than dry heat due to its greater penetrating power. There are three types of moist heat sterilization: the autoclave, pasteurization, and boiling water.

The **autoclave,** which operates by creating high temperatures under steam pressure, is the most effective, common, and practical method of sterilization (Fig. 4.1). Most modern autoclaves are equipped with a drying apparatus. They are available in appropriate sizes for physicians' offices.

Pasteurization is used primarily in the dairy industry. Pasteurization is the process whereby milk or milk products are exposed to temperature for a time

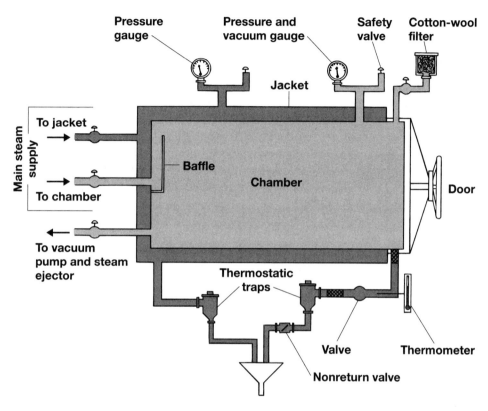

Figure 4.1.

A downward displacement autoclave. [Redrawn with permission from Russell AD, Hugo WB, Ayliffe GAJ (1982): Principles and Practice of Disinfection, Preservation and Sterilisation. Oxford: Blackwell Scientific Publications.]

which destroys pathogenic and potentially pathogenic nonspore-forming bacteria transmissible by these products, but has no or slight effect upon the flavor. The recommended temperatures and times are based upon their ability to destroy *Mycobacterium tuberculosis,* the most heat resistant of the nonspore-forming pathogenic bacteria.

Boiling water, even for as long as 30 min, is not recommended for sterilization, inasmuch as it dulls and rusts the cutting edges of instruments and does not kill bacterial spores or certain viruses such as hepatitis B.

Ultraviolet Light

Ultraviolet (UV) light is a form of radiant energy in which relatively short wavelengths are absorbed by bacterial DNA, resulting in the formation of pyrimidine dimers that interfere with normal base pairing. As a result, DNA synthesis is inhibited and the bacteria are inactivated. The DNA can be repaired by enzyme systems that hydrolyze or remove the dimers and thus allow normal synthesis to proceed. This mechanism is thought to be the major reason for the increased resistance of organisms, such as staphylococci and spore formers, to UV light. Mercury vapor lamps, which serve as a UV source, are sometimes used in enclosed areas such as operating rooms in an effort to control airborne infections; however, the ability of some potential pathogens to survive under these conditions render this procedure questionable. Ultraviolet light can cause serious **corneal damage** and is therefore never used during ophthalmological procedures.

Ionizing Radiation

Ionizing radiation is a form of radiant energy in which high energy X- and γ-rays with shorter wavelengths and greater penetrating power than UV light are absorbed by microorganisms. Ionized water within the cell results in free radicals that recombine to form peroxides damaging to the DNA. This method has been used for the sterilization and preservation of foods such as bacon, poultry, and seafood.

Filtration

Filtration is a mechanical method for eliminating bacteria from biological fluids and from the air (Fig. 4.2). **Laminar flow systems** are used to ventilate operating rooms, laboratories, and areas housing immunosuppressed and burn patients. Filtered air is pumped into the space at a pressure required to displace regular circulating air. This method creates a continual pistonlike displacement within the area that is highly effective in reducing the numbers of airborne organisms.

DISINFECTION AND ANTISEPSIS

As shown in Table 4.1, several factors influence the activity of disinfectants and antiseptic agents against microorganisms.

Surface-active agents injure the bacterial cell by damaging the cytoplasmic

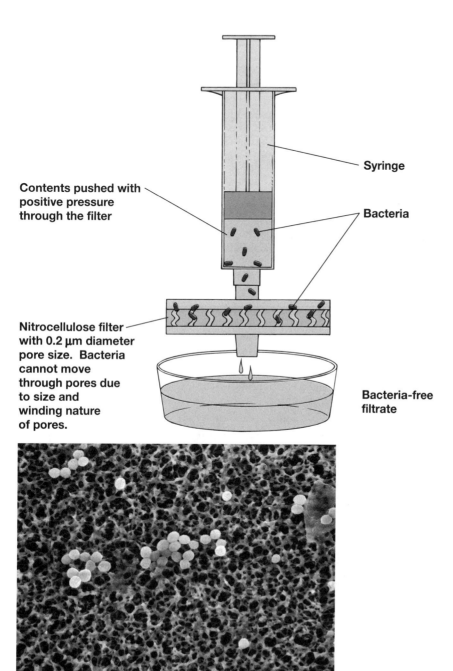

Syringe

Contents pushed with positive pressure through the filter

Bacteria

Nitrocellulose filter with 0.2 μm diameter pore size. Bacteria cannot move through pores due to size and winding nature of pores.

Bacteria-free filtrate

Figure 4.2.

Filtration. (Top) Use of filter for sterilization. (Bottom) Electron micrograph of bacteria trapped on surface of nitrocellulose filter. (Courtesy of the Millipore Corporation, Bedford, MA.)

TABLE 4.1. Factors That Influence the Activity of Disinfectants and Antiseptics Against Microorganisms

Factor	Influence upon effectiveness
Concentration	Higher concentrations are usually more effective
Exposure time	Inactivation of microorganisms requires an exposure time dependent on the organism and the agent
Temperature	Temperature required for inactivation is dependent on the chemical nature and mechanism of action of the agent; in general, bacterial inactivation occurs at double the rate for each 10°C increase in temperature
pH	Affects inactivation by influencing the degree of ionization and resultant cytoplasmic membrane penetration by the agent
Condition of the fomite	The presence of organic matter, such as blood, pus, or saliva, on hinged or nonhinged instruments may inhibit cell penetration of the agent or may result in the agent becoming inert due to nonspecific binding to protein
Type of microorganism	Most disinfectants do not kill spore formers as effectively as nonspore formers, sometimes requiring 12 h; some nonspore formers have a high degree of resistance to several disinfectants

membrane and altering cell permeability. **Cationic detergents** are quaternary ammonium compounds that dissociate to yield positively charged ions (quaternary NH_4) that disrupt cytoplasmic membrane phospholipids. **Anionic detergents** are soaps and fatty acids that dissociate to yield negatively charged ions that disrupt cytoplasmic membrane lipoproteins. Their inability to kill spores or several gram-negative organisms associated with nosocomial (hospital acquired) diseases renders them of little value as disinfectants.

Phenols are compounds that bind to and denature proteins within the bacterial cytoplasmic membrane resulting in membrane damage, leakage of cell contents, and lysis of the organism. These compounds are bactericidal for both gram-negative and gram-positive bacteria, including the spore formers. Phenolic compounds, such as **Amphyl**[R] in concentrations of 2–5%, are excellent disinfectants for washing down surfaces such as operating room floors and laboratory benches.

Halogens inactivate bacterial enzyme systems by converting functional sulfhydryl groups to the oxidized form. Chlorine and iodine compounds, like the phenols, are bactericidal for both gram-negative and gram-positive organisms, including the spore formers.

Chlorine is used as a disinfectant in treating water supplies and the hypochlorite salts are used in household cleansers. **Phisohex**[R], a bacteriostatic hexachlorophene compound containing chlorine and phenol in complex, is more effective against gram-positive than gram-negative organisms. It is used in hospital soap dispensers and as a presurgical scrub solution for physicians' hands and for the skin of patients at their operative sites. The limited effectiveness of Phisohex against gram-negative organisms, the dermatitis experienced by some adults, and the dermal absorption and fatal neurotoxicity that occurs following its use during the bathing of newborns, restrict its value. Infrequent autoclaving of soap dispensers and infrequent replacement of the compound within the dispensers contribute to the survival of potentially pathogenic organisms.

The two most frequently used iodine compounds are **Betadine**[R] and **2% tincture of iodine.** Betadine, a povidone-iodine complex, is an excellent solution for use as a presurgical scrub for physicians and patients as evidenced by its excellent bactericidal activity, minimal toxicity, and minimal allergic sensitization during human field evaluations. Both Betadine and 2% tincture of iodine are rapid and effective skin disinfectants for use prior to the removal of blood for culture.

Alcohols denature cell proteins and disorganize cytoplasmic membrane lipids resulting in a loss of membrane permeability. A **70% alcohol** solution exerts a bactericidal effect upon gram-negative and gram-positive organisms, exclusive of spore formers. Although it is most widely used as a skin disinfectant prior to the removal of blood for laboratory assays, the relatively long period of contact required for killing (e.g., 10 min for *Staphylococcus aureus*) limits its usefulness.

Heavy metals inactivate microbial enzyme systems resulting in interference with protein synthesis. Most heavy metals are too toxic for human use, but some have been employed prophylactically with success. Until relatively recently, **1% silver nitrate (AgNO$_3$)** was instilled routinely into the eyes of newborns in order to prevent gonococcal ophthalmia neonatorum; however, this has now been largely replaced by erythromycin or tetracycline ointment.

Gases are used as disinfecting agents under special circumstances.

Ethylene oxide is the most widely used of the gases. It interferes with protein synthesis by alkylating protein and thus blocking free amino groups. It is an excellent bactericidal agent against gram-negative and gram-positive organisms, including spore formers, and is used in the disinfection of heart-lung machines, polyethylene tubing, lensed instruments, biologicals, and other materials that would otherwise be damaged by heat or disinfecting solutions. Care must be taken when using ethylene oxide due to its potential tissue toxicity. Although a 24 to 72-h period of aeration is required after disinfection in order to get rid of residual fumes, a 7-day aeration has been recommended if the disinfected devices are to come in direct contact with tissues for an extended period of time (e.g., pacemakers and artificial heart valves).

Formaldehyde is a gas whose mechanism of action and bactericidal activity is identical to that of ethylene oxide. It is used to decontaminate rooms and fabrics, but causes damage to the cutting edges of instruments. Like ethylene oxide, it is irritating to the skin and leaves residual fumes which necessitate similar periods of aeration. **Formalin** is formaldehyde in aqueous form. It is used at a 10% concentration to preserve tissues for histopathological study. At appropriate concentration, formalin is valuable in the preparation of several vaccines by virtue of its ability to convert toxins to nontoxic, vaccinogenic toxoids and to inactivate certain viruses while preserving their protective immunogenic properties.

Beta-propiolactone is another gas whose mechanism of action and bactericidal activity is identical to that of ethylene oxide. Despite its poor penetrating power and potential carcinogenic property, it has been used in aqueous form to sterilize artery, bone, and cartilage grafts.

Glutaraldehyde is an alkylating agent that binds sulfhydryl or amino groups. In 2% aqueous solution, it is an excellent bactericidal agent against gram-negative and gram-positive organisms, including spore formers. Glutaraldehyde is highly effective as a ''cold'' disinfectant for lensed and other surgical instruments, as well as for respiratory therapy equipment. Because glutaraldehyde is toxic to tissues, disinfection must be followed by rinsing with sterile distilled water.

SUMMARY

1. **The autoclave, which operates by creating high temperatures under steam pressure, is the most effective, common, and practical method of sterilization in use today.**

2. **Membrane filters are effective for biological fluids, and laminar flow systems are used to ventilate operating rooms, laboratories, and areas housing immunosuppressed and burn patients.**

3. **The activity of disinfectants and antiseptic agents is influenced by several factors including concentration of the chemical agent, exposure time and temperature, pH, condition of the fomite, and type of microorganism.**

4. **Phenolic compounds, such as Amphyl, are excellent bactericidal agents and can be used effectively for washing down surfaces such as operating room floors and laboratory benches.**

5. **Chlorine is an effective disinfectant used in potable water supplies, household cleanser, and bleach, while iodine in the form of a povodone-iodine complex known as Betadine is excellent as a presurgical scrub for physicians**

and patients. Both Betadine and 2% tincture of iodine are rapid and effective skin disinfectants for use prior to the removal of blood for culture.

6. Alcohols, including 70% ethanol, are ineffective as skin disinfectants prior to the removal of blood due to the relatively long period of contact required for bacterial killing.

7. Among the gases, ethylene oxide is an excellent, frequently used disinfectant for heart-lung machines, polyethylene tubing, lensed instruments, biologicals, and other materials that would otherwise be damaged by heat or disinfecting solutions.

8. Formalin, at appropriate concentrations, is employed to preserve tissues for histopathological study and to inactivate viruses and toxins without affecting their vaccinogenic properties.

9. Glutaraldehyde in 2% aqueous solution is highly effective as a "cold" disinfectant for lensed and other surgical instruments, as well as for respiratory therapy equipment.

REFERENCES

Block SS (ed) (1983): Disinfection, Sterilization, and Preservation. 3rd ed. Philadelphia: Lea & Febiger.

Connell JF Jr, Rousselot LM (1964): Povidone-iodine. Extensive surgical evaluation of a new antiseptic agent. Am J Surg 108:849.

Gardner JF, Peel MM (1986): Introduction to Sterilization and Disinfection. Edinburgh, Scotland: Churchill Livingstone.

Joress SM (1962): A study of disinfection of the skin: a comparison of povidone-iodine with other agents used for surgical scrubs. Ann Surg 155:296.

McDade JJ, Phillips GB, Sivinski HD, Whitfield WJ (1969): Principles and applications of laminar-flow devices. In Norris JR, Ribbons DW (eds): Methods in Microbiology, Vol. 1, New York: Academic Press.

REVIEW QUESTIONS

For questions 1 and 2, choose the ONE BEST answer or completion.

1. Sterilization can best be accomplished by the use of
   a) pasteurization
   b) a bacteriostatic agent
   c) a bactericidal agent
   d) an autoclave
   e) ultraviolet light

2. The safe, effective, and practical reduction of the numbers of pathogenic airborne organisms in a hospital environment can best be accomplished by the use of
   a) dry heat
   b) membrane filters
   c) laminar flow systems
   d) ultraviolet light
   e) ionizing radiation

For questions 3 to 5, ONE or MORE of the completions given is correct. Choose the appropriate answer.

A) if only **1, 2, 3** are correct
B) if only **1 and 3** are correct
C) if only **2 and 4** are correct
D) if only **4** is correct
E) if **all** are correct

3. Factors that influence the activity of disinfectants and antiseptic agents against microorganisms include
   1) concentration of the chemical agent
   2) exposure time and temperature
   3) pH
   4) the object to be disinfected
   5) the type of microorganism

4. Effective and rapid disinfection of the skin prior to the obtaining of blood for culture is accomplished by the use of
   1) 70% ethanol
   2) Provodone-iodine compounds, such as Betadine
   3) hexachlorophene compounds, such as Phisohex
   4) 2% tincture of iodine
   5) 1% silver nitrate

5. The gas ethylene oxide
   1) is used effectively in the disinfection of heart-lung machines, polyethylene tubing, and lensed instruments
   2) functions as a bacteriostatic agent
   3) has potential tissue toxicity which necessitates aeration following its use
   4) has a poorer penetrating power than β-propiolactone
   5) can be used to inactivate toxins and certain viruses as a prelude to their use as vaccines

ANSWERS TO REVIEW QUESTIONS

1. **d** Of the methods and agents listed, only the autoclave destroys all microorganisms.

2. **c** Only the laminar flow system, with its pistonlike displacement of circulating air, is effective in reducing airborne pathogens in a hospital environment.

3. **E** All are correct statements.

4. **C** Betadine and 2% tincture of iodine are the only bactericidal agents that can rapidly and effectively disinfect the skin in preparation for the removal of blood for culture.

5. **B** Ethylene oxide functions as a bactericidal agent with excellent penetrating power in the disinfection of heart-lung machines, polyethylene tubing, and lensed instruments, but has potential tissue toxicity that necessitates aeration after its use. It cannot be used as is formalin in the preparation of vaccines.

ANTIMICROBIAL AGENTS

Until the twentieth century, there were no special agents available to treat infectious diseases, other than folk remedies and herbal concoctions. Amazingly, the hundreds of antimicrobial agents available today were developed within the last 80 years. The massive growth and profits of the antimicrobial industry have fueled interest in developing new agents; new antifungals and antivirals are important byproducts of this interest.

Criteria for a successful antimicrobial agent are listed below:

1. Displays targeted toxicity (i.e., to the offending microbe only).
2. Produces no side effects in the host.
3. Displays a narrow range of activity (i.e., does not harm normal host flora).
4. Kills the targeted microorganism (bactericidal), rather than merely inhibiting its growth (bacteriostatic).
5. Fails to induce resistance.
6. Remains stable in body fluids and retains a long period of activity (half-life, $t_{1/2}$).
7. Does not induce an allergic or toxic host response.
8. Is soluble in body fluids and tissues.

Obviously, this ideal has not yet been met. In most cases, the goal of antimicrobial therapy is to reduce the total numbers of infecting microbes to a level low enough that host defenses can destroy them. Only certain patients with extremely compromised host immune defenses, such as those receiving chemotherapy, patients with AIDS, patients whose immune systems themselves are ravaged by malignancies, those in which the infectious process is beyond the reach of internal immune mechanisms, and irradiated patients, must depend on antimicrobial agents for complete eradication of infectious agents. In many cases, these patients die as a direct result of overwhelming infection, rather than as a direct result of their underlying disease.

This chapter will discuss several aspects of antimicrobial therapy and present examples of structures and functions of the most commonly used antibacterial and antifungal agents. Antiviral agents are presented in Chapter 34. The subject of antimicrobial agents is in a state of constant flux as new agents are being developed and new therapeutic modalities are being explored.

DEFINITIONS

Antimicrobial Agent: A substance that either kills, inhibits growth of, or prevents damage due to an infectious microorganism. Antibacterial, antifungal, antiprotozoal, antihelminthic, and antiviral agents are subsets of antimicrobial agents.

Antibiotic: A substance produced by a fungus or bacterium that inhibits growth of other microorganisms. Most antimicrobial agents used therapeutically today are either wholly synthetically derived or are synthesized from precursors developed in microbes (usually fungi).

Chemotherapeutic Agent: A substance, biologically or synthetically derived, used to treat any disease, infectious or noninfectious (e.g., cancer or hypertension).

. . . cidal: Indicates that the action of the agent will kill the targeted microbe. Bactericidal, fungicidal, and virucidal are derived terms.

. . . static: Indicates that the action of the agent will inhibit growth of the targeted microbe but will not kill it. Bacteriostatic and fungistatic are derived terms.

Pharmacokinetics: The study of the concentrations and activities of chemotherapeutic agents in patients. Relevant factors include the patient's age, weight, renal function, nutritional status, other disease states; as well as the nature of the infecting organism, the site of infection, and concurrent additional therapeutic agents being administered.

Peak and Trough: Terms used to describe the highest serum concentration (peak) and the lowest (trough) of an administered antimicrobial agent. Presumably the trough occurs just before the next dose is administered.

Half-Life: The amount of time required after initial administration of an antimicrobial agent and attainment of the peak level for the serum concentration to fall by one-half. The shorter the half-life, the more often the drug will need to be given.

Empiric: Therapy chosen based on clinical impressions of the disease and its putative etiologic agent and prevalent infectious agents in the environment because specific information about the patient's organisms is not yet available. Therapy refers to delivery of an antimicrobial agent after the infection has occurred or during the course of the infection.

Prophylactic: Actions chosen to prevent development of an infectious process, before the actual development of infection or disease has occurred.

Therapeutic: Antimicrobial agent chosen specifically for its effectiveness against a particular infectious process or microbial agent.

Synergy: The antimicrobial activity of two antimicrobial agents used together is greater than the additive effect of both agents used alone (Fig. 5.1). One way in which this effect can be gained is by using two agents with different modes of action. For example, a combination of an aminoglycoside that acts on the ribosome, plasma membrane, DNA synthesis, and/or other sites and a penicillin that acts on the cell wall is often used. The penicillin's effect is to allow easier access into the bacterial cell to the aminoglycoside, which then deals the death blow. Synergy must be determined independently for each combination of bacterial agents, as results are not predictable.

Antagonism: The antimicrobial activity of one antimicrobial agent is diminished by another agent being administered concurrently. If one agent (such as a penicillin) requires cell growth to be effective, another agent (such as chloramphenicol) that inhibits cell growth will actually counteract the effects of the penicillin. As with synergy, antagonism must be determined independently for each combination of bacterial agents, as results are not predictable.

FACTORS INVOLVED IN EFFICACY

Is the Putative Pathogen Inhibited or Killed by the Antimicrobial Agent?

Some microbes are inherently resistant to certain classes of antimicrobial agents. For example, penicillins act on bacterial cell walls. Since parasites and fungi have different cell structures, penicillins have no effect upon them. Inherent

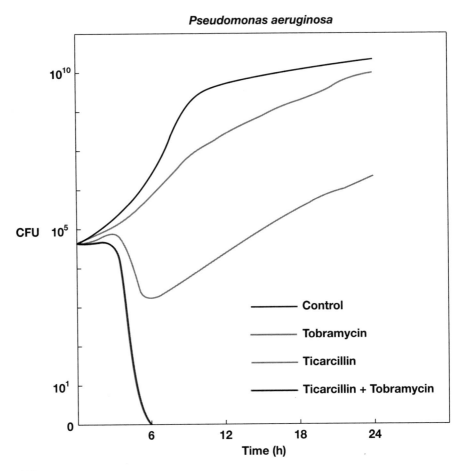

Figure 5.1.

Bacterial killing curve illustrating antimicrobial synergy. [Redrawn from Methods of Testing Combinations of Antimicrobial Agents. © 1984 Hoffman-La Roche, Inc., Nutley, NJ.]

resistance is exemplified by metronidazole, which depends on anaerobic metabolic enzymes to modify its structure to the active drug; aerobic bacteria do not possess the modifying enzymes and are not effected by metronidazole, even though it may gain entrance to the bacterial cell. Vancomycin is active only against gram-positive bacteria because the outer membrane of gram-negative organisms prevents vancomycin from reaching its active site.

Enterococci, among the most common nosocomial (hospital-acquired) pathogens are inherently resistant to several antimicrobial agents, including aminoglycosides, cephalosporins, and many penicillinase-resistant penicillins due to their structure and to chromosomally mediated enzyme production. Sulfonamides, for example, act as structural analogs of precursors in the microbial pathway of folic acid production, a step in the formation of purines. Enterococci are uniquely able to use preformed folate as a source of substrate, and thus are not susceptible to any agent that acts earlier in the synthetic pathway.

Can the Antimicrobial Agent Reach the Site of Infection With a Concentration High Enough to Inhibit or Kill the Microbe?

Several concerns are relevant.

ROUTE OF ADMINISTRATION. Available routes of administration of antimicrobial agents include: topical, aerosolized, oral, intramuscular, and intravenous, in increasing order of systemic effects.

Intravenous administration may allow high concentrations in the blood, but the agent may not pass the blood-brain barrier efficiently in some cases. Oral administration may be effective for achieving high gut levels of the agent, but systemic levels may not be adequate for treating extraintestinal sites.

PROTEIN BINDING OF THE ANTIMICROBIAL AGENT. Many agents bind to serum proteins, notably albumin. Only unbound (free) drug is able to exert antimicrobial activity.

LIPID SOLUBILITY OF THE ANTIMICROBIAL AGENT. When a drug does not efficiently cross through capillary walls into the tissues, activity may be less than expected. A highly lipid-soluble agent can more easily cross cell membrane barriers to reach the site of infection. Lipid-soluble agents include metronidazole, trimethoprim, and rifampin.

ACTIVE TRANSPORT ENZYMES IN THE HOST. Several antimicrobial agents are actively secreted by host metabolic enzymes into urine, bile, or other anatomical sites, which limits their availability at sites of infection other than those into which the agent is secreted. A second agent to inhibit this transport is sometimes given (e.g., probenicid is given to maintain high levels of penicillin after intramuscular injection for treatment of gonorrhea).

Could the Host Inactivate the Agent Enzymatically?

Certain antimicrobial agents may be hydrolyzed or destroyed by host enzymes. Imipenem, for example, is inactivated by a peptidase in the renal tubules, with concomitant loss of activity and nephrotoxicity. This problem has been addressed by administering imipenem with cilastatin, an agent that inhibits the action of the peptidase.

Is the Patient Receiving Other Agents That Might Interfere With Activity of the Antimicrobial Agent?

Cancer patients on chemotherapy may already be receiving a potentially hepatotoxic agent; the addition of pyrazinamide, an antimycobacterial agent known to be hepatotoxic, for example, would be contraindicated. Metronidazole has a disulfiram reaction with alcohol; simultaneous treatment with an alcohol-based agent would be problematic. Many other negative aspects of drug interactions exist. The pharmacologic specialist should be consulted for advice.

Are the Organisms Growing so Slowly or in a Protected Site so That the Antimicrobial Agent Will Not Be Effective?

Staphylococci may colonize a prosthetic heart valve or intravenous catheter and surround themselves with ''slime,'' a thick glycocalyx layer that inhibits penetration of host serum and cellular factors as well as antimicrobials. Once thus sequestered, the organisms exhibit very decreased metabolic rates not amenable to the action of antimicrobial agents. Microbes growing within an abscess are also protected from antimicrobial agents by their slowed growth. Some patients develop mycelial fungal infections in lung cavities created as a result of a prior tuberculosis infection. Fungi growing in such cavities are virtually impossible to treat medically and must be removed surgically. Bacteria growing in bone matrix during osteomyelitis are notoriously difficult to treat. Herpesviruses latent in nerve ganglia cannot be reached by any available antiviral agents.

Could Indigenous Bacteria Inactivate the Antimicrobial Agent?

A very controversial theory suggests that certain indigenous bacteria produce enzymes that hydrolyze antibiotics such as penicillin.

ADDITIONAL FACTORS RELATED TO CHOICE OF AN ANTIMICROBIAL AGENT

Hospital and Community Susceptibility Patterns

If a resistant strain of the putative infectious agent is prevalent in the community or the hospital, then an antimicrobial must be chosen that will be effective in the face of resistance. For example, in hospitals with numerous strains of methicillin-resistant staphylococci isolated from patients in various units, a new surgical wound infection must be treated empirically with vancomycin, which is effective against methicillin-resistant staphylococci, until the agent is identified as other than staphylococci or the susceptibility pattern of the isolate is known. Standard treatment of gonorrhea throughout the United States must be with a more expensive agent (such as ceftriaxone) that is effective against resistant strains, now that penicillin-resistant gonococci are rampant.

Dosing Schedule

Although an antimicrobial agent may be less expensive initially, if it must be delivered by intravenous (IV) infusion every 6 h, it places difficult demands on pharmacy personnel and nurses. An equally effective antimicrobial that is slightly more expensive but that can be administered every 8 h will be more cost effective in the long run. Patients on numerous chemotherapeutic regimens must be treated in such a manner as to maximize the therapies and avoid antagonisms between agents.

Cost

Not only must the cost of the antimicrobial agent be considered, but certain necessary additional tests are also important. For example, several antimicrobial agents are nephrotoxic and their serum levels must be monitored to avoid overdosing. The laboratory tests for drug levels are an expense that must be added to that of the antimicrobial agent alone. For some renally excreted agents, toxic concentrations in serum are dangerously close to the efficacy levels; thus, renal output must be monitored by creatinine clearance so that dosage modifications can be made accordingly. Other costs associated with antibiotic administration include supportive nutrients, IV sets or shunts, and lengthened hospitalization for delivery of IV agents.

Toxicities

Adverse effects of some agents are quite impressive and may not be worth the benefits accrued. For example, a drug used to treat leprosy, clofazimine, is actually a dye that can cause the skin of the patient to become orange-brown in color. Chloramphenical, active against many anaerobic and facultative gram-negative bacteria, may interfere with bone marrow function; cephalosporins, the most widely used antimicrobial agents today, often contribute to development of antibiotic-associated pseudomembranous colitis caused by overgrowth of *Clostridium difficile* in the bowel. The nephrotoxic and ototoxic effects of aminoglycosides are well documented and this very effective class of drugs is often avoided for this reason. Recently, an excellent broad-spectrum agent, moxalactam, has been virtually ignored because of its reputed association with bleeding abnormalities in patients receiving the drug.

Allergies

Patients with allergies to penicillin, for example, may exhibit allergic reactions to all β-lactam antimicrobial agents. In severe cases, the patient must be temporarily hyposensitized to allow administration of the drug of choice.

Teratogenic or Other Qualities Harmful to Developing Tissues

Metronidazole has negative effects on the developing fetus, and thus is contraindicated for treating *Trichomonas vaginalis* infections in pregnant women, where it would otherwise be the agent of choice. Tetracycline can discolor developing bones and teeth and interfere with their normal development, so it is not used for pregnant women or children younger than 8 years of age. Some quinolones may interfere with growth of long bones; thus these agents are used judiciously in young children.

Single Versus Combination Therapy

Combination therapy is chosen for one of several reasons:

1. There is a likely development of resistance, such as occurs with tuberculosis.

2. An overwhelming infection may require more effective killing than that provided by one agent alone. In such instances, a combination of two active agents is chosen to be more effective than the additive effects of each agent if used alone (synergy).

3. Polymicrobial infections cannot be treated with one agent when different classes of microorganisms are involved.

4. The poor health status of certain patients who present with a new infectious process that is not yet fully defined mandates a broad-spectrum approach to cover all possible microbial agents until laboratory testing has detected the specific etiologic agent(s). Patients receiving immunosuppressive drugs and those with immune system malignancies fall into this category.

5. Certain specific infectious disease syndromes, by virtue of the organism and the site involved, should be treated with combination therapy. One example is that of enterococcus-associated endocarditis. The enterococci are inherently resistant to penicillins and the heart valve is a difficult site for natural immune response effectors to reach; thus standards of therapy mandate a combination of an aminoglycoside and a penicillin.

ANTIBACTERIAL AGENTS

See Table 5.1 for common antimicrobial agents (grouped by mechanism of activity).

TABLE 5.1. Common Antimicrobial Agents

Mechanism of action	Examples of agents
Inhibition of cell wall synthesis	Penicillins, cephalosporins, vancomycin, bacitracin, imipenem, aztreonam
Inhibition of protein synthesis	
50S ribosomal subunit	Clindamycin, erythromycin, chloramphenicol
30S ribosomal subunit	Aminoglycosides, tetracyclines
Transcription inhibitors	Rifampin, actinomycin
Protein assembly inhibitor	Griseofulvin
Metabolic analogs	Sulfonamides, 5-fluorocytosine, isoniazid, vidarabine, acyclovir, ribavirin
Inhibitors of cell membrane activities	Colistin, polyenes, imidazoles, possibly amantadine, amphotericin B, ketoconazole
Inhibitors of DNA function	Quinolones, metronidazole, novobiocin, flucytosine

Inhibition of Cell Wall Synthesis (Penicillins, Cephalosporins and Others)

MODES OF ACTION. Penicillins and cephalosporins are members of a broad group of antimicrobial agents called "**β-lactams.**" These agents are structurally similar to the terminal peptides that participate in the final stage of cross-linking the separate structures of the peptidoglycan bacterial cell wall (Fig. 5.2). Transpeptidases and other enzymes bind the penicillin instead of the peptide side chain, the enzymes become inactive, and cross-linkage stops. The enzymes that bind penicillins, located in or on the cell membrane, are called penicillin-binding proteins (PBPs). Several types of PBPs are present in all bacteria that are susceptible to the penicillins and cephalosporins.

Once the cell wall structure is no longer stable, bacteria are killed by lysis. Either autolytic enzymes, such as those active in penicillin-mediated killing of *Streptococcus pneumoniae,* or other mechanisms that cause leaky membranes mediate cell lysis and death. Penicillins are considered to be bactericidal.

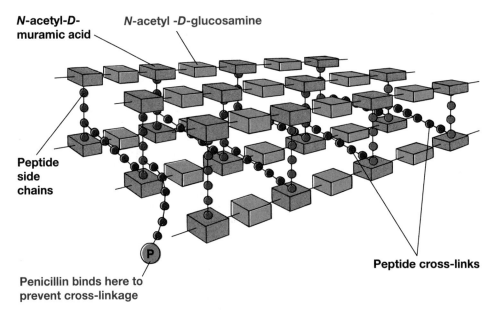

Figure 5.2.

Mechanism by which β-lactam antibiotic inhibits cell wall formation.

EXAMPLES OF AGENTS. Penicillin derivatives are achieved by adding or modifying side chains to the structure of the basic β-lactam ring (Fig. 5.3A).

1. Penicillin G.
2. Penicillinase-resistant penicillins: methicillin, oxacillin, and nafcillin. Side chains have been added to prevent, by steric interference, degradation of the β-lactam ring by penicillinase.

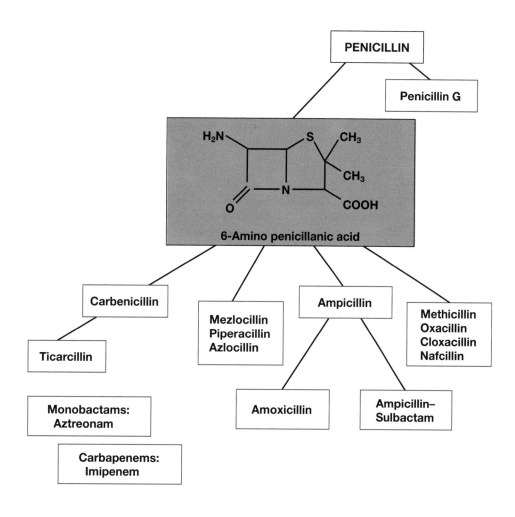

Figure 5.3A.

Diagram of ontogeny of development of penicillins.

3. Aminopenicillins: ampicillin and amoxicillin.

4. Other, more complex penicillins: carbenicillin, mezlocillin, and piperacillin.

5. Cephalosporins: The most complex group of antimicrobial agents of one type, there are now more than 25 different cephalosporin agents available in the United States alone. These antimicrobial agents are divided into "generations" based on their structure and spectrum of activity (Fig. 5.3B).

COMMON RESISTANCE MECHANISMS

1. Penicillinase and cephalosporinase production by bacteria. Penicillinases and cephalosporinases are a subgroup of a broader group of enzymes (β-lactamases) that hydrolyze the β-lactam ring of β-lactam antimicrobial agents (Fig. 5.4). The genes for β-lactamase production are usually located on plasmids or transposons, which explains why they have spread so widely among genera. Chromosomally mediated cephalosporinase and penicillinase production are also important resistance factors for some bacteria, such as anaerobic *Bacteroides* species, some *Enterobacteriaceae*, and *Pseudomonas aeruginosa*. In gram-negative bacteria, the β-lactamases reside in the periplasmic space where they contact the penicillin or cephalosporin and exert their effects before the drug reaches the membrane site of action. The most common β-lactamase among gram-negative bacteria is called TEM; it can hydrolyze the expanded spectrum penicillins, such as ampicillin and carbenicillin, and cephalosporins of all three generations. Gram-positive bacteria usually secrete the enzyme into the environment and destroy β-lactam agents before they reach the cell.

2. Alteration of penicillin-binding proteins (PBPs). An important resistance factor, particularly for methicillin-resistant staphylococci and pneumococci, is that mutational or naturally occurring modifications of standard PBPs resulting in PBPs of lower binding affinity for penicillins. Even when the other PBPs are saturated and rendered ineffective, these modified PBPs can continue to mediate cell wall cross-linking and cell growth is not diminished.

3. Permeability modifications. Changes in permeability of the outer membrane of gram-negative bacilli can prevent some penicillins from entering the periplasmic space through transmembrane channels, called **porins,** that usually provide access.

OTHER IMPORTANT CELL WALL ACTIVE AGENTS. Vancomycin is a glycopeptide antimicrobial that prevents the formation of peptidoglycan by binding to cell wall peptide precursors. This agent is active only against gram-positive

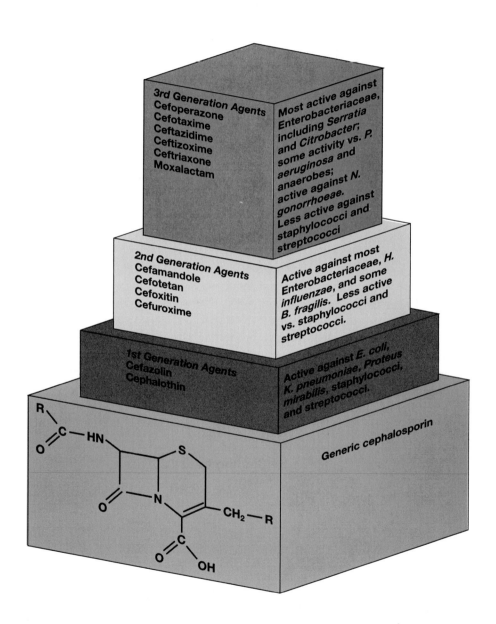

3rd Generation Agents
Cefoperazone
Cefotaxime
Ceftazidime
Ceftizoxime
Ceftriaxone
Moxalactam

Most active against Enterobacteriaceae, including *Serratia* and *Citrobacter*; some activity vs. *P. aeruginosa* and anaerobes; active against *N. gonorrhoeae*. Less active against staphylococci and streptococci

2nd Generation Agents
Cefamandole
Cefotetan
Cefoxitin
Cefuroxime

Active against most Enterobacteriaceae, *H. influenzae*, and some *B. fragilis*. Less active vs. staphylococci and streptococci.

1st Generation Agents
Cefazolin
Cephalothin

Active against *E. coli*, *K. pneumoniae*, *Proteus mirabilis*, staphylococci, and streptococci.

Generic cephalosporin

Figure 5.3B.

Diagram of ontogeny of development of cephalosporins.

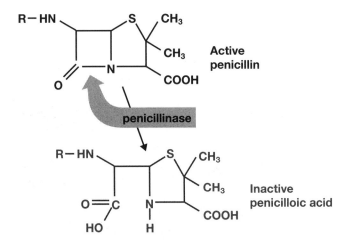

Figure 5.4.

Structure of generic β-lactam agent and illustration of hydrolysis of β-lactam ring by β-lactamase enzyme.

bacteria. Until recently, vancomycin resistance was not recognized. However, a few reports of resistant enterococcal outbreaks is a foreboding development. The resistance, clearly transmissible, seems to be due to a change in the peptide precursor structure that alters the vancomycin binding site. Daptomycin and teicoplanin are similar in structure to vancomycin and show similar spectra of activity. These agents are just being introduced for clinical use. Imipenem (a carbapenem) and aztreonam (a monobactam) are newly available β-lactam agents with efficacy against a number of otherwise resistant bacteria.

Inhibition of Protein Synthesis by Binding to the 50S Ribosomal Subunit

Since each of these agents acts at the same site in the bacterial cell, combinations of these drugs will interfere with each other and usually are antagonistic. These agents are usually considered to be bacteriostatic (Fig. 5.5).

MODES OF ACTION. Agents such as clindamycin prevent peptide chain initiation by binding to free ribosomes and preventing the binding of tRNA; chloramphenicol inhibits elongation of peptide chains on the ribosome by preventing the binding of aminoacyl-tRNA; and erythromycin and other macrolides inhibit the translocation of the growing peptide chain on the ribosome.

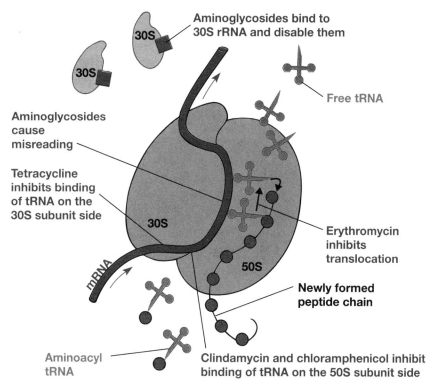

Aminoglycosides bind to 30S rRNA and disable them

30S

30S

30S

Free tRNA

Aminoglycosides cause misreading

Tetracycline inhibits binding of tRNA on the 30S subunit side

30S

mRNA

50S

Erythromycin inhibits translocation

Newly formed peptide chain

Aminoacyl tRNA

Clindamycin and chloramphenicol inhibit binding of tRNA on the 50S subunit side

Figure 5.5.

Bacterial ribosome illustrating points of inhibitory activity of antibiotics.

COMMON RESISTANCE MECHANISMS. A change in the ribosomal structure that inhibits binding of the antimicrobial agent is the most common mechanism for resistance to clindamycin. This mechanism is also important in the development of resistance to erythromycin by staphylococci. Bacterial cell wall conformational change leads to impermeability of *Pseudomonas* to chloramphenicol and of *Enterobacteriaceae* and *Pseudomonas* to erythromycin. Production of inactivating enzymes is particularly important for chloramphenicol. Certain bacteria, such as *Haemophilus influenzae* and *Salmonella,* produce an acetyltransferase that modifies chloramphenicol to an inactive derivative.

Inhibition of Protein Synthesis by Binding to the 30S Ribosomal Subunit

MODES OF ACTION. The most important agents in this group follow:

1. **Aminoglycosides** include gentamicin, amikacin, netilmicin, kanamycin, streptomycin, neomycin, and tobramycin. Due to their consistent activity against gram-negative bacilli, they are among the most useful antimicrobial agents, despite some well-known toxicities. Aminoglycosides are bactericidal by mechanisms not yet fully understood. These aminoglycosides appear to cause misreading of the codons during protein synthesis, resulting in inactive products. Aminoglycosides also seem to cause disruption of ribosomal activity by breaking up polysomes. Other activities include destabilization of the cell membrane, interference with DNA and RNA synthesis and with electron-transfer activities of the cell (Fig. 5.5).

2. **Tetracyclines** inhibit protein chain elongation by binding to the 30S ribosomal subunit and preventing attachment of the aminoacyl-tRNA.

COMMON RESISTANCE MECHANISMS. Aminoglycoside resistance is most commonly the result of the action of enzymes, often carried on plasmids, that modify the structure of the antimicrobial agent and render it inactive.

1. **Acetylases** produced by *Enterobacteriaceae, Pseudomonas aeruginosa,* and enterococci can inactivate amikacin, gentamicin, kanamycin, netilmicin, and tobramycin.

2. **Phosphorylases** produced by *Acinetobacter* spp., *Enterobacteriaceae, P. aeruginosa,* and enterococci act to destroy the activity of amikacin and kanamycin.

3. **Adenylylases,** also called **nucleotidylases,** produced by *Enterobacteriaceae*, staphylococci, and *P. aeruginosa* inactivate amikacin, kanamycin, and tobramycin.

4. **Bifunctional acetyltransferase** and **phosphotransferase enzymes** produced by staphylococci and enterococci reside on either a plasmid or a transposon.

Ribosome structural alterations, present in enterococci and gonococci, are other examples of resistance mechanisms.

Diminished permeability can result in resistance to both aminoglycosides and tetracyclines. In the case of aminoglycosides, permeability changes are usually due to chromosomal mutations. Tetracycline resistance, however, is carried on plasmids spread widely among numerous genera of gram-positive and gram-negative bacteria. In some instances, active transport of the drug into the cell is diminished and active eflux may be factor.

Inhibition of DNA and RNA Synthesis

MODES OF ACTION. The modes of action of the most important agents in this group follow:

1. **Rifampin** binds to one subunit of DNA-dependent RNA polymerase and prevents initiation of transcription. Rifampin, a bactericidal agent, is never used alone for therapy because resistance develops rapidly, but it is an effective prophylactic agent for *Neisseria meningitidis* and has synergistic or additive activity with other antimicrobial agents against staphylococci and mycobacteria.

2. **Quinolones,** including nalidixic acid and the fluoroquinolones ciprofloxacin and norfloxacin, inhibit the activity of DNA gyrase, an enzyme that participates in the coiling and nicking of DNA to form superhelices during replication and transcription (Fig. 5.6). Fluoroquinolones are especially active against the *Enterobacteriaceae* and other gram-negative bacteria, where they are considered to be bactericidal. They also have some activity against staphylococci but they exhibit poor activity against anaerobes and streptococci.

3. **Metronidazole** is taken into susceptible cells of anaerobic bacteria and parasites, such as trichomonads, where it is reduced to a cytotoxic product. It is thought that the activated cytotoxic drug interacts with DNA to cause mutations and disrupt DNA synthesis. Metronidazole is bactericidal and has excellent tissue penetration.

COMMON RESISTANCE MECHANISMS. Mutations that alter the structure of the enzyme inhibited by these drugs are the primary resistance mechanism. Such changes in RNA polymerase occur very quickly in bacteria subjected to rifampin. Fluoroquinolone resistance is mediated by mutations in the chromosome that cause altered DNA gyrase production.

The second mechanism used by bacteria resistant to the fluoroquinolones is altered permeability to the drugs, mediated by changes in outer-membrane protein (porin) expression. Additional fluoroquinolone resistance in staphylococci is mediated by reduced accumulation of drug through active transport in the membrane.

Metronidazole resistance is usually mediated by changes in membrane permeability, but changes in the intracytoplasmic enzymes that usually reduce the drug to its cytotoxic metabolite also can result in resistance.

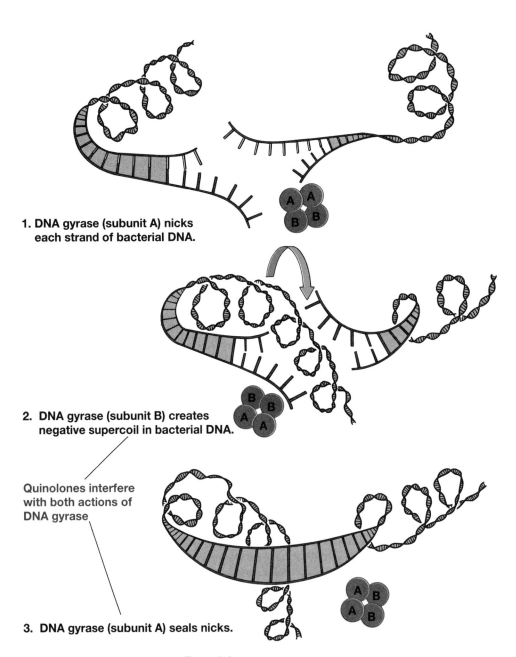

1. DNA gyrase (subunit A) nicks each strand of bacterial DNA.

2. DNA gyrase (subunit B) creates negative supercoil in bacterial DNA.

Quinolones interfere with both actions of DNA gyrase

3. DNA gyrase (subunit A) seals nicks.

Figure 5.6.

DNA gyrase activity, illustrating points of inhibition by quinolones.

Inhibition of Cell Membrane Activities

MODE OF ACTION. The mode of action of polymyxin, which includes colistin, a category of polymyxin, involves disruption of the cell membrane. Polymyxin apparently interjects itself into the lipid bilayer, opening channels and causing leakage of metabolites. Other membrane-bound enzyme functions are also inhibited. Because of the toxicity of polymyxin, it is used rarely except in topical ointments. Its spectrum includes pseudomonads resistant to other agents.

COMMON RESISTANCE MECHANISMS. Organisms rarely become resistant to polymyxins. Those that do are able to increase the cation content of their cell membranes, which can prevent some of the cellular damage.

Metabolic Analogs

The most commonly prescribed drug in this category in the United States is a combination agent, trimethoprim-sulfamethoxazole (also called cotrimoxazole). The two analog agents work synergistically to inhibit cell growth. Each acts at a different step during the microbial nucleic acid synthesis pathway. Most antiviral agents also act as metabolic analogs (see Chapter 34).

MODES OF ACTION. The modes of action of the most important agents in the group follow:

1. **Sulfonamides:** Most bacteria and some parasites convert *p*-aminobenzoic acid (PABA) to folic acid, the precursor of tetrahydrofolic acid, a coenzyme for the process of carbon utilization during purine and amino acid synthesis. Purines are essential to nucleic acid synthesis. The sulfonamides, which include sulfamethoxazole, sulfadiazine, and sulfisoxazole, because of their structural similarity to PABA, bind in its place to the enzyme that catalyzes the synthesis of dihydrofolic acid, an intermediate in the pathway to tetrahydrofolic acid (Fig. 5.7). The sulfonamides are bacteriostatic.
2. **Trimethoprim, pentamidine,** and **pyrimethamine:** Trimethoprim, a bactericidal agent, and pentamidine and pyrimethamine, used to treat protozoal infections, such as *Pneumocystis carinii* pneumonia and toxoplasmosis, act as a structural analog to dihydrofolate by binding to dihydrofolate reductase and preventing the formation of tetrahydrofolate. The ultimate result is a lack of purines for DNA and RNA synthesis and cell death.
3. **Isoniazid:** Isoniazid, usually in the form of isonicotinic acid hydrazide

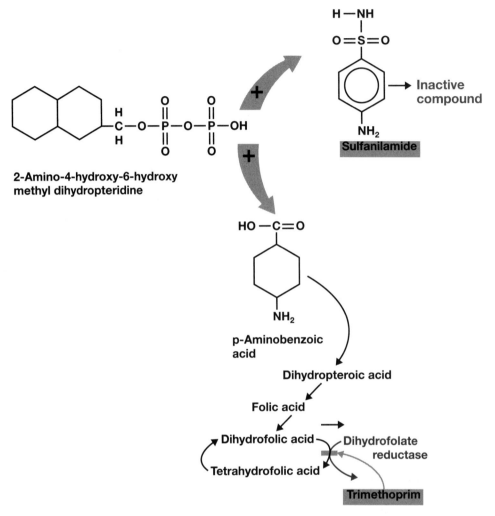

Figure 5.7.
Folic acid metabolism illustrating points of inhibition by sulfa drugs.

(INH), is the front-line antituberculosis drug. Always used in combination with at least one other antimycobacterial agent because of the rapid development of resistance in mycobacteria, INH may act as a structural analog of nicotinamide in nicotinamide adenine dinucleotide dehydrogenase. Its mechanism of action has not been fully elucidated.

COMMON RESISTANCE MECHANISMS. Acquired resistance to folic

acid pathway agents is through two mechanisms: cell wall permeability mutations, most active against sulfa drugs, and microbial acquisition of resistant enzymes that no longer bind dihydrofolate reductase enzyme. These enzymes are widespread on plasmids and transposons, especially among gram-negative bacteria. Resistance to INH by mycobacteria is usually mediated by a structural mutation, resulting in loss of activity of the drug.

β-Lactam-β-Lactamase Inhibitor Combinations

One effective strategy developed to counteract the effects of bacterial β-lactamases has been the relatively recent development of the β-lactamase inhibitor drugs clavulanic acid, sulbactam, and tazobactam, usually used in combination with a β-lactam agent. These combinations pack a double punch; the β-lactamase inhibitor binds the bacterial β-lactamase irreversibly and renders the enzyme inactive. These agents are sometimes called "suicide" inhibitors, because in trying to hydrolyze the β-lactam ring of the inhibitors, the β-lactamase is destroyed, similar to a kamakazi pilot. The second β-lactam agent, which probably would have been inactivated by the active β-lactamase enzyme, is now free to enter the cell, bind to the penicillin-binding proteins, and arrest cell growth.

The β-lactam-β-lactamase inhibitor combinations used today include amoxacillin-clavulanic acid (Augmentin[R]), ampicillin-sulbactam (Unasyn[R]), ticarcillin-clavulanic acid (Timentin[R]), and piperacillin-tazobactam (Zocin[R]). These drugs are extremely effective for treating otitis media, intraabdominal infections, and other polymicrobial infections at various sites, such as pneumonia, decubitus ulcers, sinusitis, and infections involving anaerobes. They are usually very expensive.

ANTIFUNGAL AGENTS

Table 5.2 lists some common choices of antifungal therapeutic agents.

Agents That Disrupt Membrane Integrity

Amphotericin B, the primary antifungal drug with fungicidal activity, binds to the ergosterol in the cell membrane, causing structural disturbances, leakiness, and cell death. It also appears to generate reactive oxygen radicals that contribute to cell damage. Amphotericin B is called a polyene agent because it has acidic

TABLE 5.2. Common Choices of Antifungal Therapy

Antifungal agent	Disease
Amphotericin B	Systemic disease, including cryptococcosis, aspergillosis, blastomycosis, candidiasis, coccidioidomycosis, histoplasmosis, mucormycosis, and sporotrichosis
5-Fluorocytosine	As a single agent for treating chromomycosis, and in combination with amphotericin B for treating cryptococcal meningitis and maybe candidiasis
Ketoconazole	Histoplasmosis, nonmeningeal blastomycosis, nonsystemic coccidioidomycosis, mucocutaneous candidiasis, other cutaneous fungal diseases
Clotrimazole and miconazole	Cutaneous fungal diseases, vulvovaginal candidiasis, and oropharyngeal candidiasis
Nystatin	Oropharyngeal, esophageal, and vaginal candidiasis
Fluconazole	Systemic candidiasis, cryptococcosis, aspergillosis, and histoplasmosis

and basic properties. Some binding of cholesterol in mammalian cell membranes contributes to the well-described toxicities of amphotericin B. Therapy with this agent is usually long term, as fungi react slowly.

Nystatin, the other clinically useful polyene antifungal, is too toxic for systemic use. This antifungal agent is used primarily as a topical preparation for treating vaginal and oral yeast infections.

The azoles (ketoconazole, fluconazole, miconazole, and itraconazole) prevent development of the fungal cell membrane by inhibiting the activity of certain key enzymes, including cytochromes, that mediate sterol incorporation into the membrane. These agents are similar to metronidazole, another azole type antibiotic. High concentrations of some of these agents may be fungicidal and should never be administered with amphotericin B. The activities of the two groups of antifungals are antagonistic because membrane sterol integration is necessary for amphotericin B to exert its effect. Ketoconazole is used to treat dermatophyte infections and some yeast infections. It has recently been used prophylactically in AIDS patients. Fluconazole, because of its good penetration into cerebrospinal fluid (CSF), has been particularly valuable for treating cryptococcal meningitis in AIDS patients. Miconazole is used topically for yeast infections and other localized infections.

Agents That Act as Metabolic Analogs

Flucytosine (5-fluorocytosine) is integrated into fungal RNA where it replaces cytosine. It is usually considered to be fungistatic, and is most often administered in combination with amphotericin B, which allows the dosage of the more toxic agent to be decreased. It is frequently used to treat cryptococcosis.

Agents That Destroy Protein Structure

Griseofulvin, an antifungal used exclusively to treat dermatophyte infections, seems to bind to proteins involved in tubulin synthesis. The agent is only effective against fungi with cell walls containing chitin. Mitosis is inhibited by inactive tubulin, and actively growing cells display bizarre shapes and nuclear distortion. Only cells undergoing division are affected.

Because griseofulvin is taken orally, secreted through sweat glands, and delivered systemically into actively growing skin and nail cells, it takes several months of treatment for drug-laden cells to reach the stratified corneal layer where the fungus is active.

Liposomal Complexed Antifungal Agents

One method for delivery of these toxic antimicrobial agents is to sequester the drug within a lipid bilayer vesicle (Fig. 5.8). These ''liposomes'' are then taken up by the reticuloendothelial system and somehow delivered more directly to the infecting fungi. The development of alternative delivery modes for amphotericin B and other antifungal agents is a response to the dearth of nontoxic, effective antifungals. Liposome and other nontraditional delivery systems are just beginning to be evaluated clinically.

Development of Resistance to Antifungal Drugs

Fungi rarely become resistant to polyene antibiotics. If resistance does occur, it develops by mutational changes in composition of membrane lipids. These and other resistance mechanisms of fungi have not been well characterized. Some fungi, notably *Pseudallescheria boydii,* are inherently resistant to amphotericin B. Flucytosine must be deaminated to its active metabolite within the fungal cell.

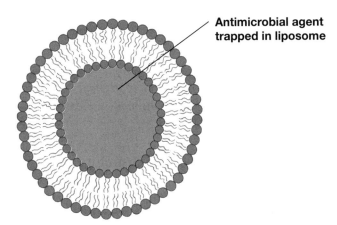

**Antimicrobial agent
trapped in liposome**

Figure 5.8.

Diagram of a liposome for
delivering amphotericin B.

Fungi that are able to alter the deamination enzyme rapidly become resistant; others that initially lack the enzyme are inherently resistant.

SUMMARY

1. Antimicrobial agents are synthetically or organism-produced (antibiotics) agents that inhibit the growth of or destroy other microbes. Subsets of antimicrobial agents include (a) antibacterial agents, (b) antifungal agents, (c) antiviral agents, and (d) antiprotozoal and antihelminthic agents.

2. Antimicrobial agents must be more toxic to the pathogenic microbe than they are to the host or they will not be acceptable.

3. Antimicrobial agents can kill (cidal) or merely inhibit growth of (static) the targeted etiologic agent.

4. Key factors to consider in determining efficacy of a given agent are (a) susceptibility of the microorganism being treated, (b) route of administration and method by which the host excretes the agent (in which body fluids does it concentrate?), (c) pharmacokinetics of the antimicrobial agent, (d) effect of concurrently administered other chemotherapeutic agents, (e) host allergies and toxicities, and (f) cost.

5. The main categories of antimicrobial agents are (a) cell wall active agents (penicillins and cephalosporins), (b) protein synthesis inhibitors (ma-

crolides and aminoglycosides), (c) metabolic analogs (sulfa drugs, isoniazid, acyclovir, and most other antiviral agents), (d) cell membrane activity inhibitors (polyene antifungal agents), and (e) DNA disruptors (quinolones and metronidazole).

6. The main strategies used by microorganisms that develop resistance to an antimicrobial agent are (a) modifications in cell wall permeability to the agent (e.g., changes in porin proteins and active transport); (b) production of antimicrobial agent–destroying enzymes (such as β-lactamases and acetyltransferases); and (c) mutation of the antimicrobial agent activity binding site, as occurs in bacteria that develop resistance to sulfa drugs or rifampin.

REFERENCES

Bartlett JG (1992): Tables of antimicrobial agents. In Gorbach SL, Bartlett JG, Blacklow NR (eds): Infectious Diseases. Philadelphia: W.B. Saunders, p 393.

Craig WA (1992): Penicillins. In Gorbach SL, Bartlett JG, Blacklow NR (eds): Infectious Diseases. Philadelphia: W.B. Saunders, p 160.

Jacoby GA, Archer GL (1991): New mechanisms of bacterial resistance to antimicrobial agents. N Engl J Med 324:601.

Kass EH, Platt R (1990): Current therapy in infectious disease—3. B.C. Toronto: Decker.

Kucers A, Bennett N (1987): The use of antibiotics: a comprehensive review with clinical emphasis. Philadelphia: J.B. Lippincott.

Lorian V (1991): Antibiotics in laboratory medicine (3rd ed.) Baltimore: Williams & Wilkins.

Murray BE (1991): New aspects of antimicrobial resistance and the resulting therapeutic dilemmas. J Infect Dis 163:1185.

Murray B (1989): Problems and mechanisms of antimicrobial resistance. Infect Dis Clin North Am 3:423.

Neu HC (1983): Considerations about the relationship of inhibitory concentrations and the pharmacologic and toxic properties of antimicrobial agents. Diagn Microbiol Infect Dis 1:41.

Stratton CW (1990): Antifungal agents: the old and the new. Infect Dis Newsletter 9:41.

Swierkosz EM (1992): Antiviral susceptibility testing: coming of age. ASM News 58:83.

REVIEW QUESTIONS

For questions 1 to 10, a list of lettered options is followed by several numbered items. For each numbered item, select the ONE lettered option that is most closely associated with it.

A) Penicillin G
B) Rifampin
C) Amphotericin B
D) Ciprofloxacin
E) Sulfonamide

For each characteristic, select the antimicrobial agent that is most closely associated.

1. Resistance to this agent is often mediated by proteins in the cell membrane that mutate to forms that no longer bind the antimicrobial.

2. A member of the fluoroquinolone group of antimicrobial agents, this agent acts at the level of DNA synthesis.

3. Similar to other polyene antimicrobial agents, this agent binds to sterols in fungal cell walls.

4. This agent acts as a competitive inhibitor of folic acid synthesis.

5. Enzymes, transferred among bacterial species on plasmids, that hydrolyze the active component of this agent are the most common resistance mechanism.

6. This agent is almost never used alone because of the ease with which bacteria develop resistance to it.

A) Ribavirin
B) Isoniazid
C) Ketoconazole
D) Vancomycin
E) Metronidazole

For each infectious disease, select the antimicrobial agent that should be used for therapy.

7. An intravenous drug abuser is diagnosed with staphylococcal endocarditis.

8. A positive tuberculin skin test develops in a healthy microbiology laboratory scientist whose skin test was negative 6 months previously.

9. The agent is chosen for long-term prophylaxis for an AIDS patient who has been successfully treated for his cryptococcal meningitis with amphotericin B and is ready to be discharged to home.

10. This agent is used to treat an anaerobic abdominal abscess.

ANSWERS TO REVIEW QUESTIONS

1. **A** Penicillin resistance may be mediated by a change in the conformation of PBPs.

2. **D** Ciprofloxacin is the most commonly used fluoroquinolone. These agents inhibit DNA gyrase and interfere with DNA coiling.

3. **C** Amphotericin B is the "gold standard" antifungal agent. None of the other agents listed have any activity against fungi.

4. **E** All of the sulfonamides act as metabolic analogs at some point in the bacterial nucleic acid synthesis pathway.

5. **A** Penicillin resistance is mediated most often by β-lactamase enzymes, ubiquitous across species and genus lines.

6. **B** Resistance to rifampin develops quickly due to mutational changes in DNA-dependent RNA polymerase, to which rifampin binds to inhibit transcription.

7. **D** Drug abusers often harbor methicillin-resistant staphylococci on their skin; thus endocarditis with a *Staphylococcus* sp. in such a patient is unlikely to respond to a penicillin, even a penicillinase resistant agent. The only agent listed that would be effective against gram-positive bacteria is vancomycin.

8. **B** Isoniazid can be used alone as a prophylactic against development of tuberculosis in someone who has just encountered the infection and developed a primary immune response if the likelihood of multidrug resistant strain acquisition is low. Isoniazid is used in combination with other agents to treat symptomatic disease.

9. **C** Ketoconazole, the only antifungal agent listed, can be given orally. It is less toxic than amphotericin B.

10. **E** Metronidazole, the only agent listed with activity against anaerobes, has good penetration into abscesses.

HOST-PARASITE INTERACTIONS

The interaction between a host and a microorganism is a dynamic process in which each protagonist acts to maximize its survival. In some instances, invasion by a microorganism results in such a mutually beneficial relationship that the microorganism becomes integral to the health of the host, such as occurs with intestinal bacteria in humans and ruminants. In other instances, the microorganism produces or induces deleterious effects in the host; the end result may be disease or even death of the host. The host, in turn, has developed numerous strategies for minimizing the damage wrought by unfriendly microorganisms. This chapter examines the nature of the interaction between humans and microorganisms.

Certain microorganisms that possess or produce specialized virulence factors often cause harm if they gain access to a human host. These ''true pathogens'' include those that cause plague, cholera, amebiasis, tuberculosis, measles, sporotrichosis, and anthrax. The dynamic interplay between a parasite and its human host determines whether (1) survival of only one entity (health vs. death), (2) a steady state (survival of both entities, i.e., infection or carrier state), or (3) disease prevails. The fascinating study of microbial pathogenesis and host immune response has developed from the need to understand and control the infectious disease process so that microorganisms do not gain the upper hand.

DEFINITIONS

Parasitism: One organism benefits at the expense of the other. The most successful parasite does not quickly destroy the host, unless it has developed a mechanism for efficient passage on to another susceptible host. If it fails to do this, then by destroying the host it also destroys itself.

Commensalism: One organism benefits without causing harm to the other. *Staphylococcus epidermidis* on intact skin represents an example of a commensal.

Symbiosis: Both organisms benefit from their association. Lactobacilli in the vagina produce acid end products that keep the vaginal pH at a relatively low level, which contributes to inhibition of growth of pathogenic organisms, such as *Neisseria gonorrhoeae.* Oropharyngeal streptococci, by colonizing the mucosal epithelium, provide a barrier to inhibit adherence of pathogenic bacteria, such as *Streptococcus pyogenes,* the agent of ''strep throat,'' in an association called ''colonization resistance.''

Certain bacteria in the human gastrointestinal (GI) tract, including *Escherichia coli* strains and others, produce vitamin K that is absorbed by the host. When antimicrobial therapy that destroys these organisms is used to treat an infectious process, the patient may require supplementation with exogenous vitamin K.

Opportunistic Infection: Certain microorganisms, notably the endogenous microbiota of the human host, are not capable of causing disease in an immunologically and physically intact host. Once the normal host defenses are breached in some way, however, these organisms can cause disease. Such organisms are called ''opportunists.''

METHODS OF TRANSMISSION OF INFECTIOUS DISEASES

Etiologic agents of infections other than those endogenous microbes that infect their hosts opportunistically must have a mechanism whereby they gain access to susceptible hosts. Several strategies have been successful and the microorganisms are rewarded by survival.

Vertical/Direct

Vertical spread occurs when a disease is transmitted from the mother to the offspring in utero, during delivery, in the mother's colostrum or breast milk, or by way of latent viruses in the germ cells. Syphilis, congenital rubella syndrome, AIDS, and viral leukemia are examples of such diseases. Infants acquire diseases, such as gonorrheal ophthalmia neonatorum and chlamydial conjunctivitis, from organisms present in the birth canal.

Horizontal/Indirect

Horizontal spread occurs when a disease is transmitted to susceptible hosts through the environment. For example, transmission can occur by way of fomites (inanimate objects on which microbes survive); in food or water; or by contact, either directly or indirectly, through a vector.

More than one susceptible individual can acquire the etiologic agent at one time by transmission from an infected patient either directly or through the environment. Two possible means of acquisition follow:

1. **By breathing in aerosols** generated by sneezing or coughing (e.g., influenzavirus and tuberculosis).

2. **By ingesting contaminated food or water,** as occurs with cholera, staphylococcal food poisoning, typhoid, and hepatitis A infection.

An infected patient can transmit the etiologic agent directly to another individual by the following means:

1. **During sexual activity,** venereal diseases such as syphilis, HIV, gonorrhea, chlamydia, and numerous others may be transmitted.

2. **By direct contact,** as often occurs with rhinovirus-associated rhinitis, which is passed by secretions on the hands; and giardiasis, which can be passed among children in a day care setting by hand-to-hand, fecal-oral transmission.

Nosocomial (hospital acquired) diseases can be transmitted from patient to patient on the hands or gloves of medical care personnel. Methicillin-resistant staphylococci are often maintained in a hospital environment in this manner.

Arthropod Vectors

An infected individual or animal host can provide an inoculum of the etiologic agent to an arthropod vector, which transmits it to susceptible hosts. For example, the etiologic agents of Lyme borreliosis, ehrlichiosis, and Rocky Mountain spotted fever are transmitted by ticks.

Environmental

The etiologic agent is present in the environment and can gain access to the susceptible host accidentally.

1. The host acquires the organism by inspiration. For example, coccidioidomycosis is acquired by susceptible hosts during travel through the desert following the breathing in of dust laden with fungal arthrospores.

2. The host is infected with the organism traumatically. For example, sporotrichosis is acquired when normal individuals prick themselves with a contaminated rose thorn.

3. The microbe enters the intact skin or surface epithelium of the host during accidental contact. *Naegleria fowleri,* a free-living soil protozoan, comes into contact with the sinus mucosa when patients swim in infested waterholes and lakes, invades normal tissue, and then travels to the central nervous system (CNS) to cause meningitis.

4. The host ingests the organism or its exotoxin. Botulism is contracted when individuals ingest food in which *Clostridium botulinum* has multiplied and released its exotoxin.

Wounds

An infected or colonized animal host can inject the etiologic agent. For example, *Pasteurella multocida* infection and cat-scratch disease occur when a normal individual is scratched by the family cat, whose claws are contaminated with the organisms (normal oral flora in cats).

Medical treatment can cause trauma that allows access for the infectious agent. Such diseases are called ''iatrogenic.'' This topic is discussed in Chapter 21.

THE INFECTIOUS PROCESS—MICROBIAL FACTORS

In host-parasite interactions there are two types of etiologic agents: exogenous and endogenous. Five critical steps are necessary for an exogenous microbe to act as an agent of disease. The organism must (1) encounter the host, (2) find a favorable environment, (3) evade normal host defense mechanisms, (4) procreate on or in the host and (5) maintain its existence in association with the host and cause an unfavorable host response—disease. As Dr. Stanley Falkow of Stanford says, "The sole aim of a bacterium is to become bacteria."

In the case of "normal flora," the organisms have already established an ecological niche and have managed to survive. If these endogenous agents find themselves in an unfamiliar environment where it is possible to cause disease, they must (a) survive host defense mechanisms, (b) multiply in the new environment, and (c) cause some kind of deleterious host response.

Encountering the Host

Factors that contribute to the ability of the organism to encounter a favorable host and selected examples follow:

1. **Survival in an arthropod vector** or other suitable nonhuman host. *Plasmodium* species, the agents of malaria, survive and multiply in mosquitoes.
2. **Survival in an aerosol droplet.** Tubercle bacilli withstand the effects of sunlight, drying, and other factors until they are inhaled by a new host.
3. **Survival in a hostile environment** until a situation favorable for growth is created. Examples include spore formation by *Bacillus anthracis* and cyst formation by *Giardia lamblia.*
4. **Production of structures** that can contribute to dissemination such as the fungal spores of *Aspergillus.*

Locating a Niche

Factors that contribute to the ability of the microbe to locate a favorable environment once it has encountered the host follow:

1. **Motility** by flagella or other mechanism allows the organism to penetrate mucous layers to reach epithelial cells (e.g., *Helicobacter pylori*). Chemotactic attractants and other features on the host encourage microbial contact with the appropriate surface.
2. **Adherence factors** (lectins, fimbriae, lipoteichoic acid, and other surface adhesins) that enhance the ability of an organism to bind to the appropriate niche once encountered.
3. **Enzymes** that modify the local environment to provide a more hospitable home. For example, hyaluronidase produced by *S. pyogenes* allows multiplication to proceed through adjacent host tissue resulting in dissemination.

4. **Previous infection and tissue damage** by one agent can predispose the host to more severe disease. For example, influenzavirus compromises lung tissue so that a superinfection by *Streptococcus pneumoniae* or *Haemophilus influenzae* is likely to be more serious than in previously healthy hosts.

5. **Ability to survive** adverse host environments until a suitable environment is reached. *Salmonella,* for example, are quite susceptible to the high acidity in the stomach and often do not survive to reach the intestine. *Shigella,* on the other hand, being more resistant, can initiate infection by means of a smaller inoculum.

6. **Ability to directly invade** host epithelium to reach a favorable environment. *Entamoeba histolytica,* trypanosomes, and other parasites enter host cells directly.

Evading Host Defenses

Factors that contribute to the ability of an organism to evade or destroy normal host defense mechanisms and multiply in the host follow:

1. **Production of extracellular matrices** that protect the organism from host immune mechanisms. For example, polysaccharide capsules produced by a number of bacteria, including *S. pneumoniae,* inhibit phagocytosis by interfering with the ability of leukocytes to attach to the microbe and then engulf it.

2. **Ability to induce "nonprofessional" phagocytic cells to engulf** the microbe. *Chlamydia trachomatis,* the etiologic agent of lymphogranuloma venereum, can be endocytosed only by squamocolumnar junction cells of the human genital tract.

3. Viruses, such as herpes simplex and HIV, have the **ability to integrate into the host's genome** in infected cells, and thus to remain latent but potentially active under appropriate circumstances.

4. Some organisms, including *Mycobacterium* spp., and many viruses, are able to survive intracellularly in macrophages. Several mechanisms promote this ability:

Inhibition of lysosomal fusion with the phagosome.
Escape from the phogosome to multiply in the cytoplasm.
Survival and growth in the phagolysosome.

5. Numerous microbes produce extracellular substances or otherwise **inactivate cellular immune responses.**

Hemolysins produced by streptococci and others directly destroy leukocyte (and erythrocyte) cell membranes.

Leukotoxins produced by clostridia and others destroy leukocytes.

The HIV virus directly infects and destroys T helper cells, thus abrogating an immune response against many infectious agents that require cell-mediated immunity for destruction.

6. Bacteria produce substances that **interfere with humoral immune responses.**

Gonococci and *H. influenzae* produce IgA proteases that destroy secretory IgA immunoglobulin.

Proteins on the surface of *S. aureus* (protein A) bind the Fc portion of antibodies and inhibit specific opsonization.

Viruses and some parasites constantly change their surface antigens, and thus force the host to continually produce new specific antibodies.

7. Some infectious agents **do not seem to invoke much of an immune response** at all, which allows them time to multiply and cause localized tissue damage. Examples are rabiesvirus and *Treponema pallidum.*

Damaging the Host

Factors that contribute to the ability of an organism to invoke a deleterious host response follow:

1. Production of **toxins** by bacteria. Bacteria produce or contain several types of toxins. Toxins produced by the bacteria and released into the environment are called **"exotoxins."** A subgroup of exotoxins are called **"enterotoxins,"** because they induce fluid release into the GI tract and cause enteric disease (see Chapter 17). **Endotoxin** is a component of the bacterial cell wall, and released only when the cell is destroyed. Endotoxin is discussed further in Chapter 16. Table 6.1 briefly characterizes the toxins associated with bacterial infections. Table 6.2 lists selected important bacterial exotoxins.

2. Production of toxins by fungi. Certain fungi produce toxins called **"aflatoxins"** that may play a role in disease, although this is speculatory. The aflatoxins of *Fusarium* spp. may cause cellular destruction and liver necrosis in systemically infected patients who are invariably immunocompromised.

3. **Direct cell and cellular function damage** by the infectious agent.

TABLE 6.1. Bacterial Toxins

Property	Exotoxin	Endotoxin
Location	Secreted extracellularly	Cell wall resident; released on cell lysis gram-negative bacteria
Source	Gram-negative and gram-positive bacteria	Gram-negative bacteria
Structure	Protein	Lipopolysaccharide
Inactivation by heat	Heat labile	Heat stable
Toxoid production	Successful, immunogenic	Not possible
Biological effects	Specific, depends on toxin	Nonspecific, general (see Chapter 17)

TABLE 6.2. Selected Important Bacterial Exotoxins

Mechanism	Organism	Toxin/disease
Cell membrane damage	*Clostridium perfringens*	Alpha toxin (lecithinase)/gas gangrene
	Staphylococcus aureus	Alpha, beta, delta toxins/abscesses, local destruction
	Streptococcus pyogenes	Streptolysins/cellulitis, inflammatory disease
Inhibition of protein synthesis	*Corynebacterium diphtheriae*	Diphtheria toxin/diphtheria
	Shigella dysenteriae	Shiga toxin/shigellosis
	Pseudomonas aeruginosa	Exotoxin A/tissue destruction, inflammatory disease
Induction of intracellular cyclic AMP (cAMP); fluid secretion in GI tract and tissue edema in respiratory tract	*Vibrio cholerae*	Choleragen/cholera
	Escherichia coli (enterotoxigenic)	Heat–labile toxin (LT)/diarrhea
	Bordetella pertussis	Pertussis toxin/whooping cough
Neurotoxin, blocks release of acetylcholine to skeletal muscle nerves	*Clostridium botulinum*	Botulism toxins A-G/botulism
Neurotoxin, blocks release of neurotransmitters to skeletal muscle nerves	*Clostridium tetani*	Tetanospasmin/tetanus
Enterotoxin acts on vomiting center of brain	*Bacillus cereus*	Emetic toxin/*B. cereus* food poisoning (emetic form)

Adherence to intestinal epithelial cells by *G. lamblia* inhibits fluid transport and induces diarrhea (Fig. 6.1).

Multiplication of viruses and chlamydiae within host cells diverts the cellular machinery away from host maintenance functions and ultimately the cells are destroyed.

Growth of *Bordetella pertussis* in the cilia of respiratory epithelial cells destroys their motility and function.

Physical presence of pathogenic organisms destroys host functions. Growth and movement of filarial worms in the eye and other infected sites directly destroys host tissue.

Production of acid by *Streptococcus mutans* decalcifies the tooth surface to which the microcolony is attached and results in cavities (caries), the most common infectious disease among humans throughout the world.

4. **Induction of a host response** that damages host tissue and function.

Endotoxin induces interleukin-1 (IL-1) and tumor necrosis factor production by macrophages and other cells, activates complement, and enhances the immune response by all host cells (see Chapter 15).

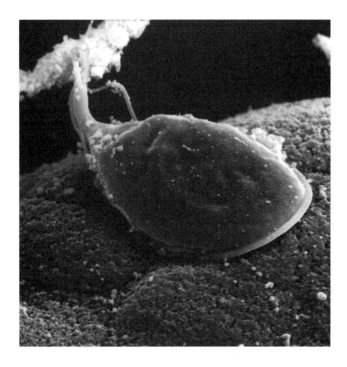

Figure 6.1.

Scanning electron micrograph of *G. lamblia* attached to intestinal mucosa. [Reproduced with permission from Garcia LS, Bruckner DA (1988): Diagnostic Medical Parasitology. New York: Elsevier.]

Polysaccharide capsules may act as a chemotactic factor to induce inflammation.

Antibodies directed against bacterial cell antigens may become self-directed against host antigens with similar structure, such as occurs in rheumatic heart disease. The antigen-antibody complexes formed when antistreptococcal antibodies bind to cross-reactive antigens on heart muscle tissue cause complement activation, inflammation, and ultimately destruction of host tissue.

Circulating soluble antigen-antibody immune complexes can become deposited in the kidneys or other sites (joints) to cause immune complex disorders including arthritis, glomerulonephritis, skin manifestations, such as erythema nodosum, petechiae, and so on.

Superantigens, molecules produced by microbes, including bacteria such as *S. aureus* and *S. pyogenes* and viruses such as HIV, and others not yet characterized, can act independently to stimulate T cell activities, including cytokine release. Superantigens are among the most potent T cell mitogens known; their stimulation of the immune system can result in anergy or, alternately, systemic immune system activation.

THE INFECTIOUS PROCESS—HOST FACTORS

Innate Host Defense Mechanisms

The first line of defense against any infectious agent, innate or nonspecific host responses must: provide an effective barrier that prevents the microorganism from penetrating, inhibit or destroy the invader if it gains access to the tissues, and eliminate or neutralize any toxic substances elaborated by the infectious agent. A list of several mechanisms that are available in the immunocompetent host follows.

MECHANICAL BARRIERS

Reflexes

The cough and gag reflex prevent particles from entering the lungs.

Sneezing works to expel explosively infectious agents from the nasal passages.

Swallowing moves potential pathogens into the stomach, where they are destroyed by stomach acidity.

Intact skin

Sebaceous gland secretions may be inhibitory.

A dry surface is not conducive to growth of microbes.

Continuously sloughing epithelial cells carry adherent microbes away.

Sweat removes microorganisms through a flushing action and contains inhibitory substances, such as lysozyme.

Conjunctiva

The flushing action of blinking and tears prevents colonization.

Lysozyme and other antibacterial substances in tears are nonspecific effectors. Lysozyme hydrolyzes a structural polysaccharide in bacterial cell walls.

Mucous membrane epithelium

Mucus layers entrap microorganisms, which are then swept by ciliary action into the throat to be swallowed.

Lysozyme in mucus secretions is antibacterial.

Cilia prevent aerosol-borne agents from entering the lungs.

Epithelial cells may not possess certain receptors necessary for adherence of infectious agents.

Nasal turbinates provide a barrier to free access into the lungs by airborne particles; such particles may impinge and stick to nasal hairs and progress no further. Particles 5 μm in diameter are best able to reach the alveoli; larger ones are stopped by protective barriers while smaller ones may not come to rest and are expired with the next breath.

Gastrointestinal tract

Saliva acts to flush away microbes that have transiently settled on the mucosa.

Lysozyme in saliva destroys bacteria.

Stomach acidity and proteolytic enzymes destroy or degrade many infectious agents and destroys enveloped viruses.

Bile secreted by the gallbladder is inhibitory to the growth of many bacteria.

Normal peristalsis forces organisms to move along the GI tract and to be excreted with fecal matter.

The mucosal layer protects epithelial cells.

Urinary tract

Flushing of urine periodically prevents bacterial population buildup.

Acidity of urine is inhibitory to some organisms.

Prostatic secretions containing spermine and zinc, which inhibit growth of some bacteria, are introduced into the urine in males.

Female vagina

Vaginal epithelium is sloughed rapidly and carries with it transient microbes.

The secretions of the vaginal tract are acidic and contain antimicrobial substances; they also promote flushing of microorganisms from the body.

SOLUBLE AND CIRCULATING NONSPECIFIC EFFECTORS

Complement: The classical pathway of the complement system, comprised of a series of at least 20 proteins and glycoproteins (labeled C1-C9), acts to lyse microbial membranes and releases inflammation-enhancing substances. Inasmuch as it is triggered by an antigen-antibody complex, initiation of this pathway cannot be considered nonspecific, although the complement effector proteins are nonspecific. The complement cascade can also be activated by the ''properdin'' or ''alternate'' pathway at the C3 stage.

Alternate pathway: The alternate pathway can be initiated by the presence of polysaccharides in bacterial or fungal cell walls, including the lipid A of endotoxin. Once initiated, the complement cascade continues from the second stage, resulting in lysis of cell membranes and release of active protein fragments that promote vasodilation, act as chemotactic factors, promote release of histamines, which also increase vascular permeability, and act as opsonins.

Acid and alkaline phosphatases can inactivate herpes viruses.

Interferon-α (IF-α) proteins are released by cells once they have been infected by a virus. The interferons protect neighboring cells from viral multiplication by inducing the production of intracellular antiviral proteins. Interferon-α also enhances killer T-cell activity.

Interferon-γ (IF-γ) activates macrophages to phagocytize and destroy intracellular parasites more effectively; IF-γ also interrupts viral replication and promotes T-cell differentiation.

Fibronectin, produced by some macrophages and epithelial cells, may act as a nonspecific opsonin for certain microbes, such as *S. aureus,* which has a natural fibronectin receptor. Inasmuch as fibronectin on cell surfaces may also act to enhance microbial adherence, its effect may not always be beneficial.

CELLULAR NONSPECIFIC IMMUNE EFFECTORS

Alveolar macrophages remove particles and organisms that enter the alveoli.

Polymorphonuclear neutrophils, the first phagocytes into an infected area, can nonspecifically phagocytize some microbes.

Eosinophils, which can phagocytize some particles, seem to be important in the removal of immune complexes.

Fixed macrophages (histiocytes) in the tonsils and Küpffer cells of the liver remove circulating particles and microorganisms.

Lactoferrin, released by activated macrophages and polymorphonuclear neutrophils, causes sequestration of iron from the plasma. This sequestration reduces the amount of iron available to invading pathogens and limits their ability to multiply.

Other **cytokines,** such as IL-1 (endogenous pyrogen), interleukin-6 (IL-6) (colony stimulating factor, hematopoietic cell stimulator), interleukin-8 (IL-8) (chemotactic factor), and tumor necrosis factor (TNF, also called cachectin), are released nonspecifically during the course of infection and modulate the response of the host.

METABOLIC OR NATURAL DEFENSES

Body temperature must be conducive for microbial growth (e.g., patients with high fevers cannot support infection with *T. pallidum*).

Specific host cell receptors must be available (e.g., distemper virus of dogs will not cause disease in humans).

The **environment** must be suitable; anaerobes cannot thrive in a highly oxygenated tissue, whereas *Mycobacterium tuberculosis* will not survive in an anaerobic environment.

The **nutritional and metabolic state of the host** are important factors in development of disease; diabetics in ketoacidosis are particularly vulnerable to yeast and other fungal infections. Low pH and high serum glucose provide a supportive environment.

Specific Immune Response Mechanisms

HUMORAL IMMUNE SYSTEM

Secretory IgA in mucus secretions can bind to infectious agents (viruses, some respiratory pathogenic bacteria) and prevent attachment.

Serum IgG acts to neutralize viruses and prevent them from entering cells; it also acts as an opsonin for bacteria, fungi, and parasites, initiates the complement cascade when bound to antigen, and neutralizes some bacterial toxins, such as diphtheria toxin.

IgM can also initiate the complement cascade and aid in phagocytosis of bound bacteria. IgM may also neutralize viruses.

CELLULAR IMMUNE SYSTEM

T lymphocytes (T helper cells) enhance antibody production by B lymphocytes.

Cytotoxic T cells can kill virus-infected host cells directly; killing of virus-infected epithelial cells is probably responsible for the various exanthems associated with viral infections.

Natural killer T cells can destroy certain bacteria and attack virus-infected cells.

Many types of cells, including T lymphocytes and monocytic cells, produce cytokines and monokines, respectively.

T suppressor cells also act to subdue the immune response.

B cells can be stimulated by the binding of T-independent antigens, such as LPS and the flagella of some bacteria, to produce specific antibodies, primarily IgM.

SUMMARY

1. Organisms that inhabit the skin and mucosa of humans perform numerous helpful functions, and are considered to be symbiotic. Some examples follow: (a) Streptococci in the respiratory tract prevent colonization of pathogens (colonization resistance). (b) Lactobacilli in the female genital tract maintain a low pH and inhibit colonization of pathogenic bacteria. (c) Bacteria in the gut produce vitamins used by the host. (d) Corynebacteria on the skin produce fatty acids that inhibit colonization by foreign bacteria.

2. Exogenous microorganisms must perform several activities successfully to cause disease. These microorganisms must (a) make contact with the susceptible host, (b) adhere to the host surface and find a favorable environment, (c) evade innate host defenses, (d) multiply on or in host tissue, and (e) induce a destructive host response.

3. Endogenous microbes cause infectious disease by (a) evading host defense mechanisms, (b) multiplying in an environment different from their natural niche, and (c) causing a destructive host response.

4. Microbial virulence factors include (a) survival in a vector, (b) environmental stability or viability, (c) adherence mechanism (motility, adhesins, fimbriae, lectins, etc.), (d) production of extracellular enzymes that destroy host tissue or lyse host immune effector cells (hemolysin, cytotoxin, etc.), (e) invasiveness, (f) avoidance of host immune mechanisms by mechanical barriers (capsule), (g) avoidance of host immune mechanisms by protected environment (intracellular survival in nonprofessional phagocyte, nonperfused site, etc.), (h) antiphagocytic capsule, (i) production of toxin that mediates an unwelcome host cell response (enterotoxin, inhibitor of protein synthesis, etc.), (j) endotoxin in gram-negative bacterial cell walls, which mediates systemic effects (fever, coagulation, fluid accumulation, etc.), and (k) invocation of a host immune response that itself results in tissue damage.

5. Innate, nonspecific host defense mechanisms include (a) intact skin and mucous membrane, (b) tears, saliva, mucus, genital secretions, (c) ciliary motility, (d) reflexes (gag, cough, etc.), (e) flushing of urine, peristalsis, and excretion of fecal matter, (f) an inhospitable local environment (vaginal pH, etc.), (g) complement (classical and alternate pathways); (h) polymorphonuclear neutrophils, alveolar, and other fixed macrophages and, (i) interferon, cytokines, and interleukins.

6. Specific host defense mechanisms include (a) humoral immunity (IgM, IgA, and IgG) and (b) cellular immune system (killer T cells, T helper cells, etc.).

REFERENCES

Gorbach SL, Bartlett JG, Blacklow NR (eds) (1992): Infectious diseases. Philadelphia: W.B. Saunders.

Mandell GL, Douglas RG, Bennett JE (eds) (1990): Principles and practice of infectious diseases. 3rd ed. New York: Churchill Livingstone.

Mims CA (1982): The pathogenesis of infectious disease, 2nd ed. London: Academic Press.

Urbaschek B (ed) (1988): Perspectives on bacterial pathogenesis and host defense. Chicago: The University of Chicago Press.

REVIEW QUESTIONS

For questions 1 to 8, choose the ONE
BEST answer or completion.

1. An alcohol-abusing person living on the
   streets of New York presents to the emergency room with fever, foul-smelling sputum, and a 4-day history of feeling ill. A
   chest X-ray reveals a cavitation in the left
   upper lobe of the lung. The host defense
   mechanism most likely to have been impaired during acquisition of his illness is
   a) colonization resistance
   b) gag and swallowing reflexes
   c) salivary IgA secretion
   d) ciliary motility
   e) stomach acidity

2. Which of the following organism's primary
   virulence factor is its ability to survive intracellularly?
   a) *Mycobacterium* spp.
   b) *Shigella dysenteriae*
   c) *Giardia lamblia*
   d) *Helicobacter pylori*
   e) *Streptococcus pyogenes*

3. Which of the following events is most likely
   to precipitate acute endotoxic shock in a patient?
   a) Staphylococcal endocarditis.
   b) Severe dental caries.

   c) Fungal infection in the bloodstream.
   d) Malaria.
   e) Gram-negative bacterial sepsis.

4. A drug that reduces the activity of intracellular cAMP would be most effective in preventing symptoms of which diseases?
   a) Malaria and urinary tract infection.
   b) Whooping cough and cholera.
   c) Neonatal meningitis and diphtheria.
   d) Botulism and tetanus.
   e) Staphylococcal food poisoning and gas
      gangrene.

5. *Haemophilus influenzae* possesses a poly-
   ribitol-phosphate polysaccharide capsule.
   An effective polysaccharide vaccine against
   this organism will be able to
   a) elicit vigorous T-cell activation in the
      vaccine recipient
   b) inhibit the primary neutrophil response to
      the infection
   c) induce strong production of opsonic IgG
      in the vaccine recipient
   d) induce strong production of circulating
      properdin in the vaccine recipient
   e) induce the formation of antigen-specific
      cytotoxic T cells

6. Which of the following organism-host pairs
   best illustrates the concept of symbiosis?

a) *Staphylococcus aureus* on the skin of a patient with severe burns.
b) Mites in the eyebrow follicles of a middle-aged man.
c) *Candida albicans* in the vagina of a pregnant woman.
d) *Lactobacillus* spp. in the vagina of a pregnant woman.
e) Nonpathogenic protozoa (*Trichomonas tenax*) in the mouth of an immunocompromised patient.

7. Which vaccine is likely to be most effective in preventing the spread of gonorrhea?
a) A killed whole cell vaccine that is injected intramuscularly.
b) A live attenuated bacterial vaccine that is ingested.
c) A live attenuated bacterial vaccine that is applied to the genital mucosa.
d) A killed whole cell vaccine that is injected intravenously.
e) A killed whole cell vaccine that is ingested.

8. Which of the following groups of microorganisms produce an exotoxin as a primary virulence factor?
a) *Legionella pneumophila, Streptococcus pyogenes, Corynebacterium diphtheriae*
b) *Bacillus anthracis, Bacteroides fragilis, Staphylococcus aureus*
c) *Vibrio cholerae, Corynebacterium diphtheriae, Streptococcus pneumoniae*
d) *Clostridium tetani, Staphylococcus aureus, Enterococcus faecalis*
e) *Corynebacterium diphtheria, Clostridium perfringens, Bacillus anthracis*

ANSWERS TO REVIEW QUESTIONS

---

1. *b* The alcoholic has aspiration pneumonia, in which his/her normal oral flora have gained access to the lung during a state of unconsciousness. The upper lobe is more likely to be seeded if the patient is supine. Thus, his/her gag and swallow reflexes were not active. Ciliary motility is active only against airborne particles. Salivary IgA does not affect the normal flora.

2. *a* Each of the other organisms possesses other virulence factors. *Shigella* produces a toxin. *Giardia* is a parasite that attaches to the intestinal epithelium within the lumen. *Helicobacter pylori* produces a urease that alkalinates its immediate environment, and *Streptococcus pyogenes* produces hyaluronidase, an enzyme that destroys host tissue.

3. *e* Only gram-negative bacteria possess endotoxin, which is a component of their cell walls. Endotoxin is released when the bacteria are destroyed, such as by the host pol-

ymorphonuclear neutrophils or, in the case of sepsis, by the action of complement through the alternate pathway.

4. **b** The exotoxins of *Bordetella pertussis* (the agent of whooping cough) and *Vibrio cholerae*, as well as the heat-labile toxin of some strains of *Escherichia coli*, act by activating intracellular cAMP, which results in various biological effects. Although toxins are virulence factors for the agents of some of the other diseases named, they do not act on cAMP.

5. **c** Defense against encapsulated bacteria entails production of specific opsonins so that phagocytic cells can adhere and engulf the pathogens. T cells may enhance B-cell activity or act as cytoxic effectors, but that is not usually the main objective of a vaccine. Additionally, only live vaccines can induce much of a T-cell response. Without opsonizing antibody, the neutrophils will not be able to phagocytize the bacteria. Properdin is nonspecific.

6. **d** The lactobacilli maintain a low pH and colonize vaginal epithelial cells, which discourages establishment of pathogenic bacteria, while they proliferate. Both parties benefit, the definition of "symbiotic." In the other cases, organisms either contribute to pathology and are considered "parasites" (*Candida albicans*, *S. aureus*), or they do not provide any positive effect for the host (*Trichomonas tenax* and the mites) and are considered "commensals."

7. **c** *Neisseria gonorrhoeae* must adhere to the epithelium by means of pili before it can cause disease. Thus, an effective preventive strategy could involve stimulation of local secretory antibodies to prevent colonization. A live bacterial strain might be able to adhere and survive long enough to stimulate a local immune response. The strain would be destroyed by stomach acidity if it were ingested. Circulating humoral immunity is probably important in preventing systemic disease, but would not be effective in the local environment early in the attachment stage.

8. **e** All three bacterial species listed produce exotoxins that play a major role in producing disease. In each other choice, at least one species either does not produce an exotoxin or relies on another, more important virulence factor. *Legionella pneumophila* is able to survive intracellularly, *B. fragilis* does not produce any prominent exotoxins, *S. pneumoniae*'s primary virulence factor is its antiphagocytic capsule, and *E. faecalis* does not produce toxins.

STAPHYLOCOCCAL INFECTION AND DISEASE

Staphylococcal disease accounts for over 80% of the suppurative diseases seen in medical practice. At present, most of the serious staphylococcal disease occurs among hospitalized patients whose normal defense mechanisms are impaired.

The major pathogen responsible for these infections is *Staphylococcus aureus,* which affects all age groups and produces a wide variety of both suppurative and nonsuppurative diseases. Other species of staphylococci, including *Staphylococcus epidermidis* and *Staphylococcus saprophyticus,* which usually exist as nonpathogens in the same habitat as *S. aureus,* may also cause human infection. *S. epidermidis* is the primary cause of opportunistic disease in hospitalized patients with an impaired host resistance. *S. saprophyticus* can cause urinary tract disease in adolescent females. *S. aureus* can be differentiated from these and other species of staphylococci by its production of coagulase, an enzyme that causes the clotting of plasma.

STAPHYLOCOCCUS AUREUS DISEASE

Habitat

S. aureus is ubiquitous, existing everywhere in nature. It constitutes part of the normal flora of the skin, nose, throat, GI tract, and genital tract of 25–50% of humans and animals. The organism is expelled into the air and onto fomites from cases or carriers.

Transmission

EXOGENOUS. In exogenous transmission of staphylococci, immunologically competent hosts as well as those with impaired host resistance may be susceptible to infection or disease. Individuals may become infected by contact with contaminated objects (such as surgical instruments) or food, by droplet nuclei in the air from a case or carrier, by skin contaminants, or by organisms contained within a lesion. Examples of settings that facilitate infection or disease with staphylococci include patients with wounds, burns, compound fractures, aortic valve replacements, protheses, other diseases (e.g., diabetes, viral disease, or tumors), and those who consume food containing staphylococcal enterotoxin.

ENDOGENOUS. Disease may result from endogenous activation of the host's own organisms as a consequence of (1) defective host resistance or (2) a disruption of the normal flora balance that leads to an establishment of a new host-parasite equilibrium that favors the organism. Immunocompromised hosts with increased susceptibility include patients on steroids or irradiation therapy, patients who have undergone extensive surgery, and patients with other diseases. Patients with an altered host-parasite balance due to either excessive antibiotic therapy (colitis) or an environment that enhances growth and toxin production by the organism (toxic shock syndrome, TSS) are also susceptible to *S. aureus* disease.

NOSOCOMIAL DISEASE. **Nosocomial** (hospital acquired) disease is most often caused by gram-negative organisms, but coagulase negative staphylococci and *S. aureus* continue to create serious problems primarily because of their resistance to multiple antibiotics. Outbreaks usually originate either from nose or throat carriers among hospital personnel (including physicians and nurses) who expel the organism into an environment in which there are susceptible sick and debilitated patients and/or from a breakdown in hospital aseptic procedures.

Properties of the Organism

Resistance to environmental, physical, and chemical agents. S. aureus is among the most resistant of the nonspore formers to adverse environmental conditions and physical and chemical agents. The organism can survive for as long as 14 weeks in dried pus and is killed by 70% ethanol only after a 10-min contact period.

Microscopic morphology. The organism is a gram-positive, nonmotile coccus occurring in grapelike clusters on solid media and singly, or in pairs, in pus. Most strains are nonencapsulated.

Macroscopic morphology. S. aureus is a facultative anaerobe that grows best on blood agar at 37°C. Although many strains are β-hemolytic and may produce a golden yellow pigment, neither property is associated with the virulence of the organism.

Antigenic structure as it relates to identification and/or virulence:

1. **Polysaccharide A** (ribitol phosphate teichoic acid) is a cell wall component covalently linked to peptidoglycan. The molecule possesses **antiphagocytic activity.**

2. **Bound protein A** is a cell wall component also covalently linked to peptidoglycan. It consists of a single polypeptide chain that is unique to *S. aureus* in its ability to bind to the Fc portion of IgG and to extracellular matrix glycoprotein. Protein A may contribute to **adherence** and possess **antiphagocytic activity.** In purified form, it is a useful reagent in the immunoserological identification of microorganisms.

3. **Bound coagulase** is an antigenic cell wall enzyme but no association with the organism's virulence has been demonstrated. It is useful in the laboratory identification of *S. aureus.* Bound coagulase catalyzes the conversion of plasma fibrinogen to a fibrin clot in the presence of a coreacting factor (CRF) thought to be prothrombin or a prothrombin derivative, resulting in the clumping of the organism.

Phage grouping. Phage grouping is commonly but erroneously referred to as phage typing. Grouping is based upon the ability of *S. aureus* strains to be lysed by specific bacteriophages. This procedure, together with restriction fingerprinting length polymorphism (RFLP) or DNA typing, is useful in the epidemiological tracing of hospital outbreaks.

Extracellular products associated with or thought to be associated with the pathogenicity of the organism:

1. **Free protein A,** in contrast to the cell wall bound component, is formed and released by the organism during its growth and multiplication. Like bound protein A, it has a putative **adherence** and **antiphagocytic function**.

2. **Lipases** are lipid-hydrolyzing enzymes. These enzymes allow the organisms to **invade cutaneous and subcutaneous tissues** by splitting fats and oils accumulating on the skin.

3. **Leucocidin** is an exotoxin that contributes to the survival of the organism. During host-parasite confrontation, it **destroys polymorphonuclear leukocytes**.

4. **Alpha and delta exotoxin (hemolysins)** molecules are **toxic to polymorphonuclear leukocytes, macrophages, and platelets**. In addition, alpha exotoxin exhibits **dermonecrotic activity** that contributes to tissue necrosis and toxemia.

5. **Free coagulase,** in contrast to the cell wall bound component, is an extracellular enzyme produced by the organism during its growth and multiplication. The mechanism of fibrin clot formation is identical to that of bound coagulase. However, free coagulase, unlike the bound form, may play a role as a virulence factor by laying down a **fibrin barrier** during abscess development. That may act to the host's advantage by walling off and **localizing the abscess**. Inasmuch as *S. aureus* is the only human-origin member of the genus containing or producing coagulase, its demonstration is essential in the laboratory identification of the organism.

6. **Exfoliative (epidermolytic) exotoxin** is produced by some strains of *S. aureus.* Synthesis is plasmid or chromosomally mediated. By causing **intraepidermal splitting of tissues and necrosis**, it is responsible for the clinical manifestations seen in scalded skin syndrome (SSS).

7. **TSST-1 (syn: pyrogenic exotoxin C and enterotoxin F).** The molecule is a protein produced by several strains of *S. aureus* and is responsible for the clinical manifestations of toxic shock syndrome (see Fig. 7.1).

8. **Enterotoxin A, B, and D** molecules are heat-stable proteins capable of withstanding boiling for 30 min and produced by one-third of *S. aureus* strains. Synthesis is plasmid or chromosomally mediated. Enterotoxin A and D are responsible for staphylococcal food poisoning by **inhibiting water absorption** from the intestinal lumen and inducing diarrhea, and by acting on the **emetic receptor sites** in the GI tract and causing vomiting. Enterotoxin B **damages the intestinal epithelium** and produces colitis.

9. **Hyaluronidase** is produced by over 90% of *S. aureus* strains. It is a mucin-splitting enzyme that hydrolyzes the hyaluronic acid constituent of connective tissue ground substance and thus facilitates the spread of the organism through the tissues.

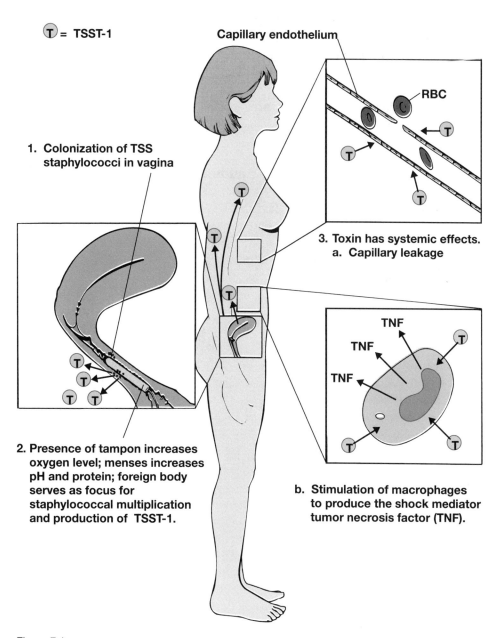

Figure 7.1.

Pathogenesis of toxic shock syndrome in menstruating woman.

10. **Staphylokinase (fibrinolysin)** is produced by several *S. aureus* strains. It dissolves fibrin clots and thus **contributes to the spread of the organism from local sites**. Those mechanisms that regulate coagulase versus staphylokinase activity are presently unknown but may be dependent on factors related to host resistance.

The structural and extracellular virulence factors, together with their location and function, are also presented in Table 7.1.

Pathogenesis and Clinical Manifestations

PRIMARY DISEASES OF THE SKIN AND SUBCUTANEOUS TISSUES. Upon entry, organisms penetrate through the skin into the subcutaneous tissues with the aid of **lipases**. Attachment to host tissue and extracellular matrices is facilitated by **bound and free protein A**. As multiplication occurs, the host responds with an acute inflammatory response characterized by polymorphonuclear leukocytic infiltration and exudate, thus initiating the confrontation between the host and the organism. Despite the antiphagocytic activity of **polysaccharide A** and both **bound and free protein A**, many organisms are phagocytized by the polymorphonuclear leukocytes following the activation of the **alternative pathway of complement** and resultant **C3b opsonification** of the bacterial surface.

Phagocytized and nonphagocytized organisms release **leucocidin** and **alpha and delta exotoxins**, which are toxic to the polymorphonuclear leukocyte and thus permit both intra- and extra-leukocytic survival. The action of the **alpha exotoxin** results in tissue necrosis and the organism, by virtue of its **coagulase** production, lays down a fibrin barrier.

The end result of the above pathogenesis process is the **furuncle** which is a painful, indurated, erythematous abscess, single or multiple, with a central area of necrosis walled off from surrounding subcutaneous tissue. Healing, if it occurs, results in sloughing of necrotic tissue with replacement by granulation tissue.

Extension of the pathogenetic process laterally and deeper into the fibrous tissues results in the formation of **carbuncles.** These lesions are characterized by multiple openings to the surface from the deeper tissues with pus discharge. Healing, if it occurs, results in sloughing of necrotic tissue and deep scars.

Other primary diseases of the skin and subcutaneous tissues, such as those involving hair follicles, paronychia (nail bed), wounds, burns, breast, and nipples, are characterized by abscesses similar to those seen in patients with furuncles. Their pathogenesis is also similar to that of a furuncle.

Table 7.1 Virulence Factors of *S. aureus* and Their Function

Virulence factor	Structure and location	Function
Polysaccharide A	Ribitol phosphate teichoic acid; cell wall component	Antiphagocytic
Protein A (bound)	Single polypeptide chain; cell wall component	Adhesin; antiphagocytic
Protein A (free)	Single polypeptide chain; extracellular	Adhesin; antiphagocytic
Lipase	Lipid-hydrolyzing enzyme; extracellular	Splits fats and oils accumulating on the skin, allowing organisms to invade cutaneous and subcutaneous tissues
Leucocidin	Exotoxin composed of two proteins; extracellular	Destroys polymorphonuclear leukocytes
Alpha and delta exotoxins (hemolysins)	Protein; extracellular	Destroy polymorphonuclear leukocytes, macrophages, and platelets; in addition, alpha toxin exhibits dermonecrotic activity that contributes to tissue necrosis and toxemia
Coagulase (free)	Enzyme; extracellular	Catalyzes the conversion of fibrinogen to a fibrin clot in the presence of a coreacting factor; lays down a fibrin barrier during abscess formation; walls off and localizes the abscess
Exfoliative (epidermolytic) exotoxin	Protein; extracellular	Produces intraepidermal splitting of tissues and necrosis seen in SSS
TSST-1 (syn: Pyrogenic exotoxin C and enterotoxin F)	Protein; extracellular	Produces chills, fever, shock, hypotension, and rash seen in SSS
Enterotoxins A and D	Protein; heat stable; extracellular	Responsible for food poisoning by inhibiting water absorption from the intestinal lumen inducing diarrhea, and by acting on emetic receptic sites in the GI tract inducing vomiting
Enterotoxin B	Protein; heat stable; extracellular	Responsible for colitis by damaging the intestinal epithelium
Hyaluronidase	Enzyme; extracellular	Hydrolyzes the hyaluronic acid constituent of connective tissue ground substance, thereby facilitating dissemination
Staphylokinase (fibrinolysin)	Enzyme; extracellular	Dissolves fibrin clots, thereby contributing to dissemination

Impetigo is a disease that is usually seen in newborns and children. It may be caused by *S. aureus* or group A streptococci, alone or in combination. It initiates on the face and may involve the eyes, nose, lips, and limbs. Although the pathogenesis is similar to that described for the furuncle, the lesions are more severe and extensive being characterized as vesicular, crusting, and/or pustular.

Scalded skin syndrome is a disease that occurs in infants and children 4 years of age or under, and in the immunocompromised adult. Again, the basic pathogenesis is similar to that described for the furuncle, except that the organisms release **exfoliative exotoxin,** which is responsible for the extensive intraepidermal splitting and bullous necrosis of the tissue.

PRIMARY DISEASE OF THE FEMALE GENITAL TRACT. **Toxic shock syndrome (TSS)** is a disease that occurs mostly in menstruating women as a result of the enhancement of growth of toxin-producing endogenous organisms. Highly absorbent tampons contribute to the initiation of the disease by providing a favorable environment for the growth of resident *S. aureus.* The basic pathogenesis relating to survival and multiplication is as described. The organisms elaborate **TSST-1** resulting in chills, fever, hypotension, shock, and a sunburnlike macular rash. Subsequent exfoliation of the skin on the feet and palms often occurs. Toxic shock syndrome may occur in men as well as in women following wound infection with *S. aureus.* A **pyrogenic exotoxin produced by group A streptococci** has been reported to be associated with a systemic toxic, shocklike syndrome with a relatively high case fatality rate.

PRIMARY DISEASE OF THE RESPIRATORY TRACT. **Bronchopneumonia with multiple abscesses** is a disease that occurs among immunosuppressed patients, the aged, infants less than 1 year of age, and frequently in children with measles, cystic fibrosis, and influenza as a result of exogenous transmission or potentiated multiplication of endogenous organisms. The pathogenesis is as described for the furuncle except that the disease initiates in the lung with resultant multiple abscesses and necrosis. The pneumonia is patchy and focal in nature.

PRIMARY DISEASE OF THE GASTROINTESTINAL TRACT. **Staphylococcal colitis** or **staphylococcal necrotizing enterocolitis** is a disease that is observed in patients whose normal bowel is altered by the oral administration of broad-spectrum antibiotics that selectively permit overgrowth by antibiotic resistant, enterotoxin-producing strains of *S. aureus.* The basic pathogenesis relating to survival and multiplication is as described. The organisms release **enterotoxin**

B, which damages the intestinal epithelium and produces fever, diarrhea, and abdominal cramps.

Staphylococcal food poisoning is the most common cause of food poisoning in the United States. The organisms are usually introduced into food, such as pastries and tuna salad, from a patient with paronychial disease. The contaminated food is kept at room temperature, during which time the organisms multiply and release heat stable **enterotoxin A or D.** The toxin-containing food may or may not look or smell unusual. Host damage is due to the ingestion of food containing pre-formed enterotoxin that acts on the emetic receptor sites to produce vomiting and inhibits water absorption from the intestine to produce diarrhea after an incubation period of only 1–6 h. The **absence of fever** is an important observation in the differential diagnosis of staphylococcal food poisoning.

DISSEMINATION BY HEMATOGENOUS SPREAD. Dissemination occurs from a primary disease focus or as an initiating disease. Predisposing factors are related to impaired host resistance induced by trauma (e.g., surgical intervention of an abscess), surgical repair or implants (e.g., aortic valve replacement), foreign bodies (e.g., catheters), or immunosuppressive disease (Fig. 7.2). **Hyaluronidase and possibly staphylokinase** facilitate dissemination by their enzymatic breakdown of connective tissue ground substance and fibrin clots, respectively, but the mechanisms responsible for production and activation of these enzymes are presently unknown.

Septicemia, or multiplication of the organisms in the circulation, is hospital acquired in 50% of the patients and usually is due to organisms with multiple antibiotic resistance. Rapid spread occurs to multiple organs including the meninges and heart valves, with resultant abscess formation.

Osteomyelitis is a disease that is usually caused by *S. aureus*. Osteomyelitis may be associated with trauma or surgery and occurs frequently in IV drug users, as well as in patients with diabetes, peripheral vascular disease, and in-dwelling catheters. The organisms spread from cutaneous lesions into the circulation and localize in the long bones where they produce abscesses.

Septic arthritis is frequently due to *S. aureus*. It may occur following orthopedic surgery or intraarticular cortisone injections.

Immunity to Reinfection

Immunity to reinfection with *S. aureus* does not exist. Recurrent disease is relatively common.

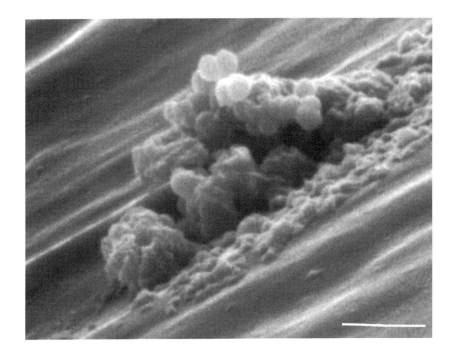

Figure 7.2.

Scanning electron micrograph of a cardiac pacemaker lead colonized by *S. aureus*. [Reproduced with permission from Costerton JW, Lappin-Scott HM (1989): Behavior of bacteria in biofilms. ASM News 55(12):653.]

Laboratory Diagnosis

SPECIMENS. Specimens obtained depend on the disease process and include lesion material, pus, sputum, blood for culture, spinal fluid, feces, and synovium. In suppurative diseases, Gram stain of pus shows single, pairs, chains, or small clumps of gram-positive cocci and numerous polymorphonuclear leukocytes.

PRIMARY ISOLATION AND IDENTIFICATION. Isolation and identification of *S. aureus* requires initial cultivation on blood agar and/or specialized media depending on the specimen. Overnight incubation under aerobic conditions at 37°C is optimal for isolation of the organism. The organism may be identified as a gram-positive, catalase-positive coccus exhibiting bound or free coagulase.

IMMUNOSEROLOGIC TESTS. An immunoserologic test for circulating teichoic acid antigen may be useful in the diagnosis of disseminated disease.

Treatment

Adequate drainage, debridement, and antibiotic therapy are essential for the treatment of localized lesions. The great majority of isolates from both the community and hospitals exhibit **multiple resistance** to antibiotics. Ninety percent of strains isolated from patients in the United States are resistant to penicillin due to the production of penicillinase (β-lactamase), which renders the β-lactam molecule inactive. Mechanisms of multiple drug resistance, including penicillinase production, are conferred upon the organism by plasmid-mediated transduction.

Multiple antibiotic resistance and a high case fatality rate exist among patients with disseminated disease due to *S. aureus*. This situation mandates initial and long-term treatment with penicillinase-resistant penicillin such as oxacillin or methicillin. At hospitals where methicillin resistance among isolated strains is high or where patients are allergic to the penicillins, long-term vancomycin should be used.

Toxic shock syndrome, with a case fatality rate of 8% even with therapy, is caused by penicillin-resistant strains and should be treated accordingly. The self-limiting nature of staphylococcal food poisoning precludes the use of antimicrobial therapy. Autogenous vaccines for treatment of *S. aureus* disease are ineffective.

Prevention and Control

In the hospital environment, recent evidence indicates that mupirocin will effectively eliminate the carrier state and significantly reduce catheter-site colonization. Proper isolation of infectious disease patients and patients at risk, along with the strict enforcement of aseptic techniques in hospitals, is essential. **Handwashing** is the most important preventive measure in the prevention and control of nosocomial disease due to *S. aureus*. Every hospital must have an Infectious Disease Committee to monitor and enforce regulations governing asepsis.

Food poisoning can be prevented by refrigeration of food. The risk of TSS in women can be reduced considerably by frequent tampon change and the use of less absorbent tampons.

DISEASE DUE TO COAGULASE-NEGATIVE STAPHYLOCOCCI

Coagulase-negative staphylococci exist as part of the normal flora on the skin and in the nose and throat. Although all species are capable of causing opportunistic nosocomial disease associated with foreign bodies and impaired resistance, *S. epidermidis* is the most important etiologic agent. Disease due to these organisms has been reported in patients with prosthetic valvular endocarditis, CSF shunts, joint and vascular prostheses, in children and elderly males who have undergone urethral instrumentation, and among IV drug users. The organism may occasionally produce disseminated disease with multiple organ damage. Multiple resistance to antibiotics, including methicillin, oxacillin, penicillin, and the cephalosporins, is common. Although vancomycin may, at times, be effective, these diseases usually have a high fatality rate even with therapy due to the underlying nature of the disease.

STAPHYLOCOCCUS SAPROPHYTICUS DISEASE

S. saprophyticus is found only occasionally on human skin and in the GI and genitourinary tracts of healthy individuals. Yet, this gram-positive coccus is the second most common cause of urinary tract disease in adolescent females. Although penicillin-resistant strains occur, the organism is susceptible to most other antibiotics.

SUMMARY

1. Staphylococci are ubiquitous, gram-positive, nonmotile, facultative anaerobic cocci that account for over 80% of the suppurative diseases seen in medical practice. The major pathogen within the genus is *Staphylococcus aureus*.

2. The basic pathogenesis process of all primary diseases of the skin and subcutaneous tissues due to *S. aureus* is similar. Organisms penetrate with the aid of lipases. Attachment is facilitated by bound and free protein A. Despite the antiphagocytic activity of polysaccharide A and bound and free protein A, many organisms are phagocytized by the polymorphonuclear leukocytes following activation of the alternative pathway of complement and resultant C3b opsonification of the bacterial surface. Organisms release leucocidin and alpha and delta exotoxins that are toxic to the polymorphonuclear leukocytes and thus permit both intra- and extra-leukocytic survival. Alpha toxin also results in tissue necrosis, and the organism, by virtue of its coagulase production, may wall off and localize the abscess. In addition, SSS is characterized by extensive intraepidermal splitting and bullous necrosis of the tissues due to exfoliative exotoxin release by the organism.

3. *S. aureus* primary disease of the (a) female genital tract manifests as toxic shock syndrome (TSS) due to TSST-1 release, (b) respiratory tract manifests as bronchopneumonia with multiple abscesses, and (c) gastrointestinal tract manifests as a colitis due to enterotoxin B release or food poisoning due to the ingestion of food containing pre-formed enterotoxin A or D.

4. Hyaluronidase and possibly staphylokinase facilitate dissemination of *S. aureus* by their enzymatic breakdown of connective tissue ground substance and fibrin clots, respectively. Hospital-acquired septicemia with rapid spread to multiple organs, osteomyelitis, and septic arthritis are pyogenic disseminated diseases frequently due to *S. aureus*.

5. The great majority of *S. aureus* isolates from both the community and hospitals are multiply resistant to antibiotics.

6. Coagulase-negative staphylococci are skin, nose, and throat commensals that can cause opportunistic nosocomial disease associated with foreign bodies and impaired host resistance. Multiple antibiotic resistance and a high case fatality rate are common.

7. *Staphylococcus saprophyticus*, an occasional skin, GI, and genitourinary tract commensal, is the second most common cause of urinary tract disease in adolescent females.

REFERENCES

Brumfitt W, Hamilton-Miller J (1989): Methicillin-resistant *Staphylococcus aureus*. N Eng J Med 320:1188.

Cohen ML (1986): *Staphylococcus aureus:* Biology, mechanism of virulence, epidemiology, J Pediatr 5:796.

Fleischer B (1991): T lymphocyte-stimulating microbial toxins as superantigens. Med Microbiol Immunol 180:53.

Hovelius B, Mardh P-A (1984): *Staphylococcus saprophyticus* as a common cause of urinary tract infections. Rev Infect Dis 6:328.

Kuhn PJ (November, 1978): Opportunistic pathogens. Microbes with a potential for violence. Diagn Med 80.

Melish ME (1992): Staphylococcal infections. In Feigin RD, Cherry JD (eds): Textbook of Pediatric Infectious Diseases, 3rd ed, Vol. 2. Philadelphia: W. B. Saunders. pp 1240–1267.

Novick RP (1990): Molecular Biology of the Staphylococci. New York: VCH.

Patrick CC (1992): Coagulase-negative staphylococci. In Feigin RD, Cherry JD (eds): Textbook of Pediatric Infectious Diseases. 3rd ed, Vol. 2. Philadelphia: W.B. Saunders.

Todd JK (1988): Toxic shock syndrome. Clin Microbiol Rev 1:432.

Wiseman GM (1975): The hemolysins of *Staphylococcus aureus*. Bacteriol Rev 39:317.

REVIEW QUESTIONS

For questions 1 to 5, choose the ONE BEST answer or completion.

1. Disease due to *Staphylococcus aureus* may be the result of
   a) consuming food containing only the organism
   b) the administration of staphylococcal human immune globulin
   c) host interaction with motile strains
   d) exogenous transmission or endogenous activation in patients whose resistance is impaired
   e) pigment production by the organism

2. The *S. aureus* virulence factors polysaccharide A (ribitol phosphate teichoic acid) and bound protein A
   a) are extracellular substances secreted by the organisms
   b) possess antiphagocytic activity
   c) are located exclusively in the cytoplasm of the organism
   d) are responsible for the clinical manifestations of staphylococcal endotoxemia
   e) are part of the capsular structure of encapsulated strains

3. A gram-positive, catalase positive, coccus was isolated from a bone spicule of a patient with osteomyelitis. The organism was identified as *S. aureus* on the basis of
   a) yellow-orange pigment production
   b) beta hemolysis
   c) its ability to grow under anaerobic conditions
   d) its ability to grow on mannitol-salt agar
   e) its ability to produce coagulase

4. Staphylococcal food poisoning
   a) is the result of enterotoxin A or D acting upon emetic receptor sites and inhibiting water absorption from the intestine
   b) produces chills and fever
   c) occurs after an incubation period of 48–72 h
   d) is the result of excessive antibiotic therapy
   e) is best treated with an autogenous vaccine

5. Essential requirements for the prevention of nosocomial disease include
   a) treatment of hospital personnel carriers with penicillin
   b) proper isolation of infectious disease patients and patients at risk, and treatment of carriers with mupirocin
   c) prophylactic antibiotic therapy for all patients admitted to the hospital
   d) administration of immune globulin to all patients prior to undergoing surgery
   e) the restriction of hospital admissions to afebrile patients

For questions 6 to 11, ONE or MORE of the completions given is correct. Choose the appropriate answer.

A) if only **1, 2, 3** are correct
B) if only **1 and 3** are correct
C) if only **2 and 4** are correct
D) if only **4** is correct
E) if **all** are correct

6. Virulence factor(s) of *S. aureus* that contribute to survival of the organism by destroying polymorphonuclear leukocytes is/are
   1) lipases
   2) leucocidin
   3) TSST-1
   4) delta exotoxin
   5) enterotoxin B

7. Virulence factor(s) thought to contribute to the dissemination of *S. aureus* from local sites is/are
   1) hyaluronidase
   2) coagulase
   3) staphylokinase
   4) TSST-1
   5) lytic phages

8. Virulence factors that contribute to the basic pathogenesis of primary diseases of the skin and subcutaneous tissues are
   1) leucocidin
   2) protein A
   3) polysaccharide A
   4) alpha and delta exotoxins
   5) coagulase

9. The exfoliative exotoxin produced by some strains of *S. aureus*
   1) causes intraepidermal splitting of tissues and necrosis
   2) is responsible for the clinical manifestations of scalded skin syndrome
   3) is plasmid or chromosomally mediated during synthesis
   4) is a mucin-splitting enzyme
   5) is an adhesin

10. Multiple antibiotic resistant strains of *S. aureus*
    1) represent the majority of hospital and community isolates
    2) may acquire their resistance by plasmid-mediated transduction
    3) produce disseminated disease with high case fatality rates
    4) produce disseminated disease that mandates long-term therapy
    5) may produce local abscesses that require adequate drainage and debridement, as well as appropriate antibiotic therapy

11. *Staphylococcus epidermidis*
    1) exists among humans as part of the normal flora of the skin, nose, and throat
    2) may produce opportunistic nosocomial disease among patients with an impaired resistance
    3) commonly exhibits multiple antiibiotic resistance
    4) is capable of producing only local abscesses
    5) produces toxic shock syndrome

ANSWERS TO REVIEW QUESTIONS

1. *d* Disease due to *Staphylococcus aureus* may be the result of either exogenous transmission or activation of endogenous organisms among patients whose resistance is impaired. The consuming of food containing only the organism (and not enterotoxin), the administration of human immune globulin, and the production of pigment by the organism, do not result in disease. Furthermore, all pathogenic cocci are nonmotile.

2. *b* Polysaccharide A and bound protein A are cell wall components that possess antiphagocytic activity. Endotoxins are not produced by gram-positive organisms.

3. *e* Coagulase production is the definitive property of a gram-positive, catalase positive coccus that characterizes organisms of human origin as *S. aureus*.

4. *a* Staphylococcal food poisoning is characterized by vomiting and diarrhea resulting from the action of enterotoxin A and D acting upon the emetic receptor sites and inhibiting water absorption from the intestine, respectively. It is further characterized by a short 1 to 6-h incubation period and the absence of fever. The disease is not the result of excessive antibiotic therapy and is self-limiting.

5. *b* Two of the most important requirements for the prevention of nosocomial disease are the proper isolation of infectious disease patients and patients at risk and the treatment of carriers with mupirocin. Prophylactic antibiotic therapy for patients admitted to the hospital, the administration of immune globulin to presurgical patients, and the restriction of hospital admissions to afebrile patients, will not succeed in preventing nosocomial disease among sick and debilitated patients.

6. *C* Leucocidin and delta exotoxin contribute to the survival of *S. aureus* by destroying polymorphonuclear leukocytes. Lipases split fats and oils accumulating on the skin, while TSST-1 and enterotoxin B are associated with the production of clinical manifestations of TSS and colitis, respectively.

7. *B* Hyaluronidase, which hydrolyzes the hyaluronic acid of connective tissue ground substance, and staphylokinase, which dissolves fibrin clots, are thought to contribute to dissemination of *S. aureus* from local sites. Free coagulase may lay down a fibrin barrier during abscess formation and wall off and localize the abscess. TSST-1 is an extracellular virulence factor that contributes to

the production of the clinical manifestations of TSS, but does not influence dissemination of the organism from local sites. While strains of *S. aureus* are susceptible to specific lytic phages, there is no known relationship between phage susceptibility and staphylococcal dissemination.

8. **E** All are correct statements.

9. **A** The exfoliative toxin produced by some strains of *S. aureus* causes the intraepidermal splitting of tissues and necrosis seen in SSS. Synthesis is both plasmid and chromosomally mediated. The toxin is neither an enzyme nor an adhesin.

10. **E** All are correct statements. Multiple antibiotic resistant strains of *S. aureus* may produce local as well as disseminated disease.

11. **A** Although *Staphylococcus epidermidis* is a common inhabitant of the skin, nose, and throat, it can produce serious opportunistic nosocomial disease among patients with an impaired resistance. Multiple antibiotic resistance contributes to a high fatality rate. This organism does not cause TSS.

CHAPTER 8

STREPTOCOCCAL AND ENTEROCOCCAL INFECTION AND DISEASE, AND LISTERIOSIS

STREPTOCOCCUS AND *ENTEROCOCCUS*

Streptococci are capable of causing a variety of suppurative and nonsuppurative diseases in both humans and animals. There are 21 groups of streptococci based upon (with the exception of the viridans group) the antigenic diversity of a cell wall carbohydrate and over 85 serotypes of a single species, *Streptococcus pneumoniae,* based upon the antigenic diversity of their capsular polysaccharides. Group A streptococci (syn: *Streptococcus pyogenes*) and *S. pneumoniae* are responsible for the great majority of human streptococcal disease. Ten million cases of septic sore throat due to group A streptococci and 500,000 cases of pneumonia due to *S. pneumoniae* occur each year in the United States. More recently, a systemic group A streptococcal toxic shocklike syndrome associated with erythrogenic (scarlet fever) toxin A production has been responsible for severe systemic manifestations resulting in a case fatality rate of up to 30%. Among the remaining streptococci, group B (*Streptococcus agalactiae*) and the viridans group are the most important with respect to their pathogenic potential for humans. *Enterococcus* species, formerly classified as members of the group D streptococci, are organisms resembling streptococci that are capable of producing disseminated disease following GI or genitourinary manipulation, and exhibit a high degree of antibiotic resistance.

GROUP A STREPTOCOCCAL DISEASE

Habitat

Group A streptococci are restricted to humans. Although their major habitats are the nose, throat, and skin of 5–15% of humans, they have also been found in the vaginal tract.

Transmission

EXOGENOUS. Exogenous infection or disease may be initiated in an immunologically normal or impaired host. Susceptible individuals may become infected by droplet nuclei from a case or carrier to the respiratory tract, from contaminated instruments or droplet nuclei into wounds, burns, or abrasions, or by ingestion of milk contaminated by a case or carrier.

ENDOGENOUS. Activation of endogenous organisms may occur from the nose, throat, or skin of a carrier to areas of impaired host resistance. Defects in host resistance may be caused, for example, by viral disease, congenitally damaged heart valves, wounds, burns, or abrasions. Those factors that determine whether an individual will become colonized (carrier), clear the organism, or develop disease following exposure, as well as those mechanisms that influence the maintenance of the carrier state versus ''activation'' and the resultant expression of endogenous disease, are not known but represent areas of intense research.

Properties of the Organism

Resistance to environmental, physical, and chemical agents. Group A, like most streptococci, are less resistant to environmental conditions than staphylococci, although they can survive on dry swabs for weeks. They are killed rapidly by physical and chemical agents.

Microscopic morphology. Group A, as well as the other grouped streptococci and members of the genus *Enterococcus,* are gram-positive, nonmotile cocci occurring in short or long chains, and occasionally singly and in pairs. Freshly isolated strains of group A streptococci are **encapsulated,** but the capsules are lost rapidly during the stationary phase of in vitro cultivation.

Macroscopic morphology. Most of the grouped streptococci, including the *Enterococcus* species, are facultative anaerobes that grow best aerobically with increased carbon dioxide on blood agar at 37°C. Depending on the group, streptococci exhibit either **α, β, or γ hemolysis** around a colony when grown on blood agar. Of the grouped streptococci to be discussed in this chapter, most species of the viridans group show α hemolysis, which is a partial lysis of the erythrocytes, and manifests as a green zone around the colony. Groups A and B streptococci exhibit β hemolysis, which is a complete lysis of the erythrocytes and manifests as a clear zone around the colony. Several species of *Enterococcus* produce γ hemolysis, which indicates that no lysis of the erythrocytes has occurred and manifests as intact erythrocytes or no change around the colony. Although not the basis for final classification or laboratory identification of the streptococci and enterococci, the type of hemolysis exhibited by these organisms assists in the accurate preliminary screening of isolates.

Antigenic structure of group A streptococci as it relates to classification and/ or virulence:

"C" carbohydrates are cell wall polysaccharides whose antigenic diversity forms **the basis for the classification of streptococci into 20 serogroups** lettered from A to V (omitting I and J). These group-specific antigens are covalently linked to peptidoglycan and are composed of a branched polymer of L-rhamnose or glycerol teichoic acid linked to a hexosamine, the latter being the determinant group responsible for group specificity. For group A streptococci, the "C" carbohydrate is composed of L-rhamnose-*N*-acetylglucosamine with the determinant being beta-linked *N*-acetylglucosamine.

Lipoteichoic acid (LTA) is a surface-exposed molecule covalently linked to cytoplasmic membrane glycolipid that extends through the cell wall and capsule. Potentially, **in concert with M protein, LTA mediates oral and skin epithelial attachment** and subsequent colonization (Fig. 8.1). The mechanism is thought to involve a fibrillar network created by the ionic interaction between negatively charged LTA and positively charged M protein. The glycolipid moiety of teichoic acid now becomes exposed to fibronectin receptors on the host cell and adherence occurs.

M proteins are surface-exposed, "fuzz" or pilus-like dimeric molecules ranging in molecular weight from 40,000 to 80,000. These proteins are anchored

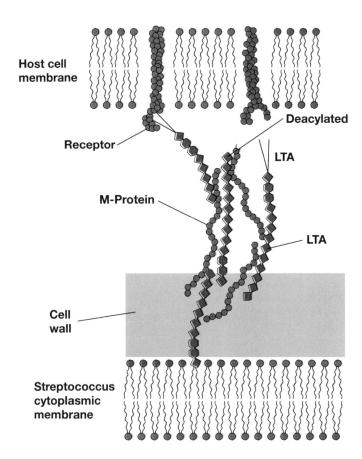

Figure 8.1.

Attachment of group A streptococci to an epithelial cell by lipoteichoic acid antigen–M protein ligands. [Redrawn from Ofek I, Simpson WA, Beachey EH (1982): Formation of molecular complexes between a structurally defined M-protein and acylated and deacylated lipoteichoic acid of *Streptococcus pyogenes.* J Bacteriol 149: 431.]

to the cytoplasmic membrane at the carboxy terminus and extend through the cell wall and capsule as a fibrillar structure composed of two alpha helical monomeric chains twisted about each other to give a coiled coil appearance. M protein is considered to be the **major virulence factor of group A streptococci.** In addition, antigenic diversity among group A streptococcal M proteins is the basis for the recognition of more than 80 serotypes. The protein possesses **antiphagocytic activity** in the absence of type-specific antibody and complement by blocking the deposition of C3b opsonin and limiting the interaction of already bound C3b with polymorphonuclear leukocyte receptors. Adherence of group A streptococci to pharyngeal and skin surfaces is much greater in M protein plus strains indicating a potential role for M protein as a **mediator of attachment in concert with LTA.** M protein stimulates type-specific protective immunity against pharyngeal but not skin diseases due to group A streptococci. Although mouse studies suggest that protection against pharyngeal colonization of heterologous M protein serotypes can be achieved with widely shared epitopes, the **cross-reactivity of anti-M protein antibody with human cardiac tissue** has raised serious questions about the possibility of vaccination with whole M protein or its determinants.

The **capsule** is composed of hyaluronic acid indistinguishable from the ground substance found in connective tissue, thus accounting for its lack of immunogenicity in the human host. It exerts **antiphagocytic activity** by a mechanism as yet unknown.

Fc receptors are unique surface proteins that bind to the Fc domain of mammalian immunoglobulin. Evidence suggests that a group A streptococcal Fc receptor for human IgG may play a role as a virulence factor in primary skin infections by **antiphagocytic** mechanisms.

C5a peptidase is a surface-bound endopeptidase found in most group A streptococci. It is thought to contribute to the virulence of the organism by specifically cleaving the C5a component of complement at lysine residue 68, which drastically inhibits the ability of C5a to bind to polymorphonuclear leukocytic surface receptors. Thus much of the ability of C5a to act as a chemoattractant of polymorphonuclear leukocytes to areas of inflammation is destroyed.

Streptolysin S (for stable) is a nonantigenic toxic protein, largely cell membrane-bound and oxygen stable, with a molecular weight of approximately 20,000. In addition to its ability to lyse human erythrocytes and phagocytic cells by direct cell-cell contact, Streptolysin S is capable of exerting a **leukotoxic effect upon polymorphonuclear leukocytes** after phagocytosis occurs by an as yet unknown mechanism. It is responsible for the surface hemolysis observed around colonies of group A streptococci grown on blood agar plates.

Extracellular products associated with or thought to be associated with pathogenicity:

Streptolysin O (for oxygen labile) is produced by most strains of group A streptococci. The molecule is an oxygen labile, immunogenic protein with a molecular weight ranging from 50,000 to 75,000 depending on the state of oxidation of the molecule. In addition to its ability to lyse human erythrocytes, the molecule can severely damage or destroy polymorphonuclear leukocytes by binding to membrane sterols and producing "slits" and "holes" that result in the release of lysosomal enzymes and degranulation. Streptolysin O is also able to destroy adjacent cells and tissues and thus **contribute to the spread of the organism from local sites.** The measurement of anti-Streptolysin O antibodies is employed diagnostically to determine recent group A streptococcal disease.

Pyrogenic (erythrogenic) exotoxins are proteins responsible for the **rash**

of scarlet fever. There are three antigenically distinct types designated A, B, and C, one or more of which are produced by more than 95% of group A streptococci strains. In addition to the rash of scarlet fever, pyrogenic exotoxin A has recently been reported to be associated with a systemic toxic shocklike syndrome with a relatively high case fatality rate. Toxin production is mediated by specific lysogenic phages that carry the *tox* gene. Those factors that control the regulation and expression of the *tox* gene are not known.

DNases are produced by most strains of group A streptococci. These molecules consist of four immunologically and electrophoretically distinct types designated A-D with molecular weights ranging from 25,000 to 30,000. DNases act by depolymerizing the viscous DNA that accumulates in thick pus as a result of polymorphonuclear leukocyte disintegration and thus **contribute to spread from local sites.** Measurement of anti-DNase B antibodies is the most useful serologic test in the diagnosis of recent group A streptococcal disease.

Hyaluronidase is produced by most strains of group A streptococci. As with *S. aureus,* hyaluronidase acts by hydrolyzing the hyaluronic acid component of connective tissue ground substance and thus **facilitates the spread of the organism through the tissues.** How the enzyme degrades the capsular hyaluronic acid of the organism to increase its susceptibility to phagocytosis remains an enigma.

Streptokinases (fibrinolysins) are produced by most strains of group A streptococci. The molecules consist of two immunologically and electrophoretically distinct types. As with staphylokinase, they act by catalyzing the conversion of plasminogen to plasmin, thus leading to fibrin digestion, the **prevention of an effective local barrier,** and spread of the organism from local sites.

The structural and extracellular virulence factors, together with their location and function, are also presented in Table 8.1.

Pathogenesis and Clinical Manifestations

PRIMARY DISEASES OF MUCOUS MEMBRANE SURFACES, SKIN, AND/OR SUBCUTANEOUS TISSUES

Septic Sore Throat and Scarlet Fever.   Both of these diseases occur in all age groups, but most often in young children. They are initiated either by droplet nuclei from a case or carrier into a susceptible host or endogenously by factors that upset host-parasite equilibrium. The organisms attach to the pharyngeal mucosa through **LTA** ligands (in concert with **M protein**) and colonize. Multiplication results in an acute inflammatory response characterized by an influx of polymor-

TABLE 8.1. Virulence Factors of Group A Streptococci and Their Function

Virulence factor	Structure and location	Function
Lipoteichoic acid	Glycolipid complex; linked to cytoplasmic membrane and extends through the cell wall and capsule	Adhesin (in concert with M protein)
M protein	Fibrillar and composed of two alpha helical monomeric chains twisted about each other (coiled coil); anchored to cytoplasmic membrane and extends through the cell wall and capsule	Adhesin (in concert with LPA); antiphagocytic; vaccinogenic
Capsule	Hyaluronic acid; external to cell wall	Antiphagocytic
Fc Receptor	Protein; cell wall component	Antiphagocytic in skin diseases
C5a Peptidase	Endopeptidase enzyme; cell wall component	Antipolymorphonuclear leukocyte chemoattractant
Streptolysin S	Oxygen-stable protein; largely cell membrane bound	Leukotoxic for the polymorphonuclear leukocyte
Streptolysin O	Oxygen-labile protein; extracellular	Toxic for the polymorphonuclear leukocyte and for tissues adjacent to site of infection
Pyrogenic (erythrogenic) exotoxins	Protein; three antigenically distinct types (A-C); extracellular	Responsible for the rash of scarlet fever; exotoxin A associated with systemic toxic shocklike syndrome.
DNases	Enzymes; four immunologically and electrophoretically distinct types (A-D); extracellular	Depolymerizes viscous DNA in pus, contributes to spread from local sites
Hyaluronidase	Enzyme; extracellular	Hydrolyzes the hyaluronic acid constituent of connective tissue ground substance, thereby facilitating dissemination
Streptokinases (fibrinolysins)	Enzymes; two immunologically and electrophoretically distinct types; extracellular	Dissolves fibrin clots thereby contributing to dissemination

phonuclear leukocytes, fluid leakage, and pus formation. During the confrontation, **M protein** is the major factor in preventing phagocytosis by polymorphonuclear leukocytes although the **capsule** appears to contribute. **C5a peptidase** may play a role in reducing the number of incoming polymorphonuclear leukocytes and thus enhance the effectiveness of those molecules with antiphagocytic activity.

Many polymorphonuclear leukocytes are destroyed by the leukotoxic activity of cell-bound **Streptolysin S** and the elaboration of **Streptolysin O** by multiplying extracellular organisms. Surviving polymorphonuclear leukocytes are able to phagocytize and destroy significant numbers of organisms although many phagocytized group A streptococci escape by way of their leukotoxic mechanism. **Septic sore throat** is the end result of this pathogenesis process and manifests as an acute, erythematous, pharyngitis and/or tonsillitis accompanied by a grayish-yellow, purulent exudate, cervical lymphadenitis, and fever. If, in addition, the organism produces a **pyrogenic exotoxin,** the end result is **scarlet fever,** in which there occurs a diffuse reddening of the skin with the rash most prominent on the trunk, neck, and extremities.

Primary Diseases of the Skin and Subcutaneous Tissues Involving Wounds, Burns, and Abrasions. These diseases are characterized by abscesses due to the same mechanism described for septic sore throat with the additional possibility that **IgG Fc receptors** may also play a role in inhibiting phagocytosis. These processes may also lead to scarlet fever due to pyrogenic exotoxin release by the organism.

Impetigo. This disease is usually seen in newborns and children. It may be caused by group A streptococci or *S. aureus,* alone or in combination. The disease initiates on the face and may involve the eyes, nose, lips, and limbs. Although the pathogenesis is similar to that described for both staphylococcal furuncles and other group A streptococcal primary diseases of the skin, the lesions are more severe and extensive as described in Chapter 7. Those strains of group A streptococci causing impetigo are frequently nephritogenic and thus may cause acute hemorrhagic glomerulonephritis.

Erysipelas. This disease can affect all age groups. The basic pathogenesis relating to survival and multiplication is thought to be similar to that described for septic sore throat and group A streptococcal impetigo. The end result is disease of the skin and subcutaneous tissues usually occurring on the face or lower extremities and characterized by a fiery red, advancing erythema.

Cellulitis, Lymphangitis, and Lymphadenitis. These clinical entities may occur in all age groups. The basic pathogenesis relating to survival and multiplication is thought to be as described for septic sore throat and group A streptococcal primary diseases of the skin. The organisms travel along lymphatic channels from cell to cell resulting in a purulent inflammation of the skin and subcutaneous tissues.

PRIMARY DISEASE OF THE FEMALE GENITAL TRACT. **Puerperal sepsis**, a disease of the uterine endometrium, is initiated in a susceptible host during or after delivery of the newborn by droplet nuclei from a case or carrier, by contaminated instruments, or by endogenous activation in pharyngeal or vaginal carriers under conditions of host-parasite imbalance. The basic pathogenesis relating to survival and multiplication is thought to be as described for septic sore throat resulting in a serosanguinous vaginal discharge.

DISSEMINATION BY DIRECT EXTENSION OR BY HEMATOGENOUS SPREAD. Dissemination most often occurs from a primary disease focus. The case fatality rate is always high when dissemination occurs. **Streptolysin O** (toxic for tissues adjacent to the site of infection), **DNases** (depolymerize viscous DNA in pus), **hyaluronidase** (breaks down connective tissue ground substance), and **streptokinases** (dissolve fibrin clots) each may contribute to the spread of the organisms from local sites by direct or downward extension or hematogenously. The organisms may spread from the pharynx by direct extension to produce abscesses in the sinuses (**sinusitis**), middle ear (**otitis media**), mastoid (**mastoiditis**), and/or meninges (**meningitis**) and by downward extension to the lungs to produce **pneumonia**. The organisms may spread by the hematogenous route from any of the primary disease sites with resultant **septicemia, acute endocarditis, purulent joint involvement, and multiple organ abscesses.** In addition, in patients with puerperal sepsis, abdominal distension can occur by direct extension. **Severe systemic shocklike disease** associated with strains of group A streptococci producing **pyrogenic exotoxin A** has been reported recently and is characterized by a scarlet feverlike rash, respiratory distress, myositis, shock, and a relatively high case fatality rate.

LATE SEQUELAE. Late sequelae refer to the nonsuppurative diseases acute rheumatic fever and acute hemorrhagic glomerulonephritis, which occur at some period of time after the onset of acute group A streptococcal disease.

Acute rheumatic fever occurs most commonly among young children during the fall and winter, and can occur only when preceded by pharyngitis caused by any of the group A streptococcal serotypes. The disease can occur in 0.1–3% of untreated patients from 1 to 5 weeks after pharyngeal onset. Although the mechanism of pathogenesis is not entirely understood, a plausible hypothesis is based upon the presence of **cross-reactive epitopes among M proteins and target tissues,** including human cardiac tissue, and the binding of anti-M protein antibody to the tissue epitopes. The major clinical manifestations are carditis, polyarthritis, and subcutaneous nodules.

Acute hemorrhagic glomerulonephritis occurs most commonly in children and can result when preceded by pharyngitis or skin disease (particularly impetigo) caused by any of 12 serotypes referred to as nephritogenic strains. The disease can occur in less than 1 to 15% of untreated patients from 1 to 5 weeks after pharyngeal or skin disease onset. Evidence supports the concept that renal damage is the result of **immune complex deposition on the glomerular basement membrane** and complement activation that generates a massive inflammatory response, membrane structural damage, and intravascular coagulation. The major clinical manifestations are renal glomerular damage, hypertension, edema, proteinuria, and hematuria (Fig. 8.2).

Immunity to Reinfection

Immunity to septic sore throat reinfection is serotype specific. Immunity to scarlet fever reinfection is only to the specific pyrogenic exotoxin that caused the rash. In skin and puerperal sepsis disease, serotype-specific antibody is minimal and immunity to reinfection does not occur. **Recurrences of rheumatic fever are frequent,** inasmuch as any of the more than 80 serotypes can initiate the preceding pharyngitis. The finding that epithelial cell receptors specific for acute rheumatic fever strains are found with a greater frequency in patients than in controls supports the concept that host factors may also play an important role as determinants of recurrence. In contrast to acute rheumatic fever, recurrences of acute hemorrhagic glomerulonephritis are rare due to the limited number of nephritogenic strains.

Laboratory Diagnosis

SPECIMENS. The specimens obtained depend on the disease process and include nose and throat swabs, lesion material, pus, sputum, blood for culture and immunoserology, urine, and spinal fluid. In suppurative diseases, a Gram stain of pus shows individual, paired or chains of gram-positive cocci and numerous polymorphonuclear leukocytes.

PRIMARY ISOLATION AND IDENTIFICATION. These procedures require initial cultivation on blood agar or specialized selective agar. Overnight incubation anaerobically or under aerobic conditions in the presence of 10% carbon dioxide at 37°C is optimal for isolation of the organism. The organism may be identified as a β-hemolytic, gram-positive, catalase-negative coccus, which hydrolyzes L-pyrrolidonyl-2-naphthylamide (PYR +) and is inhibited by bacitracin. The enzyme-linked immunosorbent assay (ELISA), latex agglutination, or

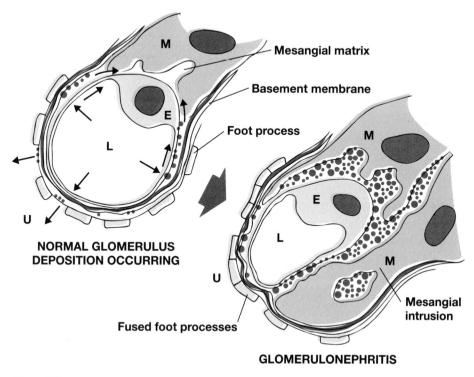

Figure 8.2.

Mechanism of autoimmune glomerulonephritis. M, mesangial cell; E, endothelial cell; L, lumen of glomerular capillary; U, urinary space. [Redrawn from Mims CA (1982): The Pathogenesis of Infectious Disease. 2nd ed. London: Academic Press.]

direct immunofluorescence assays have been used for the rapid detection of group A streptococci or antigen in throat swabs from cases or carriers during outbreaks of disease; however, these tests, while highly specific, are only 50–80% sensitive.

IMMUNOSEROLOGIC TESTS. Both the anti-Streptolysin O (ASO) and anti-DNase B (ADB) assays are useful in diagnosis.

ASO Test. This assay measures the presence of anti-Streptolysin O antibodies. A fourfold increase in titer on paired serum specimens obtained at 3 to 4-week intervals (measured in Todd units) indicates recent group A streptococcal disease. A single serum result of greater than or equal to 333 Todd units is highly suggestive. The test may also serve as a valuable aid in the diagnosis of late sequelae because the original group A infection may have subsided and cultures may be negative at this time. The sensitivity of the assay is greater for pharyngeal than for skin diseases.

ADB Test. This assay measures the presence of anti-DNase B antibodies. Interpretation is the same as that of the ASO assay. In contrast to the ASO test, the sensitivity is high for both pharyngeal and skin diseases.

Treatment

Adequate drainage, debridement, and antibiotic therapy are essential for the treatment of localized, suppurative skin lesions. Penicillin is the drug of choice for acute diseases. Penicillin has no effect upon established rheumatic heart disease and acute hemorrhagic glomerulonephritis. **Penicillin-resistant strains have not been reported.** Erythromycin is the drug of choice for penicillin-allergic patients. Rapid eradication of the organism is essential in order to prevent or reduce the occurrence of late sequelae. However, treatment of impetigo does not prevent acute hemorrhagic glomerulonephritis.

Prevention and Control

Penicillin is effective in the elimination of both cases and carriers during community outbreaks. Strict adherence to aseptic techniques in the hospital environment is essential. **Prophylactic penicillin therapy** is recommended **for the prevention of recurrent rheumatic fever.** Patients who have recovered from rheumatic fever are at risk for developing bacterial endocarditis and must be administered prophylactic antibiotics prior to and following dental, genitourinary, and GI manipulations. The efficacy of prophylactic penicillin therapy for the prevention of recurrent acute hemorrhagic glomerulonephritis is uncertain but should be attempted. Effective, practical, serotype-specific vaccines for human use have not as yet been developed due to problems related to cross-reactive M protein and target tissue epitopes and the stimulation of adequate levels of protective antibody against widely shared M protein epitopes.

GROUP B STREPTOCOCCAL DISEASE

Group B streptococci *(S. agalactiae)* are harbored in the female genital tract and male urethra of 15–25% of humans and animals, as well as in the pharynx and GI tract. The organism is transmitted from an infected mother to her infant in utero or at birth.

Group B streptococci are **encapsulated.** The capsules are polysaccharide in nature and the basis for classification into five antigenically distinct serotypes. They are also antiphagocytic and serotype-specific protective immunogens. There are no extracellular products known to be associated with the pathogenicity of the organism. These organisms (predominantly serotype III) far outnumber *Escherichia coli* K1 as **the leading cause of neonatal meningitis in the United States during the first 4 months of life.** The **antiphagocytic properties of the capsular polysaccharide** allow the organisms to survive, multiply, invade epithelial cells, and induce an acute inflammatory response. Early onset or acute stage disease occurs in utero or within 5 days of birth with resultant septicemia, meningitis, and a case fatality rate of 50%. Late onset disease occurs at age 10 days to 4 months with the same but less severe clinical manifestations and a case fatality rate of 20%. In adults, the organisms may produce pneumonia, septicemia, prosthetic joint disease, or puerperal sepsis originating from the female genital tract.

Immunity to reinfection is serotype specific. Specimens for laboratory diagnosis depend on the disease process and include blood for culture, sputum, a cervical swab, and spinal fluid. These specimens are cultured on blood agar and incubated aerobically at 37°C. Group B streptococci are β-hemolytic, gram-positive, catalase negative cocci that hydrolyze sodium hippurate. Latex agglutination or ELISA tests for the direct detection of antigen are commonly employed on serum, spinal fluid, and urine.

Early therapy with penicillin plus an aminoglycoside is essential for the prevention of progressive, fatal disease. Heavily colonized mothers can be treated with penicillin intrapartum to prevent subsequent colonization of their newborns.

DISEASE DUE TO THE VIRIDANS GROUP OF STREPTOCOCCI

The viridans group, often referred to as "oral streptococci," do not contain a "C" carbohydrate but have been grouped on the basis of rRNA cataloging and nucleic acid hybridization studies. The viridans group is comprised of 19 species on the basis of biochemical and physiological differentiation. Species within the viridans group are harbored in the nose and throat of more than 95% of humans and, with the exception of *S. mutans* and its role in the etiology of human dental caries, do not cause disease in the "normal" host.

Although adherence and colonization of *S. mutans* to tooth surfaces can be attributed to extracellular and intracellular polysaccharide synthesis from sucrose, mechanisms of attachment and adherence operative in disseminated disease caused by the viridans group are unclear. **Dental manipulation** in individuals with an **already damaged or abnormal heart valve** (usually congenital or rheumatic in origin) results in blood-borne dissemination of the organisms, adherence to the abnormal or damaged valve, and a superimposed **subacute bacterial endocarditis.**

Patients undergoing genitourinary tract manipulation can develop urinary tract disease by a similar mechanism. There is no immunity to reinfection. Specimens for laboratory diagnosis depend on the disease process and include blood for culture and urine. These specimens are cultured on blood agar and incubated aerobically at 37°C. The species of the viridans group are α or γ hemolytic, gram-positive, catalase-negative cocci that are not inhibited by optochin.

Although treatment with penicillin is effective, the occurrence of penicillin-resistant strains necessitates the use of penicillin plus an aminoglycoside. For patients with known valvular damage, prophylactic penicillin, amoxicillin, or penicillin plus aminoglycoside is essential prior to and following dental procedures. These patients must receive penicillin plus an aminoglycoside prior to and during urinary tract manipulation to cover the more resistant *Enterococcus* species.

ENTEROCOCCAL DISEASE

Enterococcus species are harbored in the GI tract of 25% of humans and animals, and do not cause disease in the ''normal'' host. Unlike streptococci, the enterococci are **highly resistant** to environmental conditions and physical and chemical agents. There are no known structural or extracellular virulence factors. Gastrointestinal or genitourinary tract manipulation can cause spread of the organisms to previously sterile sites with resultant biliary tract disease, septicemia, intraabdominal abscesses, urinary tract disease, or subacute bacterial endocarditis superimposed upon an already damaged heart valve.

There is no immunity to reinfection. Specimens for laboratory diagnosis depend on the disease process and include blood for culture and urine. These specimens are cultured on blood agar and incubated aerobically at 37°C. Enterococci are α-, β-, or γ-hemolytic, gram-positive, catalase negative cocci that grow in 6.5% salt broth, grow in bile, and hydrolyze esculin. Many biochemical properties of *Enterococcus* species are more similar to gram-negative bacilli than to other gram-positive cocci.

Enterococci are resistant to penicillin, penicillinase-resistant penicillins, and vancomycin, but penicillin plus an aminoglycoside, as well as ampicillin, are effective. Prophylactic penicillin plus an aminoglycoside should be administered to patients with valvular damage during and immediately following colonic or prostatic surgery.

STREPTOCOCCUS PNEUMONIAE DISEASE

Streptococcus pneumoniae (syn: the pneumococcus) is the most common cause of lobar and lobular (broncho) pneumonia. Approximately 500,000 cases occur each year in the United States in all age groups. This organism is the most common cause of meningitis among adults and a major cause of otitis media and sinusitis among children. The overall case fatality rate of pneumococcal disease has been reduced from 30 to 15% with the advent of antibiotics, but approaches 70% among treated patients 70 years of age and older.

Habitat

S. pneumoniae is an obligate parasite of humans and is harbored in the nasopharynx of 25–70% of the population.

Transmission

EXOGENOUS. Exogenous transmission is chiefly by droplet nuclei from a case or carrier to a susceptible host with impaired resistance due to, for example, respiratory damage by a virus, allergy, malnutrition, alcoholism, and general debilitation. Asplenic patients and patients with sickle cell anemia are particularly susceptible.

ENDOGENOUS. Endogenous activation may occur from the nasopharynx of a carrier with an impaired host resistance due to the factors described under exogenous transmission.

Properties of the Organism

Resistance to environmental, physical, and chemical agents. Pneumococci are very sensitive to environmental, physical and chemical agents. They are killed rapidly by antiseptic agents.

Microscopic morphology. S. pneumoniae is a gram-positive, nonmotile, lancet shaped coccus occurring in pairs (diplococcus). Pneumococci are **encapsulated.**

Macroscopic morphology. The organisms are facultative anaerobes that grow best aerobically on blood agar at 37°C and are α hemolytic. Colonies are often mucoid due to the capsule and tend to flatten out from the center due to an active autolytic enzyme.

Antigenic structure as it relates to classification and virulence. The **polysaccharide capsule** is the sole basis for classification and the only known virulence factor. Distinct epitopes enable the recognition of more than 85 **serotypes** of pneumococci, 23 of which are responsible for greater than 85% of pneumococcal disease in the United States. The capsule is the **single most important virulence factor** and is essential for disease to occur. It **inhibits phagocytosis** and thus allows the organisms to establish themselves in host tissue, multiply, and produce disease. The capsule stimulates serotype-specific, opsonic, protective antibody that promotes phagocytosis with resultant intracellular killing of the organisms by polymorphonuclear leukocytes.

Extracellular products associated with or thought to be associated with pathogenicity. Extracellular virulence factors are not known.

Pathogenesis and Clinical Manifestations

PRIMARY DISEASES

Nasopharyngitis. A mild-to-severe nasopharyngitis is initiated by droplet nuclei from a case or carrier or endogenously among individuals with an impaired resistance. The organisms begin to multiply in the nasopharynx with a resultant acute inflammatory response characterized by an influx of polymorphonuclear leukocytes. Phagocytosis by the polymorphonuclear leukocytes is inhibited by the **capsule** and the organisms continue to survive and multiply.

Lobar and Lobular Pneumonia. These clinical manifestations are often preceded for a few days by a nasopharyngitis. The organisms spread to the lungs, invade alveolar tissue, and multiply rapidly. The host responds with an influx of polymorphonuclear leukocytes and erythrocytes (due to capillary fragility), which accumulate in the infected alveoli. The **capsule** prevents phagocytosis by the polymorphonuclear leukocytes and allows the disease to proceed. The result is the complete consolidation (purulent exudate-filled alveoli) of one or more of the lobes (lobar) or lesions with a patchy distribution and bronchial localization (bronchopneumonia). The lobar type occurs most frequently in adults aged 30–50, while the lobular type occurs most frequently in infants, young children, and adults over 50. The clinical manifestations begin with a sudden onset after a 7 to 10-day incubation period, with chills, fever, and sharp pain during the acute inflammatory process. The disease runs an uncomplicated course for 7–10 days, during which time the organisms are transferred through the circulation to other tissues (bacteremia). During this 7 to 10-day period, **anticapsular antibody** appears and increases, resulting in what is termed "crisis," in which the patient dramatically recovers due to an adequate phagocytic defense mechanism, or dies due to overwhelming disease, an inadequate immune defense, and the absence of effective therapy.

DISSEMINATION BY DIRECT EXTENSION OR BY HEMATOGENOUS SPREAD. The organisms may spread from the nasopharynx by direct extension resulting in **otitis media** and **sinusitis**, from the nasopharynx or lungs hematogenously resulting in **septicemia, endocarditis, pericarditis, and multiple organ abscesses,** or from the nasopharynx or lungs by direct extension or hematogenously to produce **meningitis**. The basic pathogenesis process is similar to that described for nasopharyngitis and the pneumonias.

Immunity to Reinfection

Immunity to reinfection is serotype specific and permanent.

Laboratory Diagnosis

SPECIMENS AND DIRECT EXAMINATION. Specimens obtained depend on the disease process and include a nasopharyngeal swab, sputum (which may be "rusty"), blood for culture, spinal fluid, and pus. Gram stain of pus, sputum, and spinal fluid often shows gram-positive, lancet shaped, diplococci and numerous polymorphonuclear leukocytes.

PRIMARY ISOLATION AND IDENTIFICATION. These procedures require initial cultivation on blood agar or in blood culture broth. Overnight incubation under aerobic conditions at 37°C is optimal for isolation of the organism. The organism may be identified as an α hemolytic, gram-positive, catalase negative, coccus that is bile soluble and inhibited by optochin. Rapid identification of pneumococcus serotypes in spinal fluid can be accomplished by latex agglutination utilizing serotype-specific anticapsular antibody for the detection of capsular polysaccharide.

Treatment

Although penicillin is still the drug of choice, multiple-resistant strains are now appearing. Erythromycin is recommended for penicillin allergic patients, and penicillin plus vancomycin for multiple-resistant strains.

Prevention and Control

A **23-valent capsular polysaccharide vaccine** is effective in preventing more than 85% of bacteremic pneumococcal pneumonia in all age groups except children under the age of 2 years. The vaccine is recommended for patients with sickle cell anemia, asplenic patients, Armed Forces personnel, and others at special risk.

LISTERIA

LISTERIOSIS

Listeriosis, the etiologic agent of which is *Listeria monocytogenes,* is primarily a disease of animals, but can cause serious disease of the human fetus, newborn, pregnant women, immunologically normal individuals, and immunocompromised patients. In 1985, an outbreak attributable to Mexican-style cheese made from unpasteurized milk occurred in Los Angeles and Orange Counties resulting in 85 cases and 28 deaths, the latter occurring among the at-risk individuals and patients described above. The case fatality rate is 70–90% in untreated patients and 30–50% even when treated.

Although *L. monocytogenes* may be distinguished from group A streptococci by several laboratory tests, its β-hemolytic characteristic on blood agar, short rod or coccobacillary appearance, and tendency to grow in short chains, often results in an erroneous identification. For this reason, listeriosis is included in this chapter.

Habitat

L. monocytogenes is found in the GI tract, female genital tract, and throat of humans and animals. In the environment, the organism is found in water, soil, sewage, and improperly pasteurized milk.

Transmission

EXOGENOUS. Exogenous transmission can occur from the infected female genital tract in utero or at the time of delivery producing disease of the fetus or newborn, respectively. The disease is thought to be acquired by immunologically normal or compromised adult hosts by drinking contaminated water, drinking or eating raw or improperly pasteurized milk or milk products, contact with animals, or through a carrier by the oral-fecal route.

ENDOGENOUS. Activation may occur from the GI tract, female genital tract, or throat of a carrier who is immunocompromised.

Properties of the Organism

Resistance to environmental, physical, and chemical agents. L. monocytogenes multiplies and survives for years in the environment, but is killed effectively by antiseptic agents and pasteurization.

Microscopic morphology. The organism is a gram-positive, nonencapsulated short rod or coccobacillus with a characteristic ''tumbling'' motility at 22°C, and a tendency to grow in short chains. The organism is a **facultative intracellular parasite**.

Macroscopic morphology. L. monocytogenes grows best aerobically or under microaerophilic conditions (3–5% oxygen) on blood agar at 37°C. The organism produces a narrow zone of β hemolysis.

Antigenic structure. Antigenic structural components related to virulence, identification, classification, and diagnosis have not been demonstrated.

Extracellular product associated with pathogenicity. **Hemolysin** is SH dependent and both oxygen and heat labile. It functions by **lysing membrane-bound vacuoles of epithelial cells, monocytes, and macrophages.**

Pathogenesis and Clinical Manifestations

DISEASES OF THE FETUS AND NEWBORN. Organisms gain access to the fetal or newborn circulation through the mother resulting in disease. They are taken up by monocytes and macrophages, where they multiply and produce a septicemia accompanied by maculopapular lesions on the legs and trunk. **Hemolysin** release during multiplication causes lysis of monocyte and macrophage membrane-bound vacuoles. After lysis, *L. monocytogenes* enters the host cell cytoplasm and spreads from cell to cell by direct penetration and utilization of host cell actin. As a consequence, the organisms are never required to leave the intracellular environment. Organisms may be carried to the meninges to produce a **meningitis** and/or to the liver and spleen where they multiply within phagocytic and parenchymal cells and produce **multiple abscesses and granulomas** (granulomatosis infantiseptica).

DISEASES OF ADULTS. Adult disease occurs mostly in immunocompromised hosts and pregnant females, the latter often resulting in **abortion**. The disease is thought to be initiated following ingestion of contaminated milk, milk products, or water, contact with domestic animals, or by endogenous activation in an immunocompromised host. *L. monocytogenes* colonizes and multiplies in the pharynx and/or GI tract, resulting in an initial influx of polymorphonuclear leukocytes, followed by mononuclear cells and macrophages. The organisms are taken up by phagocytic and host epithelial cells, where they continue to multiply and release **hemolysin** for their survival by mechanisms described above. The end result is a **nasopharyngitis, gastroenteritis, or both**. The organisms spread to the regional lymph nodes, and enter the circulation where they multiply and survive within monocytes and macrophages after phagocytosis to produce a **septicemia**. Dissemination from the circulation produces **meningitis** (the most commonly recognized form of listeriosis), **endocarditis, pneumonia, multiple organ abscesses, and/or granulomas**. *L. monocytogenes* is the **leading cause of bacterial meningitis among adult cancer and renal transplant patients.**

Immunity to Reinfection

Patients who recover are immune to reinfection. Recovery depends on the development of an effective **cell-mediated immune (CMI)** response, whereby the organisms within mononuclear phagocytes and host epithelial cells are eliminated by macrophages activated by lymphokines (macrophage-activating factor, MAF) released by antigen-activated T cells.

Laboratory Diagnosis

SPECIMENS. Specimens obtained depend on the disease process and include blood for culture, spinal fluid, and diseased tissue. For epidemiological studies, greater success in isolation of organisms can be achieved if the specimens are stored at 4°C for 3–6 weeks prior to inoculation of the medium.

PRIMARY ISOLATION AND IDENTIFICATION. These procedures require initial cultivation on blood agar. Overnight incubation under aerobic or microaerophilic conditions at 37°C is optimal for isolation of the organism. The organism may be identified as a gram-positive, catalase positive, short rod or coccobacillus with a characteristic narrow zone of β hemolysis, "tumbling" motility at 22°C, and virulence for the rabbit conjunctiva. Tumbling motility at 22°C and rabbit virulence allow the differentiation of *L. monocytogenes* from streptococci and diphtheroids. In addition, streptococci do not produce catalase.

Treatment

Although treatment is often ineffective, early therapy offers the best chance for success. Ampicillin, penicillin plus an aminoglycoside, and erythromycin are the drugs of choice.

Prevention and Control

The prompt treatment of mothers experiencing any clinical manifestations referrable to the disease is essential. Pregnant females and immunocompromised hosts must be kept away from patients with known listeriosis and from animals. The use of pasteurized milk or milk products reduces considerably the risk of acquiring listeriosis.

SUMMARY

1. Streptococci and enterococci are gram-positive, nonmotile, facultative anaerobic cocci. Of the streptococci, groups A and B, the viridans group, and *Streptococcus pneumoniae* are the most important with respect to their pathogenic potential for humans.

2. The basic pathogenesis process of all primary diseases of the mucous membrane surfaces, skin, and subcutaneous tissues due to group A streptococci is similar. Organisms attach to host tissue through lipoteichoic ligands in concert with M protein and colonize. M protein is the major factor in preventing phagocytosis by polymorphonuclear leukocytes. Many polymorphonuclear leukocytes are destroyed by the leukotoxic activity of cell-bound streptolysin S and the elaboration of streptolysin O by multiplying extracel-

lular organisms. Surviving polymorphonuclear leukocytes are able to phagocytize and destroy significant numbers of organisms although many that are phagocytized escape by way of their leukotoxic mechanism. If, during the pathogenesis of septic sore throat, the organism produces a pyrogenic exotoxin, the end result is scarlet fever.

3. DNases, hyaluronidase, and streptokinases facilitate dissemination of Group A streptococci by the depolymerization of viscous DNA in pus, and enzymatic breakdown of connective tissue ground substance and fibrin clots, respectively.

4. Acute rheumatic fever and acute hemorrhagic glomerulonephritis are nonsuppurative late sequelae of group A streptococcal disease. Acute rheumatic fever can only occur when preceded by pharyngitis caused by any of the serotypes. In contrast, acute hemorrhagic glomerulonephritis can occur when preceded by pharyngitis or skin disease caused by any of 12 serotypes.

5. Group B streptococci (*Streptococcus agalactiae*) are the leading cause of neonatal meningitis in the United States during the first 4 months of life. The antiphagocytic properties of their capsular polysaccharide allows them to survive, multiply, and induce an acute inflammatory response with resultant septicemia and meningitis.

6. Species of the viridans group are harbored in the nose and throat as commensals. However, dental manipulation in individuals with an already damaged or abnormal heart valve may result in dissemination, adherence to the valve, and a superimposed subacute bacterial endocarditis. Patients undergoing genitourinary tract manipulation can develop urinary tract disease by a similar mechanism of dissemination and adherence.

7. *Enterococcus* species are harbored in the GI tract as commensals. However, GI or genitourinary tract manipulation can cause spread of the organism to previously sterile sites with resultant biliary tract disease, septicemia, intraabdominal abscesses, urinary tract disease, or subacute bacterial endocarditis superimposed upon an already damaged heart valve.

8. *Streptococcus pneumoniae* (the pneumococcus) is an encapsulated, lancet-shaped coccus occurring in pairs. The organism is the most common cause of lobar and lobular pneumonia and meningitis among adults, and a major cause of otitis media and sinusitis among children.

9. The single most important pneumococcal virulence factor is the polysaccharide capsule, which is essential for disease to occur.

10. The basic pathogenesis of primary pneumococcal disease begins with multiplication in the nasopharynx. The capsule inhibits phagocytosis of the organism, survival and multiplication continue, and a mild to severe nasopharyngitis results. The organisms spread to the lungs, invade alveolar tissue, and multiply rapidly. The antiphagocytic effect of the capsule allows the organisms to survive and the disease to continue. The result is the complete consolidation (purulent exudate-filled alveoli) of one or more lobes (lobar) or lesions with a patchy distribution and bronchial localization (lobular). Bacteremia occurs and anticapsular antibody increases resulting in dramatic recovery due to an adequate defense mechanism, or death due to overwhelming disease, an inadequate immune defense, and the absence of effective therapy.

11. A 23-valent pneumococcal capsular polysaccharide vaccine is effective in all age groups except children under the age of 2 years. It is especially recommended for patients with sickle cell anemia, asplenic patients, Armed Forces personnel, and others at special risk.

12. *Listeria monocytogenes*, the etiologic agent of listeriosis, is a gram-positive, nonencapsulated, short rod or coccobacillus with a characteristic "tumbling" motility at 22°C and a tendency to grow in short chains. The organism is a facultative intracellular parasite.

13. The pathogenesis of fetal and newborn listeriosis is initiated by organisms that gain access to the fetal or newborn circulation through the mother and are taken up by epithelial cells, monocytes, and macrophages, where they multiply and produce a septicemia accompanied by maculopapular lesions on the legs and trunk. Hemolysin release causes macrophage and monocyte membrane-bound vacuole disruption and allows the listeriae to survive and spread from cell to cell. Organisms may be carried to the meninges to produce a meningitis, or to the liver and spleen, where they multiply within phagocytic and parenchymal cells and produce multiple abscesses and granulomas.

14. Adult listeriosis occurs mostly in immunocompromised hosts and pregnant females, the latter often resulting in abortion. Following introduction of the organisms into the host or endogenous activation, colonization and multiplication occur in the pharynx and/or GI tract. The organisms are taken up by mononuclear phagocytes and host ephithelial cells, where they continue to multiply and release hemolysin for their survival. The result is a nasopharyngitis and/or gastroenteritis. The organisms enter the circulation through the regional lymph nodes and multiply within monocytes and mac-

rophages after phagocytosis to produce a septicemia. **Dissemination from the circulation results in meningitis, the most commonly recognized form of listeriosis and the leading cause of bacterial meningitis among adult cancer and renal transplant patients.**

15. Recovery from listeriosis depends on the development of an effective cellular immune response.

REFERENCES

Amman AJ, Addiego J, Wara DW, Lubin B, Smith WB, Mentzer WC (1977): Polyvalent pneumococcal-polysaccharide immunization of patients with sickle-cell anemia and patients with splenectomy. N Eng J Med 297:897.

Anthony BF (1992): Group B streptococcal infections. In Feigin RD, Cherry JD (eds): Textbook of Pediatric Infectious Diseases. Chap 128. 3rd ed, Vol. 2, Philadelphia: W. B. Saunders. pp 1305–1316.

Bisno AL (1990): Nonsuppurative poststreptococcal sequelae: rheumatic fever and glomerulonephritis. In Mandell GL, Douglas RG Jr, Bennett JE (eds): Principles and Practices of Infectious Diseases. Chap 177. 3rd ed. New York: Churchill Livingstone. pp 1528–1539.

Brennan RO, Durack DT (1984): The viridans streptococci in perspective. In Remington JS, Schwartz MN (eds): Current Clinical Topics in Infectious Diseases. Vol. 5, New York: McGraw-Hill Book Co.

Cossart P, Vincente MF, Mengaud J, Baquero F, Perez-Diaz JC, Berche P (1989): Listeriolysin O is essential for virulence of *Listeria monocytogenes:* direct evidence obtained by gene complementation. Infect Immun 57:3629.

Fischetti VA (June, 1991): Streptococcal M protein. Sci Am 58.

Johnston RB Jr (1991): Pathogenesis of pneumococcal pneumonia. Rev Infect Dis 13(Suppl. 6):S509.

Kaplan EL (1992): Group A streptococcal infections. In Feigin RD, Cherry JD (eds): Textbook of Pediatric Infectious Diseases. Chap 127. 3rd ed, Vol. 2. Philadelphia: W. B. Saunders. pp 1296–1305.

Murray BE (1990): The life and times of the enterococcus. Clin Microbiol Rev 3:46.

Portnoy DA, Chakraborty T, Goebel W, Cossart P (1992): Minireview: Molecular determinants of *Listeria monocytogenes* pathogenesis. Infect Immun 60:1263.

Portnoy DA, Jacks PS, Hinricks DJ (1988): Role of hemolysin for the intracellular growth of *Listeria monocytogenes.* J Exp Med 167:1459.

Schuchat A, Swaminathan B, Broome CV (1991): Epidemiology of human listeriosis. Clin Microbiol Rev 4:169.

Stevens DL (1992): Invasive group A streptococcus infections. Clin Infect Dis 14:2.

Stevens DL, Tanner MH, Winship J, Swarts R, Ries KM, Schlievert PM, Kaplan E (1989): Severe group A streptococcal infections associated with a toxic shocklike syndrome and scarlet fever toxin A. N Eng J Med 321:1.

Tilney LG, Portnoy DA (1989): Actin filaments and the growth, movement, and spread of the intracellular bacterial parasite *Listeria monocytogenes.* J Cell Biol 109:1597.

Ward J (1981): Antibiotic-resistant *Streptococcus pneumoniae:* clinical and epidemiologic aspects. Rev Infect Dis 3:254.

REVIEW QUESTIONS

For questions 1 to 15, choose the ONE BEST answer or completion.

1. Streptococci other than the viridans group and pneumococci are grouped on the basis of
   a) capsular antigenic diversity
   b) differences in biochemical reactions
   c) cell wall polysaccharide ("C" carbohydrate) antigenic diversity
   d) the type of hemolysis exhibited on blood agar
   e) surface protein antigenic diversity

2. M protein, considered to be the major virulence factor of Group A streptococci, is
   a) a surface-exposed dimeric molecule with antiphagocytic, adherence, and protective immunogenic properties
   b) a surface-exposed dimeric molecule cleaved by C5a peptidase
   c) a surface-exposed dimeric molecule that stimulates group-specific immunity
   d) a completely subsurface monomeric molecule containing no epitopes in common with human cardiac tissue
   e) a surface-exposed dimeric molecule that, in concert with LTA, binds to the Fc domain of mammalian immunoglobulin

3. A molecule which does *not* act as a virulence factor during the pathogenesis of group A streptococcal pharyngitis and scarlet fever is
   a) lipoteichoic acid
   b) "C" carbohydrate
   c) M protein
   d) Streptolysin S
   e) pyrogenic exotoxin

4. Group A streptococcal structural components and/or extracellular substances thought to act as virulence factors that contribute to their dissemination from primary disease sites include
   a) spores and flagella
   b) peptidoglycan and cytoplasmic granules
   c) Streptolysin O, DNases, and streptokinases
   d) lipopolysaccharide (LPS) and sex pili
   e) lipases and ribosomes

5. Acute rheumatic fever *differs* from acute hemorrhagic glomerulonephritis in that the former
   a) is a late sequela of group A streptococcal disease
   b) occurs most commonly among children
   c) is not amenable to penicillin therapy
   d) can occur only when preceded by pharyngitis caused by any of the group A streptococcal serotypes
   e) is a nonsuppurative disease

6. A β-hemolytic, gram-positive, catalase negative, coccus isolated from the throat of a patient with acute pharyngitis was identified as a group A streptococcus on the basis of
   a) colonial morphology on a blood agar plate
   b) its ability to grow under microaerophilic conditions
   c) its ability to form long or short chains
   d) its capsular structure
   e) its ability to hydrolyze PYR

7. The ADB assay for anti-DNase B antibodies
   a) is used specifically for the diagnosis of group A streptococcal late sequelae
   b) is a less sensitive assay than the ASO test, which measures the presence of anti-Streptolysin O antibodies
   c) is best conducted on a single serum specimen obtained from patients during the acute stage of their illness
   d) is a measure of recent group A streptococcal disease and may serve as an aid in the diagnosis of late sequelae
   e) is an accurate measurement of group B streptococcal carriers

8. An effective and practical serotype-specific vaccine against group A streptococcal disease has not as yet been developed because
   a) the protective immunogen has not been identified
   b) M protein and human cardiac tissue contain cross-reactive epitopes
   c) the immunogenic capsule cannot be purified
   d) the organisms undergo extensive antigenic variation
   e) M protein cannot be purified

9. Group B streptococci
   a) rarely cause neonatal meningitis
   b) stimulate immunity to group A streptococcal disease
   c) produces disease following transmission by droplet infection
   d) are strict anaerobes
   e) are able to survive and multiply in the host due to the antiphagocytic property of their polysaccharide capsule

10. The members of the viridans group of streptococci and *Enterococcus* species
    a) are not capable of producing disease
    b) are capable of producing disseminated disease under appropriate circumstances
    c) exhibit little or no resistance to penicillin
    d) stimulate a high degree of immunity to reinfection during the course of their initial disease process
    e) are exclusively α hemolytic

11. The single most important virulence factor of *Streptococcus pneumoniae* is
    a) its polysaccharide capsule
    b) its peptidoglycan layer
    c) its spores
    d) an extracellular substance
    e) its common pili

12. Pneumococcal vaccine
    a) is usually ineffective in preventing pneumococcal pneumonia
    b) is recommended for patients with sickle cell anemia, asplenic patients, and others at special risk
    c) is prepared from the serotype responsible for producing more than 85% of the

pneumococcal disease in the United States

d) is composed of heat-killed organisms

e) is effective in children under the age of 2 years

13. A major step in the pathogenesis of listeriosis is

a) the formation of antigen-antibody complexes with resultant complement activation and tissue damage

b) the release of hyaluronidase by *Listeria monocytogenes,* which contributes to its dissemination from local sites

c) the antiphagocytic activity of the *L. monocytogenes* capsule

d) the ability of polymorphonuclear leukocytes to phagocytize and destroy *L. monocytogenes* early in the course of the disease

e) the survival and multiplication of *L. monocytogenes* within mononuclear phagocytes and host epithelial cells

14. Among renal transplant and adult cancer patients, *L. monocytogenes* is the leading cause of

a) tonsillitis

b) otitis media

c) bacterial meninigitis

d) sinusitis

e) conjunctivitis

15. Recovery from and immunity to listeriosis depend on the development of

a) an effective IgG response by the host

b) an effective IgA response by the host

c) an effective IgM response by the host

d) an effective cell-mediated immune response by the host

e) an effective humoral and cell-mediated immune response by the host

ANSWERS TO REVIEW QUESTIONS

1. *c* "C" carbohydrates are composed of a branched polymer of L-rhamnose or glycerol teichoic acid linked to hexosamine, the latter being the determinant group responsible for group specificity.

2. *a* M protein is a pilus-like, surface-exposed molecule composed of two alpha helical monomeric chains twisted about each other to give a coiled coil appearance. In addition to its antiphagocytic and protective immunogenic properties, it acts in concert with LTA as a mediator of attachment and is the basis for group A streptococcal serotyping.

3. *b* There is no evidence to implicate "C" carbohydrates as virulence factors in the

pathogenesis of group A streptococcal disease. As indicated in Question 2, M protein is antiphagocytic and, in concert with LTA, acts as a mediator of attachment during the pathogenesis of these streptococcal syndromes. Streptolysin S exerts a leukotoxic effect upon PMNLs and pyrogenic exotoxins are responsible for the rash of scarlet fever and a systemic toxic shocklike syndrome.

4. *c* Streptolysin O, DNases, and streptokinase are extracellular substances that contribute to dissemination of group A streptococci from local sites. Streptolysin O, an oxygen-labile protein, is able to destroy adjacent cells and tissues, DNases are able to depolymerize viscous DNA in pus, and streptokinases act by catalyzing the conversion of plasminogen to plasmin leading to fibrin digestion and the prevention of an effective local barrier. Lipases, LPS, flagella and spores are not group A streptococcal products or structural components, and peptidoglycan, cytoplasmic granules, sex pili, and ribosomes do not appear to be associated with mechanisms of dissemination.

5. *d* While acute rheumatic fever can occur only when preceded by pharyngitis caused by any of the group A streptococcal serotypes, acute hemorrhagic glomerulonephritis can occur when preceded by pharyngitis or skin disease caused by any of 12 nephritogenic serotypes. The remaining statements apply to both syndromes.

6. *e* Because the organism is a β-hemolytic, gram-positive, catalase negative coccus, its ability to hydrolyze PYR or to be inhibited by bacitracin establishes it as a group A streptococcus (*S. pyogenes*). The remaining phenotypic characteristics cannot be used as a means for final identification.

7. *d* The ADB assay is more sensitive than the ASO test as a measure of recent group A streptococcal disease and as an aid in the diagnosis of late sequelae A positive result is best demonstrated by a four-fold rise in titer on paired serum specimens contained at 3 to 4-week intervals.

8. *b* Although M proteins have been purified and identified as protective immunogens, the fact that acute rheumatic heart disease is thought to be the result of the binding of anti-M protein antibody to M protein cross-reactive epitopes on cardiac tissue precludes their use as effective vaccinogens.

9. *e* The polysaccharide capsule of group B streptococci is antiphagocytic, thereby allowing the organisms to survive and multiply. It is also the basis for serotype classification of the organisms and a protective immunogen. Group B streptococci are the leading cause of neonatal meningitis during the first 4 months of life, are transmitted from an infected mother to her infant, and stimulate serotype-specific immunity. The organisms are facultative anaerobes.

10. ***b*** Both members of the viridans group and *Enterococcus* species are capable of producing a subacute bacterial endocarditis superimposed upon an already damaged heart valve following dental and GI or genitourinary tract manipulation, respectively. Enterococci are uniformly resistant to penicillin and penicillinase-resistant penicillins, and significant numbers of penicillin resistant viridans group strains are being reported. There is no immunity to reinfection. Members of the viridans group are α or γ hemolytic while *Enterococcus* species may exhibit α, β, or γ hemolysis.

11. ***a*** The major and only known pneumococcal virulence factor is the polysaccharide capsule.

12. ***b*** Pneumovax is a 23-valent pneumococcal capsular polysaccharide vaccine recommended for patients with sickle cell anemia, asplenic patients, and others at special risk. It protects individuals 2 years and older against pneumococcal pneumonia.

13. ***e*** The key step in the early pathogenesis of listeriosis is the survival and multiplication of phagocytized *Listeria monocytogenes* within mononuclear phagocytes and host epithelial cells. Polymorphonuclear leukocytes phagocytize the organisms early in the course of the adult disease but do not destroy them. Antigen-antibody complexes play no role in pathogenesis. The organism is not encapsulated and does not produce hyaluronidase.

14. ***c*** *L. monocytogenes* is the leading cause of bacterial meningitis among renal transplant and adult cancer patients. Tonsillitis, otitis media, sinusitis, and conjunctivitis due to listeriae have not been reported.

15. ***d*** Recovery from and immunity to listeriosis is dependent on an effective CMI response by the host. Humoral mechanisms, alone or in concert with CMI, are not known to be involved.

DIPHTHERIA, ANTHRAX, AND *BACILLUS CEREUS* DISEASE

DIPHTHERIA

Diphtheria, the etiologic agent of which is *Corynebacterium diphtheriae,* is a disease that occurs mostly in infants and children, but may be seen in adults who fail to maintain protective levels of circulating antitoxin through toxoid boosters. Like the clostridial diseases described in Chapter 10, the clinical manifestations are due exclusively to exotoxin produced by the organism. In contrast to the Unites States, in which the prevalence is relatively low due to effective vaccination, diphtheria occurs with a high frequency in many other areas of the world as a result of incomplete or no immunization. With the advent of effective antitoxin and antimicrobial therapy, the overall case fatality rate has been reduced from 30–50% to 5–10%. *C. diphtheriae* is considered the most important pathogen of this genus. "**Diphtheroids,**" which are corynebacteria that occupy the skin, nose, throat, nasopharynx, urinary tract, and conjunctiva of normal individuals can, in rare instances, infect immunosuppressed hospitalized individuals (e.g., patients with prosthetic heart valves), and produce septicemia with a high case fatality rate due in large part to their oftentimes multiple antibiotic resistance.

Habitat

C. diphtheriae is an obligate parasite of humans. Together with diphtheroids, they are harbored in the nose, throat, and nasopharynx and on the skin of cases and carriers.

Transmission

EXOGENOUS. Transmission appears to be exclusively by the exogenous route. Classic diphtheria is usually thought of as a disease that initiates in the upper respiratory tract of a susceptible host as a result of droplet nuclei from a case or carrier. However, cutaneous disease can occur as a result of organisms from a case or carrier colonizing the skin and entering through a minor or major wound. Occasionally, transmission may occur by drinking milk contaminated by a case or carrier. Factors that determine whether diphtheria or a carrier state will develop following exposure are unknown.

Properties of the Organism

Resistance to environmental, physical, and chemical agents. C. diphtheriae can survive for as long as 14 weeks in pseudomembranous lesions and is readily destroyed by most physical and chemical agents.

Microscopic morphology. The organism is a gram-positive, nonmotile, non-encapsulated, slender, straight, or curved rod. The irregular distribution of deeply staining metachromatic granules within the cytoplasm gives the organisms a "beaded," "barred," or "clubbed" appearance after the use of a simple stain, such as methylene blue. Furthermore, the sharp angles and parallelism that they create with each other cause the organisms to appear like "Chinese letters" and "palisades." These typical microscopic characteristics are responsible for their **pleomorphic** appearance.

Macroscopic morphology. C. diphtheriae is a facultative anaerobe that grows best aerobically on most media at 37°C. It is best characterized on a cysteine-tellurite agar plate, a selective medium in which potassium tellurite is reduced to tellurite within the organism during its growth, resulting in a gray-black colony. For epidemiological purposes, the organisms can be classified into three types on the basis of their colonial appearance or size, namely, gravis (rough colonies), mitis (smooth colonies), and intermedius (small colonies). The growth of organisms on a Loeffler's coagulated serum slant, a starvation medium toxic to many other bacteria, accentuates the formation of metachromatic granules.

Diphtheroids. These organisms occur in the same habitat and may have the same morphological and biochemical properties as *C. diphtheriae.* The major phenotypic difference is their **inability to produce exotoxin.**

Antigenic structure as it relates to virulence. A heat-labile protein is located at the surface of the cell wall and referred to as a **K antigen.** The **antiphagocytic property** of the K antigen allows the organisms to colonize prior to multiplication and exotoxin production.

Extracellular product associated with pathogenicity. The active **diphtheria exotoxin** molecule is a heat-labile protein consisting of two polypeptide fragments held together by a disulfide bond. The toxin acts by **inhibiting protein synthesis** at the ribosome level. Fragment B has no independent activity but is required for transport into the mammalian cell of enzymatically active fragment A, which catalyzes the adenosine diphosphate (ADP) ribosylation and resultant inactivation of the peptidyl-tRNA elongation factor-2 (EF-2). As a result, the ribosomes cannot form polypeptides, protein synthesis is halted, and the cell dies. The reaction may be represented as follows:

$$EF\text{-}2 + NAD \underset{}{\overset{fragment\ A}{\rightleftharpoons}} ADPR.EF\text{-}2 + Nicotinamide + H^+$$

Lysogeny with a beta-prophage carrying the *tox* gene is essential for toxin production (Fig. 9.1). In vitro, maximum production of toxin occurs in the presence of relatively low concentrations of iron, which allows maximum expression of the phage *tox* gene by preventing the activity of repressors.

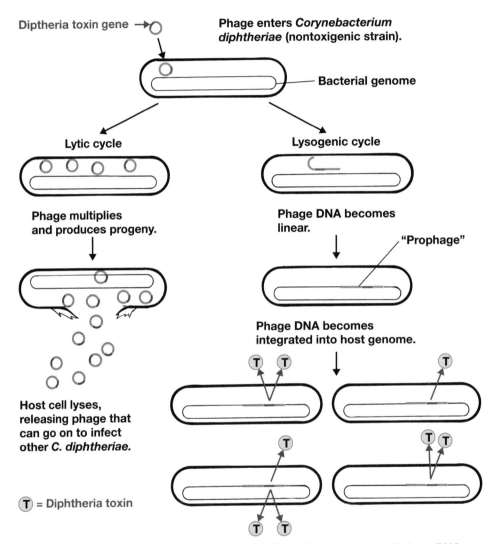

Figure 9.1.

Lysogeny of phage that causes *C. diptheriae* to produce toxin.

Pathogenesis and Clinical Manifestations

INITIATION IN THE UPPER RESPIRATORY TRACT

Tissue area of susceptible host
(nose, throat, nasopharynx)
↓
Colonization due to K antigen antiphagocytic activity
↓
Growth of *C. diphtheriae* on superficial layers
of mucous membrane surfaces and epithelial cells
↓
Exotoxin production

Toxin absorption
by adjacent cells   ↙   ↘

Tissue necrosis   Acute inflammatory response
(nidus of necrotic tissue,   (polymorphonuclear leukocytes,
extension laterally and   damaged red cells, fibrin
deeper into tissues)   deposition)

↓

Local toxic   Fibrinous exudate
manifestations   (grayish and inconspicuous; fibrin mesh for
polymorphonuclear leukocytes, red cells,
necrotic epithelial cells, and *C. diphtheriae*)
↓
Continued exotoxin production
↓
Extension of process
↓
Diphtheritic pseudomembrane
(extensive fibrinous exudate)
↓
Continued exotoxin production
↓
Exotoxin absorption by blood and lymphatics

↓

Systemic toxic   Toxemic degeneration
manifestations   (viscera—particularly myocardium
and peripheral motor neurons)

The incubation period is 1–7 days. The onset is abrupt with fever, chills, pharyngitis, cervical lymphadenitis, massive edema of the neck in severe cases, and the characteristic thick, closely adherent, dirty gray pharyngeal, tonsillar, or laryngeal **pseudomembrane.** Death is usually due to respiratory paralysis or myocarditis.

INITIATION IN THE SKIN (CUTANEOUS DIPHTHERIA). Colonization, growth and exotoxin production, absorption, and extension in the subcutaneous tissues occur as described above following entry through the skin resulting in the development of an ulcerative lesion with a dirty gray pseudomembrane. As with the upper respiratory type, toxin absorption by the blood and lymphatics can occur with resultant toxemic degeneration and death.

Immunity to Reinfection

Recovery from diphtheria does not necessarily confer immunity to reinfection. Patients who recover must be vaccinated with diphtheria toxoid.

Laboratory Diagnosis

SPECIMENS. Specimens obtained depend on the disease process and include a nose, throat, nasopharyngeal, and wound swab. The laboratory must be notified that diphtheria is suspected so that special media can be made available for inoculation. Diagnosis must be prompt, and thus presumptive, based upon history, clinical manifestations, and the use of a simple staining technique with an aniline dye, such as methylene blue, on exudate smears. Inasmuch as *C. diphtheriae* and some diphtheroids may appear the same microscopically when stained in this manner, the demonstration of exotoxin by culture isolates as described below must be performed.

PRIMARY ISOLATION AND IDENTIFICATION. These procedures require initial cultivation on cysteine-tellurite agar and Loeffler's coagulated serum. In addition, differential diagnosis necessitates primary cultivation on blood and chocolate agar. Identification of gray-black colonies on cysteine-tellurite agar, the typical Chinese letter, beaded, barred, and/or palisading arrangement of pleomorphic rods with accentuated metachromatic granules by methylene blue staining of colonies on cysteine-tellurite agar, and growth on Loeffler's coagulated serum, constitute presumptive evidence for *C. diphtheriae*. Definitive identification of the organism is based upon the demonstration of exotoxin production by a virulence test in guinea pigs or by a modified in vitro gel diffusion assay utilizing specific antitoxin (the Elek test).

Treatment

Specific antitoxin must be administered immediately. Inasmuch as the antitoxin is generated in horses, a skin test to ensure the absence of hypersensitivity to horse protein is essential prior to its use. Although antibiotics have no effect upon the toxemic disease process, penicillin or erythromycin is effective in killing *C. diphtheriae* and thus preventing further toxin production. In addition, these antibiotics eliminate or reduce both the carrier state and secondary invaders, such as group A streptococci.

Prevention and Control

THE CARRIER. The carrier continues to pose a serious threat to the initiation of diphtheria outbreaks. In addition to the existence of healthy carriers who acquire *C. diphtheriae* from a case or another carrier, 1% of patients continue to harbor the organism indefinitely after therapy.

THE SCHICK TEST. This procedure has been used during outbreaks of diphtheria to determine which case contacts are susceptible to the disease, and thus in need of immunization. A small amount of diphtheria toxin is injected intradermally into one forearm and a heated toxin control into the other. Susceptibility versus immunity is dependent on the amount of circulating diphtheria antitoxin. Redness and induration within 1–2 days at the test site only, or their appearance at both sites with persistence at the test site but disappearance from the control site in 4–7 days, signifies susceptibility due to lack of sufficient antitoxin. In contrast, no reaction at both the test and control sites, or redness and induration at both sites within 1 day, reaching a maximum in 2–3 days, and fading rapidly from both sites, signifies immunity due to the presence of sufficient neutralizing antitoxin.

ACTIVE IMMUNIZATION WITH FORMALIN-INACTIVATED TOXOID. Vaccination is highly effective. It is first administered early in infancy along with tetanus toxoid and killed *Bordetella pertussis* (DTP) and must be followed by periodic toxoid boosters throughout childhood and adulthood (see Chapter 10, under Tetanus Prevention and Control, for the recommended primary immunization and booster schedules).

REGULATIONS DURING DIPHTHERIA OUTBREAKS. Cases and contacts are quarantined until two nose and throat cultures are negative not less than 24 h apart. Cultures cannot be taken less than 7 days after the termination of penicillin therapy.

ANTHRAX

Bacillus anthracis, the etiologic agent of anthrax, is the major pathogen of the genus. The organism was the first to be established as the causative agent of an infectious disease by Koch in 1877. In 1881, Pasteur became the first to develop a successful vaccine against a bacterial disease when he protected sheep against anthrax utilizing live, attenuated *B. anthracis.* Anthrax is usually an occupational disease occurring, for example, among veterinarians, butchers, farmers, and mill workers. The disease is rare in the United States, but does occur frequently in other parts of the world. The case fatality rate among patients with cutaneous anthrax has been reduced from 50 to less than 25% with antibiotic therapy. In contrast, the case fatality rate among treated patients with the inhalation form (woolsorters' disease) remains at 80%.

Habitat

Spores of *B. anthracis* gain access to the soil from the carcasses of large animals, such as sheep, goats, horses, and cattle, that die of disseminated disease. The organism is harbored in the GI tract of those animals that do not develop or survive the disease.

Transmission

EXOGENOUS. Transmission appears to be exclusively by the exogenous route. Cutaneous anthrax is the result of infection with spores that gain access to humans through small abrasions or scratches in the skin while handling diseased animals or animal products, such as meats, hides, shaving brushes made from infected horse hair, piano keys made from infected ivory tusks, and drums constructed of infected goat skins. Inhalation anthrax or woolsorters' disease is the result of transmission by droplet nuclei from a patient with respiratory disease or by the inhalation of spores from infected animals or animal products.

Properties of the Organism

Resistance to environmental, physical, and chemical agents. Spores of *B. anthracis* survive in the soil for as long as 30 years and, like spores of the clostridia (Chapter 10), are highly resistant to physical and chemical agents.

Microscopic morphology. B. anthracis is a gram-positive, spore-forming, encapsulated, nonmotile rod with characteristic square cut ends. The organism occurs singly, in pairs, or in long chains with a ''string of pearls'' appearance and is **encapsulated.** Spores are oval and centrally located.

Macrocopic morphology. The organism is a facultative anaerobe that grows best aerobically on blood agar at 37°C and is nonhemolytic. Colonies appear rough with an irregular edge that gives a ''Medusa head'' appearance.

Antigenic structure as it relates to virulence. A **polypeptide capsule** made up exclusively of D-glutamic acid exhibits **antiphagocytic activity** but does not stimulate protective antibody.

Extracellular product associated with pathogenicity. The **exotoxin** is a heat-labile protein composed of three components referred to as protective antigen (PA), lethal or toxic factor (LF), which is responsible for most of the toxicity, and edema factor (EF). Although the mechanism of action is not well understood, maximal biological activity occurs only when all components are present together with the capsule.

Pathogenesis and Clinical Manifestations

CUTANEOUS ANTHRAX. Cutaneous anthrax is both a toxemic and invasive disease. Spores are introduced into the skin through abrasions or cuts and germinate. The vegetative cells multiply locally and the host responds with an acute inflammatory response characterized by an influx of polymorphonuclear leukocytes. Phagocytosis by the polymorphonuclear leukocytes is inhibited by the **capsule** and the organisms continue to survive and multiply. The organisms release **exotoxin** locally and begin to invade adjacent tissue rapidly producing extensive damage. Within 2–5 days, this process manifests as a **malignant pustule**— a necrotic, black lesion surrounded by a ring of vesicles containing dark, bluish-black, serosanguinous fluid and exotoxin. Rapid dissemination occurs by way of the lymphatics to the circulation resulting in **septicemia** and tissue invasion, including the lungs. Profound toxemia and necrosis may result in death despite therapy.

INHALATION ANTHRAX OR WOOLSORTERS' DISEASE. This syndrome is also both toxemic and invasive. The disease is acquired either by inhalation of vegetative cells in droplet nuclei from a patient with respiratory disease or by the inhalation of spores from infected animals or animal products. When spores are introduced, they germinate to vegetative cells in the trachea, bronchi, and/or lungs. Vegetative cells undergo multiplication in these organs with the host response, mechanism of survival, and **exotoxin** release as described for the cutaneous form of the disease. Within 24 h, **pulmonary necrosis, septicemia,** and **meningitis** occur, which is most often and rapidly fatal despite therapy.

Immunity to Reinfection

Immunity to reinfection is permanent upon recovery.

Laboratory Diagnosis

Rapid presumptive diagnosis based upon history and clinical manifestations is essential.

SPECIMENS AND DIRECT EXAMINATION. Specimens obtained depend on the disease process and include material from lesions, blood for culture, spinal fluid, and sputum. Gram stain of the specimen will reveal characteristic gram-positive rods with square cut ends and often in pairs or long chains; spores appear as an oval unstained ''space'' in the center of the organism. The presence of spores may be confirmed by the use of a special spore stain. A direct immunofluorescence assay on smears prepared from the specimen utilizing specific fluorescein-tagged anti-*B. anthracis* immunoglobulin is useful in the identification of the organism.

PRIMARY ISOLATION AND IDENTIFICATION. These procedures require initial cultivation on blood agar. Overnight incubation under aerobic conditions at 37°C is optimal for isolation of the organism, which is identified as a nonhemolytic, gram-positive, nonmotile, spore-forming rod with square cut ends and occurring singly, in pairs, or in long chains. A direct immunofluorescence assay on the isolated organism or a virulence test in animals is used for definitive identification.

Treatment

Penicillin and tetracycline are effective in the treatment of cutaneous anthrax only when given early in the course of the disease. The effectiveness of antimicrobial therapy among patients with inhalation anthrax is minimal.

Prevention and Control

Carcasses of dead animals must be disposed of by incineration or deep underground burial. Commercial products prepared from potentially infected animals must be decontaminated. Those at risk must wear masks and gloves and be clothed appropriately. A live, attenuated spore vaccine, used alone or in conjunction with a PA vaccine, has been found to be highly effective and relatively long lasting for large animals, such as cattle.

The **PA vaccine** alone is effective for humans and should be used by those in high risk occupations, such as mill workers. Such individuals should be made aware that the efficacy of protection drops from 100 to 52% in 3.5 months even when boosters are administered.

BACILLUS CEREUS DISEASE

Bacillus cereus exists as a saprophyte in water and soil. The organism differs from *B. anthracis* in that it is motile, nonencapsulated, and β hemolytic. The organism may cause a self-limiting type of food poisoning, usually resulting from the ingestion of contaminated rice or meat dishes containing enterotoxins. The incubation period and clinical manifestations resemble those seen in staphylococcal food poisoning. *B. cereus* may occasionally cause a disseminated, usually fatal, disease in immunocompromised individuals as a result, for example, of colonization of postoperative wounds or colonization during prosthetic device surgery.

SUMMARY

1. Diphtheria is a disease whose clinical manifestations are due exclusively to exotoxin produced by *Corynebacterium diphtheriae*.

2. *C. diphtheriae*, like other corynebacteria, are gram-positive, non-

spore-forming, nonmotile, nonencapsulated slender, straight, or curved rods. However, only *C. diphtheriae* produces exotoxin. The antiphagocytic property of a K (surface) antigen allows *C. diphtheriae* to colonize prior to multiplication and exotoxin production.

3. The extracellular product associated with the pathogenicity of *C. diphtheriae* is an exotoxin consisting of two polypeptide fragments held together by a disulfide bond. It inhibits protein synthesis and results in death of the cell.

4. The pathogenesis of diphtheria initiating in the upper respiratory tract begins with the colonization of the nose, throat, and/or nasopharynx due to the antiphagocytic action of the K antigen. *C. diphtheriae* multiplies and produces exotoxin, which is absorbed by adjacent cells causing tissue necrosis, and elicits an acute inflammatory response. Continued exotoxin production results in an extensive fibrinous exudate referred to as a diphtheritic pseudomembrane. Absorption of the toxin by the blood and lymphatics produces toxemic degeneration.

5. The pathogenesis of diphtheria initiating in a wound follows a similar pattern of colonization, growth and exotoxin production, absorption, and extension in the subcutaneous tissues as with the upper respiratory type.

6. Active immunization with diphtheria toxoid is highly effective and is administered to normal infants and children together with tetanus toxoid and killed *Bordetella pertussis* (DTP).

7. Anthrax is an occupational disease occurring, for example, among veterinarians, butchers, farmers, and mill workers.

8. *Bacillus anthracis*, the etiologic agent, is a gram-positive, spore-forming, encapsulated, nonmotile rod with square cut ends and occurs singly, in pairs, or in chains. The polypeptide capsule of *B. anthracis*, made up exclusively of D-glutamic acid, exhibits antiphagocytic activity.

9. The extracellular product associated with the pathogenicity of *B. anthracis* is an exotoxin composed of three components referred to as protective antigen (PA), lethal or toxic factor (LF), and edema factor (EF).

10. The pathogenesis of cutaneous anthrax is both toxemic and invasive. Spores introduced into the skin germinate and vegetative cells multiply locally. Phagocytosis is inhibited by the capsule and the organisms continue to survive, multiply, and release exotoxin that invades adjacent tissue rapidly

producing extensive damage. Rapid dissemination occurs by way of the lymphatics to the circulation resulting in septicemia and tissue invasion including the lungs.

11. The pathogenesis of inhalation anthrax is also both toxemic and invasive. Spores germinate to vegetative cells in the trachea, bronchi, and/or lungs and multiply. The mechanism of survival and exotoxin release are as described for the cutaneous form. Pulmonary necrosis, septicemia, and meningitis occur rapidly and are most often fatal despite therapy.

12. *Bacillus cereus* exists as a saprophyte in water and soil, but may cause a self-limiting type of food poisoning or a disseminated and usually fatal disease in immunocompromised individuals.

REFERENCES

Brachman PS (1980): Inhalation anthrax. Ann N Y Acad Sci 353:83.

Collier RJ (1975): Diphtheria toxin: Mode of action and structure. Bacteriol Rev 39:54.

Davey RT Jr, Tauber WB (1987): Posttraumatic endophthalmitis: The emerging role of *Bacillus cereus* infection. Rev Infect Dis 9, 110.

Feigin RD, Stechenberg BW, Strandgaard BH (1992): Diphtheria. In Feigin RD, Cherry JD (eds): Textbook of Pediatric Infectious Diseases. Chap 109. 3rd ed, Vol. 1. Philadelphia: W. B. Saunders. pp 1110–1116.

Freeman VJ (1951): Studies on virulence of bacteriophage-infected strains of *Corynebacterium diphtheriae*. J Bacteriol 61:675.

Ivins BE, Welkos SL (1986): Cloning and expression of the *Bacillus anthracis* protective antigen gene in *Bacillus subtilis*. Infect Immun 54:537.

Karzon DT, Edwards KM (1988): Diphtheria outbreaks in immunized populations. N Eng J Med 318:41.

Larsson P, Brinkhoff B, Larsson L (1987): *Corynebacterium diphtheriae* in the environment of carriers and patients. J Hosp Infect 10:282.

Lund BM (1990): Foodborne disease due to *Bacillus* and *Clostridium* species. Lancet, 336:982.

Rappuoli R, Perugini M, Falsen E (1988): Molecular epidemiology of the 1984–1986 outbreak of diphtheria in Sweden. N Eng J Med 318:12.

Turnbull PCB (1981): *Bacillus cereus* toxins. Pharmacol Ther 13:453.

Turnbull PCB (1990): Anthrax. In Smith GR, Easmon CR (eds): Bacterial Diseases. Topley and Wilson's Principles of Bacteriology, Virology, and Immunity, Vol. 3, Sevenoaks, England: Edward Arnold, p 364.

REVIEW QUESTIONS

For questions 1 to 12, choose the ONE BEST answer or completion.

1. Diphtheria is usually the result of
   a) endogenous activation in immunologically compromised patients
   b) exogenous transmission from a case or carrier by droplet nuclei or by entrance of *Corynebacterium diphtheriae* through a wound
   c) drinking pasteurized milk
   d) tissue invasion by *C. diphtheriae* spores
   e) infection with a diphtheroid

2. The definitive identification of *C. diphtheriae* isolated from a throat swab
   a) is based upon the demonstration of typical pleomorphic rods in methylene blue stained smears
   b) is based upon gray-black colony formation on cysteine-tellurite agar plates
   c) necessitates the demonstration of exotoxin by the organism
   d) must be done before therapy can be initiated
   e) is based upon the demonstration of typical pleomorphic rods in Gram-stained smears

3. Colonization of *C. diphtheriae* in a susceptible host is the result of

a) the antiphagocytic property of a surface K antigen
b) exotoxin production by the organism
c) adherence by pili
d) the antiphagocytic property of the organism's capsule
e) the antiphagocytic property of its flagella

4. One of the following statements relating to the exotoxin responsible for the clinical manifestations of diphtheria is NOT true.
   a) The toxin molecule consists of two polypeptide fragments held together by a disulfide bond.
   b) Fragments A and B are enzymatically active.
   c) Fragment A catalyzes the ADP ribosylation and resultant inactivation of EF-2.
   d) Lysogeny with a beta-prophage carrying the *tox* gene is essential for toxigenicity.
   e) The toxin acts by inhibiting protein synthesis at the ribosome level.

5. The pseudomembrane that results from *C. diphtheriae* toxin production and absorption by mucous membrane surfaces and epithelial cells
   a) occurs only in cutaneous diphtheria
   b) is characterized predominantly by the presence of macrophages
   c) is a systemic toxic manifestation
   d) occurs only in nasopharyngeal diphtheria

e) is essentially an extensive fibrinous exudate

6. Vaccination against diphtheria
   a) has had only limited success in the United States
   b) must be done in concert with vaccination against pertussis and tetanus to be effective
   c) should always be preceded by a Schick test to determine susceptibility
   d) is highly effective in preventing the disease
   e) utilizes heat-killed *C. diphtheriae* as the protective immunogen

7. Diphtheroids
   a) can infect immunosuppressed individuals and produce a fatal septicemia
   b) produce a powerful exotoxin responsible for the pathogenesis of disease by these organisms
   c) are usually susceptible to antibiotics
   d) never produce disease
   e) are always distinguishable from *C. diphtheriae* on the basis of their microscopic morphology following methylene blue staining.

8. Cutaneous anthrax *differs* from inhalation anthrax in that the *former*
   a) is both a toxemic and invasive disease
   b) is usually fatal even when treated
   c) manifests initially as a characteristic malignant pustule
   d) can disseminate rapidly resulting in septicemia and tissue invasion
   e) never involves the lungs

9. The two known virulence factors of *Bacillus anthracis* are
   a) extracellular substances produced by the organism
   b) produced only by spores
   c) structural components of the organism
   d) operative only in the respiratory form of anthrax
   e) the antiphagocytic polypeptide capsule and the three-component exotoxin

10. Gram-stain of a blood smear from a patient with anthrax septicemia will usually reveal
    a) gram-positive rods with square cut ends
    b) gram-positive cocci
    c) gram-positive rods with pointed ends
    d) numerous organisms resembling diphtheroids
    e) gram-negative, spore-forming cocci

11. Anthrax in humans can often be prevented by
    a) refrigerating meat from potentially infected animals
    b) immunization with a capsular vaccine
    c) immunization with killed *B. anthracis* vegetative cells
    d) immunization with the protective antigen (PA) component of *B. anthracis* exotoxin
    e) immunization with a flagellar vaccine

12. Disease due to *Bacillus cereus*
    a) never occurs, inasmuch as the organism exists only as a saprophyte in water and soil
    b) may manifest as a type of food poisoning with clinical manifestations resembling those of botulism

c) may manifest as a highly fatal, disseminated disease in immunocompromised patients

d) is preventable by immunization with *B. cereus* spores

e) is common in cattle and goats

ANSWERS TO REVIEW QUESTIONS

---

1. *b* Diphtheria is transmitted exclusively by the exogenous route from a case or carrier by droplet nuclei or entrance of *Corynebacterium diphtheriae* through a wound. The organism does not produce spores, is killed by pasteurization, and is not a diphtheroid.

2. *c* *C. diphtheriae* can only be identified definitively by the in vivo (guinea pig) or in vitro (Elek test) demonstration of exotoxin production. The demonstration of typical pleomorphic rods by methylene blue staining and gray-black colony formation on cysteine-tellurite agar represents only presumptive identification; Gram staining often fails to accentuate the characteristic metachromatic granules and is not used for presumptive identification. Therapy must be initiated promptly and is based upon history, clinical manifestations, and presumptive diagnosis.

3. *a* The antiphagocytic activity of the surface K antigen of *C. diphtheriae* allows the organism to colonize prior to multiplication and exotoxin production. The organism does not have pili, a capsule, or flagella.

4. *b* *C. diphtheriae* exotoxin consists of two polypeptide fragments held together by a disulfide bond. Fragment B has no enzymatic activity but is required for transport into the mammalian cell of enzymatically active fragment A, which catalyzes the ADP ribosylation and resultant inactivation of EF-2. As a result, protein synthesis is inhibited at the ribosome level. Lysogeny with a beta-prophage carrying the *tox* gene is essential for toxin production.

5. *e* The diphtheritic pseudomembrane is essentially an extensive fibrinous exudate resulting from *C. diphtheriae* toxin production and absorption by mucous membrane surfaces and epithelial cells. This thick, closely adherent, dirty gray pseudomembrane is a local toxic manifestation that occurs in both nasopharyngeal and cutaneous diphtheria. The pseudomembrane is characterized essentially by

the presence of necrotic cells, erythrocytes, *C. diphtheriae,* and polymorphonuclear leukocytes trapped in a fibrin mesh.

6. *d* Diphtheria toxoid is a highly effective immunizing agent that is combined with tetanus toxoid and killed *Bordetella pertussis* vaccine (DTP) or with tetanus toxoid (Td) alone as a matter of ease and convenience. As a result of vaccination, the prevalence of diphtheria in the United States is relatively low. Schick testing to determine susceptibility as a prelude to vaccination is used during diphtheria outbreaks.

7. *a* Diphtheroids can, in rare instances, infect immunosuppressed individuals and produce a septicemia with a high case fatality rate due in large part to their oftentimes multiple antibiotic resistance. The organisms do not produce exotoxin and are often morphologically indistinguishable from *C. diphtheriae.*

8. *c* The malignant pustule is characteristic of cutaneous anthrax. Both cutaneous and inhalation anthrax are toxemic and invasive, and can disseminate rapidly resulting in septicemia and tissue invasion. The lungs are a primary target in inhalation anthrax and may be involved in the cutaneous disease. The case fatality rate among patients with cutaneous anthrax has been reduced from 50 to less than 25% with antibiotic therapy.

9. *e* The two known virulence factors of *Ba-*

cillus anthracis are the antiphagocytic polypeptide capsule and the extracellular three component (PA, LF, and EF) exotoxin. These factors are operative in the pathogenesis of both cutaneous and inhalation anthrax.

10. *a* Gram stain of a blood smear from a patient with anthrax septicemia will usually reveal gram-positive rods with square cut ends typical of *B. anthracis.* Spores appear as an oval, unstained ''space'' in the center of the organism.

11. *d* The PA vaccine is of some value in preventing anthrax in humans and should be administered to those in high risk occupations, such as mill workers, despite the fact that the efficiency of protection drops from 100 to 52% in 3.5 months. Vaccines composed of killed *B. anthracis* vegetative cells have not been shown to be effective. The capsule does not stimulate protective antibody. The organism is nonmotile and by definition does not have flagella. Refrigeration of meat from infected animals will not kill *B. anthracis* spores; such products can be a source of transmission and should be decontaminated and discarded.

12. *c* Disease due to *Bacillus cereus* may manifest as a highly fatal, disseminated disease in immunocompromised patients. It may also manifest as a type of food poisoning resembling staphylococcal food poisoning in terms of incubation period and clinical manifestations. There is no vaccine for the disease and it has not been reported in animals.

CLOSTRIDIAL DISEASES

CLOSTRIDIUM

The genus *Clostridium* consists of gram-positive, spore-forming, anaerobic rods. Pathogens of the genus produce disease by virtue of their ability to elicit powerful **exotoxins** responsible for the clinical manifestations and, additionally, by their invasiveness in clostridial myonecrosis and anaerobic cellulitis. In addition to exotoxins, as yet undetermined structural virulence factors may be operative in immunocompromised patients who develop septicemia and organ abscesses due to the invasive clostridia.

Habitat

Clostridial spores are widely distributed in nature, particularly the soil. The organisms are also present in the GI tract of animals and humans.

Properties of the Organism

Resistance to environmental, physical, and chemical agents. Clostridial spores, like those of the members of the genus *Bacillus,* survive for years in the soil and are highly resistant to physical and chemical agents.

Microscopic morphology. The organisms are gram-positive, spore-forming, motile or nonmotile rods. A capsule, which is not associated with virulence, is produced by only one of the many species capable of causing disease, *Clostridium perfringens.* All pathogens in the genus, with the exception of *Clostridium tetani,* produce oval, subterminal spores. *C. tetani* produces round, terminal spores that give the organism a characteristic ''drumstick'' or ''tennis racket'' appearance (Fig. 10.1).

Macroscopic morphology. The organisms are **strict anaerobes** that multiply only in the absence of oxygen or in an environment of low oxidation-reduction

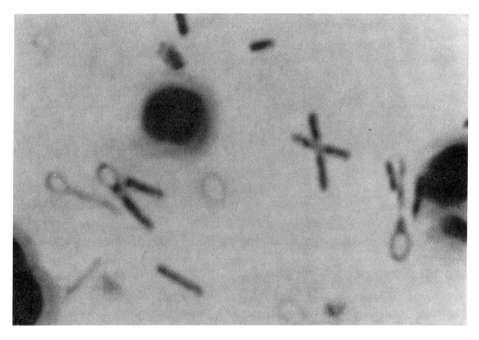

Figure 10.1.

Gram stain of a culture of *C. tetani.* Note that the spore does not stain. [Reproduced with permission from Bottone EJ, Girolami R, Stamm JM (eds)(1984): Schneirson's Atlas of Diagnostic Microbiology, 9th ed. Abbott Park, IL: Abbott Laboratories, p. 7]

potential. Clostridia grow best at 37°C on blood agar under anaerobic conditions or in liquid medium containing reducing agents under aerobic conditions. Several species are β hemolytic. On solid media, most pathogens produce colonies that appear as a compact center with irregular edges surrounded by a loose meshwork of filaments spread delicately over the surface like a "sprig of maidenhair fern"; some pathogens like *C. perfringens* produce colonies with entire edges. Those pathogenic species that ferment carbohydrates with the production of acid and gas are referred to as **saccharolytic**. This fermentative characteristic is an important virulence factor operative in the pathogenesis of clostridial myonecrosis.

Antigenic structure. Antigenic structural components related to virulence, identification, classification, and diagnosis, is unknown.

TETANUS

Tetanus, the etiologic agent of which is *C. tetani,* is a disease preventable by vaccination, yet 30–50 cases are reported each year in the United States and thousands more in other countries throughout the world as a result of incomplete or no vaccination. During World War II, when vaccination of Armed Forces personnel against tetanus was mandatory, there were over 3,000,000 military hospital admissions due to wounds, but only 12 cases of tetanus with 5 deaths. In the civilian population during this time, there were several thousand cases with 2574 deaths among those with incomplete or no vaccination. The seriousness of the disease and the importance of early diagnosis is signified by a case fatality rate of 60% in the untreated disease and 20–30% in the treated disease.

Transmission

EXOGENOUS. Transmission appears to be exclusively by the exogenous route. Spores are introduced from soil-contaminated objects or surgical instruments into major injuries, such as deep wounds and compound fractures. Spores may also be introduced as a result of minor injuries produced, for example, by contaminated rose thorns and slivers. Superficial minor wounds account for more cases than major injuries, inasmuch as they go unnoticed and thus untreated. Cases occur mostly among farmers and gardeners, drug addicts who use contaminated needles, surgical patients treated with contaminated dressings, and newborns infected through a contaminated umbilicus at birth.

Extracellular Product Associated With the Pathogenicity of the Organism

Tetanospasmin or neurotoxin, one of the most powerful exotoxins known, is a heat-labile protein produced by vegetative cells and released during autolysis. A plasmid gene is thought to be responsible for controlling production of the toxin. The toxin acts by **blocking presynaptic inhibition** that results in excitation of the central nervous system (CNS). An uncontrollable spread of impulses initiates in the CNS and produces hyperreflexia of the skeletal muscles (Fig. 10.2).

Pathogenesis and Clinical Manifestations

Spores are introduced into injured tissue
↓
A lowered oxidation-reduction potential in the damaged tissue results in germination of the spores to vegetative cells
↓
Vegetative cells multiply locally, tetanospasmin is produced within the bacterial cell and released during autolysis
(Organisms do not spread from the local site)
↓
Released tetanospasmin travels along the axis cylinders of the motor neurons of the spinal cord and medulla and becomes fixed to nerve cells

The incubation period averages 10 days but can vary from 2 to 50 days. The earliest sign is stiffness of the jaw due to spasmic contraction of the masseter muscles (trismus). Later signs include sustained contraction of the facial muscles (risus sardonicus) with extension of the spasmic contractions to the back (opisthotonus), neck, and respiratory muscles. As the disease progresses, **intermittent convulsive seizures** are brought on by the slightest stimulus. Death is due to respiratory complications, usually pneumonia or asphyxiation.

Immunity to Reinfection

Recovery from tetanus does not necessarily confer immunity to reinfection. Patients who recover must be vaccinated with tetanus toxoid.

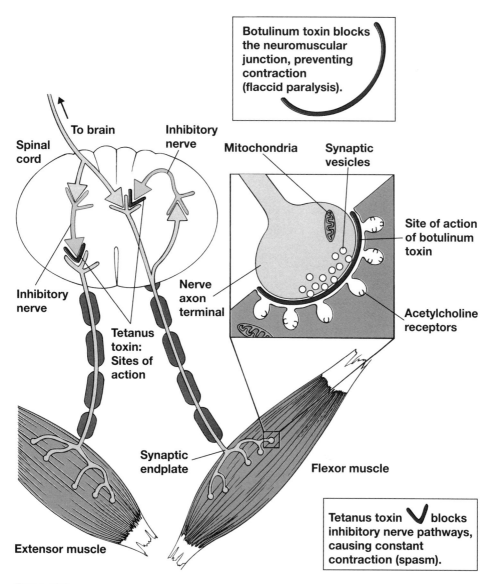

Figure 10.2.

The action of tetanus and botulism toxin on nerve cell receptor.

Laboratory Diagnosis

Diagnosis must be prompt and thus presumptive based upon history of injury and clinical manifestations. Therapy must be instituted immediately. Suspicion should be aroused if stiffness of the jaw is present.

PRIMARY ISOLATION AND IDENTIFICATION. If a wound is present, initial anaerobic cultivation is required on blood agar and in liquid media such as thioglycollate and cooked meat broth, in which the oxidation-reduction potential is low. Definitive identification of the organism is based upon the demonstration of a gram-positive rod with a round and terminal spore that gives the organism a ''drumstick'' appearance and by its production of tetanospasmin as determined by a mouse virulence assay. The wound must also be cultured aerobically for secondary pyogenic invaders such as staphylococci and streptococci.

Treatment

If a wound is present, debridement is essential. Human tetanus immune globulin must be administered as soon as possible after onset to prevent additional toxin from fixing to nerve cells. Although antibiotics have no effect upon the toxemic disease process, penicillin and/or broad spectrum antibiotics are effective in inhibiting the growth of C. tetani and secondary pyogenic invaders. Mechanical ventilation (hyperbaric O_2) to support breathing may be useful when used early in the course of the disease. Tracheostomy is required in patients with laryngeal obstruction.

Prevention and Control

ACTIVE IMMUNIZATION BEFORE INJURY. Active immunization is effective in the prevention of tetanus. **Tetanus toxoid,** which is formalin-inactivated toxin, is administered to normal infants and children together with diphtheria toxoid and killed *Bordetella pertussis* (diphtheria, tetanus, pertussis; **DTP vaccine**) at 2, 4, and 6 months with booster doses at 15 months and 4–6 years. Tetanus toxoid combined with a reduced dose of diphtheria toxoid (Td) should be administered as a booster every 10 years thereafter. The recommended schedule for individuals 7 years of age and older not immunized at the recommended time is an initial injection of Td followed by one primary injection of the Td vaccine at 2 months, and a booster 6–12 months later and every 10 years thereafter. For infants and children less than 7 years of age not immunized at the recommended time, the schedule is similar to that described above except that DTP should be employed until the individual reaches age 7, at which time Td should be used.

PROPHYLACTIC TREATMENT AFTER INJURY. If a wound is present, debridement, as well as penicillin and/or broad spectrum antibiotic therapy, is essential. The approach to prophylactic treatment after injury depends on the extent and nature of the wound and the history of tetanus immunization at the time of injury. Table 10.1 is the recommended summary guide to tetanus prophylaxis in routine wound management.

CLOSTRIDIUM PERFRINGENS DISEASE

Clostridial myonecrosis (gas gangrene), anaerobic cellulitis, septicemia, and organ abscesses are caused by several species of clostridia, but the most common etiologic agent is *C. perfringens,* which is also capable of producing food poisoning. Although there are five types of *C. perfringens* based upon exotoxin production, the great majority of human disease is caused by the alpha toxin producing type A. Prior to the days of antisepsis and asepsis, clostridial myonecrosis and anaerobic cellulitis were the inevitable outcome of surgery. During World War I, 1 out of every 35 wounded developed either of these syndromes with a case fatality

TABLE 10.1. Summary Guide to Tetanus Prophylaxis in Routine Wound Management[a]

History of tetanus immunization	Clean, minor wounds		All other wounds	
	Tetanus and diphtheria toxoids (for adult use)	Human tetanus immune globulin	Tetanus and diphtheria toxoids (for adult use)[b]	Human tetanus immune globulin
Uncertain	Yes	No	Yes	Yes
0–1	Yes	No	Yes	Yes
2	Yes	No	Yes	No[c]
3 or more	No[d]	No	No[e]	No

[a] Values are from Immunization Practices Advisory Committee, Centers for Disease Control (CDC).
[b] For children younger than 7 years of age, DTP vaccine adsorbed (or diphtheria and tetanus toxoids adsorbed for pediatric use if pertussis vaccine is contraindicated) is preferred to tetanus toxoid alone. For persons 7 years of age and older, tetanus and diphtheria toxoids for adult use is preferred to tetanus toxoid alone.
[c] Yes, if wound is more than 24 h old.
[d] Yes, if more than 10 years since last dose.
[e] Yes, if more than 5 years since last dose. (More frequent boosters are not necessary and can accentuate side effects.)

rate of 25%, mostly among those with clostridial myonecrosis. Although the number of cases has been reduced considerably with the advent of antibiotics and improved surgical techniques, the case fatality rate remains the same despite therapy. The seriousness of septicemia and organ abscesses due to the clostridia is evidenced by the 80% case fatality rate in both the untreated and treated disease. In contrast to the invasive clostridial disease syndromes, *C. perfringens* food poisoning is self-limiting.

Transmission

EXOGENOUS. Clostridial myonecrosis and anaerobic cellulitis are the result of transmission by means of massive injury with soil contaminated objects or by contaminated surgical instruments. Food poisoning is the result of transmission by the ingestion of improperly cooked food contaminated with *C. perfringens* vegetative cells and left at room temperature.

ENDOGENOUS. Septicemia and organ abscesses occur as a result of extraintestinal growth of organisms from the GI tract. These diseases occur in hosts immunocompromised by drugs and/or other diseases.

Extracellular Products Associated With the Pathogenicity of *C. perfringens*

Lecithinase C (alpha toxin) hydrolyzes lecithin-containing lipoprotein complexes in red cell and tissue membranes and mitochondria, causing **cell membrane disruption and lysis, tissue necrosis, and edema.**
Collagenase (kappa toxin) digests and liquefies the collagen in connective tissue.
Hyaluronidase (mu toxin) hydrolyzes the hyaluronic constituent of connective tissue ground substance.
DNase depolymerizes DNA, resulting in **tissue liquefaction.**
Enterotoxin is a heat labile protein responsible for diarrheal food poisoning by **inhibiting fluid absorption** from the gut.

Pathogenesis and Clinical Manifestations

CLOSTRIDIAL MYONECROSIS OR GAS GANGRENE. This syndrome is both an invasive and toxemic disease. Upon introduction of spores into a wound, germination to vegetative cells results due to the lowered oxidation-reduction potential created by the damaged tissue. Vegetative cells multiply and produce **lecithinase C (alpha toxin),** which diffuses into surrounding healthy tissue, particularly muscle, causing red cell lysis, interference with the blood supply, and necrosis (gangrene) (Fig. 10.3). The process of tissue destruction is enhanced by **collagenase, hyaluronidase, and DNase.** Continuous and rapid multiplication occurs as the organisms advance into the areas of tissue destruction and red cell lysis created by the release of the exotoxins (enzymes). During the invasive process, large amounts of **gas** form due to the **saccharolytic** action of the organisms on muscle carbohydrate. The exotoxins are absorbed into the circulation from damaged tissue and carried to a multiplicity of organs with resultant toxemic degeneration and death. The gangrenous process occurs 12–48 h after injury followed by toxemia and death 24–48 h later.

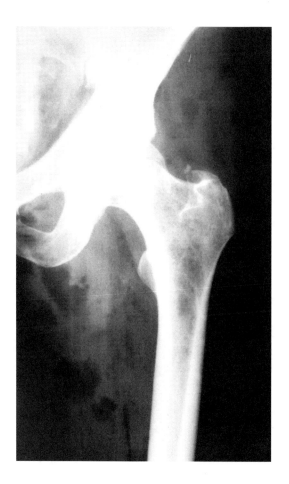

Figure 10.3.

Radiograph of the right hip of a patient with necrotizing fasciitis. The view shows gas in the soft tissues. (Courtesy of William A. Schwartzman, UCLA.)

ANAEROBIC CELLULITIS. The pathogenesis of anaerobic cellulitis is essentially the same as for clostridial myonecrosis except that the organisms spread along fascial planes between muscle and do not invade muscle. Gas is prominent and tissue necrosis extensive, yet there is **no systemic exotoxin absorption** and the prognosis is better than for myonecrosis.

SEPTICEMIA AND ORGAN ABSCESSES. These syndromes are produced by endogenous organisms that invade the circulation of immunocompromised hosts (e.g., cancer patients and those on steroids) and are carried to the tissues. The mechanisms of pathogenesis are unknown.

FOOD POISONING. Food poisoning is the result of ingesting improperly cooked meat, fish, or poultry containing greater than or equal to 10^8 *C. perfringens* vegetative cells. As the organisms sporulate, **enterotoxin** is produced in the GI tract. After an incubation period of 6–18 h, diarrhea occurs as a result of the inhibition of fluid absorption in the gut by the enterotoxin. **Fever and vomiting are absent** and the disease is self-limiting.

Immunity to Reinfection

Immunity to reinfection does not occur.

Laboratory Diagnosis

CLOSTRIDIAL MYONECROSIS AND ANAEROBIC CELLULITIS. As for tetanus, the diagnosis of clostridial myonecrosis and anaerobic cellulitis must be immediate and thus presumptive based upon history of injury and clinical manifestations. The potential necessity for amputation points to the importance of a rapid and accurate diagnosis. Wounds must be cultured anaerobically for clostridia to confirm the diagnosis and aerobically for the presence of secondary pyogenic invaders, such as staphylococci and streptococci, that may facilitate extended growth of the organisms by further damaging tissue. Direct Gram stain of the leading edge of a necrotic process or exudate will usually reveal the typical boxcar-shaped *C. perfringens;* leukocytes are often absent or sparse due to destruction by clostridial toxins.

SEPTICEMIA AND ORGAN ABSCESSES. Gram stain of a blood smear may reveal gram-positive rods consistent with the morphology of *C. perfringens.*

The organism is often isolated from the blood of asymptomatic patients. Positive blood cultures from symptomatic patients are essential for a definitive diagnosis.

PRIMARY ISOLATION AND IDENTIFICATION. Specimens from patients with the above clinical syndromes require initial anaerobic cultivation on blood agar and in liquid media, such as thioglycolate and cooked meat broth, in which the oxidation-reduction potential is low. Presumptive identification of the organism is based upon the demonstration of a gram-positive, boxcar-shaped rod with no visible spores, and production of a "double zone" of hemolysis on blood agar, "stormy fermentation" in iron milk medium, and **lecithinase** on egg yolk medium. Definitive identification is based upon the inhibition of hemolysis by specific antitoxin (Nagler test).

Diagnosis of *C. perfringens* food poisoning is based upon history and clinical manifestations.

Treatment

CLOSTRIDIAL MYONECROSIS AND ANAEROBIC CELLULITIS. For patients with clostridial myonecrosis and anaerobic cellulitis, prompt and extensive debridement of the wound is essential. Penicillin and/or broad spectrum antibiotics are effective against *C. perfringens* and secondary pyogenic invaders. Mechanical ventilation (hyperbaric O_2) is effective in "detoxifying" patients rapidly and has reduced the necessity for early radical amputation. Polyvalent antitoxin against several invasive clostridia, including *C. perfringens,* is available but rarely used due to lack of evidence for its effectiveness.

SEPTICEMIA AND ORGAN ABSCESSES. Penicillin may be useful if given early to patients with septicemia and organ abscesses. However, these syndromes are not usually recognized early enough for the antibiotic to be effective. The self-limiting and mild nature of *C. perfringens* food poisoning precludes the use of antimicrobial therapy.

Prevention and Control

Early and adequate debridement of the wound, together with penicillin and/or broad spectrum antibiotic therapy is essential. Surgical instruments must be clean and sterile. Awareness that clostridia can cause septicemia and organ abscesses in immunocompromised patients can sometimes result in early, effective therapy. Clostridial food poisoning can be prevented by **refrigerating** meats, fish, and poultry after cooking.

CLOSTRIDIUM DIFFICILE DISEASE

Clostridium difficile, an important nosocomial pathogen, is the most common cause of **pseudomembranous colitis.** The organism may also produce a milder form of diarrheal disease in which the pseudomembranous manifestations are absent.

Transmission

EXOGENOUS. Noncolonized patients may become colonized (carriers) from *C. difficile* patients or carriers by hospital personnel transmission. Patients who move into a hospital room previously occupied by a *C. difficile* patient are 30% more likely to become colonized with the organism. Alternatively, noncolonized patients who have undergone abdominal or intestinal surgery may develop *C. difficile* disease upon exogenous exposure. In particular, disease may occur among those patients whose GI flora has been altered by the use of certain antibiotics, such as penicillin, ampicillin, clindamycin, and the cephalosporins, that upset host-parasite balance and allow unrestricted multiplication of the organism.

ENDOGENOUS. The disease can occur as a result of endogenous activation after abdominal or intestinal surgery when, as previously mentioned, certain antibiotics, such as penicillin, ampicillin, clindamycin, and the cephalosporins, are employed. Again, this results in an upset in host-parasite balance that allows the unrestricted multiplication of *C. difficile* in the GI tract.

Extracellular Products Associated With the Pathogenicity of the Organism

Enterotoxin A and cytotoxin B are antigenically distinct, heat-labile proteins produced by the vegetative cells. These proteins are both responsible, in concert, for the **epithelial necrosis and stimulation of host fibrinous exudate** leading to toxic manifestations. Although an enterotoxin is thought to cause the mild diarrheal colitis that may occur due to *C. difficile,* its association has not been established unequivocally.

Pathogenesis and Clinical Manifestations

The vegetative cells multiply in the GI tract and release **toxins A and B,** which together cause necrosis of the mucosal surface of the colon. The host responds with a fibrinous exudate which, together with the area of necrosis, results in the formation of a **pseudomembrane.** The patient exhibits fever, bloody diarrhea, and abdominal cramps. Colitis in the absence of a pseudomembrane often occurs with resultant diarrhea. The most serious complication is **toxic megacolon**.

Immunity to Reinfection

Immunity to reinfection does not occur.

Laboratory Diagnosis

The ELISA is considered the ''gold standard'' procedure for toxin detection. The demonstration of toxin B in stool specimens utilizing a tissue culture assay for cytotoxicity is useful in establishing the diagnosis.

PRIMARY ISOLATION AND IDENTIFICATION OF THE ORGANISM. Isolation and identification of the organism from stool specimens, together with the demonstration of toxin by a pure culture of the organism, requires initial cultivation on selective agar medium. However, positive cultures and toxin demonstration must be interpreted with caution, inasmuch as 20% of hospitalized patients are colonized asymptomatically with either toxin- or nontoxin-producing strains.

Treatment

Vancomycin is highly effective in the treatment of *C. difficile* pseudomembranous colitis. Metronidazole is an alternate, but less effective therapy. Retreatment may be necessary due to the occasional occurrence of relapses. Toxic megacolon may require emergency colostomy.

Prevention and Control

Awareness of the circumstances under which the disease can occur can be useful in the initiation of early therapy. These patients should be isolated and hands should be thoroughly washed after examining patients. Terminally clean the hospital rooms of *C. difficile* patients to rid the area of spores. When suspected, discontinue the antibiotics being used or substitute alternate antibiotics believed to be less frequently associated with the disease.

BOTULISM

The two types of botulism, food borne and infant, are caused by *Clostridium botulinum* and occur sporadically. Most cases of the food-borne type occur during the winter months when canned foods are eaten and in the western states where the spore count in the soil is high. The case fatality rate among patients with food-borne botulism is 70% in the untreated disease and 25% when treated early. In contrast, and for unknown reasons, infant botulism is self-limiting.

Transmission

EXOGENOUS. Both types of botulism are transmitted exclusively by the exogenous route.

FOOD-BORNE BOTULISM. In food-borne botulism, spores gain access to foods such as vegetables and some fruits grown in close association with the soil and maintained at a slightly alkaline or neutral pH during the canning process. The suitable pH, anaerobiasis, and a faulty canning process, provide the favorable conditions necessary for spore germination and multiplying vegetative cells that produce neurotoxin intracellularly and release it into the food during cell autolysis. Transmission then occurs when individuals taste and ingest improperly prepared and improperly cooked canned foods containing the pre-formed neurotoxin. Transmission may occur in a similar fashion from the ingestion or tasting of fish improperly vacuum packed or smoked and containing neurotoxin.

INFANT BOTULISM. In infant botulism, infants aged 2 days to 6 months ingest food containing spores that germinate in the GI tract. Vegetative cells then produce neurotoxin intracellularly and release it into the gut. The foods re-

sponsible for transmission are unknown, but **contaminated honey** has been suspected.

Extracellular Product Associated With the Pathogenicity of the Organism

Neurotoxin, the most powerful exotoxin known, is a protein that is inactivated in food by boiling for 20 min. There are eight specific serotypes (A-H) based
upon their antigenic diversity; four produce human disease, but the most common
are serotypes A, B, and E. The toxin is produced intracellularly over a narrow pH
range of 7.0–7.3 by vegetative cells and released during autolysis. A prophage
carrying the *tox* gene is required for toxin expression. The toxin acts by **suppressing or blocking the presynaptic release of acetylcholine** responsible for muscle
tone (see Fig. 10.1).

Pathogenesis and Clinical Manifestations

FOOD-BORNE BOTULISM. Food-borne botulism is initiated following
the ingestion or tasting of food containing **pre-formed neurotoxin** as a result of
faulty canning, vacuum packing, or smoking, and improper heating of the canned
food prior to consumption. The toxin is so potent that it **is only necessary to
touch the tongue to the neurotoxin-containing food to acquire a fatal disease.**
Neurotoxin is absorbed by the mucosa of the stomach and upper GI tract, taken
up by the blood stream, and selectively absorbed by peripheral neurons at the
myoneural junctions, where it acts as described causing **paralysis most often of
the pharyngeal, ocular, and respiratory muscles.** After an incubation period of
12–46 h, the most common clinical manifestations are diplopia (double vision),
dysphagia (difficulty in swallowing), and dysphonia (thickness of speech) commonly referred to as the "3 d's." Death occurs in 12–24 h due to respiratory
paralysis.

INFANT BOTULISM. Infant botulism is initiated following the ingestion
of spore-contaminated food (honey?). Spores germinate in the GI tract. The vegetative cells multiply and produce **neurotoxin** intracellularly, which is released
into the gut during autolysis. The mechanism of action of the neurotoxin following
absorption by the GI mucosa is similar to that described for the food-borne type.
After an incubation period of 8–22 days, ptosis (droopy eyelids), dysphagia, and

fever result. The infant appears **"floppy"** due to loss of neck and limb muscle strength.

Immunity to Reinfection

Immunity to reinfection is type specific and permanent.

Laboratory Diagnosis

The rapidity with which death can occur with the food-borne type of botulism necessitates an immediate diagnosis based upon history (if possible) and clinical manifestations. For epidemiological purposes, serum specimens and food are analyzed for neurotoxin by mouse virulence assays. The infant type is usually diagnosed on clinical grounds, but may be confirmed by demonstrating the neurotoxin in the stool.

Treatment

FOOD-BORNE BOTULISM. Mechanical ventilation must be maintained. Immediate IV use of equine polyvalent antitoxin against serotypes A, B, and E, obtainable from the CDC, is essential. However, tests must be conducted to determine hypersensitivity to the antitoxin and the potential necessity for desensitization prior to its administration.

INFANT BOTULISM. Infant botulism requires only supportive therapy.

Prevention and Control

FOOD-BORNE BOTULISM. Large outbreaks of food-borne botulism have been largely prevented by strict regulation of commercial canning, although occasionally sporadic outbreaks occur. Most cases result from the improper preparation of home canned foods, smoked fish, and vacuum-packed fresh fish in plastic bags. Wherever possible, education on proper home canning techniques should be publicized. The risk of food intoxication can be reduced by boiling canned foods for at least 20 min, but this is seldom done due to loss of flavor.

Although toxic foods may be rancid or spoiled and cans may appear swollen, it is essential to note that **both the food and the can may appear normal.**

INFANT BOTULISM. Recommendations for the prevention of infant botulism include the careful inspection of jars or cans of baby food for evidence of spoilage. Despite the lack of definitive evidence for its role in transmission, **honey should not be fed to infants.**

SUMMARY

1. The genus *Clostridium* consists of gram-positive, spore-forming anaerobic rods widely distributed in the soil and present in the GI tract of humans and animals.

2. The sole virulence factor of *Clostridium tetani*, the etiologic agent of tetanus, is tetanospasmin (neurotoxin), an extracellular protein that blocks presynaptic inhibition.

3. Following introduction of *C. tetani* spores into injured tissue, germination to vegetative cells occurs. Vegetative cells multiply locally and tetanospasmin is produced, which travels along the axis cylinders of the motor neurons of the spinal cord and medulla and becomes fixed to nerve cells. The earliest clinical manifestation is due to contraction of the masseter muscles. Later signs result from sustained contraction of the facial muscles with extension of the spasmic contractions to the back, neck, and respiratory muscles. Intermittent convulsive seizures occur with slight stimulus as the disease progresses.

4. Active immunization with tetanus toxoid prior to injury is effective in preventing tetanus and is administered to normal infants and children together with diphtheria toxoid and killed *Bordetella pertussis* (DTP vaccine).

5. Clostridial myonecrosis (gas gangrene), anaerobic cellulitis, septicemia, and organ abscesses are caused by several species of clostridia, but the most common etiologic agent is *Clostridium perfringens*, which is also capable of causing food poisoning.

6. Clostridial myonecrosis is both an invasive and toxemic disease. Germination to vegetative cells occurs following introduction of spores into a wound. Vegetative cells of *C. perfringens* multiply and produce lecithinase C, which causes cell membrane disruption, lysis, tissue necrosis, and edema

(gangrene). The process of tissue destruction is enhanced by collagenase, hyaluronidase, and DNase. Large amounts of gas form due to the saccharolytic action of the organisms on muscle carbohydrate. The exotoxins are absorbed into the circulation and carried to a multiplicity of organs with resultant toxemic degeneration and death.

7. The pathogenesis of clostridial anaerobic cellulitis is essentially the same as for clostridial myonecrosis except that the organisms spread along fascial planes between muscle and do not invade muscle. There is no systemic toxin absorption and the prognosis is better than for myonecrosis.

8. Clostridial septicemia and organ abscesses are produced by endogenous organisms that invade the circulation of immunocompromised hosts and are carried to the tissues.

9. *C perfringens* food poisoning is the result of ingesting greater than or equal to 10^8 vegetative cells.

10. Disease due to *Clostridium difficile* may occur in patients who have undergone abdominal or intestinal surgery and in patients whose GI flora has been altered by the use of antibiotics that upset the host-parasite balance.

11. *C. difficile* vegetative cells multiply in the GI tract and release toxins A and B, which act in concert to cause necrosis of the mucosal surface of the colon. The host responds with a fibrinous exudate which, together with the area of necrosis, results in the formation of a pseudomembrane. Colitis without a pseudomembrane with resultant diarrhea often occurs.

12. Food-borne and infant botulism are caused by *Clostridium botulinum.* The food-borne type is acquired as a result of tasting or eating sporecontaminated foods. The infant type is acquired at age 2 days to 6 months as a result of ingesting food containing spores that germinate in the GI tract, then produce neurotoxin.

13. The sole virulence factor of *C. botulinum* is a neurotoxin produced intracellularly by vegetative cells over a narrow pH range and released during autolysis of the organism. The neurotoxin acts by suppressing or blocking the presynaptic release of acetylcholine.

14. In the food-borne type of botulism, pre-formed neuroxin is ingested with the food. The toxin is absorbed by the mucosa of the stomach and upper GI tract, taken up by the blood stream, and selectively absorbed by peripheral neurons at the myoneural junctions, where it causes paralysis mostly of the

pharyngeal, ocular, and respiratory muscles. Death occurs in 12–24 h due to respiratory paralysis. In the infant type of botulism, following ingestion of spore-contaminated food, germination occurs in the GI tract. Vegetative cells multiply and produce neurotoxin intracellulary, which is released into the gut during autolysis. Recovery occurs with supportive therapy.

REFERENCES

Arnon SS (1990): Infant botulism. In Boriello SP (ed): Clinical and Molecular Aspects of Anaerobes. Petersfield, England: Wrightson Biomedical Publishing, pp 41–48.

Bartlett JG (1982): Virulence factors of anaerobic bacteria. Johns Hopkins Med J, 151:1.

Bizzini B (1979): Tetanus toxin. Microbiol Rev 43:224.

Finegold SM (1991): Anaerobic infections: An overview. Korean J Clin Pathol 11:507.

Finegold SM, George WL (eds) (1989): Anaerobic Infections in Humans. San Diego, CA: Academic Press.

George WL (1984): Antimicrobial agent-associated colitis and diarrthea: Historical background and clinical aspects. Rev Infect Dis 6 (Suppl. 1):S208.

Hathaway CL (1990): Toxigenic clostridia. Clin Microbiol Rev 3:66.

Lyerly DM, Krivan HC, Wilkins TD (1988): *Clostridium difficile:* Its disease and toxins. Clin Microbiol Rev 1:1.

Mills DC, Arnon SS (1987): The large intestine as the site of *Clostridium botulinum* colonization in human infant botulism. J Infect Dis 156:997.

Simpson LL (1986): Molecular pharmacology of botulinum toxin and tetanus toxin. Ann Rev Pharmacol Toxicol 26:427.

Smith LDS (1979): Virulence factors of *Clostridium perfringens.* Rev Infect Dis 1:254.

Stanfield JP, Galazaka A (1984): Neonatal tetanus in the world today. Bull WHO 62:647.

REVIEW QUESTIONS

For questions 1 to 12, choose the ONE
BEST answer or completion.

1. Tetanus and clostridial myonecrosis
   a) have a very similar pathogenesis
   b) are caused by organisms that produce virulence factors with identical mechanisms of action
   c) are caused by organisms that may be transmitted to humans by soil-contaminated objects
   d) are invasive and toxemic diseases
   e) are caused by organisms that produce round, terminal spores

2. The pathogenesis of tetanus
   a) is initiated following introduction of *Clostridium tetani* vegetative cells into injured tissue
   b) results from the activity of *C. tetani* produced hyaluronidase on the hyaluronic acid of connective tissue ground substance
   c) is always the result of a major injury with a heavily contaminated object
   d) is due to the action of fibrinolysin produced by *C. tetani*
   e) is the result of the blocking of presynaptic inhibition by tetanospasmin, which is released by autolysing *C. tetani* vegetative cells

3. The prevention and control of tetanus include
   a) the administration of heat-killed *C. tetani* vegetative cells as a booster to previously immunized infants
   b) active immunization of infants, children, and adults with tetanus toxoid
   c) passive immunization of patients with clean, minor wounds
   d) elimination of ticks that harbor the organism in their midgut
   e) active immunization of adults with *C. tetani* spores

4. Virulence factors operative during the pathogenesis of clostridial myonecrosis include
   a) enterotoxin
   b) the capsule of *Clostridium perfringens*
   c) lecithinase C
   d) erythrogenic toxin
   e) pili

5. Anaerobic cellulitis due to *C. perfringens* *differs* from clostridial myonecrosis in that the *former*
   a) is characterized clinically by gas formation due to the in vivo saccharolytic properties of the organisms
   b) is characterized by tissue necrosis
   c) is caused by an anaerobic, spore-forming rod

d) is characterized by an absence of systemic exotoxin absorption and a good prognosis

e) occurs as a result of massive injury with soil contaminated objects

6. Clostridial septicemia and organ abscesses
   a) occur as a result of exogenous transmission
   b) are produced by endogenous organisms that invade the circulation of immunocompromised hosts
   c) can be diagnosed conclusively by demonstrating gram-positive organisms consistent with *C. perfringens* in a blood smear
   d) can be treated effectively with penicillin
   e) are self-limiting diseases

7. Staphylococcal and *C. perfringens* food poisoning are similar in that
   a) they are initiated following the ingestion of pre-formed enterotoxin
   b) they are caused by gram-positive, spore-forming rods
   c) the diarrhea that is produced is the result of the inhibition of water absorption from the intestinal lumen
   d) they result in vomiting
   e) they can be prevented by vaccination

8. Disease due to *Clostridium difficile*
   a) may be the result of endogenous activation or exogenous transmission from a colonized to a noncolonized patient who has undergone abdominal or intestinal surgery
   b) is the result of vancomycin therapy
   c) occurs following the inhalation of spores

d) results in a significant degree of immunity to reinfection

e) always results in the formation of a pseudomembrane

9. The epithelial necrosis and fibrinous exudate observed in patients with *C. difficile* disease
   a) can be prevented by vaccination
   b) are the direct result of tissue invasion by clostridial spores
   c) must be treated with penicillin
   d) is due to the combined activity of enterotoxin and cytoxin produced by *C. difficile* vegetative cells
   e) is found only in patients injured by soil-contaminated objects

10. Food-borne botulism is acquired
    a) by ingesting food containing 10^9 *Clostridium botulinum* spores
    b) by ingesting food containing pre-formed botulinum neurotoxin
    c) by ingesting highly acid fresh fruit left at room temperature for 24 h
    d) by ingesting food containing a potent enterotoxin
    e) exclusively by immunocompromised patients

11. Infant botulism *differs* from food-borne botulism in that the *former*
    a) is due to the action of a neurotoxin
    b) is usually fatal
    c) requires treatment with polyvalent antitoxin
    d) occurs as a result of a faulty home canning process
    e) is initiated by the ingestion of food containing *C. botulinum* spores

12. One of the following statements relating to botulinum neurotoxin is false. Botulinum neurotoxin
    a) acts by suppressing or blocking the presynaptic release of acetylcholine responsible for muscle tone
    b) is produced by *C. botulinum* vegetative cells
    c) is produced by either *C. botulinum* spores or vegetative cells
    d) is the cause of muscle paralysis in patients with food-borne botulism
    e) can be inactivated at 100°C for 20 min

ANSWERS TO REVIEW QUESTIONS

1. *c* Tetanus and clostridial myonecrosis can both be initiated following injury with soil-contaminated objects containing spores. However, the tetanospasmin produced by the vegetative cells of *Clostridium tetani* and the lecithinase C, collagenase, hyaluronidase, and DNase produced by the vegetative cells of *Clostridium perfringens* differ markedly in their function. As a result, the pathogenesis of the two diseases are different, including the fact that tetanus is a strictly toxemic disease, while clostridial myonecrosis is both toxemic and invasive. *C. tetani* is the only pathogenic member of the genus that produces round and terminal spores.

2. *e* Following the introduction of *C. tetani* spores into a major or minor wound, germination to vegetative cells occur, and tetanospasmin is produced and released following autolysis of the organism. The toxin is the only known virulence factor of the organism and acts by blocking presynaptic inhibition.

3. *b* Active immunization of infants, children, and adults with tetatus toxoid is highly effective in preventing tetanus. Infants and children are given tetanus toxoid with diphtheria toxoid and killed *Bordetella pertussis* vaccine (DTP) at designated intervals until age 6, and appropriate boosters with Td thereafter. Neither vegetative cells nor spores are effective vaccinogens. Passive immunization with human tetanus immune globulin could provide immediate protection against the disease but is not necessary if the patient has a clean, minor wound. Tetanus is not a tick-borne disease.

4. *c* Of the structures and extracellular products given, lecithinase C is the only *C. perfringens* virulence factor. It hydro-

lyzes the lecithin-containing lipoprotein complexes in red cell and tissue membranes and mitochondria causing cell membrane disruption and lysis, tissue necrosis, and edema.

5. *d* In contrast to clostridial myonecrosis, anaerobic cellulitis is characterized by an absence of systemic exotoxin absorption and a good prognosis. Both syndromes are characterized by gas formation in vivo and tissue necrosis and can occur as a result of massive injury with objects contaminated with soil containing *C. perfringens,* an anaerobic spore-forming rod.

6. *b* Clostridial septicemia and organ abscesses occur exclusively as a result of the extraintestinal growth of endogenous organisms that invade the circulation of immunocompromised hosts. Inasmuch as *C. perfringens* can be isolated from the blood of asymptomatic patients, the demonstration of organisms consistent with *C. perfringens* in blood smears is not conclusive. Positive blood cultures must be obtained. These syndromes are usually fatal despite penicillin therapy.

7. *c* Both staphylococcal and *C. perfringens* food poisoning occur as a result of enterotoxin production by their respective etiologic agents resulting in inhibition of water absorption from the intestinal lumen. However, in contrast to clostridial food poisoning, staphylococcal food poisoning is caused by a gram-positive, nonspore-forming coccus, occurs follow-

ing the ingestion of food containing pre-formed enterotoxin, and results in clinical manifestations that include vomiting. There are no vaccines for either syndrome.

8. *a* *Clostridium difficile* disease can occur as a result of either endogenous activation or exogenous transmission, but only when vegetative cells multiply, produce, and release enterotoxin and cytotoxin. Vancomycin is the treatment of choice, there is no immunity to reinfection, and colitis in the absence of a pseudomembrane can occur.

9. *d* The epithelial necrosis and fibrinous exudate seen in patients with *C. difficile* disease is the result of the combined action of enterotoxin and cytotoxin produced by vegetative cells. Spores do not produce the toxins nor do they cause the disease syndromes. Penicillin is one of the antibiotics that can upset host-parasite balance and allow *C. difficile* vegetative cells to multiply in the GI tract and release the toxins. Susceptible patients are those who have had abdominal and intestinal surgery.

10. *b* Ingestion of food containing pre-formed botulinum neurotoxin by immunologically normal or immunocompromised hosts results in food-borne botulism. Infant botulism is initiated by eating food containing *Clostridium botulinum* spores that germinate in the GI tract; the vegetative cells then produce neurotoxin. Neurotoxin can be produced as a result

of fruit grown in close association with soil, maintained at a slightly alkaline or neutral pH during canning, and held under anaerobic conditions during a faulty canning process. Enterotoxin is not produced.

11. *e* As indicated above, infant botulism is initiated by the ingestion of food containing *C. botulinum* spores rather than preformed toxin. It is self-limiting, does not require treatment with polyvalent antitoxin, and does not occur as a result of a faulty home canning process.

12. *c* Botulinum neurotoxin acts by suppressing or blocking the presynaptic release of acetylcholine responsible for muscle tone, is produced *only* by vegetative cells, is the cause of muscle paralysis in patients with food-borne botulinum, and can be inactivated at 100°C for 20 min.

NONSPORE-FORMING ANAEROBIC BACTERIAL DISEASES

ANAEROBIC DISEASES

The nonspore-forming anaerobic bacteria are the most common cause of anaerobic diseases in humans. These bacteria are normal flora of the mucous membranes, GI tract, and numerous other environmental niches of humans and other animals. These organisms outnumber the aerobic bacterial colonizers by 1000:1 and exist in numbers as high as 10^{11} bacteria per cubic centimeter. When a break in host defenses allows these inhabitants of our lumens access to normally sterile tissue, disease almost always follows. Although they are of low virulence, they can act synergistically to invoke an inflammatory response. Certain anaerobes seem to induce abscess formation in the host.

Because these organisms are unable to survive in the presence of atmospheric oxygen (the reason for their name *anaerobes*), they cannot be passed easily from patient to patient. Thus, these organisms cause disease almost exclusively in their original hosts. Most diseases with nonspore-forming anaerobes are endogenous in origin. Notable exceptions are clenched fist and bite wound infections, in which the oral flora of one individual is traumatically implanted into the tissue of another.

It was not until practical anaerobic microbiological laboratory techniques became widely available during the 1960s that most clinicians gained an appreciation for the variety and seriousness of anaerobic diseases. Even today, many hospital laboratories lack the time and the resources necessary to perform complete anaerobic microbiological studies. In almost all cases, **diseases due to the nonspore-forming anaerobes are polymicrobial** (multimicrobial). This fact makes it difficult to determine a ''predominant organism,'' as is practiced commonly with aerobic bacteria isolated from clinical specimens, and demands expanded laboratory services. In addition, the ''pathogens'' are also normal human flora from the adjacent mucous membrane, and any compromises in specimen collection techniques will render the results uninterpretable. Because final microbiological results may require several days, clinicians must choose initial therapy based on rapid laboratory results, such as Gram stain, and clinical considerations. For this reason, it is important to know the etiology of various infectious processes due to nonspore-forming anaerobes so that appropriate empiric therapy can be chosen.

Nature of the Organism

ANAEROBIC METABOLISM. A universal definition of *anaerobe* has not been determined, as the oxygen tolerance of ''anaerobic bacteria'' varies greatly among species. For practical purposes, **anaerobic bacteria are those that require reduced oxygen tension for growth.** Room air contains approximately 18% oxygen; oxygen pressures greater than 0.4% may inhibit growth of some pathogenic anaerobes. A small group of investigators feels that the oxidation-reduction potential (E_h), which is dependent on pH, may be of equal importance. Interestingly, the more common etiologic agents of anaerobic diseases seem to be more aerotolerant. It has been suggested that the **enzyme superoxide dismutase, which protects bacteria from the toxic effects of the superoxide radical,** may be produced in greater amounts by the more virulent anaerobic species.

A few species of anaerobes, notably some spore-forming species, clostridia, are aerotolerant. Although they grow better in an anaerobic atmosphere, they are able to grow, albeit poorly, on fresh agar medium in air with increased carbon dioxide. The *Bacteroides fragilis* group, the most common pathogens among the nonspore-forming anaerobes, are not aerotolerant but are able to survive some period of oxygen exposure in the original specimen and on an agar plate once colonies have matured. In all probability, this is the reason that these species are recovered more frequently than any others by clinical microbiology laboratories performing minimal anaerobic techniques.

SPECIFIC GENERA. Nonspore-forming anaerobes are classified by Gram-stain morphology in the same manner as are the aerobic bacteria. Several genera are important in human diseases (Table 11.1).

1. Gram-negative bacilli: The most important pathogens in this group are the **B. fragilis group,** of which there are 10 species. These organisms are **normal flora of the GI tract** and are involved in infectious processes disproportionate to their numbers in the bowel flora. Several virulence factors account for their presence in diseases.

The genus **Fusobacterium** is common in the **oral cavity** and is an important pathogen in neighboring anatomic sites.

Several other genera, including *Prevotella, Porphyromonas,* and *Bilophila,* are less commonly isolated.

2. Gram-negative cocci: *Veillonella* species make up part of the normal oral and vaginal flora and are occasionally involved in genital and other diseases.

3. Gram-positive bacilli: **Propionibacterium acnes, a normal inhabitant of the skin,** is a frequent cause of **prosthetic joint diseases** and occasionally enters the bloodstream to cause endocarditis. This species is also involved in diseases following ophthalmic surgery. **Actinomyces,** an inhabitant of the oral mucosa, can invade into the surrounding tissue and cause **actinomycosis.** Members of this genus are also involved in female genital tract diseases, lung abscesses, and other processes. *Lactobacillus* spp., members of the normal female vaginal flora and normal oral flora, although of low pathogenicity, nevertheless have been

TABLE 11.1. Prevailing Disease Syndromes That Involve Nonspore-forming Anaerobes and Their Commonly Associated Bacteria

Disease	Predominant anaerobes
Brain abscess	*Peptostreptococcus, Fusobacterium, Prevotella, Porphyromonas,* oral flora
Bacteremia	*Bacteroides fragilis* group, *Propionibacterium acnes* (as a contaminant)
Eye diseases	*Actinomyces, Propionibacterium, Peptostreptococcus, Veillonella*
Periodontal disease, oral abscesses	*Porphyromonas, Prevotella, Peptostreptococcus,* oral flora
Aspiration pneumonia	*Fusobacterium, Prevotella, Peptostreptococcus,* oral flora
Intraabdominal disease	*Bacteroides fragilis* group, *Bilophila, Fusobacterium, Porphyromonas, Peptostreptococcus, Eubacterium*
Infected prostheses	*Propionibacterium acnes*
Wound diseases, decubitus ulcers	*Bacteroides fragilis* group, *Fusobacterium, Peptostreptococcus*
Gynecologic diseases	*Prevotella, B. fragilis* group, *Peptostreptococcus, Actinomyces, Veillonella*

reported numerous times as an etiologic agent of endocarditis. *Eubacterium* spp., a gram-positive rod found in the oral and GI tracts, is occasionally found in intraabdominal processes and wound diseases.

4. Gram-positive cocci: These bacteria, present on all mucous membranes and primarily of the genus *Peptostreptococcus,* are involved in **aspiration pneumonia, brain abscess, genital tract diseases,** and **wound infections.**

Habitat

The human body is host to innumerable bacteria, predominantly anaerobic (Fig. 11.1). All mucous membranes have a diverse flora, as do the GI tract and the female genital tract. Other ecological niches where the oxygen tension is low, even on the skin (such as deep within hair follicles), support anaerobic bacteria.

A few species of the spore-forming anaerobic bacteria *Clostridium* spp. live in the cecal contents. Some, such as *Clostridium difficile, Clostridium septicum,* and *Clostridium perfringens,* are capable of causing endogenously acquired disease. These bacteria are discussed in Chapter 10 on clostridial diseases. Nonsporeforming anaerobes produce a much larger number of diseases than do the clostridia and, thus, are of much greater significance.

Transmission

ENDOGENOUS. **Endogenous infections** occur in the following circumstances:

1. **A traumatic loss of integrity to the mucosal epithelium,** such as occurs from a gunshot wound or automobile accident; or a surgical procedure that accidentally allows luminal contents surrounded by a mucous membrane, such as the vagina, GI tract, and gingiva, to spill into adjacent normal tissue, permitting anaerobes to become pathogens.

2. **Hematogenous seeding of anaerobes to a distant focus from an infected site,** such as diverticulitis or periodontal disease, can occur. This mechanism accounts for anaerobic involvement in disseminated diseases, including brain abscesses, endocarditis, and spinal osteomyelitis.

3. There may be **contamination of a surface wound** or incision with the patient's own fecal flora.

4. **Direct extension** from a heavily colonized mucous membrane to adjacent tissue can result, such as occurs with diseases that include peritonitis associated

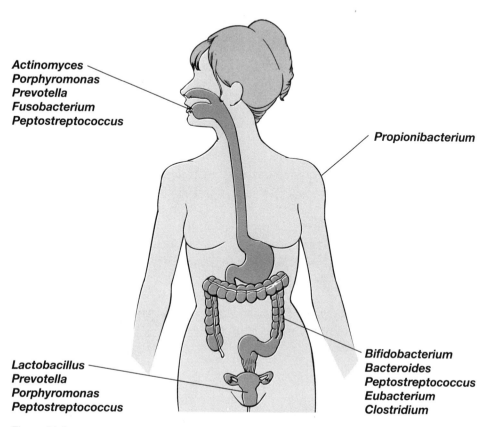

Actinomyces
Porphyromonas
Prevotella
Fusobacterium
Peptostreptococcus

Propionibacterium

Lactobacillus
Prevotella
Porphyromonas
Peptostreptococcus

Bifidobacterium
Bacteroides
Peptostreptococcus
Eubacterium
Clostridium

Figure 11.1.

Anaerobes found as part of the normal flora that are often involved in disease processes.

with appendicitis, actinomycosis of the uterus in women with intrauterine devices (IUDs), and mandibular osteomyelitis.

5. **Necrosis of the membrane tissue,** such as occurs during ischemic bowel syndrome, can also allow spillage of anaerobes from the normally protected lumen into surrounding tissues and the bloodstream.

6. **Overgrowth of a subpopulation of anaerobes** can occur in a site with a normal anaerobic population, such as in bacterial vaginosis and contaminated small bowel syndrome.

7. **Inoculation of oral flora into sterile lungs by aspiration** may occur.

8. There may be **injection** of a patient's oral flora into the tissue, such as happens when IV drug users inject ''contaminated'' saliva as a diluent along with their drugs.

EXOGENOUS. **Exogenous infections** include bite wound or clenched fist wound infections and disease acquired by the neonate in utero from the vaginal anaerobic flora of the mother.

Properties of the Organism

Resistance to environmental, physical, and chemical agents. As indicated by their name, **anaerobic bacteria are susceptible to oxygen.** Exposure to air and drying will kill them rapidly. Specimens must be collected and transported in such a manner as to minimize exposure to air, or anaerobic bacteria will not be recovered in culture.

The organisms are somewhat protected in the original specimen; pus, for example, contains a very low oxidation-reduction potential (E_h) and allows survival of anaerobes for several hours. Necrotic tissue also provides good protection.

Most chemical disinfectants, heat, and sunlight are effective in killing these fragile bacteria.

Microscopic morphology. The microscopic morphology of nonspore-forming anaerobic bacteria encompasses the following:

1. Gram-negative bacilli

Bacteroides fragilis group. These organisms are **highly pleomorphic, gram-negative bacilli** that often show vacuoles, swellings, and long filaments on the initial Gram stain.

Fusobacteria. These bacteria are characterized by diverse morphologies. *Fusobacterium nucleatum,* one of the most common isolates, displays **long, thin, fusiform gram-negative rods with pointed ends.** Its appearance is quite pathognomonic for the genus.

Other fusobacteria, such as *Fusobacterium mortiferum* and *Fusobacterium necrophorum* may show bizarre, swollen and misshapen forms, or, like *Fusobacterium naviforme,* small boat-shaped fusiforms. Many species of fusobacteria are nondescript.

2. Gram-negative cocci. *Veillonella* species are very small gram-negative diplococci that resemble members of the genus *Neisseria.*

3. Selected gram-positive bacilli. Examples of the morphology of gram-positive bacilli follow:

Propionibacterium acnes and related genera are seen as **pleomorphic co-**

ryneform gram-positive rods or coccobacilli. These organisms display all the characteristics of aerobic corynebacteria, including clubbing, palisading, and snapping forms.

Actinomyces species are characterized by **branching, pleomorphic, irregular staining gram-positive rods** that may form intertwining nestlike groups.

Lactobacilli are usually very straight-sided, long, blunt-ended gram-positive rods, but some curly forms and other bizarre shapes may be seen occasionally.

4. Gram-positive cocci. Like streptococci, their aerobic counterparts, the anaerobic *Peptostreptococcus* species are **spherical or elongated cocci,** often occurring in chains or pairs. Cell size is used to differentiate among some species.

Macroscopic morphology. The anaerobic nonspore-forming bacteria must be cultivated in an anaerobic atmosphere. Large laboratories perform anaerobic studies in plastic, self-contained anaerobic chambers that contain an atmosphere of 5% hydrogen, 10% carbon dioxide, and 85% nitrogen. Materials are manipulated in a chamber with rubber gloves that are attached and inserted through ports for use by the technologist. Oxygen is removed by catalyzing the reaction of $2H_2 + O_2 \rightarrow H_2O$.

Specialized incubation systems, including plastic pouches and gas-impermeable jars, are used in clinical laboratories that do not use chambers (Fig. 11.2).

Because several important genera require the growth factors hemin and menadione (vitamin K_1), they are usually added to all anaerobic media. Primary media usually contain blood. Laked blood, frozen and thawed, with its damaged red cell membranes enhances the formation of fluorescence and pigments that are characteristic of several genera of nonspore formers.

In colonial morphology a few species of nonspore-forming anaerobes have very distinctive colonies that aid in their identification on the culture. The *B. fragilis* group yield large, shiny, opaque colonies on blood agar. **All species of** *Porphyromonas* and some species of *Prevotella,* a gram-negative bacillus, **are pigmented.** They use the heme component of RBCs in the medium to generate porphyrin compounds, which become components of various dark pigments. Colonies containing porphyrins will fluoresce under UV light before the pigments have developed. After several more days, the colonies appear beige, brown, or black on blood agar plates as a result of production of porphyrin-containing pigments. Colonies of some strains of *F. nucleatum* show typical bread-crumb appearance or another characteristic morphotype, the internally speckled colony. *P. acnes* colonies are shiny white and opaque. *Actinomyces israelii* colonies take several days to develop but often resemble molar-tooth structures.

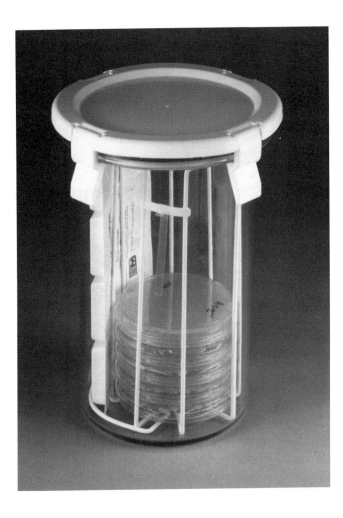

Figure 11.2.

Self-contained, self-sealing anaerobic jar incubation system, containing inoculated agar plates in a rack and gas-producing packet (includes gas-producing chemicals, catalyst, and oxygen indicator). (Courtesy of EM Diagnostic Systems, Gibbstown, New Jersey.)

Anaerobes are identified by morphology, enzymatic and biochemical tests, the production of specific end products of glucose metabolism as detected using gas-liquid chromatography (GLC) of spent culture medium, and by cell wall fatty acid composition. Definitive identification of many species of anaerobes can only be performed in specialized laboratories. However, rapid 2-day presumptive identification is within the capabilities of any clinical microbiology laboratory.

Antigenic structure. The gram-negative bacilli, presumably because of their pathogenic significance, have been the most extensively studied of the nonspore-forming anaerobes. Little information on the antigenic structure of gram-positive nonspore-forming anaerobes or the anaerobic cocci is available for discussion here. Each of the anaerobic species have adherence factors that allow them to multiply on mucous membrane surfaces and many of them produce proteolytic and lipolytic enzymes.

The gram-negative anaerobes contain lipopolysaccharide (LPS) in their cell walls. The lipopolysaccharide of fusobacteria appears similar to that of aerobic gram-negative bacteria, but the LPS of members of the *B. fragilis* group is distinctly different. This unusual LPS does not possess many of the toxic properties of aerobic gram-negative LPS. *Bacteroides* endotoxin is still thought to be a virulence factor, however, since it contributes to abscess formation.

Several species of anaerobic gram-negative bacilli have been shown to possess pili or fimbriae, which mediate attachment to epithelial cells. The pili of some gram-negative anaerobes mediate adherence to polymorphonuclear leukocytes and enhance phagocytosis.

The **polysaccharide capsule of B. fragilis** has been extensively studied as **the principal virulence factor** of these strains. In the presence of cofactors, such as cecal contents, **purified capsular polysaccharide can induce abscess formation** in animal models. Other genera, such as *Fusobacterium* and *Prevotella,* also include encapsulated species.

B. fragilis possesses a surface hemagglutinin, which may aid in invasion of host tissues.

Extracellular products associated with pathogenicity. The **superoxide dismutase** produced by *B. fragilis* and other anaerobes contributes to their survival in the presence of oxygen and may be a virulence factor that allows the organisms to persist in an infected site until the oxygen tension is lowered enough to permit multiplication. The capsular polysaccharide of *B. fragilis* described previously is secreted into the surrounding environment during growth. The capsule not only enhances abscess formation but also inhibits phagocytosis of the bacteria by polymorphonuclear leukocytes. Production of enzymes, such as phospholipases, by *Prevotella melaninogenica* and *Prevotella intermedia,* two pigmenting strains found in the oral cavity, contributes to the ability of these organisms to colonize the gingival crevices. *Porphyromonas gingivalis* produces collagenase, which aids in the induction of necrosis in infected tissues. Some fusobacteria produce lipases. Several anaerobes produce proteases that may cleave immunoglobulins and thus inhibit opsonization. Additional enzymes produced by several nonspore-forming anaerobes include hyaluronidase and fibrinolysin.

Pathogenesis and Clinical Manifestations

ABSCESS FORMATION. **Abscesses are the predominant feature of many diseases due to the nonspore-forming anaerobes.** Intraabdominal abscesses illustrate the progression of disease.

The infectious process begins typically with a breakdown in the mucosal tissue that allows bowel flora to escape into the peritoneal cavity. In some cases, phagocytic cells carry bacteria across the intact mucosal tissue without overt loss of integrity of the mucosa (translocation). **Anaerobes can invade intact tissue** by means of the fibrinogen-degrading enzymes, lipases, and collagenases. Rarely is one species of bacteria isolated from an abscess process. The **anaerobes seem to work synergistically with facultative bacteria,** notably *Escherichia coli* and *Enterococcus* species, when bowel flora gain entry to the peritoneal cavity. Colonization of host tissue, mediated by pili or fimbriae, is the first step in the infectious process.

The capsule of *B. fragilis* group organisms acts to promote abscess formation. **It is thought that T lymphocytes are critical to the establishment of abscesses;** mice treated with anti-T lymphocyte antibodies or with cyclophosphamide, which depletes lymphocytes, cannot form abscesses after challenge with *B. fragilis.* However, T lymphocytes from donor mice can restore the abscess-forming ability to cyclophosphamide-treated mice.

As the bacteria multiply and induce an inflammatory response, the host produces a layer of fibrin to contain the dead bacteria and phagocytic cell debris that are generated. This walled-off site is an abscess, within which bacteria continue to multiply and produce enzymes. The abscess contents, together with the proteolytic products of phagocytes, becomes liquefied.

The low E_h in an abscess and oxygen utilization by both the facultative coinfectors and the phagocytic cells serve to enhance growth of anaerobic strains. The anaerobes promote the growth and virulence of coexisting aerobic flora by inhibiting phagocytosis, producing essential growth factors, activating complement, and inhibiting neutrophil chemotaxis. The abscess itself is a very difficult site for antimicrobial agents and internal immune response effectors to breach.

NECROTIZING, INVASIVE DISEASES. The nonspore-formers can cause devastating disease that resembles classical clostridial "gas gangrene." The names of these syndromes, including **necrotizing fasciitis,** Fournier's gangrene (necrotizing fasciitis of the scrotum), and **synergistic nonclostridial anaerobic myonecrosis,** reflect the polymicrobial and destructive nature of these diseases. Patients presenting with the signs and symptoms of acute onset of pain, swelling, erythema or discoloration of skin, foul odor, thin gray pus exudate, and possible crepitation (crackling sound heard when the tissue is lightly compressed) indicating gas formation in the tissues, should be treated as **true surgical emergencies.** The necrotic tissue must be debrided extensively or removed entirely, depending on the extent of the damage.

To begin the process, anaerobic bacteria are somehow inoculated into subcutaneous tissue. If the tissue is damaged or anoxic, the organisms multiply rapidly, producing factors, such as hyaluronidase and collagenase, that allow destruction of tissue planes and extensive spread of the organisms.

Areas of cellulitis and bullae due to gas formation may appear. Tissue may be crepitant, but often gas quantity is too small to detect clinically and detection relies on radiologic studies.

Emergent surgical debridement or even amputation may be necessary to stop the rapid spread of infection. Without treatment, the case fatality rate approaches 50%. Clinical clues to an anaerobic infection include the following:

1. A foul or putrid odor.
2. Location of the infection near a mucosal surface.
3. Gas in infected tissue.
4. Necrotic tissue and destructive process.
5. Presence of ''sulfur granules'' in exudate (indicates actinomycosis).
6. Failure of organisms seen on Gram stain to grow on routine aerobic cultures.

Immunity to Reinfection

There is virtually no immunity to reinfection. These organisms are part of the normal flora of the host, who has grown effectively ''tolerant.''

Laboratory Diagnosis

Certain specimens contain normal anaerobic flora and should *never* be cultured for anaerobic bacteria in clinical laboratories. These include sputum, oropharyngeal swabs, skin surface swabs, vaginal material, fecal contents or fecally contaminated sources, voided or catheterized urine, and oral or gingival swabs.

SPECIMENS. **Tissue biopsy material is the best specimen.** If it is large enough, it can be transported in a sterile container in which anaerobes will survive for several hours. If it is small, it should be placed into a transport vial with a protected anaerobic environment. Aspiration of abscess contents is the next best specimen. Specimens should be obtained from intact, disinfected skin with a needle and syringe. The material should be inoculated into an **anaerobic transport vial** for maintenance during transport to the laboratory (Fig. 11.3). Sterile body fluids, such as blood, thoracentesis, empyema, and peritoneal fluid, are collected by transcutaneous aspiration and transported in an anaerobic transport vial, sterile tube, or blood culture broth bottle. If anaerobic urinary tract disease is suspected, a suprapubic bladder aspirate is the only acceptable specimen.

Intrauterine specimens can be obtained using a triple-lumen suction catheter device. Vaginal swabs are not acceptable because of the high degree of contamination by normal vaginal anaerobic flora. A swab is the least desirable specimen, since surface drainages are contaminated by colonizing and resident skin flora. If necessary, the surface should be decontaminated by debridement or by extensive washing with an iodophore before the specimen is collected. The swab must be transported in a special anaerobic transport medium.

Respiratory secretions in cases of suspected aspiration pneumonia **must be collected by a protected bronchial brush, transtracheal aspiration, or special bronchoalveolar lavage protocols.** Expectorated sputum, bronchial washings, and bronchial lavages are not useful because of the extensive anaerobic oral flora that always contaminates such specimens. Periodontal and subgingival exudates can be collected on sterile paper points that are placed immediately into a reduced transport broth.

PRIMARY ISOLATION AND IDENTIFICATION. Direct Gram stains should always be performed; typical organism morphology may be present and provide a very early clue to the etiologic agents. Specimens are inoculated onto special media supplemented with hemin and menadione. Standard media include

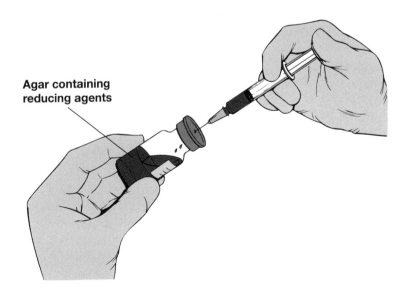

Agar containing reducing agents

Figure 11.3.

Injection of an aspirated specimen into an anaerobic transport vial.

anaerobic blood agar; a laked blood agar to enhance pigment formation; a selective agar containing antibiotics to suppress facultative gram-negative bacilli; *Bacteroides*-bile-esculin agar, a selective and differential plate for rapid identification of the *B. fragilis* group; and a broth enrichment backup culture. **All cultures are incubated anaerobically for 48 h** before they are examined for the first time. Additional incubation for as long as 1 week is standard in some laboratories. Isolates are identified based on colony morphology, Gram-stain morphology, susceptibility to antibiotics, constitutive enzymes, biochemical reactions, and by the end products of glucose metabolism. A few rapid tests can identify most isolates to genus within 2 days of observing isolated colonies.

Gas-liquid chromatographic analysis of volatile and nonvolatile fatty acids produced by metabolic processes of anaerobes is the definitive identification method. End product production is genus and occasionally species specific. The cumbersome nature of the methods and the expense of the apparatus precludes the use of these tests in most clinical laboratories.

IMMUNOSEROLOGIC TESTS. Although fluorescent antibody stains directed against several genera of anaerobes have been evaluated in experimental studies, none is available commercially.

GENETIC METHODS. New molecular technology methods have been applied to the diagnosis of periodontal disease caused by synergistic combinations of anaerobic gram-negative bacilli. A DNA probe directed against each of three bacterial species involved in the process is added to test samples directly. If the appropriate target bacterial genetic sequences are present, the probes bind to the sequence. Bound, double-stranded DNA hybrids are removed from the test sample and enzymatic markers are used to visualize binding. Assays of this type may become the standard for the detection and characterization of mixed bacterial infections, including those caused by anaerobic nonspore formers.

Treatment

Surgical drainage and debridement are key factors in successful treatment of anaerobic diseases. Only a few types of diseases, including liver and brain abscesses, can be treated medically with antibiotics alone.

Antimicrobials that have activity within abscesses are most effective for anaerobic diseases. Ampicillin-sulbactam, ticarcillin-clavulanic acid, and amoxicillin-clavulanic acid are effective against β-lactamase producing anaerobes. **Metronidazole has good penetration into abscesses** and is effective for most nonspore-forming anaerobes. Imipenem is quite active against most anaerobes, although some limited resistance has been reported. Ceftizoxime, cefoxitin, and cefotetan are still useful in limited situations, although resistant strains, especially among the *B. fragilis* group, are becoming more common. Clindamycin and chloramphenicol are effective and may be useful in some circumstances, but in general they are less desirable.

Prevention and Control

Drain collections of pus and debride necrotic tissue immediately. Clean surgical wounds and any other areas showing loss of skin integrity scrupulously and act to prevent fecal contamination. Prevent loss of consciousness if possible, in order to avoid the development of aspiration pneumonia. Maintain good oral hygiene.

SUMMARY

1. **Nonspore-forming anaerobic bacteria are the principal endogenous bacterial inhabitants of our GI tract and mucous membranes, outnumbering the aerobic and facultative bacteria by 1000:1.**

2. **As anaerobes, they are unable to survive prolonged exposure to atmospheric oxygen and they require a very low oxygen concentration for growth. Special laboratory methods are used to isolate and identify these organisms.**

3. **These bacteria cause infections when they gain access to a sterile environment, usually through trauma. Necrotic tissue and lack of adequate perfusion serve to enhance their ability to cause infections.**

4. **The *Bacteroides fragilis* group of gram-negative anaerobic bacilli are the most important. These organisms cause intraabdominal infections by an abscess-promoting virulence factor associated with the capsule. These species are also the most important agents of bacteremia among this diverse group of endogenous bacteria.**

5. **Other important nonspore-forming anaerobes involved in infectious diseases are (a) *Fusobacterium* spp.: oral abscesses, aspiration pneumonia, and brain abscesses. (b) *Propionibacterium acnes*: prosthetic device infections, and endocarditis. (c) *Actinomyces*: actinomycosis and uterine infections (IUD**

associated). (d) *Peptostreptococcus* spp.: brain abscess, female genital tract abscesses, intraabdominal infectious processes, aspiration pneumonia, and bite wound infections. (e) Pigmented anaerobic gram-negative bacilli, *Porphyromonas* spp. and *Prevotella* spp.: oral abscesses, aspiration pneumonia, brain abscesses, and bite wound infections. (f) Nonpigmenting *Prevotella* spp., *Mobiluncus* spp., and *Peptostreptococcus* spp. are involved in bacterial vaginosis.

6. Extracellular enzyme production and induction of a host inflammatory response are the key pathogenic mechanisms of nonspore-forming anaerobes other than the *B. fragilis* group.

7. Specimens must be collected to avoid contamination by normal mucosal flora, which can reach numbers up to 10^{11}/g, and to avoid exposure to oxygen during collection, transport, and laboratory manipulation.

REFERENCES

Appelbaum PC (1987): Anaerobic infections, nonsporeformers. In Wentworth BB (ed): Diagnostic procedures for bacterial infections. 7th ed. Washington, DC: American Public Health Association, pp 45–109.

Finegold SM, George WL (eds) (1989): Anaerobic infections in humans. San Diego: Academic Press, 851 pp.

Finegold SM, Wexler HM (1988): Therapeutic implications of bacteriologic findings in mixed aerobic-anaerobic infections. Antimicrob Agents Chemother 32:611.

Rodloff AC, Appelbaum PC, Zabransky RJ (1991): Cumitech 5A. Practical anaerobic bacteriology. In Rodloff AC (ed): American Society of Microbiologists Washington, DC, 17 pp.

Styrt B, Gorbach SL (1989): Recent developments in the understanding of the pathogenesis and treatment of anaerobic infections, Parts 1 and 2. N Engl J Med 321:240; 321:298.

Summanen P, Baron EJ, Citron DM, Strong CA, Wexler HM, Finegold SM (1993): Wadsworth Anaerobic Bacteriology Manual. 5th ed. Belmont, CA: Star Publishing, 180 pp.

REVIEW QUESTIONS

> For questions 1 to 6, choose the ONE
> BEST answer or completion.

1. The main virulence factor of *Bacteroides fragilis,* the most important agent of infection among the nonspore-forming anaerobes, is
   a) adherent capsular material
   b) antiphagocytic capsular material
   c) abscess inducing capsular material
   d) resistance to penicillins
   e) production of a potent cytotoxin

2. Superoxide dismutase enzyme may act as a virulence factor by
   a) acting as a powerful leukocidin that destroys host macrophages and other phagocytes
   b) reducing harmful oxygen radicals to allow survival in well-perfused tissue
   c) inhibiting abscess formation in the abdominal cavity
   d) dissolving host tissue collagen and allowing spread of the organisms
   e) lysing RBCs (hemolysin)

3. Which of the following is NOT a feature important in the development of mixed flora anaerobic-aerobic abscesses?
   a) Production of elastase by anaerobes within the abscess.
   b) Lowered oxygen tension in the abscess.

   c) Production of pigments by oral anaerobes.
   d) Inhibition of phagocytosis mediated by capsular polysaccharide.
   e) Fibrin and other host tissue deposits around periphery of abscess limit access by host immune factors and antimicrobial agents.

4. Gram stains of vaginal discharge are rarely accepted for definitive diagnosis of gonorrhea because
   a) anaerobic bacteria in the vagina prevent adherence of *Neisseria gonorrhoeae,* so they cannot be seen on Gram stain
   b) the numerous lactobacilli mask the presence of *N. gonorrhoeae*
   c) *Veillonella* species, normal female genital tract flora, are also gram-negative diplococci and may result in false-positive results
   d) there are so many bacteria in the vagina that gonococci are virtually impossible to identify independently based on Gram-stain morphology alone
   e) organisms may have been introduced externally and are only transiently colonizing the patient

5. Isolation of nonspore-forming anaerobes in the microbiology laboratory demands that one

a) inoculate laked blood agar plates and incubate at 35°C
b) inoculate special supplemented media and incubate in an atmosphere of less than 0.5% oxygen
c) inoculate special supplemented media and a backup broth and incubate in an atmosphere of 18% oxygen
d) inoculate laked blood agar plates and incubate at 35°C in 10% oxygen
e) inoculate special supplemented media and incubate at 37°C in an atmosphere of 10% oxygen

6. What characteristic of the aspirated contents of an abscess suggests an anaerobic infection?
a) Bright red color of aspirated material.
b) Presence of fat globules.
c) Gram stain showing large gram-negative bacilli.
d) Foul odor.
e) Gray-green color, anchovy-pastelike consistency of aspirated material.

For questions 7 to 11, a list of lettered options is followed by several numbered items. For each numbered item, select the ONE lettered option that is most closely associated with it.

A) *Actinomyces israelii*
B) *Porphyromonas gingivalis*
C) *Fusobacterium nucleatum*
D) *Propionibacterium acnes*
E) *Peptostreptococcus anaerobius*

Choose the bacterial species most likely to be associated with the following infectious processes.

---

7. A woman with a 10-year history of an IUD visits her gynecologist because of abdominal pain and a foul-smelling discharge from her vagina.

8. A Gram stain of material from a brain abscess shows numerous gram-positive cocci in chains.

9. A prosthetic hip develops signs of infection 8 months after the patient has gone home from the hospital.

10. A Gram stain of pus aspirated by needle and syringe from the lung of a patient who acquired aspiration pneumonia shows pale, narrow, gram-negative bacilli with pointed ends.

11. A patient has an endodontal (at the root of the tooth) abscess drained. Cultures yield a pure culture.

ANSWERS TO REVIEW QUESTIONS

1. **c** Capsular polysaccharide of *Bacteroides fragilis,* even in the absence of viable bacteria, can induce the formation of abscesses when appropriate cofactors are present.

2. **b** Superoxide dismutase seems to be possessed in higher amounts by more virulent anaerobes than in the less virulent species. By breaking down toxic oxygen radicals, it allows prolonged survival in air of anaerobes that possess this enzyme compared to the survival time of those anaerobes deficient in the enzyme.

3. **a** Elastase is not produced by anaerobes in abscesses.

4. **c** Only this statement is true. Although veillonellae are usually smaller than gonococci, they may fool inexperienced workers.

5. **b** Anaerobes grow only in a very low E_h ($< 0.5\%$ or less). The use of more than one medium, all of which must be supplemented with vitamin K and hemin, and the special atmosphere at 35–37°C, will improve isolation of anaerobes from specimens.

6. **d** Foul odor is a strong clue suggestive of anaerobic infection. Aerobic and facultative anaerobic bacteria do not produce the short-chain fatty acids responsible for the odor that are produced during anaerobic metabolism.

7. **A** The woman probably has an actinomycotic infection of her IUD.

8. **E** *Peptostreptococcus* species are very common in brain abscess. Other species named (*Prevotella,* and *Porphyromonas*), although they are also involved in brain abscess, are gram-negative rods.

9. **D** *Propionibacterium acnes,* because it is normal skin flora, is the most common anaerobic bacterium associated with prosthetic device infections. It is also a common contaminant in blood cultures, and must be distinguished from a real infectious agent.

10. **C** *Fusobacterium nucleatum,* normal oral flora and thus a common agent in aspiration pneumonia, displays a characteristic gram morphology: pale, thin, pointed-ended gram-negative bacilli.

11. **B** *Porphyromonas gingivalis,* a pigmenting gram-negative bacillus, is among the most common etiologic agents of endodontal infections (see Table 11.1).

HAEMOPHILUS INFECTION AND DISEASE, AND PERTUSSIS

Several genera of pleomorphic gram-negative bacilli are inhabitants of the respiratory tract and other mucosal surfaces of humans and diverse mammals. Under certain circumstances, they cause disease. The two genera discussed in this chapter, *Haemophilus* and *Bordetella,* both require special growth factors for in vitro cultivation and both produce an extracellular capsule that serves as an antiphagocytic virulence factor. These genera initiate disease by colonizing the respiratory tract epithelium, although they adhere to different cell types.

Haemophilus influenzae, the most important species in the genus, is an agent of **sepsis and meningitis** (especially in children), **otitis media, contagious conjunctivitis** (pink-eye), **epiglottitis, pneumonia, cellulitis,** and urinary tract infections. *Haemophilus ducreyi* is responsible for **chancroid,** a highly contagious sexually transmitted disease that seems to place victims at increased risk of acquiring HIV infection from sexual intercourse. Other *Haemophilus* species occasionally cause respiratory tract infections, sepsis, and endocarditis in immunocompromised humans. As with all opportunistic pathogens, normally commensal *Haemophilus* species can cause a variety of infections if they encounter a susceptible host.

Bordetella pertussis, an obligate parasite of humans, is the etiologic agent of **whooping cough.** Other species of *Bordetella* are important agents of respiratory disease in animals and occasionally infect humans as well. Unusual presentations of whooping cough in previously vaccinated individuals are gaining recognition in the United States.

HAEMOPHILUS SPECIES

Haemophilus species were first isolated during a viral pandemic of influenza in the 1890s, hence the species name *influenzae.* The bacterium was thought to be the cause of the pandemic. The organism was probably a secondary invader of epithelial tissues damaged by the virus. The association of secondary bacterial pneumonia as a sequel to primary viral respiratory tract disease is now well established.

Eight species of *Haemophilus* can cause human disease. The most important are listed in Table 12.1. **Species are differentiated by their requirements for hemin** (growth factor X) and **nicotinamide adenine dinucleotide (NAD;** growth factor V). *H. influenzae,* the most important species, contains six biotypes that can be differentiated biochemically and by the types of disease they cause. This species is the worldwide major etiologic agent of meningitis in infants and children aged 2 months to 5 years. A subgroup of *H. influenzae, H. influenzae* biogroup *aegyptius,* is responsible for a fulminant and occasionally fatal disease in Brazilian children called Brazilian purpuric fever. A less virulent form of the *aegyptius* strain is associated with acute contagious conjunctivitis (pink-eye) in the United States.

Because of its importance as the major pathogen in the genus, the bulk of the discussion to follow will center on *H. influenzae.*

TABLE 12.1. Most Common Species of *Haemophilus* That Infect Humans

Species	Growth factors		Associated infection
	X	V	
aphrophilus	+?	—	Rare cause of respiratory tract infections, endocarditis, and others
ducreyi	+	—	Chancroid
haemolyticus	+	+	Rare abscesses and endocarditis
influenzae	+	+	Sepsis, meningitis, pneumonia, epiglottitis, urinary tract infection, otitis, sinusitis, and conjunctivitis

HAEMOPHILUS INFLUENZAE INFECTIONS

Along with *Streptococcus pneumoniae* and *Neisseria meningitidis*, *H. influenzae* is one of the three major etiologic agents of meningitis (see Fig. 12.1). Paradoxically, the same organism is part of the normal flora in the upper respiratory tract of as many as 80% of humans. **A major virulence factor is the polysaccharide capsule; capsule type b** is responsible for greater than 90% of all serious infections. Only 5% of asymptomatic persons carry *H. influenzae* type b. Nonencapsulated strains cause infections, but they rarely disseminate beyond localized sites. Since the introduction and widespread use of the very effective polysaccharide vaccine in 1987, invasive *H. influenzae* type b disease has decreased dramatically (reported decreases of 70–90%) in the United States.

Antibody to the capsule is protective; thus infants less than 2 months old are unlikely to become infected because of passively transferred maternal antibody. As adults age and the immune system becomes less active or during other immunocompromised states, they are again at risk for *H. influenzae* infection, notably pneumonia. Other types of infections seen are cellulitis and purulent infections at diverse sites. There is also increasing interest in *H. influenzae* as a cause of urinary tract infections.

Habitat

H. influenzae is part of the normal upper respiratory tract flora of humans. It colonizes the mucosal layer of pharyngeal epithelial cells. There is no other known reservoir. Nontypable, often unencapsulated strains are more likely to be isolated from healthy humans, but capsular polysaccharide type b strains do appear. The organisms do not cause pharyngitis, but multiplication and subsequent invasion almost always are initiated from a respiratory tract focus.

Transmission

EXOGENOUS. *H. influenzae* **is transmitted on secretions,** either by aerosol droplets or **on the hands.** Once acquired, the organisms colonize the nasopharyngeal epithelium. Virulent, encapsulated strains are often colonizers in asymptomatic children, who develop antibodies over time. The presence of antibodies, including secretory IgA, against capsular polysaccharide selects for nonencapsulated strains as children grow older. By age 5 years, most children have

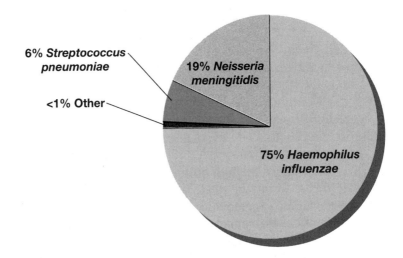

6% *Streptococcus pneumoniae*

19% *Neisseria meningitidis*

<1% Other

75% *Haemophilus influenzae*

Figure 12.1.
Pie chart showing relative contribution of *H. influenzae, S. pneumoniae,* and *N. meningitidis* to causes of meningitis in 5-year-old children prior to widespread use of vaccine in the United States.

antibody to type b polysaccharide, so that colonizing strains of *H. influenzae* are likely to be nonencapsulated.

ENDOGENOUS. Carriers develop disease after a breakdown of normal host defenses. Organisms colonizing the nasopharynx begin to multiply and invoke a host response. Encapsulated strains are most likely to cause disease in children without actively acquired antibody. Adults with impaired immunity are more likely to develop disease associated with a nonencapsulated (nontypable) strain.

Properties of the Organism

Resistance to environmental, physical, and chemical agents. The *Haemophilus* species are highly susceptible to drying, sunlight, and disinfectants, and die rapidly on inanimate objects (fomites).

Microscopic morphology. The organisms are **pleomorphic, nonmotile gram-negative bacilli,** ranging from tiny coccobacilli to long filamentous forms within the same specimen or culture. The strains that cause disseminated infections are usually encapsulated.

Macroscopic morphology. H. influenzae is a facultative anaerobe **requiring 3–10% carbon dioxide (capnophilic)** for initial isolation. Its growth in broth is unusual in that organism density may never reach a point that allows visual detection of turbidity. Both X and V growth factors (Table 12.2) must be present

TABLE 12.2. Growth Factors Required by *H. influenzae*

Factor	Description
X	Heme portion of hemoglobin; required for synthesis of essential enzymes
V	Nicotinamide adenine dinucleotide (NAD) or NAD phosphate (NADP); co-enzymes. Present in erythrocytes but unavailable for some erythrocyte types, such as sheep RBCs, unless the cell membrane is lysed. Intact horse and rabbit RBCs provide V factor

for growth of the organism in vitro. However, other bacteria growing in mixed culture with *Haemophilus* species may provide the missing growth factor; e.g., *H. influenzae* cannot grow on sheep blood agar, which contains only X factor, most of which is unavailable in intact RBCs. When a *Staphylococcus aureus* is cocultured on the medium, *H. influenzae* can grow as tiny satellite colonies close to the staphylococcal colonies. This reaction occurs because the staphylococci secrete V factor (NAD) into the medium surrounding their colonies and because red cell lysis induced by staphylococcal hemolysins releases both heme and NAD from blood cells in the medium. *H. influenzae* grows best on chocolate agar (red cells are heated to release X factor and enzymes are inactivated to prevent destruction of V factor).

Antigenic structure. The **polysaccharide capsule is the primary virulence factor;** it has antiphagocytic activity. Six capsular antigenic types are known, but only type b is important in disease. *H. influenzae* capsule type b consists of polyribose-ribitol phosphate (PRP). Typing of isolates in the laboratory is accomplished easily using one of many commercially available systems. Practically speaking, laboratories only type isolates for type b; all others are reported as ''nontypable'' or ignored.

Outer-membrane proteins are present but have no known pathogenic significance. Like other gram-negative bacilli, *H. influenzae* cell walls contain lipopolysaccharides (LPS); in this case it is a variant called lipooligosaccharide (LOS). Its role in pathogenicity has not been determined. Fimbriae or pili may mediate attachment but this aspect of colonization is not well characterized.

Extracellular products associated with pathogenicity. No extracellular products are known to act as virulence factors. Capsular polysaccharides are released into the surrounding tissue and can be detected in serum and urine, however, which is useful for noninvasive diagnosis by immunoserological tests for these antigens.

Pathogenesis and Clinical Manifestations

H. influenzae **colonize the mucous membranes of the upper respiratory tract.** In many cases, there is no local disease. However, host factors may allow the organisms to produce a localized purulent infection, usually manifested as otitis, sinusitis, or cellulitis.

Epiglottitis is a life-threatening type of cellulitis that starts at the epiglottis and spreads into surrounding tissues. The most immediate risk is for complete airway obstruction. Procuring a throat culture is not recommended in cases of epiglottitis because of the possibility of spasm. Although epiglottitis is not common in the United States, it should be diagnosed quickly and accurately because of its high morbidity. Children often sit with chin protruded to breathe more clearly and may drool because they are unable to swallow.

Even in the absence of local disease, the capsule allows *H. influenzae* to evade phagocytosis and multiply. After achieving an essential mass 2–4 days later, the organisms invade the epithelium and are carried to regional lymph nodes. Once they have invaded through the mucosa, the organisms lose their pili; bacteria recovered from systemic sites are nonpiliated. From the lymph nodes, the bacteria are seeded into the bloodstream, causing septicemia, characterized by fever and other common manifestations of sepsis. Alternatively, septicemia can follow a local respiratory tract infection, such as otitis media. **If untreated, septicemia can progress within hours to fatal septic shock.**

Bacteria in the bloodstream show an affinity for the central nervous system (CNS). Meningitis caused by *H. influenzae* is indistinguishable clinically from that of the other acute bacterial meningitides, with signs of fever, vomiting, lethargy, and nuchal rigidity. If inadequately treated, and often even when adequately treated, complications of *Haemophilus* meningitis may develop, including subdural effusions, seizures, and **long-term neurologic defects.** It is estimated that as many as 50% of children retain some functional abnormality after recovering from *H. influenzae* meningitis.

Other infections caused by *H. influenzae* are listed below:

1. Pneumonia. Pneumonia is the most common serious disease in adults caused by *H. influenzae* occuring both as community-acquired cases and as nosocomial disease. *H. influenzae*-associated pneumonia is rare in children.

2. Septic arthritis. *H. influenzae* can infect a joint after hematogenous seeding. This is a common infection both in children and adults.

3. Osteomyelitis. Also acquired during septicemia, osteomyelitis is caused by *H. influenzae* type b strains.

4. Infections caused by nonencapsulated, nontypable strains. Nonencapsu-

lated strains are usually responsible for localized, purulent infections such as chronic bronchitis, otitis, sinusitis, and cellulitis. These infections are more common in adults than children.

Immunity to Reinfection

Antibody against capsular polysaccharide type b is protective. Secretory IgA may exert some protection against mucosal colonization, but its role is unclear. Reinfection with other capsular types and with nontypable strains is not prevented by the antitype b antibody.

Laboratory Diagnosis

SPECIMENS. In order **to diagnose meningitis, cerebrospinal fluid (CSF) and blood cultures** should be obtained. Insasmuch as the polysaccharide capsular antigen is concentrated in the kidneys and collects in the urine, this specimen may be tested for antigen. In pyogenic infections, purulent exudate is collected by aspiration or on a swab, as indicated. Isolation of *H. influenzae* from patients with pneumonia is not an easy task. Sputum is never a very satisfactory specimen, since the oropharynx is usually contaminated with the same organisms that may be pathogenic. **Bronchoalveolar lavage is the specimen of choice** for diagnosis of nosocomial pneumonia. Blood cultures may reveal the etiologic agent in 20% of the cases. In cases of epiglottitis, direct culture collection from the affected throat is not recommended, since the trauma may cause airway obstruction. Blood cultures are often positive.

PRIMARY ISOLATION AND IDENTIFICATION. Direct microscopic visualization of organisms in CSF should be attempted for all suspected cases of bacterial meningitis. Gram stains prepared using a cytocentrifuge to concentrate cells and organisms are the most sensitive, but centrifuged sediment is also an excellent specimen to examine.

Rapid tests for polysaccharide antigens, such as latex particle agglutination assays, are useful for CSF and urine specimens, especially those from children. Of the tests available, those testing for *H. influenzae* type b seem to yield the most clinically useful results. Older formats for direct antigen detection, such as counterimmunoelectrophoresis and coagglutination, are less sensitive and specific than the newer commercial products. Although the Gram stain is usually as sensitive and more conclusive than the antigen tests, polysaccharide antigen detection assays play a useful role in the diagnosis of disease in patients with partially treated infections and in validating a tentative morphologic identification of an organism seen on a Gram stain.

Culture of all specimens must be carried out on a medium containing X and V factors. If chocolate agar or other suitable medium is not available, 5% sheep blood agar may be cross-streaked with *S. aureus* to provide the V growth factor. The organism is capnophilic, i.e., 5–10% carbon dioxide enhances growth of *H. influenzae.*

Human blood contains sufficient X and V factors to support growth of this organism in blood cultures. Since blood cultures may not show any visible turbidity, if they are not being monitored instrumentally, they should be subcultured blindly before being discarded as negative. Because the carriage rate of *H. influenzae* is so high among uninfected individuals, culture of the nasopharynx or throat is never recommended.

Identification of isolates is based on requirement for X and V factors (Fig. 12.2), enzymatic and biochemical test results, hemolytic activity on rabbit blood, and possibly serotype. *Haemophilus haemolyticus* and *Haemophilus parahaemolyticus* are β hemolytic on rabbit blood, whereas the other species are nonhemolytic. Encapsulated strains can be serotyped using specific antisera. Since only type b has epidemiologic and pathogenic implications, most laboratories have only type b antiserum available for typing isolates.

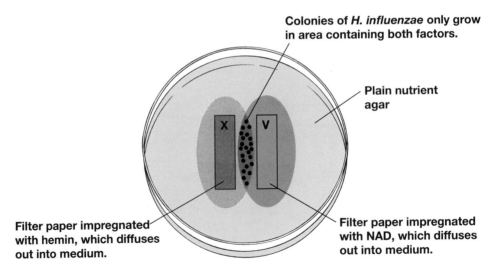

Colonies of *H. influenzae* only grow in area containing both factors.

Plain nutrient agar

Filter paper impregnated with hemin, which diffuses out into medium.

Filter paper impregnated with NAD, which diffuses out into medium.

Figure 12.2.

Enhancement of the growth of *H. influenzae* on nutrient agar plate with X and V factor strips.

Treatment

The current treatment recommendations for meningitis are either **a combination of ampicillin and chloramphenicol** (classic therapy) or **cefotaxime** (new therapy). Otitis and sinusitis are usually treated with amoxicillin-clavulanic acid. Ampicillin is the drug of choice for pneumonia and urinary tract infections. Alternative therapies include cefuroxime, trimethoprim-sulfamethoxazole, and doxycycline.

Prevention and Control

H. influenzae type b polyribose-ribitol phosphate (PRP) capsular conjugate vaccines are available for children age 2 months and older. These vaccines combine the poorly immunogenic capsular antigen with a more immunogenic protein antigen, hence the term ''conjugate.'' Efficacy is approximately 93%. All children should now be vaccinated before they enter day care, and should preferably begin their vaccination series at age 6 weeks. Widespread vaccination has profoundly decreased the number of invasive *H. influenzae* type b infections in the United States and prevented much of the severe and common sequelae of meningitis.

Adults at risk of acquiring *H. influenzae* b disease, such as patients infected with HIV, those with sickle cell disease or leukemia, splenectomized patients, and the elderly with chronic lung disease, may benefit from the conjugate vaccine, but no large-scale trials have examined the issue.

Rifampin should be administered as a **prophylactic agent** to close household contacts of an index case who may be at risk of developing meningitis. Rifampin can also be used to eradicate the carrier state if susceptible individuals are present in a household to which an infected patient returns following hospitalization. Rifampin susceptibility should be verified with a susceptibility test, since resistant strains of *H. influenzae* have been described.

HAEMOPHILUS DUCREYI DISEASE (CHANCROID)

H. ducreyi disease (chancroid, or soft chancre) has been a common sexually transmitted disease (STD) primarily of tropical, undeveloped areas of the world. However, since 1985 several large outbreaks have occurred in the United States, principally in California. In the last 6 years, approximately 4000 cases have been reported annually in the United States. Males are the predominant victims, although female prostitutes have been the vehicle of transmission.

The organism, *H. ducreyi,* inhabits the genital tract of humans only. Organisms enter the susceptible host through breaks in the skin or genital epithelium during sexual intercourse and multiply locally for up to 1 week, forming a small erythematous papule. The papule develops into a painful, friable ulcer that may be confused with a primary syphilitic chancre by inexperienced clinicians. Organisms are carried to the inguinal lymph nodes where they multiply and produce a lymphadenopathy prone to rupture. Exudates from the primary chancre and nodes are highly contagious.

Although Gram stain of the exudate of an ulcerative lesion may show the typical small, pleomorphic gram-negative bacilli in characteristic clusters (*school of fish* morphology), this is unusual. Culture should be attempted. Exudate must be inoculated onto fresh media containing X growth factor, serum, and vancomycin as a selective agent. Better recovery is obtained when two different media are employed. The organism grows best in an atmosphere with increased carbon dioxide and high humidity.

Treatment with ceftriaxone, erythromycin, ciprofloxacin, amoxicillin-clavulanic acid, or trimethoprim-sulfamethoxazole has been effective.

INFECTIONS CAUSED BY OTHER *HAEMOPHILUS* SPECIES

Haemophilus influenzae Biogroup *aegyptius*

H. influenzae biogroup *aegyptius* has historically been called the Koch-Weeks bacillus. This organism, closely related to *H. influenzae,* is the **agent of acute contagious conjunctivitis, or pink-eye.** Humans are the only host for this organism and the infection is spread by hands and objects contaminated with eye secretions.

One related group of *H. influenzae* biogroup *aegyptius* is also the agent of Brazilian purpuric fever, a fulminant, occasionally fatal systemic febrile disease that begins as a hemorrhagic conjunctivitis. The strain responsible for this disease is currently confined to areas of South America.

Other Species of *Haemophilus*

There are other species of *Haemophilus* that are of low virulence and rarely cause infections. Occasionally, however, they enter the bloodstream from oral sites, and if they encounter a damaged heart valve they may colonize it and cause endocarditis. Hematogenous seeding is also responsible for septic arthritis and osteomyelitis of extremities and spine. Immunocompromised adults and elderly patients are at risk for developing cellulitis and pneumonia from normally non-pathogenic *Haemophilus* species.

BORDETELLA PERTUSSIS

PERTUSSIS

Whooping cough or pertussis (*Bordetella pertussis* disease) was one of the most important infectious diseases of children in the United States. As many as 265,000 cases and 7500 deaths each year were attributed to *B. pertussis* infections during the 1930s. After use of the vaccine became widely adopted in the late 1940s, pertussis declined to its present low incidence. Approximately 4500 cases were reported in the United States in 1990. The true incidence is likely to be much higher, however, inasmuch as many cases go unrecognized because the presentation of disease in previously vaccinated patients is not typical. It is estimated by some that only 11% of cases are reported.

The term "pertussis" refers to the intensive cough experienced by patients. The whooping stage is not universal, but has given the disease its name. Bouts of coughing can last so long that patients are deprived of oxygen; at the end of a coughing bout, they forcefully draw air back into the lungs with the characteristic "whoop."

Currently there are three named species that can cause respiratory disease in humans (see Table 12.3). *B. pertussis* is the most important human pathogen; the others cause milder disease and will not be mentioned further.

TABLE 12.3. *Bordetella* **Species Recovered From Humans**

Species	Normal host
bronchiseptica	Wild and domestic animals: rabbits, dogs, swine
parapertussis	Humans only (may be a nonvirulent variant of *B. pertussis*)
pertussis	Humans only

Habitat

***B. pertussis* colonizes the ciliated epithelial cells of the human respiratory tract.** It is the only pathogenic bacterium known to colonize this cell type exclusively. All colonized individuals are considered as having the disease; there is **no asymptomatic carrier state.**

Transmission

EXOGENOUS. The organism is **highly contagious.** Attack rates among close contacts vary from 50 to 100%. Transmission occurs via **aerosol droplets** that are breathed in by the susceptible host. Because the disease may develop slowly and secretions are contagious during both the early catarrhal and the paroxysmal phases, an infected person may transmit disease for several weeks.

Properties of the Organism

Resistance to environmental, physical, and chemical agents. Bordetella are easily killed by desiccation, heat, and chemical agents. These organisms do not survive on fomites for any length of time.

Microscopic morphology. ***Bordetella* are very small gram-negative, non-motile coccobacilli.** These organisms possess fimbriae, but their role in adherence is not well characterized. Some strains produce an extracellular polysaccharide capsule that has been used in serotyping schemes, but no role in pathogenicity has been demonstrated for this component.

Macroscopic morphology. Bordetella is a **strict aerobe.** It does not ferment carbohydrates; its metabolism is based on the oxidization of amino acids. The growth of *Bordetella* on artificial media is slow, taking up to 10 days for its initial isolation. Recovery of *B. pertussis* requires specialized media containing factors to neutralize the inhibitory effects of fatty acids, sulfides, and peroxides.

Bordet-Gengou medium, formulated with potatoes, glycerol, and added sheep RBCs, has been traditionally the medium of choice. For optimal isolation of the organism, the medium must be freshly prepared. Today, newer media without blood containing charcoals and ion-exchange resins are recommended. On permissive media, colonies are shiny and have a characteristic metallic or pearly sheen. On blood agar, they show a small zone of hemolysis.

Antigenic structure. The antigenic structure of this organism is shown in Figure 12.3. A single cell wall somatic O protein antigen is common to all three

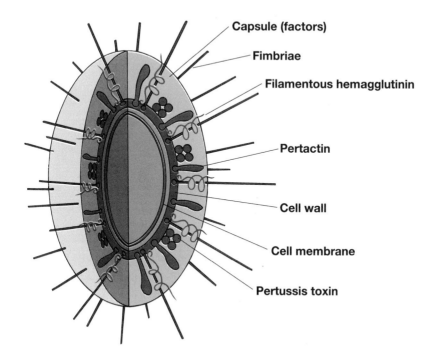

Capsule (factors)

Fimbriae

Filamentous hemagglutinin

Pertactin

Cell wall

Cell membrane

Pertussis toxin

Figure 12.3.
B. pertussis showing structural antigens.

species of *Bordetella*. Fourteen capsular polysaccharide types (called **Factors**) exist. Factor 7 is common to the entire genus and Factors 1–6 are found on *B. pertussis* only. Factor 1 may be an agglutinating antigen with some role in attachment. The Factor antigens are used in vaccine preparation, not because antibodies against them are protective, but because presence of anti-Factor antibody is one marker used to evaluate vaccine effectiveness.

Filamentous hemagglutinin (FHA), a surface protein associated with the fimbriae, **is the major adhesin associated with colonization.** This protein mediates binding of *B. pertussis* to the cholesterol-containing receptors of respiratory cilia. The presence of antibody against FHA is the best predictor of vaccine efficacy in children.

The fimbriae (pili) of *B. pertussis* may also play a role in adherence to epithelial cells. Changes in the proteins expressed on fimbriae during growth cycles are designated "Phases." Freshly recovered isolates usually express Phase I and exhibit smooth, shiny colonies. After passage in vitro, progression to less virulent Phases II, III, and IV are seen. When the organisms reach Phase IV, the colonies have passed through intermediate morphologic stages and are now rough. Another protein, an outer membrane protein (OMP) called "pertactin," may act as an additional adhesin. The pertussis toxin (described below) is also a cell wall associated protein hemagglutinin, known variously as lymphocyte-promoting factor (LPF), histamine-sensitizing factor, and pertussigen.

Extracellular products associated with pathogenicity:

1. Pertussis toxin. **Pertussis toxin (pertussigen) is a four polypeptide toxin with diverse activities.** Pertussigen's biological activities include its actions as a histamine-sensitizing factor; as a lymphocytosis-promoting factor, with polyclonal activation of T lymphocytes and inhibition of lymphocyte migration from blood vessels; and as an islet-activating protein that alters insulin secreting functions. The toxin has two structural domains. As with most other subunit toxins, the B subunit mediates binding of the toxin and induces internalization while the A subunit carries out the biological activities. The toxin seems to act by **ribosylating a glycoprotein in the cell membrane,** using nicotine adenine dinucleotide (NAD) as a cofactor. The final result of toxin action is **activation of adenylate cyclase** and increased cyclic AMP (cAMP) in the host cell. Cholera and diphtheria toxins act in a similar manner.

2. Adenylate cyclase toxin. Once inside the target cell (often a leukocyte), this toxin is activated by calmodulin to catalyze the formation of cAMP from ATP. The increased cAMP interferes with cell function and may cause death. The toxin is also thought to be the hemolysin of the organism, since no specific hemolysin has been identified.

3. Tracheal cytotoxin. This toxin, considered to be a component of the bacterial cell wall peptidoglycan, inhibits ciliary motility, inhibits DNA synthesis, and ultimately causes death of ciliated epithelial cells. The dead ciliary cells are sloughed from the mucosal surface. Interestingly, a similar toxin is produced by many gram-negative bacteria.

4. Dermonecrotic toxin. Dermonecrotic toxin (mouse-lethal toxin or heat-labile toxin) is a heat-labile toxin that causes vascular smooth muscle contraction and results in necrotic lesions at the site of bacterial multiplication.

5. Lipopolysaccharide (LPS). Although the biological effects of *B. pertussis* LPS are similar to those of the lipopolysaccharides of other gram-negative bacteria, the former differs in that the activities are distributed between two separate structural entities with the core region appearing to possess greater toxicity.

Pathogenesis and Clinical Manifestations

B. pertussis enters the nasotracheal turbinates on aerosols and attaches to ciliated respiratory epithelial cells in the bronchi and trachea. Adherence is mediated by FHA, and probably by the fimbriae proteins and pertactin OMP. As the organism multiplies, it produces adenylate cyclase toxin, which inhibits phago-cytosis; tracheal cytotoxin, which prevents ciliary motion and mucociliary clear-ance; and pertussis toxin, which disrupts epithelial cell function.

Local tissue damage is caused by the dermonecrotic toxin resulting in clinical symptoms of the first stage of disease (catarrhal). During this stage, which is manifested 6–20 days after infection, the disease is highly communicable. Patients exhibit red eyes, runny nose, mild cough, and sneezing. During the next week, the cough progresses to a more severe, hacking cough (paroxysmal stage). Cough-ing spasms occur as often as 1/h; vomiting often follows. Any stimulus, such as a loud noise, air current, or even suggestion, can initiate a coughing paroxysm. The characteristic whoop is heard at this stage as the patient struggles to breathe at the end of a long, anoxic coughing fit. Hypoxia during coughing spasms can lead to death. After a paroxysm, patients are exhausted and lethargic, but otherwise not in much distress. Patients are much less contagious during the paroxysmal stage, which can last from 1 to 4 weeks.

Convalescence extends for 1–6 months. Paroxysms slowly regress and be-come less severe. Recovery is slow. Complications are not common, but they may be severe. These complications can include (a) pneumonia caused by secondary bacterial infection (bronchiectasis); (b) seizures, encephalopathy, and coma; and (c) hemorrhagic events due to the high blood pressure exerted during coughing.

For some unknown reason, this disease is more common and morbidity more severe in females than males.

Immunity to Reinfection

Most people are immune after convalescence from pertussis, but second at-tacks have been reported. Insasmuch as protective antibody does not cross the placenta, neonates are highly susceptible. **Immunization with the current vac-cine** of whole killed cells of *B. pertussis* in a trivalent vaccine containing diph-theria and tetanus toxoids **confers a high degree of protection.** Vaccine efficacy is 80–90% but appears to disappear after some years (10–12 years). Vaccinated adults may contract mild, atypical disease, but still serve as reservoirs of infection for susceptible hosts.

In rare instances, adverse reactions to immunization include convulsions and encephalopathy. More common adverse reactions involve fever, erythema and swelling at the inoculation site, anorexia, and vomiting. Some vaccinated babies cry fretfully for days. Because of adverse reactions and inner city populations that fall outside of normal health care delivery modes, vaccination compliance is waning in the United States, contributing to an increase in the numbers of cases of pertussis. Large unvaccinated populations present a stage for epidemic outbreaks.

Laboratory Diagnosis

SPECIMENS. Secretions collected on **nasopharyngeal swabs** consisting of calcium alginate or Dacron on wire handles **are the best specimen.** The wire can be bent to conform to the nasal passage and the swab should be inserted deep into the nostril until it touches the pharynx and be allowed to remain there for 30 s, if possible (Fig. 12.4). The swab must be inoculated immediately onto media at the patient's bedside or transported in a moist, protective medium to the laboratory for immediate culture. Two swabs, one from each nostril, are ideal. Cough plates are not recommended. If transport of the swab is required, it should be placed immediately in charcoal-blood transport or Amies charcoal transport medium. For short transport times, the specimen may remain at room temperature. For longer transport times, it is probably best to refrigerate the sample unless selective antibiotics in the transport medium allow enrichment of *B. pertussis.* In the latter case, incubation is recommended. Nasopharngeal washings might be a useful specimen, but the predilection to initiate a paroxysm renders this method unacceptable.

PRIMARY ISOLATION AND IDENTIFICATION. Direct fluorescent antibody (DFA) stains for the organism are the fastest diagnostic tool. Although this

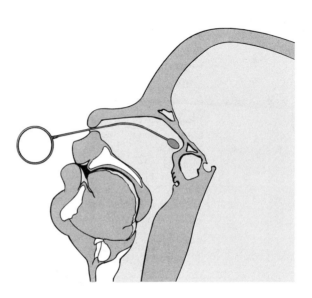

Figure 12.4.
Diagram illustrating collection of pertussis specimen with a nasopharyngeal swab.

method is only 60% sensitive, it is very specific. Nasopharyngeal swabs are rolled directly onto slides and stained for presence of the bacteria. Because of its low sensitivity, the DFA test should never be performed without concommitant cultures.

Specimens are inoculated onto special media, such as Regan-Lowe agar, Jones-Kendrick charcoal agar, or freshly made Bordet-Gengou agar. Cultures are incubated in a humidified atmosphere without added carbon dioxide for a minimum of 10 days. Once the characteristic colonies appear, they can be identified using a fluorescent antibody stain. *B. pertussis* is oxidase positive and microscopic examination should reveal very tiny gram-negative coccobacilli.

IMMUNOSEROLOGIC TESTS. Enzyme-linked immunosorbent assay (ELISA) tests specific for IgM and IgG in serum and IgA in respiratory secretions have been evaluated favorably for early diagnosis of pertussis. They have not yet gained widespread use or availability.

Treatment

Primary treatment is supportive. **Erythromycin,** because of its higher penetration into the respiratory tract, is the antibiotic of choice for cases that require therapy. Treatment ameliorates severity of the disease. During the paroxysmal phase, some patients may benefit from steroids to reduce symptoms. **Close contacts at risk** of acquiring infection **should be treated with erythromycin prophylactically.**

Prevention and Control

Vaccination is the key to control; all susceptible populations should be immunized. Immunization of unvaccinated children older than 7 years of age or adults is not recommended at this time because of the decreased severity of disease among these age groups. Acellular vaccines are in the development stage. Because of the multipronged pathogenesis of pertussis, component vaccines are essential. Such vaccines are more difficult to prepare and evaluate.

SUMMARY

1. *Haemophilus* **species are pleomorphic, capnophilic (grows best in enhanced CO_2 atmosphere) gram-negative bacilli that require one or both growth factors: (a) hemin (X factor) or (b) NAD (V factor).**

2. These organisms are part of the normal respiratory mucosal flora in mammals. Infections are acquired by aerosol and occasionally by contact transmission of respiratory secretions.

3. *Haemophilus influenzae*, the most important species, causes acute bacterial meningitis in children 2 months to 5 years of age after maternal protective antibody has dissipated and before colonization has induced active antibody development.

4. Other infectious syndromes caused by *H. influenzae* include septicemia, pneumonia (older adults), epiglottitis, otitis, sinusitis, cellulitis, and contagious bacterial conjunctivitis (pink-eye).

5. The most important virulence factor is the polysaccharide capsule, which aids the bacterium in evading phagocytosis. Polysaccharide vaccine is extremely effective.

6. Up to 80% of asymptomatic persons carry nontypable *H. influenzae* as part of the normal flora in the respiratory tract. Only 5% of asymptomatic persons carry *H. influenzae* capsular type b, the virulent strain.

7. *Haemophilus ducreyi* is the agent of chancroid, a sexually transmitted disease characterized by ulcerative lesions of the genital tract and inguinal lymphadenopathy.

8. *Bordetella pertussis*, a gram-negative aerobic coccobacillus, is the agent of whooping cough.

9. *B. pertussis*, an obligate parasite of the human respiratory epithelium, adheres only to ciliated epithelial cells, from which it elaborates the primary virulence factor, a potent polypeptide toxin.

10. Pertussis toxin activates adenylate cyclase with resulting effects of histamine-sensitization, lymphocyte activation, and multiple metabolic defects in the host cell.

11. Another adenylate cyclase toxin also activates adenylate cyclase in epithelial cells; the increased cAMP interferes with cellular function and inhibits phagocytosis of the organism. Other toxins, including a cytotoxin that decreases ciliary motility and a heat-labile toxin that induces smooth muscle contraction, may contribute to pathogenesis.

12. An effective killed whole cell vaccine is administered to most infants in the United States, but decreases in vaccinated native populations and in-

fluxes of unvaccinated immigrants have resulted in an increased incidence of whooping cough.

13. An atypical form of pertussis is seen in older patients whose vaccine-induced protection is waning with time.

REFERENCES

Brenner DJ, et al. (1988): Biochemical, genetic, and epidemiologic characterization of *Haemophilus influenzae* biogroup Aegyptius *(Haemophilus aegyptius)* strains associated with Brazilian purpuric fever. J Clin Microbiol 26:1524.

Broome CV (1987): Epidemiology of *Haemophilus influenzae* type b infections in the United States. Pediatr Infect Dis 6:779.

Centers for Disease Control (1991): Diphtheria, tetanus, and pertussis: recommendations for vaccine use and other preventive measures: recommendations of the Immunization Practices Advisory Committee. MMWR 40:1.

Centers for Disease Control (1991): *Haemophilus* b conjugate vaccines for prevention of *Haemophilus influenzae* type b disease among infants and children two months of age and older: recommendations of the Immunization Practices Advisory Committee. MMWR 40:1.

Cherry JD, Brunnel PA, Golden GS, Karzon DT (1988): Report of the task force on pertussis and pertussis immunization—1988. Pediatrics 81(Suppl.):939.

Crowe HM, Levitz RE (1987): Invasive *Haemophilus influenzae* disease in adults. Arch Intern Med 147:241.

Schmid GP, Sanders LL Jr, Blount JH, Alexander ER (1987): Chancroid in the United States: reestablishment of an old disease. JAMA 258:3265.

Thomas MG (1989): Epidemiology of pertussis. Rev Infect Dis 11:255.

Weinstein AJ (1985): *Hemophilus influenzae* infections in older adults. Geriatr Med Today 4:xx.

REVIEW QUESTIONS

For questions 1 to 7, lists of lettered options are followed by several numbered items. For each numbered item, select the ONE lettered option that is most closely associated with it.

A) Exotoxin
B) Antiphagocytic capsule
C) Fimbriae
D) Intracellular multiplication
E) Filamentous hemagglutinin

For each organism, select the most important virulence mechanism.

1. *Haemophilus influenzae* type b

2. *Bordetella pertussis*

A) *Haemophilus influenzae*
B) *Haemophilus influenzae* biogroup *aegyptius*
C) *Haemophilus ducreyi*
D) *Haemophilus aphrophilus*
E) *Haemophilus parainfluenzae*

For each infectious syndrome, select the most commonly associated organism.

3. Epiglottitis

4. Chancroid

5. Endocarditis

6. Brazilian purpuric fever

7. Pink-eye

For questions 8 to 12, choose the ONE BEST answer or completion.

8. Specimens from which *Haemophilus influenzae* is being sought must be cultured onto chocolate agar because
   a) this medium inhibits the growth of *Haemophilus haemolyticus,* which will interfere with detection of *H. influenzae*
   b) this medium does not contain NAD, which is toxic to *H. influenzae*
   c) this medium contains both growth factors required by *H. influenzae*, NAD and heme.
   d) this medium inactivates red cell enzymes, such as peroxidase, that inhibit growth of *H. influenzae*
   e) this medium does not require incubation in increased carbon dioxide to support growth of *H. influenzae*

9. A 3-year-old girl presents to the Emergency

Room with fever, lethargy, and a stiff neck. Which of the following includes the first diagnostic test requests that you should make?

a) Nasopharyngeal culture.
b) Urinalysis, peripheral blood white cell count and differential.
c) Peripheral blood complete blood count (CBC) and cerebrospinal fluid white blood cell count and differential.
d) Cerebrospinal fluid white blood cell count (WBC), differential, protein, and glucose.
e) Blood culture; cerebrospinal fluid white blood cell count, differential, protein, glucose, Gram stain, and culture.

10. Why is the *H. influenzae* PRP capsular conjugate vaccine recommended for first administration to babies only 6-weeks old?

a) Levels of protective IgM antibody that crossed the placenta from the mother begins to decrease at 6 weeks.
b) Levels of protective IgG antibody that crossed the placenta from the mother begins to decrease at 6 weeks.
c) Babies' ability to produce a humoral immune response is nonexistent before 6 weeks of age.
d) Babies' ability to produce a cellular immune response is nonexistent before 6 weeks of age.
e) After 6 weeks, many mothers return to work and place the babies in daycare, where they are likely to contract the infection.

11. What is the factor most likely to be responsible for the restriction of *Bordetella pertussis* to humans?

a) The specific targeting of the action of the tracheal cytotoxin to human respiratory epithelium.
b) The specific targeting of the action of the dermonecrotic toxin to human respiratory epithelium.
c) The ability of the organism to survive on droplet nuclei created during the spasmodic coughing phase of pertussis.
d) A specific receptor site on the surface of human squamous respiratory epithelial cells.
e) A specific receptor site on the surface of human ciliated respiratory epithelial cells.

12. A 6-year-old child, newly arrived from El Salvador, develops a paroxysmal cough with a terminal expiratory whoop. What is the first test you should order for diagnosis?

a) Gram stain of nasopharyngeal exudate.
b) Direct fluorescent antibody stain of nasopharyngeal exudate.
c) Culture of nasopharyngeal exudate onto Bordet-Gengou agar.
d) Culture of nasopharyngeal exudate onto buffered charcoal yeast extract agar.
e) Serologic test for specific antibody.

ANSWERS TO REVIEW QUESTIONS

1. **B** Antibody to capsular polysaccharide protects against disease.

2. **E** Vaccine containing only killed cells is protective; the organism must adhere before it can produce disease.

3. **A**

4. **C**

5. **D**

6. **B**

7. **A** or **B** Both typical *Haemophilus influenzae* and the subtype, *H. influenzae* biogroup *aegyptius* are important etiologic agents of conjunctivitis (pink-eye).

8. **c** Chocolate agar contains heme (X factor) released from erythrocytes and NAD (V factor), both of which are required by *H. influenzae*. Initial preparation of this medium was by heating red blood cells to release heme and inactivate the red cell enzymes that might have otherwise destroyed the NAD present in the medium. Today, chocolate agar is made by adding exogenous heme and NAD (no RBCs) to a nutrient agar base.

9. **e** The girl is most likely presenting with meningitis. At age 3, *H. influenzae* is the most common etiologic agent. The blood culture is important because as many as 50% of patients with meningitis also have concurrent septicemia. The Gram stain is probably the single most important rapid diagnostic test; almost 80% of patients with *H. influenzae* meningitis have positive Gram stains. Because a large number of normal individuals carry *H. influenzae* in the respiratory tract, nasopharyngeal cultures are of no discriminatory value.

10. **b** The vaccine induces a humoral immune response, which replaces the falling levels of circulating IgG that the baby passively received from the mother in utero.

11. **e** Because adherence is the first requirement for establishment of infection, the tropism of *Bordelella pertussis* for humans is dependent on specific binding of human ciliary cell walls by a fimbriae-associated protein (FHA).

12. **b** The direct fluorescent antibody stain for *B. pertussis* organisms is rapid and specific. Although the serologic tests are the next best choice, they usually require a day or more before results are available, and antibody may not be present early in the disease.

YERSINIAL DISEASE, TULAREMIA, PASTEURELLOSIS, AND BRUCELLOSIS

YERSINIA

The genus *Yersinia* contains three important invasive species that produce diseases transmissible from animals to humans. *Yersinia pestis* causes plague, while diarrheal disease due to *Yersinia enterocolitica* and *Yersinia pseudotuberculosis* is referred to as yersiniosis.

PLAGUE

Plague, sometimes referred to as the Black Death, has been responsible for over 150 major epidemics and pandemics throughout the years. During a pandemic in the fourteenth century, the disease spread by way of rat-infested ships from a Central Asia focus to Europe, where it killed 25,000,000 people including two-thirds of the population of Great Britain. In 1924, a plague outbreak occurred in

Los Angeles, originating in the rat-infested slum area of the East side and resulting in 32 cases of pneumonia and 6 cases of bubonic plague with 32 deaths. The major enzootic areas today are Southeast Asia, India, Africa, the Middle East, and North and South America. In the United States, the disease is endemic mostly but not exclusively in the western states.

Habitat

The major reservoir hosts throughout the world are wild rodents. In the United States, the three major groups of wild rodents that serve as primary reservoirs are ground squirrels on the West Coast, wood rats in the South, and prairie dogs in Arizona, Utah, and New Mexico. Wild and domestic rodents may acquire fatal disease or become carriers upon exposure, shedding the organisms into the circulation intermittently. The carrier state ensures the endemicity of the disease.

Transmission

EXOGENOUS. Transmission is exclusively exogenous. Although most commonly transmitted to humans by the bite of the oriental rat flea, *Xenopsylla cheopis,* there are more than 38 flea species capable of transmitting the organisms.

The flea vector becomes infected by feeding upon the blood of a carrier or diseased rodent and by ingesting considerable numbers of *Y. pestis* (Fig. 13.1). The ingested organisms multiply in the stomach and, at temperatures of **less than or equal to 27°C, produce coagulase** that clots the blood and traps the organisms in a fibrin matrix. The fibrin matrix containing the organisms then occludes the proventriculus so that more food is prevented from entering the stomach. The flea becomes very hungry and attempts to feed upon a new rat or, if none is available, a human. The new, aspirated blood becomes contaminated with *Y. pestis* at the occluded site and is regurgitated back into the bite wound, thus initiating the bubonic form of the disease. At temperatures above 27°C, the organisms do not produce coagulase or may produce fibrinolysin, which dissolves an already-existing fibrin network due to coagulase and thus prevents blockage and regurgitation. As a result, flea transmission is low or absent during the hot and dry seasons.

Epizootics among wild and domestic rodents usually precedes human outbreaks resulting in disease and death or a carrier state among the animals. When the rat population is depleted the flea feeds upon humans. In the United States,

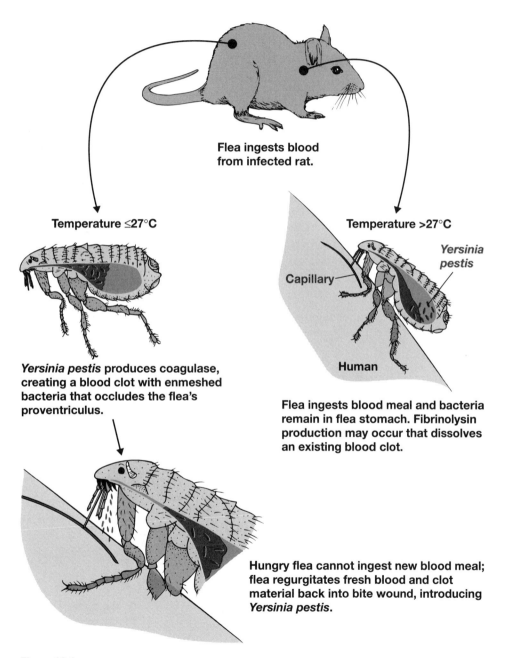

Flea ingests blood
from infected rat.

Temperature ≤27°C

Temperature >27°C

*Yersinia
pestis*

Capillary

Human

Yersinia pestis produces coagulase,
creating a blood clot with enmeshed
bacteria that occludes the flea's
proventriculus.

Flea ingests blood meal and bacteria
remain in flea stomach. Fibrinolysin
production may occur that dissolves
an existing blood clot.

Hungry flea cannot ingest new blood meal;
flea regurgitates fresh blood and clot
material back into bite wound, introducing
Yersinia pestis.

Figure 13.1.

Pathogenicity and transmission of *Y. pestis* in the rat flea.

sporadic cases occur among individuals, such as hunters or Indian populations, who come in close contact with rodent reservoirs. Transmission may occur by droplet nuclei from patients with the pneumonic forms of the disease.

Properties of the Organism

Resistance to environmental, physical, and chemical agents. Y. pestis survives several months in infected carcasses, sputum, and flea feces, but is readily destroyed by physical and chemical agents.

Microscopic morphology. The organism is a gram-negative, nonmotile, ellipsoidal rod that exhibits characteristic **bipolar staining** (safety pin appearance) with special polychromatic stains. Freshly isolated strains are surrounded by an **"envelope"** (capsule?). The organism is a **facultative intracellular parasite.**

Macroscopic morphology. Y. pestis is a facultative anaerobe that grows best aerobically on blood agar at 28°C and is nonhemolytic.

Antigenic structure as it relates to virulence (Fig. 13.2):

F-1 antigen is an **envelope (capsular?) antigen** produced maximally at

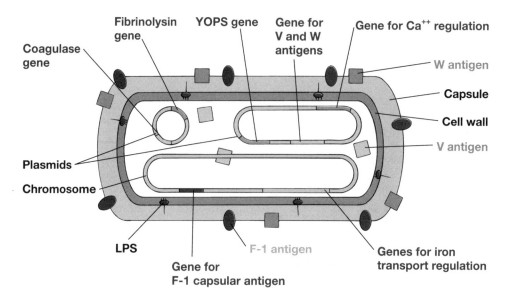

Figure 13.2.

Genetic location and expression of virulence factors in *Y. pestis.*

37°C. This antigen consists of a protein and protein-polysaccharide complex, exerts **antiphagocytic** activity, and appears to be capable of inducing **some protection** in humans.

V-W antigens and *Yersinia* **outer membrane proteins (YOPs)** are plasmid-mediated gene products **coordinately expressed only at 37°C in the presence of low Ca²⁺** concentration. Although essential for virulence, the mechanisms of action are not completely understood. The expression of these proteins at low Ca^{2+} levels may play a dual role by contributing to **extracellular survival through antiphagocytic activity and to intracellular survival and multiplication within macrophages** by a mechanism in which they are able to acquire lysosomal enzyme resistance. Although the V antigen is a cytoplasmic protein and the W antigen is an envelope protein, they are always expressed together.

The role of **LPS** in the pathogenesis of plague is not clearly understood. It appears to be responsible, at least in part, for the **clinical manifestations of hemorrhage, vascular collapse, and focal necrosis.**

Extracellular products associated or thought to be associated with pathogenicity. These products are not well understood. Although coagulase and fibrinolysin are produced by the organisms (Fig. 13.2), their role has been established only with respect to pathogenesis in the rat flea (Fig. 13.1).

Pathogenesis and Clinical Manifestations

PRIMARY DISEASE OR BUBONIC PLAGUE. Bubonic plague is initiated following the bite of an infected flea, usually on the lower extremities. *Y. pestis* is regurgitated into the bite of the wound as described earlier. Within a few hours, the organisms are carried to the regional lymph nodes, usually in the groin, where rapid multiplication occurs. The organisms, through their **F-1 antigens** and, to some extent, **V-W and YOPs antigens under Ca²⁺** regulation, are able to resist phagocytosis by the early response polymorphonuclear leukocytes, which are ultimately destroyed. Macrophages phagocytize the organisms but are not able to kill them. **Intracellular survival** and multiplication are thought to be the result of plasmid-mediated mechanisms of **coordinate expression involving V-W, YOPs, and intracellular Ca²⁺** regulation already described.

Y. pestis may exit macrophages and continue to multiply both extracellularly and intracellularly by these mechanisms. **LPS** release by the organisms is thought to be responsible for the hemorrhagic necrosis produced in the affected lymph node. The host-parasite interaction results in a sudden onset with chills, fever, and an acute regional lymphadenitis referred to as a **"bubo."**

PRIMARY PULMONARY PLAGUE. Primary pulmonary plague is initiated by droplet nuclei from a patient with pulmonary disease. The organisms proceed directly to the lung parenchyma where they multiply rapidly and unrestricted both extracellularly and intracellularly within alveolar macrophages by mechanisms already described. Death is rapid, occurring in less than 2 days in almost all patients, treated or untreated.

DISSEMINATION. Dissemination by mechanisms not as yet known may occur from the regional lymph nodes of patients with acute regional lymphadenitis to one or more organs and tissues through the circulation, producing **hemorrhagic necrosis** putatively as a result of **LPS** release. Death is rapid in the untreated disease occurring in 3–4 days. In 2–5% of patients, the organisms disseminate to the lungs and initiate a rapidly progressive and **fatal secondary pneumonic** process by mechanisms already described for the primary disease.

SEPTICEMIC PLAGUE. Septicemic plague, which usually occurs in children, results when the organisms gain immediate access to the circulation following the bite of the infected flea. Again, *Y. pestis* multiplies rapidly both extracellularly and intracellularly within phagocytic monocytes as described. **LPS** release is thought to result in extensive **intravascular coagulation with vascular and renal collapse.** As with the pneumonic forms of the disease, death occurs in most patients and is rapid.

Immunity to Reinfection

Immunity to reinfection occurs but is not permanent. Mechanisms of acquired resistance are not well understood, but appear to involve both the humoral and cellular arms of the immune response.

Laboratory Diagnosis

A rapid, presumptive diagnosis on the basis of history and clinical manifestations is essential.

SPECIMENS. Specimens obtained depend on the disease process and include bubo aspirates, blood for smear and culture, sputum, and cerebrospinal fluid. Direct smears prepared from specimens must be Gram stained for the presence of gram-negative ellipsoidal rods, Wayson (polychromatic) stained for bipolar (safety-pin) appearance, and stained by direct immunofluorescence for specific identification of *Y. pestis.*

PRIMARY ISOLATION AND IDENTIFICATION. These procedures require initial cultivation on blood agar and MacConkey's agar. Overnight incubation under aerobic conditions at 28°C is optimal for isolation of the organism. Definitive identification is made by direct immunofluorescence of the cultured organisms, which is usually available only at regional Public Health Laboratories.

Treatment

Early treatment with streptomycin, tetracycline, or chloramphenicol is essential. Despite poor success in the treatment of patients with pulmonary, disseminated, and septicemic disease, prompt recognition and treatment of bubonic plague without respiratory complications in the United States has reduced the case fatality rate from 50 to 6%. Streptomycin resistance has been reported, but not in the United States. Treatment with large doses of bactericidal antibiotics in the late stages of septicemic plague may result in death due to the massive destruction of *Y. pestis* with subsequent release of potent LPS.

Prevention and Control

Flea and rat control through surveys and strictly enforced Federal regulations, such as rat-proofing, ship and airplane inspections, and judicious use of insecticides, is essential. Quarantine and prophylactic antimicrobial therapy of contacts of pneumonic plague patients are mandatory. An **effective formalin-killed vaccine** is available against bubonic, but not pneumonic plague and is recommended for those traveling to endemic areas, as well as for high-risk groups in the field and in the laboratory.

YERSINIOSIS

Yersiniosis is the term given to a primary ulcerative ileitis and mesenteric adenitis resembling acute appendicitis caused by *Y. enterocolitica* and *Y. pseudotuberculosis.* Primary septicemia has also been reported. The organisms are harbored in the GI tract of wild and domestic animals and birds and may be found in water contaminated by animal and bird feces. Transmission occurs mostly by ingestion of contaminated food or water. Recently, several cases of *Yersinia* septicemia occurred in patients receiving transfusions with blood containing large numbers of organisms as a result of growth during refrigeration storage for more than 25 days. *Y. enterocolitica* and *Y. pseudotuberculosis* are gram-negative, non-encapsulated coccobacilli that are motile only at 25°C, do not exhibit bipolar staining, and are facultative anaerobes. As with *Y. pestis,* both species **coordinately express V-W and YOPs antigens, which are essential for virulence, only at 37°C and in the presence of low Ca²⁺** concentrations. A functional *inv* **(invasin) chromosomal gene** codes for a large molecular weight rare outer membrane protein present on the surface of both yersinial species that mediates adherence and cell invasion. A functional *ail* **(adherence invasion locus) chromosomal gene** codes for a small molecular weight outer membrane protein present on the surface of *Y. enterocolitica* that contributes to adherence and cell entry. There are no known extracellular virulence factors.

Y. enterocolitica and *Y. pseudotuberculosis* gain entrance to the GI tract, **adhering mostly to the ileal mucosa by mechanisms involving inv and/or ail proteins,** multiplying, and inducing an acute inflammatory response. The organisms **invade mucosal cells, Peyer's patches, and macrophages by the same mechanism, where they survive and multiply, presumably by V-W and YOPs coordinate expression** at low Ca²⁺ concentration. The result is a gastroenteritis (mostly with *Y. enterocolitica*) followed by ulcerative ileitis **mimicking acute appendicitis** and mesenteric lymphadenitis. Gastrointestinal disease manifests as fever, headache, diarrhea, and abdominal pain. Dissemination may sometimes occur through the circulation, resulting in septicemia, liver abscesses, and a reactive polyarthritis mostly in HLA-B27 positive individuals. Primary septicemia resulting from blood transfusion manifests as **septic shock.** There is no known immunity to reinfection.

Specimens for laboratory diagnosis depend on the disease process and include stool, rectal swab, ulcerative material, and blood for culture and serology. The specimens are cultured on blood agar, MacConkey's agar, and CIN (cefsoludin, irgasan, novobiocin) agar, a special selective medium. Incubation is carried out aerobically at room temperature for 48 h. Stool and rectal swab cultures suspected of containing relatively small numbers of organisms may be placed in the refrigerator for 2 weeks prior to media inoculation. Many organisms constituting the normal flora of the GI tract die in contrast to the enhanced growth of the yersiniae. Differentiation between the two species is based upon biochemical reactions. Agglutination titers of greater than or equal to 1:160 on a single serum specimen or a fourfold rise in titer on paired specimens are indicative of yersiniosis.

Although the GI disease is usually self-limiting, trimethoprim-sulfamethoxazole and IV aminoglycosides, such as gentamicin, have been used successfully in the treatment of severe primary disease. The case fatality rate is at least 50% in both treated and untreated patients with primary or disseminated septicemia. Prevention and control are best practiced by educating the population as to the dangers of oral-fecal spread from domestic animals and birds, and the potential for water and food contamination. Physicians must be made aware of the striking similarities between yersiniosis and acute appendicitis. There are no vaccines available against this disease.

FRANCISELLA

TULAREMIA

Francisella tularensis, the etiologic agent of tularemia (rabbit fever), was first isolated in 1912 from a ''plaguelike disease'' among ground squirrels in Tulare County, CA. The organisms are harbored in the blood and tissues of wild and domestic animals, including rodents. In the United States, the chief reservoir hosts are wild rabbits and ground squirrels. Transmission is through the skin and/ or conjunctiva from handling infected animals, through the skin from the bite of infected blood-sucking deer flies and wood ticks, through the GI tract from the ingestion of improperly cooked meat or contaminated water, and through the respiratory tract by aerosol inhalation. *F. tularensis* is a gram-negative, nonmotile, coccobacillary or pleomorphic rod. Virulent organisms appear to be **encapsulated** and are **facultative intracellular parasites.** These fastidious organisms are strict aerobes that grow best on blood-glucose-cysteine agar at 37°C. The role of structural or extracellular virulence factors has not been clearly defined despite the presence of a capsule and LPS.

Organisms entering through the unbroken or abraded skin, GI tract, or conjunctiva, establish residence locally and in the regional lymph nodes. They enter **macrophages and mononuclear phagocytes with intracellular multiplication** resulting in ulcer formation, and regional lymphadenopathy (ulceroglandular or oculoglandular) accompanied by fever, nausea, vomiting, and/or abdominal pain. Disease may occur with only lymphadenopathy (glandular) or with clinical manifestations similar to typhoid fever (typhoidal). Hemorrhagic necrosis of pulmonary and other tissues may result from septicemic dissemination of the above disease processes or as a result of aerosol inhalation. Immunity to reinfection is permanent and is the result of a **CMI mechanism** in which macrophages activated by MAF released from antigen-sensitized effector T cells destroy the phagocytized organisms.

Because this organism is one of the most easily acquired in the laboratory, most clinical laboratories send specimens to the regional Public Health Laboratory for culture. Specimens for laboratory diagnosis depend on the disease process and include lesion and lymph node aspirates, blood for culture and serology, and sputum. The requirement for a special medium, as well as the slow-growing and highly infectious nature of the organism, has resulted in relatively few isolations of the organism in the laboratory. Primary isolation and identification require initial cultivation on blood-glucose-cysteine medium and aerobic incubation at 37°C. It may require 3 weeks for growth to occur. Organisms are identified as *F. tularensis* on the basis of specific immunofluorescent or agglutination tests utilizing specific antisera. By far, the most common assay utilized to establish a diagnosis is an agglutination test utilizing killed *F. tularensis* antigen. Although single titers greater than or equal to 1:160 and a fourfold rise in titer on paired specimens are considered diagnostic, cross-reactivity with *Brucella* antigens necessitate performance of agglutination tests with both antigens. *Brucella* titers are at least twofold and usually fourfold less than *F. tularensis* titers in patients with tularemia. An ELISA test under evaluation is proving of value in the serologic diagnosis of this disease.

Streptomycin and gentamicin have been effective in reducing the case fatality rate to 1% except among patients with pneumonia, where a 50% fatality rate prevails. Prevention and control include avoiding infected animals, such as ''lazy'' rabbits, taking the proper precautions in handling animals, and proper clothing and protection from arthropod vectors. A **live, attenuated vaccine** capable of generating complete or partial immunity is available from the CDC for use among high-risk groups, such as laboratory personnel.

PASTEURELLA

PASTEURELLOSIS

Of the several members of the genus *Pasteurella,* the major human pathogen is *Pasteurella multocida.* The organisms are harbored in the upper respiratory and GI tracts of wild and domestic animals and birds. Disease in the United States is most commonly initiated by the bite or scratch of infected cats or dogs. Septicemia in immunocompromised patients and superimposed disease in patients with chronic lung disease have been reported but the portal of entry and method of transmission are not well understood. *P. multocida* is a gram-negative, nonmotile, **encapsulated, piliated** coccobacillus that exhibits bipolar staining. The organisms are facultative anaerobes that grow best aerobically on blood agar at 37°C. Identified virulence factors are the hyaluronic acid **capsule** that exhibits antiphagocytic activity **and pili** that function as adhesins.

After entry of the organism through the skin following an animal bite, **cellular adhesion by means of their pili** results in local colonization of the organisms. Multiplication occurs with frequent spread to the regional lymph nodes. An acute inflammatory response is elicited, but the organisms are able to resist phagocytosis by polymorphonuclear leukocytes as a result of the **antiphagocytic property of the capsule.** The disease manifests within 24 h as a painful red lesion at the bite site with regional lymphadenopathy. Severe bites with extension of the disease process may result in cellulitis, synovitis, and osteomyelitis. Both septicemic and pulmonary superimposed disease may produce hemorrhagic necrosis and abscesses in the lung as well as other organs and tissues. There is no known immunity to reinfection.

Specimens for laboratory diagnosis depend on the disease process and include lesion and lymph node aspirates, blood for culture, and sputum. Primary isolation and identification requires initial cultivation on blood agar and aerobic incubation at 37°C. Differentiation from other organisms within the genus and from similar organisms in other genera is accomplished by means of biochemical reactions. Penicillin, tetracycline, and chloramphenicol are effective in the treatment of the disease. Adequate cleaning of the animal bite wound is essential. There are no effective vaccines against pasteurellosis. The disease may be prevented by avoiding contact with wild and domestic animals and birds.

BRUCELLA

BRUCELLOSIS

Brucellosis (undulant fever, Malta fever) is an acute or chronic recurrent disease transmissible from animals to humans. Although a wide range of animal reservoir hosts exist for each of the four species capable of producing human disease, they exhibit significant animal-host specificity. The major reservoir hosts are cattle for *Brucella abortus*, goats and sheep for *Brucella melitensis*, swine for *Brucella suis,* and dogs (particularly beagles) for *Brucella canis.*

Upon contact with the organisms, pregnant animals develop either an asymptomatic infection or uterine and mammary gland disease that culminates in abortion. Erythritol, an alcohol present in the placenta and fetal fluids of animals but not humans, serves both as a growth factor for virulent brucellae and enhances intracellular phagocytic growth, thereby accounting for the occurrence of fetal predilection and abortion only in animals. The animals shed organisms in their milk for weeks or months during the carrier state and after recovery.

Transmission to humans is from the ingestion of contaminated raw milk or dairy products in most parts of the world, but in the United States, disease most commonly results from the handling of infected animals by high risk individuals, such as veterinarians, butchers, meat packers, and farmers.

The brucellae are gram-negative, nonmotile, encapsulated coccobacilli and are **facultative intracellular parasites.** They are strict aerobes, but *B. abortus* requires 5–10% carbon dioxide for growth. Optimal growth occurs at 37°C in or on serum or blood enriched complex media. The role of structural or extracellular virulence factors has not been well defined, despite the presence of LPS and the identification of outer membrane proteins.

Brucellae gain entry through the broken or unbroken skin, by ingestion, or through the conjunctiva. They are carried to the liver, spleen, and bone marrow by the lymphatics and circulation, where they **enter fixed macrophages and parenchymal host cells. Intracellular multiplication** induces a chronic inflammatory response characterized by a mononuclear infiltration and resultant granuloma and giant cell formation. Spread from these foci of infection to other organs and tissues may occur by septicemic dissemination. After a variable incubation period of a few days to several weeks or months, the acute phase is ushered in and is characterized by an **undulant fever,** chills, sweating, and often times fatigue. Regional lymphadenopathy, hepatosplenomegaly, septicemia, osteomyelitis and an acute arthritis sometimes occur. In most cases, the acute manifestations generally subside within a few weeks as the result of a **CMI mechanism** that appears to involve the activation of macrophages by MAF released from antigen-sensitized effector T cells during the course of the disease. However, the intracellular persistence of some organisms result in chronic manifestations characterized by low-grade intermittent fever, joint pain, and poorly defined aches and pains that may persist for years.

Some degree of acquired resistance to reinfection develops during the course of the disease, again presumably due to a **CMI response** involving activated macrophages as described above. However, reexposure can result in an exacerbation of the disease due to a delayed-type hypersensitivity (DTH) reaction on already sensitized tissues.

Specimens for laboratory diagnosis depend on the disease process and include lymph node and bone marrow aspirates and blood for culture and serology. As with *F. tularensis,* the requirement for a special medium as well as the slow-growing and highly infectious nature of the organisms have resulted in relatively few isolations of the organisms in the laboratory. Primary isolation may be enhanced by using a biphasic blood culture system containing trypticase soy enriched broth and agar incubated aerobically under 5–10% carbon dioxide at 37°C for a minimum of 4 weeks or by using one of the newer automated blood culture systems. Subcultures are made to trypticase soy enriched blood agar and incubated under the same conditions. Organisms are identified as *Brucella* on the basis of biochemical reactions and are speciated on the basis of hydrogen sulfide production, dye inhibition, carbon dioxide requirement for growth, and agglutinin absorption assay. By far, the greatest number of cases of brucellosis is diagnosed on the basis of the **agglutination reaction** utilizing phenolized, heat-killed *B. abortus*, which also reacts with *B. melitensis* and *B. suis* antibodies, and *B. canis* antigen. As in tularemia, although single titers of greater than or equal to 1:160 and a fourfold rise in titer on paired specimens are considered diagnostic, cross-reactivity with *F. tularensis* antigens necessitates performance of the agglutination test with each of the antigens. *F. tularensis* titers are at least twofold and usually fourfold less than those of *Brucella* titers in patients with brucellosis. An ELISA test under evaluation is proving of value in the serologic diagnosis of the disease.

Prolonged treatment with combined doxycycline and rifampin, trimethoprim-sulfamethoxazole or doxycycline and gentamicin, or with streptomycin, or gentamicin alone depending on the extent of the disease and the age of the patient, is essential due to the intracellular location of the organisms. Even under these circumstances, the organisms may not be completely eradicated, relapse may occur, and retreatment becomes necessary.

Since the routine use of pasteurization in the United States, imported milk and cheese products, as well as products from local ''natural food'' dairies, account for the relatively few cases of brucellosis initiated from raw milk or dairy products. Although effective immunization of cattle, sheep, and goats with live, attenuated vaccine along with test and slaughter control methods has reduced considerably the number of cases of brucellosis in the United States, the disease still occurs among high risk groups, such as meat packers, butchers, farmers, and veterinarians who handle infected animals or animal products. Education of these individuals with respect to the wearing of special gloves and clothing is essential.

SUMMARY

1. Plague, the etiologic agent of which is *Yersinia pestis*, is a worldwide disease. It occurs in the United States and is endemic mostly in the western states.

2. The major worldwide reservoir hosts for *Y. pestis* are wild rodents.

3. *Y. pestis* is a gram-negative, nonmotile, "enveloped," ellipsoidal, facultative intracellular rod that exhibits bipolar staining.

4. The basic pathogenesis process of primary disease (bubonic plague) is initiated following the bite of an infected flea, whereby *Y. pestis* is regurgitated into the bite wound. Organisms are carried to the regional lymph nodes and multiply rapidly. The organisms, through their F-1 antigens and, to some extent, V-W and *Yersinia* outer membrane protein (YOP) antigens under Ca^{2+} regulation, are able to resist phagocytosis by polymorphonuclear leukocytes, which are ultimately destroyed. Macrophages phagocytize the organisms but they undergo intracellular survival and multiplication thought to be the result of plasmid-mediated mechanisms of coordinate expression involving V-W, YOPs, and intracellular Ca^{2+} regulation. *Y. pestis* may exit macrophages and continue to multiply both extracellularly and intracellularly. LPS release is thought to be responsible for the hemorrhagic necrosis seen in lymph nodes.

5. The basic pathogenesis of primary pulmonary plague is initiated by droplet nuclei from a patient with pulmonary disease.

6. Dissemination may occur in patients with bubonic plague through the circulation, producing hemorrhagic necrosis presumably due to LPS release. Organisms may disseminate to the lungs and initiate a rapidly progressive secondary pneumonic process. Septicemic plague results when the organisms gain immediate access to the circulation following the bite of the infected flea. LPS is thought to cause extensive intravascular coagulation with vascular and renal collapse.

7. Yersiniosis, caused by *Yersinia enterocolitica* and *Yersinia pseudotuberculosis,* is a primary ulcerative ileitis and mesenteric adenitis resembling acute appendicitis; primary septicemia also may occur.

8. Both agents of yersiniosis coordinately express V-W and YOPs antigens, which are essential for virulence, only at 37°C and in the presence of low Ca^{2+} concentrations. A functional *inv* (invasin) chromosomal gene codes for a rare outer membrane protein (OMP) that mediates attachment and invasion. A functional *ail* (adherence invasion locus) chromosomal gene codes for an OMP on the surface of *Y. enterocolitica* that contributes to adherence and cell entry.

9. Tularemia (rabbit fever) is caused by *Francisella tularensis,* an organism harbored in the blood and tissues of wild and domestic animals, in-

cluding rodents. The major reservoir hosts in the United States are wild rabbits and ground squirrels.

10. *F. tularensis* is a gram-negative, nonmotile, coccobacillary or pleomorphic, facultative intracellular, strict aerobic, fastidious rod that grows best on blood-glucose-cysteine agar.

11. *Pasteurella multocida,* the major human pathogen in this genus, causes pasteurellosis, which is commonly initiated by the bite or scratch of infected cats or dogs in the United States.

12. *P. multocida* is a gram-negative, nonmotilie, encapsulated, piliated, facultative anaerobic coccobacillus that exhibits bipolar staining.

13. Brucellosis (undulant fever and Malta fever) is an acute or chronic disease transmissible from animals to humans. The major reservoir hosts are cattle for *Brucella abortus,* goats and sheep for *Brucella melitensis,* swine for *Brucella suis,* and dogs (particularly beagles) for *Brucella canis.*

14. Transmission is usually by ingestion of contaminated raw milk or dairy products, and handling infected animals by high risk individuals, such as veterinarians, butchers, meat packers, and farmers.

15. Brucellae are gram-negative, nonmotile, encapsulated, facultative intracellular, strict aerobic, coccobacilli that require serum or blood-enriched complex media for growth.

REFERENCES

Adlam C, Rutter JM (1989): *Pasteurella* and pasteurellosis. London, England: Academic Press.

Barnes AM (1990): Plague in the U.S.: present and future. In Davis LR, Marsh RE. (eds): Proceedings of the 14th Vertebrate Pest Conference, Davis, California: The Vertebrate Pest Council of the Vertebrate Pest Conference. pp 43–45.

Bolin I, Portnoy DA, Wolf-Watz H (1985): Expression of the temperature-inducible outer membrane proteins of yersiniae. Infect Immun 48:234.

Butler T (1972): A clinical study of bubonic plague. Am J Med 53:268.

Cornelis G, Laroche Y, Balligand G, Sory MP (1987): *Yersinia enterocolitica,* a primary model of invasiveness. Rev Infect Dis 9:64.

Cover TL, Aber RC (1989): *Yersinia enterocolitica.* N Eng J Med 321:16.

Evans ME, Gregory DW, Schaffner W, McGee ZA (1985): Tularemia: A 30-year experience with 88 cases. Medicine 64:251.

Miller VL, Farmer JJ III, Hill WE, Falkow S (1989): The *ail* locus is found uniquely in *Yersinia enterocolitica* serotypes commonly associated with disease. Infect Immun 57:121.

Perry RD, Harmon PA, Bowmer WS, Straley SC (1986): A low-Ca^{2+} response operon encodes the V antigen of *Yersinia pestis*. Infect Immun 54:428.

Portnoy DA, Falkow S (1981): Virulence-associated plasmids from *Yersinia enterocolita* and *Yersinia pestis*. J Bacteriol 148:877.

Sanford JP (1988): Landmark perspective: tularemia. JAMA 250:3225.

U.S. Department of Health and Human Services (1982): Multi-state outbreak of yersiniosis. MMWR 31:505.

U.S. Department of Health and Human Services (1984): Plague pneumonia-California. MMWR 33:481.

Weber DJ, Hansen AR (1991): Infections resulting from animal bites. Infect Dis Clin N Am 5:663.

Weber DJ, Wolfson JS, Swartz MN, Hooper DC (1984): *Pasteurella multocida* infections. Reports of 34 cases and a review of the literature. Medicine 63:133.

Young EJ (1983): Human brucellosis. Rev Infect Dis 5:821.

REVIEW QUESTIONS

For questions 1 to 14, choose the ONE BEST answer or completion.

1. *Yersinia pestis* is usually transmitted to humans
   a) by droplet nuclei from an infected rat
   b) by an infected flea vector during the taking of a blood meal
   c) by the inhalation of spores from patients with the pneumonic form of the disease
   d) because the organisms are able to dissolve a fibrin matrix by the action of a fibrinolysin
   e) when their immune system is impaired

2. One of the following statements relating to *Y. pestis* is NOT TRUE.
   a) The organisms are facultative intracellular parasites.
   b) Freshly isolated strains are surrounded by an "envelope".
   c) The organisms produce coagulase at temperatures greater than 27°C.
   d) The organisms exhibit characteristic "bipolar" staining with special polychromatic stains.
   e) The organisms are gram-negative ellipsoidal rods.

3. The V-W antigens and *Yersinia* outer membrane proteins (YOPs) are plasmid-mediated gene products that may function as virulence factors of *Y. pestis* by
   a) contributing to extracellular survival through antiphagocytic activity and intracellular survival and multiplication within macrophages by acquiring lysosomal resistance

b) coordinate expression in the presence of high salt concentrations

c) coordinate expression in the presence of high concentrations of Ca^{2+}

d) coordinate expression at 25°C in the presence of low Ca^{2+} concentrations

e) causing vascular collapse

4. Primary pulmonary plague *differs* from bubonic plague in that the *former*

a) disseminates through the circulation

b) is characterized by ''bubo'' formation

c) is the result of extracellular and intracellular multiplication

d) is usually fatal, even when treated

e) is the result of endogenous activation of organisms among immunosuppressed carriers

5. A presumptive diagnosis of bubonic plague may be confirmed by

a) the inguinal inoculation of rabbits, subsequent culture on blood agar and MacConkey's agar, and identification by biochemical testing

b) Gram-staining bubo aspirates

c) culturing on blood agar and MacConkey's agar and identification by Gram staining and Wayson staining for the characteristic ''bipolar'' appearance

d) demonstrating on direct smears from bubo aspirates gram-negative ellipsoidal rods, ''bipolar'' appearance utilizing a polychromatic stain, and *Y. pestis* by direct immunofluorescence with specific fluorescein labeled anti-*Y. pestis* globulin

e) history and clinical manifestations

6. The pathogenesis of yersiniosis due to *Yersinia enterocolitica*

a) is the result of initial adherence to the ileal mucosa and cell invasion mediated by inv and/or ail outer membrane proteins

b) does not include invasion of host tissues by the organisms

c) manifests as an acute appendicitis

d) does not include intracellular survival and multiplication by a putative mechanism involving the coordinate expression of V-W and *Yersinia* outer membrane protein antigens

e) never disseminates through the circulation

7. Yersiniosis may be diagnosed by

a) history and clinical manifestations

b) a fourfold rise in agglutination titers on paired serum specimens taken at 3-week intervals

c) the demonstration of gram-negative coccobacilli in direct smears prepared from rectal swabs

d) an agglutination titer of 1:20 on a single serum specimen obtained during the acute phase of the disease

e) the demonstration of gram-negative coccobacilli in direct smears prepared from stool specimens

8. *Francisella tularensis,* the etiologic agent of tularemia,

a) is harbored mostly in cattle and swine in the United States

b) is a facultative, intracellular parasite

c) is rarely transmitted by handling infected animals

d) can be isolated from clinical specimens on blood agar

e) is a facultative anaerobe

9. One of the following statements relating to the pathogenesis of tularemia is NOT TRUE.
   a) *F. tularensis* multiplies within macrophages and mononuclear phagocytes.
   b) Septicemic dissemination occurs with resultant hemorrhagic tissue necrosis.
   c) After entrance into the host, the organisms establish residence locally and in the regional lymph nodes.
   d) Powerful exotoxins released by the organisms during multiplication are responsible for the clinical manifestations.
   e) The role of structural components as virulence factors has not been clearly defined.

10. Pasteurellosis in the United States is most commonly initiated
   a) by the accidental inhalation of contaminated bird droppings
   b) by handling infected rodents
   c) by droplet nuclei from infected dogs
   d) in immunocompromised patients
   e) by the bite or scratch of infected cats or dogs

11. Adherence of *Pasteurella multocida* and its resistance to phagocytosis during the pathogenesis of pasteurellosis ultimately permit the development of a painful red lesion and regional lymphadenopathy. The responsible virulence factors are
   a) LPS and exotoxins
   b) V-W and YOPs antigens
   c) pili and capsules
   d) coagulase and fibrinolysin
   e) flagella and spores

12. The brucellae
   a) are obligate intracellular parasites
   b) can be transmitted to humans by ingesting contaminated raw milk or dairy products and by handling infected animals
   c) produce only asymptomatic infection in their reservoir hosts
   d) have well-defined structural virulence factors
   e) are easily cultured on chocolate agar

13. The pathogenesis or clinical manifestations of acute brucellosis is characterized by
   a) the absence of fever
   b) the formation of humoral immune mechanisms responsible for the ultimate subsiding of the acute manifestations
   c) an infiltration of polymorphonuclear leukocytes during an acute inflammatory response
   d) intracellular multiplication within fixed macrophages and parenchymal host cells
   e) persistence of intracellular brucellae following a CMI response

14. In the United States, human brucellosis is usually diagnosed on the basis of
   a) specific agglutination titers greater than or equal to 1:160 on a single serum specimen or a fourfold rise in titer on paired serum specimens taken at 3-week intervals, provided reactivity with *F. tularensis* antigen is at least twofold less in titer
   b) a positive skin test utilizing brucellergen
   c) isolation and speciation of brucellae using a biphasic blood culture system con-

taining trypticase soy enriched broth and agar and biochemical reactions

d) RNA-DNA hybridization

e) lymphadenopathy in guinea pigs follow-

ing inguinal inoculation with lymph node aspirates, and a positive delayed-type hypersensitivity (DTH) response by the animal to brucellergin

---

ANSWERS TO REVIEW QUESTIONS

---

1. **b** *Yersinia pestis* is usually transmitted to humans by an infected flea vector during the taking of a blood meal. Infection by droplet nuclei from a rat does not occur, the organism does not produce spores, and susceptible hosts can have a normal or impaired immune system. It is the coagulase-mediated fibrin clot that serves as a requirement for transmission and not fibrin dissolvement by fibrinolysin.

2. **c** *Y. pestis* produces coagulase at temperatures less than or equal to 27°C. The organisms are gram-negative, ellipsoidal rods that exhibit bipolar staining with polychromatic stains, are surrounded by an "envelope," and are facultative intracellular parasites.

3. **a** The V-W antigens and YOPs of *Y. pestis* are plasmid-mediated gene products that contribute to extracellular survival through antiphagocytic activity and intracellular survival and multiplication within macrophages by acquiring lysosomal resistance. Vascular collapse is

thought to be due to LPS. Coordinate expression of these gene products occurs only at 37°C in the presence of low Ca^{2+} concentration.

4. **d** The case fatality rate of bubonic plague without respiratory complications, in contrast to primary pulmonary plague, has been reduced to 6% as a result of treatment. Both forms of the disease are the result of extracellular and intracellular multiplication of the organism and may disseminate. The bubonic form is characterized by "bubo" formation. Endogenous activation has not been reported in either normal or immunologically suppressed individuals.

5. **d** The definitive diagnosis of bubonic plague can be made by first demonstrating the presence of gram-negative, "bipolar," ellipsoidal rods in direct smears from bubo aspirates, and then confirming *Y. pestis* by direct immunofluorescence. The latter technique is essential to confirmation. Rabbits or other animals

are never used for definitive diagnosis. A rapid presumptive diagnosis is required and made on the basis of history and clinical manifestations.

6. *a* The pathogenesis of yersiniosis due to *Yersinia enterocolitica* is the result of initial adherence to the ileal mucosa and cell invasion mediated by inv and/or ail OMPs. The pathogenesis does, indeed, include intracellular survival and multiplication by a putative mechanism involving the coordinate expression of V-W and YOPs antigens. The organism is invasive to tissues, may disseminate through the circulation, and produces a disease that simulates but does not manifest as an acute appendicitis.

7. *b* The demonstration of greater than or equal to fourfold rise in agglutination titers on paired serum specimens taken 3-weeks apart provides a definitive diagnosis of yersiniosis. A titer of greater than or equal to 1:160 on a single specimen would also be indicative of the disease. The diversity of gram-negative rods and coccobacilli in the stool precludes use of the Gram stain on direct smears prepared from a stool or rectal swab specimen. Again, history and clinical manifestations may be used to establish only a presumptive diagnosis.

8. *b* *Francisella tularensis* is a facultative, intracellular parasite. The organism is a strict aerobe that requires a blood-glucose-cysteine agar for best growth. The organism is harbored in the blood and tissues of wild rabbits and ground squirrels in the United States, and is often transmitted by handling infected animals.

9. *d* Exotoxins are not produced by *F. tularensis*. However, the organism does establish residence locally and in the regional lymph nodes, *F. tularensis* does multiply within macrophages and mononuclear phagocytes, septicemic dissemination with hemorrhagic necrosis does occur, and the virulence factors have not been well defined.

10. *e* Pasteurellosis in the United States is most commonly initiated by the bite or scratch of infected cats or dogs. The inhalation of contaminated bird droppings or droplet nuclei from dogs, and the handling of infected rodents have not been established as methods of transmission. Septicemia in immunocompromised patients has been reported but is rare.

11. *c* Adherence of *Pasteurella multocida* is mediated by pili and resistance to phagocytosis by the capsule during the pathogenesis of pasteurellosis. The organism is nonmotile and does not produce spores, exotoxin, coagulase, or fibrinolysin. A role for LPS has not been demonstrated.

12. *b* Pathogenic members of the genus *Brucella* can be transmitted to humans by ingesting raw milk or dairy products and by handling infected animals. These organisms are facultative intracellular parasites and require serum or blood en-

riched complex media for optimal growth. Virulence factors have not been well defined. The organisms may produce abortion in their reservoir hosts.

13. *d* Acute brucellosis is an undulant febrile disease whose pathogenesis is characterized by intracellular multiplication within fixed macrophages and parenchymal host cells. An acute inflammatory response is either not induced or insignificant. Cell-mediated immunity and not humoral immune mechanisms appears to be responsible for the subsiding of the acute manifestations of brucellosis, following which there is an intracellular persistence of some brucellae.

14. *a* In the United States, brucellosis is usually diagnosed in febrile patients suspected of having the disease. A specific agglutination titer of greater than or equal to 1:160 on a single serum specimen or an greater than or equal to fourfold rise in titer on paired serum specimens taken 3-weeks apart is confirmatory, provided cross-reactivity with *F. tularensis* antigen is at least twofold less in titer. Isolation from blood cultures and speciation is the best method for the definitive diagnosis of brucellosis but is done relatively infrequently in the United States. RNA-DNA hybridization has not been developed and animal inoculation techniques are not utilized for identification of brucellae. A positive skin test with brucellergen establishes present or past infection and not necessarily active disease.

NEISSERIAL INFECTION AND DISEASE

THE FAMILY *NEISSERIACEAE*

The *Neisseriaceae* are related gram-negative cocci or coccobacilli consisting of the genera *Neisseria, Moraxella, Acinetobacter,* and *Kingella,* each of which contains nonpathogens, as well as potentially pathogenic organisms. *Neisseria meningitidis* (syn: the meningococcus), the etiologic agent of meningococcal disease, and *Neisseria gonorrhoeae* (syn: the gonococcus), the etiologic agent of gonorrhea, are the two major pathogens of the family and will be considered at some length in this chapter. However, several members of the other genera are capable of causing disseminated disease among individuals with a lowered host resistance in both a community and nosocomial environment. Of particular recent interest is the pathogenic potential of *Moraxella catarrhalis,* a former member of the genera *Neisseria* and *Branhamella.* This organism has now been shown to cause a wide diversity of clinical manifestations, such as acute suppurative otitis media and sinusitis, among children with normal immune mechanisms, as well as septicemia, endocarditis, meningitis, and lower respiratory infections among immunosuppressed and immunodeficient children and adults. The organisms in the family *Neisseriaceae,* many of which exist in the upper respiratory tract or on other mucous membrane surfaces, can be distinguished from each other on the basis of biochemical reactions.

MENINGOCOCCAL DISEASE

N. meningitidis causes endemic or epidemic disease of worldwide prevalence. All age groups may be affected, but the prevalence is greatest among infants, children, and young adults. In the United States, about 2000–3000 cases are reported each nonepidemic year and as many as 20,000 cases during epidemics, which tend to occur in cyclic waves and may last for several years. As an example, an epidemic began in Sao Paulo, Brazil in 1971, and spread throughout the entire country over a 3-year period, resulting in thousands of cases. The initial outbreak was due to *N. meningitidis,* serogroup C, but shifted to serogroup A in 1974, at which time over 20,000 cases were reported with a case fatality rate of 15%.

Epidemic and endemic cases in the Western Hemisphere during the last few years have been caused mainly by serogroups A, B, C, W-135, and Y. Epidemics in the United States, which have occurred in both the military and civilian populations, have been markedly reduced as a result of vaccination. The most commonly recognized form of this disease is **meningitis.** The high prevalence and case fatality rates among untreated patients, together with the epidemic nature of the disease, points to the importance of this syndrome among the bacterial meningitides.

Habitat

N. meningitidis is an obligate parasite of humans. The organisms are harbored in the nasopharynx of cases and carriers. Several nonpathogenic species of *Neisseria* are normal inhabitants of the human nasopharynx and must be differentiated from the pathogens in clinical disease.

Transmission

EXOGENOUS. Exogenous transmission is by droplet nuclei from or direct contact with a case or carrier. Factors that contribute to the origin of outbreaks include opportunities for intimate contact with carriers, such as exist in military barracks, schools, institutions, and day care centers, and conditions, such as fatigue and exposure to inclement weather, which lower host resistance.

The nasopharyngeal carrier rate in the normal United States population is 2–8% during interepidemic years and increases to 40–90% in the affected community just preceding and during epidemics. However, the percentage of individuals who develop disseminated disease during an outbreak is less than 1%. As seen in the Brazil epidemic, a shift in the serogroup responsible for disease may occur at any time during an outbreak for as yet undetermined reasons.

ENDOGENOUS. Endogenous activation from the nasopharynx of a carrier is thought to occur infrequently. Those factors that are responsible for a breakdown in host resistance may be the same as those described for exogenous transmission (e.g., fatigue and exposure to inclement weather).

Properties of the Organism

Resistance to environmental, physical, and chemical agents. Meningococci are destroyed rapidly in the environment and are highly susceptible to physical and chemical agents.

Microscopic morphology. N. meningitidis is a gram-negative, nonmotile, diplococcus with the appearance of a "kidney bean" or "coffee bean" because it is flattened on one side. The flattened sides occur adjacent to one another when the organisms are in pairs. The organisms are **encapsulated and piliated.**

Macroscopic morphology. The organisms are strict aerobes that grow best on chocolate agar at 35–37°C in the presence of 3–10% carbon dioxide. The several morphologically similar nonpathogenic and potentially pathogenic members of the genera *Moraxella, Acinetobacter,* and *Kingella* that are normal inhabitants of the upper respiratory tract or other mucous membrane surfaces, can be distinguished from the *Neisseria* in general on the basis of oxidase production, catalase production, glucose fermentation, and/or nitrite reduction.

Within the genus *Neisseria,* it is essential to be able to differentiate not only the pathogens from the nonpathogens that occupy the nasopharynx, but also the two pathogenic species from each other, inasmuch as *N. gonorrhoeae* can produce pharyngeal disease and the meningococcus has been isolated from homosexuals with proctitis and urethritis. The organisms can only be identified as members of the *Neisseria* genus on the basis of their Gram-stain morphology and oxidase production. However, differentiation can be accomplished by determining their ability to ferment glucose, maltose, sucrose, and lactose and is summarized in Table 14.1.

Antigenic structure as it relates to virulence and/or classification:

TABLE 14.1. Differentiation of *Neisseria* Species on the Basis of Sugar Fermentation Reactions

Neisseria sp.	Glucose	Maltose	Sucrose	Lactose
meningitidis	+	+	−	−
gonorrhoeae	+	−	−	−
lactamica	+	+	−	+
Other nonpathogens	±	±	±	−

Pili mediate **attachment** of the organism to nasopharyngeal mucosa and enable the organisms to colonize.

The **polysaccharide capsule** is antigenically diverse, which forms the basis for the classification of the meningococci into 13 serogroups. The great majority of meningococcal disease is caused by serogroups A, B, C, W-135, and Y. The capsules are **antiphagocytic and may facilitate meningeal invasion.** They stimulate **serogroup-specific protective immunity** against disease due to several of the key serogroups and form the basis for effective vaccination. The serogroup B capsule is immunologically identical to the capsule of *Escherichia coli* K1, a leading cause of neonatal meningitis in which the presence of the capsule correlates with invasiveness of the organism.

Outer membrane proteins (OMPs) of the organism are also antigenically diverse, which enables serotyping of meningococci within each serogroup. In addition, OMPs act as **porins** (see Chapter 1).

Lipooligosaccharide (LOS), which is an abundant component of the organism, is released upon multiplication and autolysis. LOS differs from LPS in that the former has shorter, nonrepeat, O-antigenic side chains and thus has a lower molecular weight. LOS is responsible for many of the toxic manifestations of disseminated meningococcal disease.

Extracellular product thought to be associated with pathogenicity. An **IgA1 protease** is produced by both neisserial pathogens but not by the nonpathogens. The enzyme **inactivates local secretory IgA** and thus may play a role in facilitating the **adherence** of meningococci to the nasopharyngeal mucosa.

Pathogenesis and Clinical Manifestations

PRIMARY DISEASE. Primary disease is initiated in the nasopharynx by droplet nuclei from or direct contact with a case or carrier. Adherence to the mucosal surface with resultant colonization is mediated by **pili** and possibly facilitated by cleavage of secretory IgA by **IgA1 protease**. Factors that determine whether the colonized organisms will remain quiescent (carrier state) or initiate mild-to-severe nasopharyngeal disease are unknown. In the susceptible host, the organisms multiply and induce an acute inflammatory response characterized by an influx of polymorphonuclear leukocytes and leakage of fluid containing immunoglobulin and complement. Phagocytosis by the polymorphonuclear leukocytes is inhibited by the **capsule** and the organisms continue to multiply producing a mild to severe nasopharyngitis. The great majority of these patients produce **complement-dependent bactericidal antibody, predominantly of the IgM type, and opsonic antibody,** both of which restrict the organisms to the mucosal surface of the nasopharynx (carrier state) and eventually cause their riddance. Occasionally, *N. meningitidis* may cause proctitis or urethritis among homosexuals by similar mechanisms.

DISSEMINATED DISEASE. Disseminated disease occurs by hematogenous spread among a relatively few number of exposed individuals. The onset of disseminated disease correlates with **(1) the absence of complement-dependent bactericidal antibody (predominantly IgM) and opsonic antibody or (2) the presence of serum IgA antibody that blocks the initiation of immune lysis.** Dissemination may also occur in patients with complement component deficiencies. Those factors that cause the absence or blockage of the serum protective antibodies and complement deficiencies are unknown.

Septicemia. In septicemia (meningococcemia), the organisms invade the blood stream from the nasopharynx, multiply unrestricted in the blood and, during multiplication and autolysis, release **LOS**, which is responsible for the ensuing clinical manifestions. After an incubation period of 3–6 days, chills, fever, and petechial hemorrhages appear. The rash may either disappear in a few days or, as a result of further capillary thrombosis and extravasation of erythrocytes, assume a purple, splotchy appearance known as **"purpura."** In some instances, usually in infants, a fulminating disease known as the Waterhouse-Friderichsen syndrome may occur, characterized by massive hemorrhage and necrosis of the adrenals resulting in vascular collapse, shock, and death within 6–8 h.

Meningitis. Meningitis (meningococcal meningitis) is the most common complication of meningococcemia. The organisms cross the blood-brain barrier and reach the meninges, where they multiply and induce an acute inflammatory response characterized by an influx of polymorphonuclear leukocytes and a leakage of fluid. The end result is a purulent meningitis with fever, stiff neck, vomiting, severe headache, convulsions, bulging of the fontanelles, and progression to a coma within a few hours. Sequelae, if they occur, include eighth nerve deafness and brain damage.

Less commonly, the organisms may disseminate from the circulation to the joints, lungs, and heart valves to produce arthritis, pneumonia, and endocarditis, respectively.

Immunity to Reinfection

Some serogroup-specific protection is provided for up to 3 months in newborns by means of transplacental transfer of protective antibody from the mother. Immunity to reinfection is serogroup specific, but not always permanent. The degree of immunity is dependent on the amounts of functional protective antibodies present.

Laboratory Diagnosis

SPECIMENS AND DIRECT EXAMINATION. Specimens obtained depend on the disease process and include petechial or purpuric aspirates, blood for culture, cerebrospinal fluid, and joint fluid; nasopharyngeal swabs are useful for the detection of carriers. Gram stain of skin lesion exudates, joint fluid, the buffy coat of blood, and cerebrospinal fluid may show gram-negative, intracellular and extracellular diplococci in association with polymorphonuclear leukocytes. It should be noted, however, that failure to demonstrate the organisms does not rule out their presence.

PRIMARY ISOLATION AND IDENTIFICATION. Primary isolation requires initial blood cultures and culture on either chocolate agar plates or, if a mixed flora is anticipated, Thayer-Martin medium, which is an enriched chocolate agar medium containing vancomycin (to inhibit gram-positive organisms), colistin (to inhibit gram-negative rods), nystatin (to inhibit yeasts), and trimethoprim (to inhibit *Proteus* species). Incubation for 48 h at 35–37°C under aerobic conditions in the presence of 3–10% carbon dioxide is optimal for isolation of the organism, which may be identified as a gram-negative, oxidase-positive, diplococcus that ferments glucose and maltose, but not sucrose or lactose (Table 14.1) and agglutinates in the presence of serogroup-specific anticapsular antibody. Rapid presumptive identification of serogroup-specific meningococci in cerebrospinal fluid can be accomplished by latex agglutination utilizing serogroup-specific anticapsular antibody for the detection of capsular polysaccharide; confirmation by culture, subsequent Gram-staining, biochemical testing, and latex agglutination of the isolate with serogroup-specific anticapsular antibody, is essential, inasmuch as false positive and false negative results can occur.

Treatment

Early treatment with penicillin has reduced the case fatality rate in disseminated disease from 40–90% to 10–15%, but the antibiotic is **ineffective in eradicating the carrier state.** Chloramphenicol and ceftriaxone are effective in penicillin-allergic individuals.

Prevention and Control

An **effective capsular polysaccharide vaccine** is available in monovalent, bivalent, or polyvalent form against serogroups A, C, W-135, and Y meningococci. The effectiveness of this vaccine is based upon the stimulation of protective complement-dependent and opsonic antibodies. The vaccinogen is used in selected population groups, such as the military, and during both military and civilian epidemics to control the outbreak. In general, these vaccines, like other unconjugated polysaccharide vaccines, are ineffective in children under the age of 2 years. A vaccine against serogroup B meningococci is not available because the capsule is easily degraded and poorly immunogenic in humans.

The control of outbreaks is accomplished by the use of rifampin or minocycline. Both of these antimicrobial agents eradicate the carrier state and serve as effective prophylactic agents for those who come in contact with cases or carriers. The emergence of **rifampin-resistant strains,** together with **the vestibular dysfunction associated** with **minocycline,** points to the potential limitations of these antimicrobials.

GONORRHEA

Gonorrhea (the clap) is primarily a sexually transmitted, worldwide disease of both epidemic and endemic proportions. Between 500,000 and 1,000,000 new cases are reported each year to the National Centers for Disease Control. The prevalence is thought to be significantly greater due to the under reporting of cases and contacts. The disease occurs in all age groups but most often among sexually active, young adults whose sexual preference characterizes them as heterosexual, bisexual, or male homosexual. The organism has no special predilection for race, creed, color, or socioeconomic class. Significantly, about 8–10% of gonococcal strains isolated in the United States exhibit single or multiple resistance to antibiotics with the great majority being **penicillinase-producing *N. gonorrhoeae* (PPNG)** (Fig. 14.1). **The gonococcus is second only to *Chlamydia trachomatis* as a leading cause of sterility in females** (see Chapter 23).

Habitat

N. gonorrhoeae is an obligate parasite of humans. The organisms are harbored in the male and female genital tracts (urethra and/or cervix), rectum, and/or pharynx of cases or asymptomatic carriers.

Transmission

EXOGENOUS. Transmission is exclusively exogenous by either sexual contact (including fellatio, anal sex, and sexual abuse) or from an infected pregnant female to the newborn as a result of passage through an infected birth canal resulting most commonly in ophthalmia neonatorum. Transmission from fomites, such as toilet seats and doorknobs, does not occur.

Properties of the Organism

Resistance to environmental, physical, and chemical aspects. Gonococci are destroyed rapidly in the environment and are highly susceptible to physical and chemical agents.

Microscopic morphology. Like the meningococcus, the organism is a gram-negative, nonmotile, diplococcus with the appearance of a "kidney bean" or "coffee bean" because it is flattened on one side. The flattened sides occur adjacent to one another when the organisms are in pairs. The organisms are **nonencapsulated but piliated**, the latter being associated with the virulence of genital strains.

Macroscopic morphology. The organisms are strict aerobes that grow best on chocolate agar at 35–37°C in the presence of 3–10% carbon dioxide. On primary isolation and subculture, five distinct types of colonies are recognized. The T-1 and T-2 colonies are relatively small, contain piliated organisms, and are

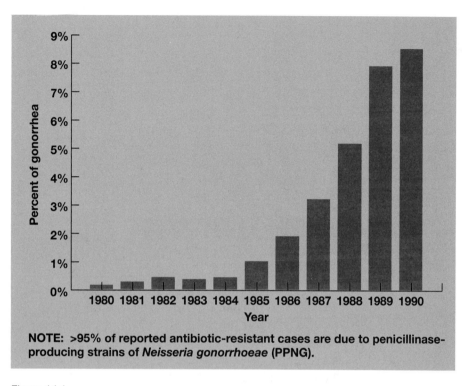

NOTE: >95% of reported antibiotic-resistant cases are due to penicillinase-producing strains of *Neisseria gonorrhoeae* (PPNG).

Figure 14.1.

Gonorrhea. Percentage of reported cases caused by antibiotic-resistant strains, United States, 1980–1990. [Redrawn with permission from U.S. Department of Health and Human Services (1990): Summary of notifiable diseases, United States, 1991. MMWR 39:no. 53.]

associated with virulence, while T-3, T-4, and T-5 colonies produced by subculture on nonselective medium are larger, nonpiliated, and avirulent. Differentiation of the gonococcus from other members of the genus *Neisseria,* as well as from members of the genera *Moraxella, Acinetobacter,* and *Kingella,* has been described previously (Macroscopic morphology, p. 273) and in Table 14.1. However, it is worth noting that the gonococcus is the only member of the genus *Neisseria* that ferments **only glucose** among the sugars utilized in differentiation. **Most strains that require arginine, hypoxanthine, and uracil (A⁻H⁻U⁻ auxotrophs)** are associated with **dissemination.**

Antigenic structure as it relates to virulence:

Pili mediate **attachment** of the organism to epithelial and mucosal cell surfaces and are **antiphagocytic.** The expression of the pili is turned on and off by

DNA rearrangement. The antigenically variable domains of pili are immunodominant and not associated with attachment, while the conserved immunorecessive domains are critically involved in adherence. The high frequency with which **antigenic variation** occurs during natural infection accounts for the antigenic heterogeneity and resultant numerous pili types among strains. This provides a possible explanation for one mechanism that may contribute to the ability of the gonococcus to **evade the immune response** and to cause **repeated infection in the same host.** Pilus antigenic variation involves intragenic recombination and gene conversion in which each gonococcal cell carries different DNA sequences representing portions of the pilus that vary among the different possible antigenic types.

Three **OMPs** have been studied extensively:

1. **Protein I.** This protein is considered to be the **major OMP,** is antigenically diverse among different strains, and functions as a **porin in complex with Protein III.** Although the mechanism is unknown, gonococci that contain high molecular weight Protein I molecules are serum sensitive (see below) and associated with primary genital disease. In contrast, serum-resistant organisms with low molecular weight Protein I are most often associated with disseminated disease.

2. **Protein II.** This protein is often referred to as the "opacity" protein because of its presence in opaque gonococcal colonies, and **mediates attachment to host cells along with pili.** The ability of Protein II to undergo extensive **antigenic variation** may also contribute to the ability of the gonococcus to **evade the immune response,** as well as **cause repeated infection.**

3. **Protein III.** This protein is in complex with Protein I, and acts as a **porin.** In addition, it appears to be the binding site for IgG blocking antibody that **prevents complement-mediated bactericidal antibody function and thus may contribute to dissemination of the disease.** Protein III shows no evidence of antigenic diversity or variation.

LOS of the gonococci, like that of the meningococci, differs from LPS in that the former has shorter, nonrepeat, O-antigenic side chains and thus a lower molecular weight. LOS has been implicated as a potential cause of **fallopian tube damage** in patients with salpingitis and may be a contributing factor in the toxicity exerted upon other cells during the course of the disease. LOS also **attracts polymorphonuclear leukocytes to the primary site of infection.** The antigenic diversity of LOS is the result of the unique epitope structure of the O-antigenic side chains of the molecule among different gonococcal strains.

Primary and invasive (direct extension) disease strains. Primary and invasive disease is usually caused by gonococcal strains **sensitive to killing by normal human serum and relatively resistant to penicillin.**

Disseminated gonococcal infection (DGI) strains. In contrast, **serum-resistance and a high degree of penicillin susceptibility are usually seen in strains isolated from patients with DGI.**

Surface-modifying factors and mechanisms of action. Although the gonococcal structural targets, surface-modifying factors, and mechanisms of action are unknown, these characteristics undoubtedly contribute in some way to the **pathogenicity of the organism and the outcome of the disease process (primary disease vs. dissemination).**

Extracellular product thought to be associated with pathogenicity. As with the meningococcus, the organism produces an **IgA1 protease.** The enzyme **inactivates local secretory IgA** and thus may play a role in facilitating the **adherence** of gonococci to mucosal surfaces.

Pathogenesis and Clinical Manifestations

ASYMPTOMATIC INFECTION. Asymptomatic infection occurs in about 10% of males and in about 20-80% of females following the introduction of the organism into a susceptible host. **Pili** and **Protein II** mediate adherence of the gonococci to mucosal cells of the urethra, cervix, rectum, and/or pharynx depending on the portal of entry, with resultant colonization. Adherence may be facilitated by cleavage of secretory IgA by **IgA1 protease. Pili** enable the organisms to resist phagocytosis. Those factors that determine the asymptomatic versus disease state are not known. However, asymptomatic individuals are both **communicable and capable of developing disseminated disease.**

PRIMARY DISEASE. Primary disease manifests as an acute urethritis, proctitis, pharyngitis, and/or ophthalmia neonatorum in both the male and female, and in the female as an acute cervicitis or vulvovaginitis.

Acute Male Urethritis. The organisms come in contact with the stratified columnar epithelium of the urethra and periurethral ducts and glands. As described for the initiation of asymptomatic infection, pili mediate antiphagocytic activity while adherence to the mucosal cells is mediated by **pili, Protein II, and IgA1 protease.** The organisms now penetrate the columnar epithelium through the intercellular spaces and reach the subepithelial connective tissue, where they multiply and induce a severe acute inflammatory response characterized by an influx of polymorphonuclear leukocytes attracted to the primary site by gonococcal **LOS and host complement components. Both pili and Protein II** mediate attachment of the gonococci to the surface of the polymorphonuclear leukocytes with eventual **phagocytosis and killing of many or all of the organisms.** The result of this confrontation is a sudden onset after a 2 to 8-day incubation period characterized by **burning and frequency of urination, and a purulent, creamy-yellow discharge.** The extent of the phagocytic process influences cure or subsequent invasion.

Acute Cervicitis and Female Urethritis. Colonization and primary disease initiates in the endocervix and urethra, respectively. The mechanisms of pathogenesis are similar to those described above for acute male urethritis. In addition to burning and frequency of urination, and vaginal mucopurulent discharge, **females experience fever and abdominal pain.**

Acute Proctitis and Pharyngitis. Colonization and primary disease can occur in either the rectum or pharynx of the male or female as a sole or accompanying primary syndrome in which the mechanisms of pathogenesis are similar to those described above for acute urethritis. In the male, acute proctitis occurs almost exclusively among bisexuals and homosexuals, while acute pharyngitis can occur irrespective of sexual preference. Clinical manifestations include purulent discharges, pharyngeal erythema, and sore throat.

Vulvovaginitis. Vulvovaginitis occurs in children 2–8 years of age following sexual abuse. Colonization and primary disease initiate in the alkaline vagina. The mechanisms of pathogenesis are similar to those already described.

Ophthalmia Neonatorum. Ophthalmia neonatorum occurs when gonococci gain access to the conjunctiva of the newborn during **passage through an infected birth canal.** An **acute conjunctivitis** results through the mechanisms of pathogenesis already described and progresses to **blindness** if not treated. This syndrome is entirely preventable through prophylaxis at birth.

INVASION (DIRECT EXTENSION) FROM THE PRIMARY DISEASE FOCUS.   This situation occurs in 1% of male and 15% of female patients.

In the Male. The organisms spread from the anterior to the posterior urethra and Cowper's glands with subsequent fibrosis leading to **urethral strictures.** They may spread from a primary urethral focus to the prostate and epididymis, colonizing, multiplying, and producing **prostatitis and/or epididymitis** by the mechanisms already described. Subsequent fibrotic obstruction of the lumen of the epididymis results in **permanent sterility.**

In the Female. The organisms spread from the primary urethral or cervical foci to the fallopian tubes and pelvic peritoneum, causing **salpingitis and pelvic inflammatory disease (PID)** by the mechanisms of pathogenesis already described with **LOS** providing an additional operative mechanism by contributing to fallopian tube damage. Subsequent fibrosis of the fallopian tubes leads to **permanent sterility or ectopic pregnancy** in 20% of salpingitis patients.

DISSEMINATED GONOCOCCAL INFECTION. Dissemination occurs in about 1% of male or female patients, usually those with asymptomatic genital infection. As indicated earlier, while the virulence factors responsible for dissemination are poorly understood, it is known that **most DGI strains,** in contrast to those that produce only primary and/or invasive disease, **are resistant to killing by normal serum, are of the $A^-H^-U^-$ auxotype,** and have **surface Protein III binding sites for IgG blocking antibody that prevents complement-mediated bactericidal antibody function.**

Septicemia results when the organisms gain access to the circulation, usually from primary genital sites, but occasionally from invasive sites. As the organisms multiply unrestricted, **LOS toxicity** contributes to the clinical manifestations of chills, fever, malaise, and characteristic petechial or papular skin lesions with central necrosis.

Arthritis and tenosynovitis result when gonococci disseminate from the circulation to the joints and synovium and multiply unrestricted. Both these forms of the disease are accompanied by fever and may or may not occur with skin lesions.

Endocarditis and meningitis are the rarest of the disseminated disease syndromes and are the result of dissemination from the circulation to the heart valves and meninges. If unrecognized, they are usually fatal.

Immunity to Reinfection

Immunity to reinfection does not exist, probably due to the considerable antigenic variation or diversity that exists among the key surface components of the organism. Multiple repeat infections are common.

Laboratory Diagnosis

SPECIMENS AND DIRECT EXAMINATION. Specimens obtained depend on the disease process and include urethral, cervical, rectal, pharyngeal, and/or conjunctival exudates, blood for culture, skin scrapings, joint fluid, and cerebrospinal fluid. The coexistence of syphilis in 2% of patients with gonorrhea necessitates the obtaining of a blood specimen for serological testing.

The correct choice of specimens is critical to successful isolation and identification of the gonococcus.

1. The culturing of rectal specimens in addition to cervical specimens from all female patients in whom asymptomatic infection or primary or invasive genital disease is suspected, results in a significant increase in the number of positive isolates.

2. Rectal and pharyngeal specimens must be obtained from bisexuals, male homosexuals, and both male and female heterosexuals when oral and/or anal sex is suspected.

3. In patients with DGI, the urethra or cervix should be cultured along with blood, skin lesions, joint fluid, and/or cerebrospinal fluid.

The direct demonstration of gram-negative intracellular diplococci within polymorphonuclear leukocytes is diagnostic only when observed in the urethral exudates of males with characteristic clinical manifestations.

1. Culture is required when gram-negative intracellular diplococci are not observed in the exudate (is it gonorrhea or chlamydial disease?), a high prevalence of PPNG occurs in the community, and tests for cure are required due to antimicrobial resistance.

2. Gram stains of smears from female urethral and cervical exudates, from rectal, pharnygeal, and conjunctival exudates of males and females, and from specimens obtained from asymptomatic patients, are unreliable due to the potential presence of nonpathogens resembling gonococcal morphology, and lack of sensitivity. In addition, *Neisseria* species present in pharyngeal exudates may be meningococcal. All such specimens must be cultured and the isolated organism identified.

The direct demonstration of gram-negative, intracellular diplococci is demonstrable in 30–50% of smears from the skin scrapings, joint fluid, and cerebrospinal fluid of patients with DGI, is diagnostic for the pathogenic *Neis-*

seria, **and must be differentiated from the meningococcus by culture and biochemical reactions.** Thus, culture of these specimens is always required.

RNA-DNA hybridization techniques on urethral and cervical smears are available and proving valuable in the rapid identification of the gonococcus. However, under circumstances already described, follow-up culture may be required.

PRIMARY ISOLATION AND IDENTIFICATION. These techniques require initial cultivation on Thayer-Martin medium. Incubation for 48 h at 35–37°C under aerobic conditions in the presence of 3–10% carbon dioxide is optimal for isolation of the organism, which may be identified as a gram-negative, oxidase positive, diplococcus that ferments glucose, but not maltose, sucrose, or lactose (Table 14.1).

Treatment

The latest treatment regimen recommended by the United States CDC is based upon the rapid development of **PPNG, tetracycline-resistant gonococci, strains with chromosome-mediated resistance to multiple antibiotics,** the relatively high frequency (up to 45%) and serious complications of coexisting chlamydial infection and disease, and the absence of a practical and reliable test for the diagnosis of chlamydial infection and disease. The PPNG strains, which represent the greatest concern, contain two plasmids, 3.4 or 4.7 MDa in size, which contain genes that code for β-lactamase production transmissable by conjugation.

The recommended regimen for patients with uncomplicated urethritis, cervicitis, or proctitis is 250 mg of ceftriaxone IM in a single injection plus 100 mg of doxycycline orally twice a day for 7 days for potential coexisting chlamydial infection. For patients who cannot take ceftriaxone, the recommended alternate is 2 g of spectinomycin IM in a single dose plus the doxycycline. For pregnant females, 500 mg of erythromycin base or stearate orally 4 times daily for 7 days is recommended as a substitute for doxycycline. The above ceftriaxone regimen is recommended for uncomplicated pharyngitis, but the alternate therapy is 500 mg of ciprofloxacin orally as a single dose.

Patients with DGI must be hospitalized and treated aggressively IM or IV with either ceftriaxone, ceftizoxime, or cefotaxime. If allergic to these antimicrobials, spectinomycin is used. Ceftriaxone or cefotaxime, in doses depending on the disease process, is recommended for the treatment of gonorrhea in infants and children including ophthalmia neonatorum. Children weighing less than 45 kg should be treated with one-half the dose of ceftriaxone required for adults or, if not tolerated, 40 mg/kg of spectinomycin IM in a single dose.

Prevention and Control

Tests for cure following therapy, identification and treatment of case contacts, the use of condoms, and education and screening of high risk populations are essential prevention and control measures. Although the reporting of cases and contacts to health authorities by physicians is required by law, compliance is less than satisfactory. The **instillation of 0.5% erythromycin, 1% tetracycline, or 1% silver nitrate into the conjunctiva of newborns at birth is required by law** and prevents gonococcal ophthalmia neonatorum.

SUMMARY

1. *Neisseria meningitidis* **is an obligate parasite of humans, harbored in the nasopharynx, and transmitted by droplet nuclei from or direct intimate contact with a case or carrier. Factors contributing to susceptibility include fatigue and exposure to inclement weather.**

2. The meningococcus is a gram-negative, nonmotile, encapsulated, piliated, strict aerobic diplococcus flattened on one side to give the appearance of a ''kidney bean'' or ''coffee bean.'' The antigenic diversity of the capsule forms the basis for classification of the meningococci into 13 serogroups.

3. The basic pathogenesis process of primary meningococcal disease is initiated in the nasopharynx from a case or carrier. Adherence to the mucosal surface with resultant colonization is mediated by pili and possibly facilitated by secretory IgA cleavage by IgA1 protease. Phagocytosis is inhibited by the capsule and the organisms continue to multiply, producing nasopharyngitis. Most patients produce complement-dependent bactericidal antibody, predominantly of the IgM type, and opsonic antibody, both of which restrict the organisms to the mucosal surface of the nasopharynx (carrier state) and eventually cause their riddance.

4. Disseminated meningococcal disease manifests most often as septicemia (meningococcemia) and meningitis. Onset may correlate with the absence of complement-dependent bactericidal antibody and opsonic antibody, the presence of serum IgA antibody that blocks the initiation of immune lysis, or complement component deficiencies. The clinical manifestations of septicemia are the result of LOS release by the organisms.

5. Effective capsular polysaccharide vaccines against meningococcal serogroups A, C, W-135, and Y are available for use in selected population

groups, such as the military. These vaccines are ineffective in children under the age of 2 years.

6. *Neisseria gonorrhoeae* is an obligate parasite of humans, harbored in the male and female genital tracts, rectum, and pharynx of cases and carriers, and transmitted exogenously by either sexual contact or from an infected female to the newborn at birth.

7. Like the meningococcus, *N. gonorrhoeae* is a gram-negative, non-motile, piliated, strict aerobic diplococcus flattened on one side so as to give the appearance of a kidney bean or coffee bean.

8. Asymptomatic infection occurs mostly, but not exclusively, in the female following introduction of *N. gonorrhoeae* from a case or carrier into a susceptible host. Adherence to the mucosal surface with resultant colonization is mediated by pili and Protein II and possibly facilitated by secretory IgA cleavage by IgA1 protease. Pili enable the organisms to resist phagocytosis. Asymptomatic individuals are communicable and capable of developing disseminated disease.

9. In acute male gonococcal urethritis, the pili mediate antiphagocytic activity and adherence to the urethral mucosal cells is mediated by pili, Protein II, and IgA protease. Polymorphonuclear leukocytes are attracted to the primary site by LOS and host complement components. Pili and Protein II mediate attachment to the surface of the polymorphonuclear leukocytes with phagocytosis and killing of many or all of the organisms. These events manifest as a sudden onset characterized by burning, frequency of urination, and a purulent, creamy-yellow discharge.

10. In acute gonococcal cervicitis, female urethritis, acute proctitis, and acute pharyngitis, colonization and primary disease can occur by the same mechanisms of pathogenesis as those seen in patients with acute male urethritis.

11. Invasion or direct extension from a primary gonococcal disease focus occasionally occurs in both males (1%) and females (15%). In the male, this results in urethral strictures, prostatitis, and/or epididymitis with fibrotic obstruction of the lumen causing permanent sterility. In the female, extension occurs from the primary urethral or cervical sites to the fallopian tubes and pelvic peritoneum resulting in salpingitis and pelvic inflammatory disease (PID).

12. Disseminated gonococcal infection (DGI) occurs in about 1% of

male or female patients, usually those with asymptomatic genital infection. Most DGI strains are resistant to killing by normal serum, are of the A⁻ H⁻ U⁻ auxotype, and have surface Protein III binding sites for IgG blocking antibody.

REFERENCES

Blake MS, Gotschlich EC (1987): Functional and immunogenic properties of pathogenic *Neisseria* surface proteins. In Inouye M (ed): Bacterial Membranes as Model Systems. New York: Wiley. pp 377–399.

Britigan BE, Cohen MS, Sparling PF (1985): Gonococcal infection: a model of molecular pathogenesis. N Eng J Med 312:1683.

Broome CV (1986): The carrier state: *Neisseria meningitidis*. J Antimicrobial Chemother 18 (Suppl A):25.

Catlin BW (1990): *Branhamella catarrhalis:* an organism gaining respect as a pathogen. Clin Microbiol Rev 3:293.

DeVoe IW (1982): The meningococcus and mechanisms of pathogenicity. Microbiol Rev 46:162.

Feldman HA (1986): The meningococcus: a twenty year perspective. Rev Infect Dis 8:288.

Frasch CE (1989): Vaccines for prevention of meningococcal disease. Clin Microbiol Rev 2:S134.

Knapp JS, Holmes KK (1975): Disseminated gonococcal infections caused by *Neisseria gonorrhoeae* with unique nutritional requirements. J Infect Dis 132:204.

Olyhoek T, Crowe BA, Achtman M (1987): Clonal population structure of *Neisseria meningitidis* serogroup A isolated from epidemics and pandemics between 1915 and 1983. Rev Infect Dis 9:665.

Roberts MC (1989): Plasmids of *Neisseria gonorrhoeae* and other *Neisseria* species. Clin Microbiol Rev 2:S18.

Rothenberg R (1979): Ophthalmia neonatorum due to *Neisseria gonorrhoeae:* prevention and treatment. Sex Trans Dis 6 (Suppl 2):187.

Sparling PF, Cannon JG, So M (1986): Phase and antigenic variation of pili and outer membrane protein II of *Neisseria gonorrhoeae*. J Infect Dis 153:196.

U.S. Department of Health and Human Services (1982): Global distribution of penicillinase-producing *Neisseria gonorrhoeae* (PPNG). MMWR 31:1.

U.S. Department of Health and Human Services (1990): Plasmid-mediated antimicrobial resistance in Neisseria gonorrhoeae—United States 1988 and 1989. MMWR 39:284.

REVIEW QUESTIONS

For questions 1 to 15, choose the ONE BEST answer or completion.

1. The initiation of disease due to *Neisseria meningitidis*
   a) is usually the result of endogenous activation
   b) never occurs in the rectum or genital tract
   c) can occur when conditions, such as fatigue, lower host resistance and the opportunity for intimate contact with a case or carrier is provided
   d) occurs following impairment of nasopharyngeal host resistance by *Moraxella catarrhalis*
   e) is restricted to the military population

2. Disseminated meningococcal disease
   a) occurs only among infants and children
   b) occurs in a relatively low percentage of nasopharyngeal carriers
   c) rarely results in meningitis
   d) is usually fatal, even when treated early
   e) is the result of an impaired cellular immune mechanism

3. The meningococcus *differs* from the gonococcus in that the *former*
   a) is a gram-negative diplococcus
   b) is piliated
   c) contains outer membrane proteins
   d) ferments glucose, maltose, sucrose, and lactose
   e) is encapsulated

4. The virulence factors of *N. meningitidis* responsible for or thought to facilitate adherence to the nasopharyngeal mucosa are
   a) pili and IgA1 protease
   b) outer membrane proteins (OMPs)
   c) capsules and lipooligosaccharide (LOS)
   d) exotoxins and enterotoxins
   e) flagella and spores

5. One of the following statements relating to meningococcemia (septicemia) and/or meningococcal meningitis is NOT TRUE.
   a) These syndromes are the most common forms of disseminated meningococcal disease.
   b) The development of these syndromes may correlate with the absence of complement-dependent bactericidal antibody and opsonic antibody.
   c) The development of these syndromes may correlate with the presence of serum IgA antibody that blocks the initiation of immune lysis.
   d) The clinical manifestations of meningococcemia are due to a powerful exotoxin.
   e) The capsule of the meningococcus is antiphagocytic and may facilitate meningeal invasion.

6. Rapid presumptive identification of the meningococcus in patients with meningitis
   a) is accomplished by the demonstration of gram-negative diplococci in nasopharyngeal swab cultures
   b) is accomplished by the use of a latex agglutination assay on spinal fluid utilizing serogroup-specific anticapsular antibody
   c) is accomplished by culturing spinal fluid on Thayer-Martin medium, and demonstrating the presence of gram-negative diplococci on isolated colonies
   d) is accomplished by conducting a direct oxidase test on spinal fluid
   e) is rarely necessary, inasmuch as the clinical manifestations are mild

7. Meningococcal vaccines
   a) are prepared from the cell wall of *N. meningitidis*
   b) rarely prevent dissemination of organisms from the primary site
   c) are serogroup-specific, capsular polysaccharides
   d) are effective for all age groups
   e) are particularly effective in the prevention of disease due to serogroup B

8. One explanation for the ability of the gonococcus to evade the immune response and to cause repeated infection in the same host is
   a) the high frequency with which pili and Protein II undergo antigenic variation during natural infection
   b) the presence of an antigenically diverse capsule
   c) the high frequency with which Protein III undergoes antigenic variation during natural infection

   d) the ability of Protein I to function as a porin in concert with Protein III
   e) its unique ability to ferment glucose

9. Asymptomatic gonococcal infection
   a) occurs exclusively in females
   b) cannot be transmitted to a susceptible host
   c) results in the development of immunity to disseminated disease
   d) is the result of pili, Protein II, and (putatively) IgA1 protease mediated adherence of the organism to mucosal cells followed by colonization
   e) never progresses to disseminated disease

10. Primary gonococcal disease
   a) occurs only as an acute male or female urethritis
   b) results in an acute inflammatory response characterized by polymorphonuclear leukocytes attracted to the primary site by LOS and host complement components
   c) is usually treated with penicillin
   d) never coexists with chlamydial or syphilitic infection
   e) never initiates in the pharynx or rectum

11. One of the following statements relating to salpingitis and/or pelvic inflammatory disease (PID) due to *Neisseria gonorrhoeae* is NOT TRUE.
   a) LOS contributes to fallopian tube damage.
   b) Subsequent fibrosis of the fallopian tubes leads to permanent sterility or ectopic pregnancy.

c) Pelvic inflammatory disease is due mainly to a powerful exotoxin.

d) These syndromes result from the spread of gonococci from a primary urethral or cervical focus to the fallopian tubes and pelvic peritoneum.

e) The mechanisms of pathogenesis are similar to those operative in the primary disease.

12. Most gonococcal strains that produce disseminated disease
   a) are sensitive to killing by normal human serum
   b) are relatively resistant to penicillin
   c) are of the T-3 or T-4 colonial type
   d) do not contain LOS
   e) are $A^-H^-U^-$ auxotrophs

13. A gram-negative diplococcus was isolated on Thayer-Martin medium from the cervix of a patient with asymptomatic infection. The organism was identified as *N. gonorrhoeae* on the basis of
   a) a positive oxidase test
   b) an agglutination test with specific antiserum
   c) a positive oxidase test and its ability to ferment glucose, but not maltose, sucrose, and lactose
   d) colonial morphology

e) a positive oxidase test and its ability to ferment glucose and maltose, but not sucrose and lactose

14. One of the following statements relating to gonococcal ophthalmia neonatorum is NOT TRUE.
   a) The untreated disease may progress to blindness.
   b) The disease can occur when the organisms gain access to the conjunctiva of the newborn during passage through an infected birth canal.
   c) The disease usually occurs as a result of transplacental passage.
   d) The disease is entirely preventable by the instillation of 0.5% erythromycin, 1% tetracycline, or 1% silver nitrate into the conjunctiva of the newborn at delivery.
   e) Ceftriaxone or cefotaxime is the treatment of choice.

15. Measures to prevent and control gonorrhea do NOT include
   a) vaccination
   b) tests for cure following therapy
   c) reporting of cases and contacts to health authorities by physicians
   d) the use of condoms
   e) treatment of case contacts

ANSWERS TO REVIEW QUESTIONS

1. **c** Factors, such as fatigue, lower host resistance so that intimate contact with a case or carrier can initiate disease. Endogenous activation rarely occurs. Proctitis or urethritis may occasionally occur in homosexuals. While *Moraxella catarrhalis* can cause a wide diversity of clinical manifestations among both normal, immunosuppressed, and immunodeficient individuals, it is usually a nonpathogenic inhabitant of the nasopharynx and *does not cause* impairment of nasopharyngeal host resistance. Meningococcal disease occurs in both the civilian and military population.

2. **b** Disseminated meningococcal disease occurs in a relatively low percentage of nasopharyngeal carriers and may occur among all age groups. The most commonly recognized form of meningococcal disease is meningitis, which can be successfully treated if recognized early. Disseminated disease is thought to be the result of impaired or inoperative humoral rather than cellular immune mechanisms.

3. **e** The meningococcus differs from the gonococcus in being encapsulated. Both are gram-negative, piliated, and contain OMPs. Neither ferments glucose, maltose, sucrose, and lactose.

4. **a** Pili are responsible for adherence of *Neisseria meningitidis* to the nasopharyngeal mucosa and IgA protease is thought to facilitate the process. Outer membrane proteins act as porins, capsules are antiphagocytic, and LOS is responsible for many of the toxic manifestations of disseminated meningococcal disease. Meningococci do not have flagella or spores and do not produce exotoxins or enterotoxins.

5. **d** As already indicated, meningococci do not produce exotoxins. However, meningococcemia and meningococcal meningitis are the most common forms of the disseminated disease, and correlate with the absence of complement-dependent bactericidal antibody and opsonic antibody or with the presence of serum IgA antibody that blocks the initiation of immune lysis. The meningococcal capsule is antiphagocytic and may facilitate meningeal invasion.

6. **b** Rapid presumptive identification of the meningococcus in patients with meningitis is essential and is accomplished by the use of a latex agglutination assay on spinal fluid utilizing serogroup-specific anticapsular antibody. The potential occurrence of both false positive and false negative results necessitates culture,

Gram-staining of the culture isolate, biochemical testing, and serogroup-specific latex agglutination testing of the isolate for definitive identification. Nasopharyngeal culture isolates of gram-negative diplococci could be nonpathogenic *Neisseria* or members of other genera. Furthermore, gram-negative diplococci cultured from spinal fluid may be pathogenic members of other genera, such as *M. catarrhalis.* In either case, culturing is not considered a "rapid" method for identification, either presumptive or definitive. Biochemical determinations are never conducted on spinal fluid specimens, inasmuch as they contain exudative components that interfere with the accuracy of the procedures. Furthermore, many genera of bacteria contain organisms that are oxidase positive.

7. *c* Meningococcal vaccines are serogroup-specific, capsular polysaccharides. Serogroup A, C, W-135, and Y vaccines are highly effective in the prevention of disseminated meningococcal disease in adults and children, age 2 years and older; under the age of 2 years, the vaccines are ineffective. Furthermore, a vaccine against serogroup B is unavailable because the capsule is easily degraded and poorly immunogenic.

8. *a* The high frequency of antigenic variation among pili and Protein II has been offered as an explanation for the ability of the gonococcus to evade the immune response and to cause repeated infection in the same host. Protein III does not undergo antigenic variation. Its function as a porin in concert with Protein I has no relationship to the mechanisms of immune response evasion or repeated infection. The organism is nonencapsulated, and its ability to ferment glucose is neither unique among bacteria nor relevant to the mechanisms operative in gonococcal evasion or reinfection.

9. *d* Asymptomatic gonococcal infection occurs in both males and females, can be transmitted to susceptible hosts, and is the result of pili, Protein II, and (putatively) IgA1 protease mediated adherence of the organism to mucosal cells followed by colonization. Disseminated disease usually occurs in patients with asymptomatic genital infection.

10. *b* Primary gonococcal disease results in an acute inflammatory response characterized by polymorphonuclear leukocytes attracted to the primary site by LOS and host complement components. It can initiate in the urethra, cervix, vagina, rectum, pharynx, or conjunctiva and may coexist with chlamydial or syphilitic infection. The rapid emergence of PPNG strains has precluded the recommendation of penicillin in the treatment of primary gonococcal disease.

11. *c* The gonococcus does not produce an exotoxin. However, LOS does contribute to fallopian tube damage and fibrosis of the fallopian tubes leads to permanent sterility or ectopic pregnancy. Salpingitis and PID result from the spread of gonococci

from a primary urethral or cervical focus to the fallopian tubes and pelvic peritoneum, and occur by mechanisms of pathogenesis similar to those operative in primary disease.

12. *e* Most DGI strains are A⁻H⁻U⁻ auxotrophs, serum resistant, susceptible to penicillin. All strains contain LOS and are of the virulent T-1 or T-2 colonial type.

13. *c* A gram-negative diplococcus may be identified definitively as *Neisseria gonorrhoeae* on the basis of a positive oxidase test *and* the ability of the organism to ferment glucose but not maltose, sucrose, and lactose. Neither a positive oxidase test nor colonial morphology would be specific for the gonococcus. Agglutination tests are nonspecific.

14. *c* Ophthalmia neonatorum does not occur in utero as a result of transplacental passage, but rather during passage through an infected birth canal. Blindness may occur if therapy is not instituted. Ceftriaxone or cefotaxime is the recommended treatment of choice. Ophthalmia neonatorum is entirely preventable by the instillation of 0.5% erythromycin, 1% tetracycline, or 1% silver nitrate into the conjunctiva of the newborn at delivery.

15. *a* There is no vaccine for gonorrhea. However, prevention and control measures do include tests for cure following therapy, reporting of cases and contacts to health authorities by physicians, the use of condoms, and the treatment of case contacts.

ENTEROBACTERIACEAE AND NONENTERIC INFECTIONS

The *Enterobacteriaceae* comprise a large and diverse family of gram-negative bacilli. They are facultative anaerobes and grow quite well in the human GI tract. These organisms are the most common of the nonanaerobic bacteria found in the human gut. For this reason, they are sometimes given the nickname "enteric" organisms, meaning "living in the GI tract." Other bacteria, such as pseudomonads (see Chapter 18), can and do live in the GI tract, but historically they have not been considered "enterics." In addition to the GI tracts of mammals, members of the family *Enterobacteriaceae* are found in the GI tracts of all other types of animals, fish, and insects, as well as in plants, soil, and water. These organisms can cause disease in each of their living hosts, even though most species are considered to be harmless parasites or commensals.

Enterobacteriaceae are usually characterized by **three key properties:**

1. *Enterobacteriaceae* **do not possess the cytochrome oxidase enzyme** and are thus "oxidase negative."

2. *Enterobacteriaceae* possess enzymes that enable them to **reduce nitrate to nitrite.**

3. *Enterobacteriaceae* are able to **ferment glucose.**

In addition, the motile organisms possess peritrichous flagella. There are now more than 100 species in at least 27 genera, with more species being named every year. As human pathogens, they cause disease by a number of different virulence mechanisms. Some examples are given in Table 15.1.

ENTEROBACTERIACEAE IN THE HUMAN GI TRACT

Many members of the *Enterobacteriaceae* are **inhabitants of the human GI tract.** Under normal circumstances, they do not cause disease in the GI tract, but **they can cause disease in other organ systems.** The presence of these organisms may even help to prevent the colonization of pathogenic bacteria that gain entry to the GI tract when the host ingests them. Other members of the *Enterobacteriaceae*, however, no matter how few are recovered, are **always** considered to be **pathogens in humans.** Diseases due to these agents originate in the GI tract, often with diarrhea as a presenting sign. These diseases are called ''enteric'' diseases and the etiologic agents are called the ''enteric pathogens.'' *Yersinia* (as an enteric pathogen), *Salmonella*, and *Shigella* species will be discussed in greater detail in Chapters 16 and 17.

Methods for Identification

COLONY MORPHOLOGY ON SELECTIVE MEDIA.   These organisms can be identified in several ways. Specimens are usually cultured on at least two types of microbiological media; the growth patterns and colony morphologies of *Enterobacteriaceae* are so characteristic that experienced microbiologists can rec-

TABLE 15.1. Virulence Mechanisms and Representative Diseases of Selected *Enterobacteriaceae*

Virulence mechanism	Type of infection	Examples of species
Enterotoxin	Diarrhea	*Escherichia coli*
Antiphagocytic capsule	Pneumonia	*Klebsiella pneumoniae*
Adherence	Urinary tract infection	*Escherichia coli*
Endotoxin	Fatal septicemia	*Serratia marcescens*
	Endotoxic shock	*Escherichia coli*
Invasiveness	Typhoid fever	*Salmonella typhi*
	Dysentery	*Shigella dysenteriae*
Intracellular survival	Plague	*Yersinia pestis*

ognize them easily. The *Enterobacteriaceae* are able to grow well on selective and differential agar, such as MacConkey agar, and they exhibit a negative oxidase test.

BIOCHEMICAL REACTIONS. Once the isolate has been initially identified as a member of the *Enterobacteriaceae* based on colonial morphology on selective agar and blood agar and positive nitrate, negative oxidase, and glucose fermentative reactions, an additional large and diverse series of biochemical reactions are tested to determine the genus and species.

Enterobacteriaceae are inoculated into tubes of media containing carbohydrate substrates and pH indicators. If they are able to utilize the carbohydrate, they will form acid products of metabolism and lower the pH of the medium. The resulting color change in the pH indicator signifies the enzymatic capabilities of the strain being tested. **Carbohydrates** important for identifying *Enterobacteriaceae* include lactose, sucrose, and mannitol. Other types of biochemical tests used to differentiate among these bacteria include tests for the presence of **enzymes,** such as the ''indole test'' for tryptophanase, the urease test, tests for the presence of dehydrogenase and dihydrolase enzymes, and the Methyl Red, Voges-Proskauer (MRVP) test for end products of glucose metabolism. The ability of an organism to produce **hydrogen sulfide (H_2S) gas** and **motility** are also important differentiating characteristics.

ANTIGENIC CHARACTERIZATION. Biochemical reactions, however, are very similar for large groups of *Enterobacteriaceae* that are different genetically or are different based on the type of disease that they cause. For example, some *Escherichia coli* are harmless inhabitants of the bowel, whereas others possess either K1 capsular structure, genes that encode for toxins, or invasive capabilities that allow them to cause disease. Each of these organisms is biochemically identical, but it is important for epidemiologic and pathogenetic reasons to be able to differentiate among them. The second identification step includes **antigenic classification** of the strain based on serologic reactivities.

To create specific antibodies, known strains are injected into animals. Three antigenic structures associated with the complex bacterial cell structure seem to elicit the strongest and most useful antibody response in experimental animals (Fig. 15.1):

Flagellar Antigens (H Antigens). The most external is the flagellar protein antigen [called H for the German word for breath (*hauch*), which the growth of a motile strain on a plate is said to resemble].

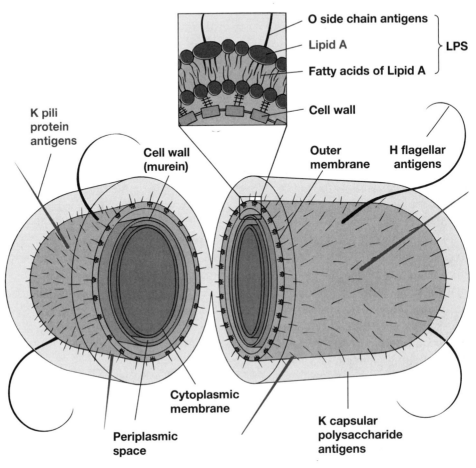

Figure 15.1.

General antigenic structure of *Enterobacteriaceae.*

Capsular Antigens (K Antigens). Capsular **polysaccharide** or **protein,** called K (for the German *kapsule*), is external to the cell wall structure. Specific polysaccharide K antigens of *Salmonella typhi* are called Vi (for virulence). In some other genera, K antigens are proteins that participate in bacterial adherence. The K88 antigen of *E. coli,* for example, comprises the structure of pili or fimbriae responsible for adherence to intestinal epithelial cells (see Chapter 1).

Somatic Antigens (O Antigens). O **polysaccharide** antigens compose the outer region of lipopolysaccharides (LPSs) in the cell wall.

Table 15.2 summarizes some important characteristics of these antigens. If the organism is not motile (e.g., *Shigella*), it will not possess flagella or flagellar H antigens. The extensive use of classical serologic typing schemes for identification of *Salmonella* spp. is discussed in Chapter 17 and the serologic identification of *Shigella* species is discussed in Chapter 18.

Species can be serotyped using whole cell agglutination tests, gel immunodiffusion, fluorescent stains linked to specific antibodies, and ELISA assays.

NONENTERIC INFECTIONS CAUSED BY *ENTEROBACTERIACEAE*

When these organisms gain access to a previously sterile site, such as the bloodstream, subcutaneous tissues, urinary tract, or when they colonize a site that is usually able to rid itself of unwelcome bacteria, such as the urethra and lung parenchyma, *Enterobacteriaceae* that are not classical enteric pathogens can cause a **destructive host response.** The type of infectious process is determined by the virulence mechanism and by the host immune status (Table 15.1). Certain *Enterobacteriaceae* are important causes of specific syndromes that will be discussed in more detail later, such as some nosocomial infections (see Chapter 21) and plague, which is caused by *Yersinia pestis,* another member of the *Enterobacteriaceae* (Chapter 13).

Endotoxin-Mediated Gram-Negative Septic Shock

Endotoxin, a term for a component of gram-negative bacterial cell walls, is one of the most important biological response mediators among the *Enterobacteriaceae*. Endotoxin is the primary contributor to their ability to cause infections with systemic complications once the bacteria escape their normal GI tract habitat. The endotoxin in bacterial cell walls is composed of and synonymous with LPS. This component is only released on destruction of the bacterial cell wall, either during autolysis or when the microbe is killed by antimicrobial agents or the immune system.

STRUCTURE OF LPS

Basic Structural Components. Lipopolysaccharide is a very long, heat-stable molecule arranged into three regions (Fig. 15.2). Region III, also called "lipid A," is integrated into the outer membrane section of the gram-negative cell wall.

TABLE 15.2. **Characteristics of Bacterial Surface Antigens**

Antigen category	Key features
Flagella (H)	Heat labile Externally located protein Elicit IgG antibody
Capsule (K or Vi)	Heat labile Protein or polysaccharide No specific antibody class elicited
Somatic cell wall (O)	Heat stable (resists boiling for 2 h) Linked to a common core structure Elicits IgM antibody

It is responsible for the biologic ''toxic'' properties of LPS. Attached to and distal to the lipid A is Region II, the ''core polysaccharide.''

Variable Region. The outer region, Region I, called ''O-specific side-chain polysaccharide,'' is different among different species and even among different ''serovars'' (serologic variants) within the same species of bacteria. The arrangement of the carbohydrates in this section of the chain determines serologic reactivity of the strain and allows microbiologists to differentiate among strains of the

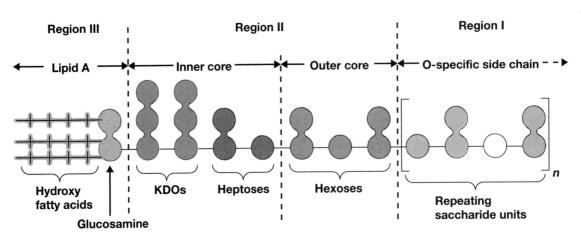

Figure 15.2.
Structure of LPS. KDO, 2-Keto-3-deoxyoctonate.

same species for epidemiologic purposes. Serologic typing based on O-specific side chain structures can be used to characterize serotypes or serovars of several genera of *Enterobacteriaceae,* including *Klebsiella, Escherichia, Shigella,* and *Salmonella.* The use of serotyping for identification of *Salmonella* species is discussed in Chapter 17.

ACTIVITIES OF LIPID A. The biologically active component of endotoxin, lipid A, mediates a number of processes in the infected host, not all of which are destructive. Some of the activities of endotoxin include:

1. Inducement of a **febrile response** in the host by two mechanisms: (a) **activation of the hypothalamus** directly and (b) action on host cells to induce synthesis of **endogenous pyrogens,** such as Interleukin-1 (IL-1) and prostaglandins.
2. Activation of **complement, granulocytes,** and **macrophages.**
3. Induction of **interferon** production.
4. Induction of **tumor necrosis factor** (cachectin) production, which reduces capillary endothelial cell permeability and promotes development of shock.
5. Induction of **colony stimulating factor** production.
6. Activity as a **B-cell mitogen.**

TREATMENT OPTIONS. **Endotoxic shock** is often fatal because of its systemic effects, particularly in debilitated patients. For this reason, vigorous research is ongoing to develop nonantibiotic therapies. Since release of bacterial cell wall components, including LPS, is one effect of antibiotic activity, antibiotic treatment is problematic. Possible candidates in the human trial stages include two slightly different types of antiendotoxin antibody preparations. These immunogenic modulators bind to endotoxin and prevent it from carrying out its biologic activities. Treatment with these new agents is still being evaluated.

Urinary Tract Infections

HOST FACTORS. Host factors, such as susceptible urinary tract epithelial cells, in combination with organism factors, such as pilial or fimbriael adhesins, some of which are also K antigen proteins, allow seemingly ''normal'' individuals to develop urinary tract infections (UTIs). These infections are much more common in women than in men for several reasons:

1. Short, moist distance (perineum) between the anal opening and the urethral meatus.

2. Sexual activity in women can disturb delicate urethral epithelium and increase chances for fecal contamination.

3. Pregnancy distorts normal anatomy and encourages some bladder retention.

4. Changes in hormonal influence on genital tract epithelium and mucosa may enhance development of urinary tract infection.

CATEGORIES OF UTI. Urinary tract infection usually falls within one of three categories. (1) **Cystitis** (confined to the bladder), (2) **Pyelonephritis** (extending to the kidney), and (3) **Acute urethral syndrome** in sexually active women, involving both an inflamed urethra and colonization of the bladder.

The number of organisms required to invoke a host inflammatory cell response, the hallmark of an infectious process, varies depending on the syndrome (Table 15.3). For this reason, clinical microbiology laboratories perform quantitative cultures of urine. Small numbers of organisms are often present in the urethra in the absence of disease; they can multiply in unrefrigerated urine and cause confusion when they are isolated in the laboratory. In the absence of mitigating circumstances, the numbers of colonies isolated from their urine must surpass a defined threshold for patients to be considered ''infected.''

ORGANISM FACTORS. The most common organism found in UTIs is *E. coli,* some of which possess special fimbriae that allow the organisms to adhere to urinary tract epithelial cells. Acute urethral syndrome is most often caused by *E. coli.*

Hospitalized patients may develop UTI with *Proteus* spp., *Providencia* spp., *Enterobacter* spp., *Klebsiella* spp., *Citrobacter* spp., or *Serratia* spp., among the *Enterobacteriaceae*. Their urinary tracts are compromised by surgery, catheters, bladder retention due to posture or neurologic problems, and other factors, discussed further in Chapter 21.

TABLE 15.3. Definition of Urinary Tract Infection[a]

Sexually active female with pyuria and symptoms (pain, burning, urgency)	> 100 CFU pure culture *Enterobacteriaceae*
Asymptomatic female	> 100,000 CFU/ml
Male	> 1000 CFU/ml

[a] Definition based on numbers of colony forming units (CFU) isolated per milliliter of urine.

Pneumonia

HOST FACTORS. Most patients who develop pneumonia due to a member of the *Enterobacteriaceae* are compromised. Hospitalized patients are often prone, with diminished cough reflexes, and anesthesia and respiratory manipulations may have damaged some of their innate immune responses, such as ciliary motility and mucus. This aspect of infectious diseases will be discussed further in Chapter 21.

Nonhospitalized patients who have lost consciousness for some time, such as alcoholics and drug addicts, elderly victims of falls or cerebrovascular accidents (strokes), are also at risk.

ORGANISM FACTORS. Among the *Enterobacteriaceae, Klebsiella pneumoniae,* historically called ''Friedlander's bacillus,'' is the most common etiologic agent of pneumonia. Like *Streptococcus pneumoniae* (see Chapter 8), this organism produces an **extracellular polysaccharide capsule** that inhibits phagocytosis of the organisms by alveolar macrophages in the lung and by other phagocytic cells.

PATHOGENESIS AND CLINICAL MANIFESTATIONS. After gaining a foothold in the lung, *K. pneumoniae* multiplies to large numbers and induces a vigorous **inflammatory response** by the host, even though the recruited phagocytic cells are not efficient at destroying the invader. The host response, consisting of an influx of polymorphonuclear leukocytes, fluids, and breakdown products of spent host cells, obstructs the free flow of oxygen between capillaries and alveolar spaces. Thus, patients actually drown in their own fluids. The characteristic X-ray picture of a patient with lobar pneumonia due to *K. pneumoniae* shows obliteration or ''white-out'' of the air-containing spaces in that section of the lung. Other *Enterobacteriaceae*, particularly those with polysaccharide capsules (*Enterobacter* and *Serratia* spp.) can also cause pneumonia.

Neonatal Meningitis and Sepsis

E. coli is second only to group B streptococci as an important etiologic agent of **neonatal meningitis and sepsis.**

ORGANISM FACTORS. *E. coli* most often implicated in neonatal sepsis are those possessing the **K1 capsular polysaccharide,** which consists partially of sialic acid and affords the organism some protection from phagocytosis and complement-mediated lysis. The K1 polysaccharide structure is very similar to the sialic acid component of mammalian cells such that the immature immune system of a newborn may not recognize the organism as being "foreign." Thus, an effective immune response is not mounted.

PATHOGENESIS AND CLINICAL MANIFESTATIONS. The neonate becomes colonized in the nose and ears and swallows material containing *E. coli* as it passes through the birth canal contaminated with fecal bacteria from the mother. Because the baby's immune response is not as yet developed, organisms gain relatively easy access to the bloodstream and, hence, to the CNS, producing septicemia and meningitis. Clinical manifestations may be subtle, including failure to eat, minimal movement, and weak cry.

OTHER INFECTIONS

Wound Infections

Enterobacteriaceae are important causative agents in wound diseases. Environmental strains may infect contaminated wounds such as *Enterobacter agglomerans* infections in farmers who injure themselves on dirty equipment used in the fields. Although such diseases may be serious and often are complicated by mixed bacterial species, the organisms acquired in the external environment are usually quite susceptible to antibiotics. This is not the case with infectious diseases acquired by hospitalized patients, such as postsurgical wound disease. The species resident in the hospital environment have usually responded to the selective pressure of surviving in the presence of multiple antibiotics by developing antibiotic resistance, often to several classes of antibiotics. Diseases involving these "hospital strains" are usually more difficult to eradicate, as discussed in Chapter 21.

Peritonitis

A patient's own endogenous bowel flora may be the source of disease. If the bowel integrity is compromised during abdominal surgery or when the GI mucosa is damaged by diseases, such as cancer or enterocolitis, the normal intestinal flora can spill into the peritoneal cavity and multiply, causing a very serious peritonitis.

Alternatively, contamination with the patient's bowel contents of an IV catheter insertion site, a shunt used for chronic ambulatory peritoneal dialysis, a postoperative wound, or simply damaged skin, can rapidly lead to infection. If *Enterobacteriaceae* gain entry to a vulnerable site, such as a necrotic ulcer on the extremity of a diabetic, or a pressure sore on a paralyzed patient, they are often able to colonize, thrive, produce toxic products, and initiate a vigorous immune response from the host, which results in tissue damage. The endotoxin released from damaged and destroyed bacterial cells contributes further to the disease process.

SUMMARY

1. The *Enterobacteriaceae* are a large and diverse group of gram-negative, facultatively anaerobic bacteria that live in mammalian GI tracts.

2. These organisms can cause disease using several virulence mechanisms: (a) toxin production (Example: *Shigella*), (b) antiphagocytic capsule (Example: *Klebsiella pneumoniae*), (c) adherence (Example: *Escherichia coli* UTI), (d) invasiveness (Example: *Salmonella typhi*), (e) intracellular multiplication (Example: *Yersinia pestis*), and (f) Endotoxin (Example: *Serratia marcescens* bacteremia).

3. The cell walls of *Enterobacteriaceae*, as for all gram-negative bacteria, contain endotoxin (LPS, syn: lipopolysaccharide), the active lipid A component of which mediates several biologic effects, including induction of host febrile response by production of IL-1 and prostaglandins, activation of complement, induction of interferon production, production of tumor necrosis factor, production of colony stimulating factor, and activity as a B-cell mitogen.

4. *Enterobacteriaceae* cause many kinds of diseases, including urinary tract, septicemia, wound, pneumonia, gastrointestinal, and bubonic and pneumonic plague.

5. Antigens significant as virulence factors and in classification of the *Enterobacteriaceae* are (a) capsular (K), (b) cell wall or somatic (O) and (c) flagellar (H).

REFERENCES

Baron EJ, Peterson LR, Finegold SM (1994): *Enterobacteriaceae*. In Bailey & Scott's Diagnostic Microbiology. 9th ed. St. Louis: C.V. Mosby. pp 362–385.

Brenner DJ (1984): *Enterobacteriaceae* Rahn 1937. In Krieg NR, Holt JG, (eds): Bergey's manual of systematic bacteriology, Vol. 1. Baltimore: Williams & Wilkins.

Ewing WH (1986): Edwards and Ewing's identification of *Enterobacteriaceae*. 4th ed. New York: Elsevier.

Starr MP, Stopl H, Truper HG, Balows A, Schlegel HC (eds) (1981): The prokaryotes: a handbook on habitats, isolation and identification of bacteria. New York: Springer-Verlag.

REVIEW QUESTIONS

For questions 1 to 6, a list of lettered options is followed by several numbered items. For each numbered item, select the ONE lettered option that is most closely associated with it.

A) Fimbriae
B) Antiphagocytic capsule
C) Enterotoxin
D) Endotoxin
E) Invasiveness

For each infectious disease syndrome caused by *Escherichia coli,* select the associated virulence mechanism.

1. Septic shock

2. Recurrent cystitis

3. Neonatal meningitis

4. Travelers' diarrhea

   A) 200 CFU/ml of *E. coli*
   B) 1000 CFU/ml of *E. coli*
   C) 10,000 CFU/ml of mixed *E. coli* and *Klebsiella* species
   D) 100,000 CFU/ml of *E. coli*

   E) 80 CFU/ml of mixed *E. coli* and *Klebsiella* species

5. A sexually active young woman presents with urgency and pain on urination. In the presence of more than 10 WBCs/mm³, what is the minimum number of colony forming units of bacteria per milliliter of urine that is still consistent with your diagnosis of acute cystitis?

6. A male patient hospitalized for orthopedic surgery develops a new fever and his urine shows moderate RBCs and a few WBCs. What is the minimum number of colony forming units of bacteria per milliliter of urine that will encourage you to treat him for a urinary tract infection?

For questions 7 and 8, choose the ONE BEST answer or completion.

7. A controversial new treatment for patients in septic shock is the administration of a genetically engineered monoclonal antibody. Against which gram-negative bacterial cell feature should this antibody be directed to have the most immediate effects in ameliorating the morbidity and perhaps the mortality of shock?
   a) The extremely outer portion of the O poly-

saccharide side chains in the bacterial cell wall.

b) The entire O polysaccharide side chain in the bacterial cell wall.

c) Region II, the core polysaccharide of the LPS.

d) Region III, the lipid A component of the LPS.

e) The major outer membrane protein (MOMP) of the bacterial cell wall.

8. Which statement is most applicable to the pathogenesis of pneumonia caused by a member of the *Enterobacteriaceae*?

a) The strong urease enzyme of *Proteus* species alkalinates the local milieu in the lung and prevents the killing of the organisms by polymorphonuclear neutrophils.

b) The adherence of *E. coli* to respiratory cell epithelium is mediated by K88 fimbriae.

c) The resistance to desiccation of *Enterobacter aerogenes* allows it to survive in droplet nuclei and evade innate host defenses until it reaches the alveoli, where it colonizes.

d) The polysaccharide capsule of *Klebsiella pneumoniae* allows it to grow to critical numbers in the lung while evading destruction by host phagocytic cells.

e) The endotoxin of *Klebsiella pneumoniae* allows it to grow to critical numbers in the lung by destroying host phagocytic cells.

ANSWERS TO REVIEW QUESTIONS

---

1. **D** Endotoxin, a lipopolysaccharide component of all gram-negative bacterial cell walls, induces fever, the activation of cytokines, and other effectors of septic shock.

2. **A** Recent studies have shown that women with recurrent urinary tract infections (UTIs) have specific receptors for sites on the fimbriae (particularly K88 antigens) of certain strains of *Echerichia coli,* which are more likely to be the etiologic agents of UTIs in these women.

3. **B** *E. coli* strains possessing the K1 capsular polysaccharide predominate among those associated with neonatal meningitis.

4. **C** One enterotoxin of diarrheal strains of *E. coli* is almost identical to that of *Shigella,* the agent of dysentery. Others cause milder forms of diarrhea.

5. **A** In the presence of pyuria, very low numbers of a pure culture of a species of *Enterobacteriaceae*, predominantly *E. coli,*

cause the "acute urethral syndrome," a form of cystitis.

6. **B** In males, the significant colony count required for entertainment of the diagnosis of a urinary tract infection is low (1000 CFU/ml), since the male anatomy discourages the entry of fecal organisms into the urethra. Relatively low numbers of mixed cultures may be indicative of overgrowth of contaminants during transport, but should be investigated, particularly if the patient has significant pyuria.

7. **d** Only lipid A, which is common to all bacterial endotoxins (LPS), mediates the biological effects of endotoxic shock.

8. **d** The antiphagocytic capsule of *Klebsiella pneumoniae,* the most common *Enterobacteriaceae* associated with pneumonia, allows this species to establish an infection once the organism gains access to the lung.

ENTEROINVASIVE AND ENTEROTOXIGENIC DIARRHEAS: SHIGELLOSIS, CHOLERA, AND OTHERS

Diarrhea may be defined as a higher volume and frequency of bowel movements than normal. It can result from numerous insults to the GI tract, but two primary mechanisms are recognized: (1) **invasion and destruction of mucosal epithelial cells** with subsequent loss of reabsorptive function, and (2) production of an exotoxin that mediates fluid secretion from intestinal epithelial cells and thus is called an **enterotoxin.** Three genera of *Enterobacteriaceae, Shigella, Escherichia,* and *Yersinia,* and a member of the *Vibrionaceae* family, *Vibrio cholerae,* are representative of agents that cause these types of diarrheas. Members of these genera also produce other kinds of infections, which are discussed in Chapters 13, 15, 17, and 18.

The genera *Shigella* and *Escherichia* are genetically similar by DNA homology and could be combined into one genus. The separate genus designations have been retained for historical reasons and for more precise conveyance of information, because *Shigella* spp. are all associated with a similar disease process and are always treated as pathogens.

Although the most important member of the genus *Yersinia* historically has been *Yersinia pestis,* the etiologic agent of plague (see Chapter 13), *Yersinia enterocolitica* is being recognized as an increasingly common etiologic agent of gastroenteritis in temperate climates. The organism can survive and multiply in cold groundwater. Unlike shigellae, *Y. enterocolitica* inhabits a well-defined environmental niche.

V. cholerae has served as a model of enterotoxigenic diarrhea production for many years. The 1990s are witness to yet another epidemic of cholera, carried to South America from China in early 1991. Now established throughout northern and central South America, more than 300,000 cases and 3000 deaths have been associated with the current epidemic.

SHIGELLOSIS

Shigella species are pathogenic members of the *Enterobacteriaceae* family. The four members of the genus (Table 16.1) cause **bacillary dysentery,** characterized by bloody diarrhea with pus, often accompanied by cramping and abdominal pain. Almost 30,000 cases of shigellosis were reported in the United States in 1990. ***Shigella sonnei* is the most common etiologic agent in the United States,** associated with 80% of cases. Shigellosis often occurs in areas of crowding and poor hygiene, such as institutions for the mentally impaired, child day care settings, or dormitories. Sporadic cases are also recognized.

TABLE 16.1. Characteristics of *Shigella* Species

Species	Serogroup	Key features
dysenteriae (Shiga bacillus)	A	12 Serotypes; serotype 1 most important worldwide; major cause of epidemic dysentery; produces a potent toxin (Shiga)
flexneri	B	14 Serotypes; does not produce Shiga toxin, therefore causes less severe disease
boydii	C	18 Serotypes
sonnei	D	1 Serotype; most common serogroup in United States

Habitat

Shigella is confined to humans and some higher primates; most infections are passed by the **fecal-oral** route. *Shigella dysenteriae,* the most virulent species, is usually acquired by Americans during foreign travel. It is endemic in developing countries where standards of hygiene are low.

Transmission

EXOGENOUS. *Shigella* is transmitted by contamination of food, fingers, feces, flies, and fomites (the five ''F''s). The infective dose is extremely low, less than 200 organisms. The organisms are transmitted during ingestion of contaminated water or food. Bathing, washing clothes, and playing in water sources used for sewage are high risk activities. In areas of good sanitation, infection is usually acquired by poor handwashing practices. Food handlers, young children, teachers, and health care workers are at risk.

Properties of the Organism

Resistance to environmental conditions and physical and chemical agents. Shigellae can remain viable in food and water and on fomites for as long as 6 months. Paradoxically, shigellae are very fragile in human feces collected for laboratory studies. These organisms die rapidly, usually within 30 min, in feces exposed to cold, drying conditions, or simply in feces placed in clean collection containers. Shigellae are readily killed by chlorination of water, heat, and chemical agents.

Microscopic morphology. *Shigella* species are **gram-negative, nonspore-forming nonmotile bacilli** without a demonstrable capsule.

Macroscopic morphology. *Shigella* are facultative anaerobes and grow well on ordinary laboratory media. On selective media, such as Hektoen enteric agar and MacConkey agar, they form distinctive colonies. The four species cannot be distinguished biochemically, definitive identification must be performed with specific antisera.

Antigenic structure. **Polysaccharide somatic O antigens** are used for serogroup and serotype classification and assist the organism in avoiding phagocytosis and killing by serum. *Shigella* LPS is thought to be responsible for necrosis of epithelium in terminal ileum and colon, superficial necrosis, hemorrhage, fever, and in severe cases, vascular collapse. The *Shigella* LPS core is similar, if not identical, to LPS of other *Enterobacteriaceae.*

Extracellular products associated with pathogenicity:

1. Shiga toxin. This toxin, produced by *S. dysenteriae*, possesses **cytotoxin, neurotoxin,** and **enterotoxin activity,** and consists of two chains: a single A subunit responsible for biologic activity and five B subunits responsible for binding the toxin to susceptible cells. The A subunit inhibits protein synthesis, and thus alters the ability of epithelial cells to transport electrolytes, leading to fluid accumulation in the intestinal lumen. The A subunit also mediates neurotoxic activity, which may be responsible for the severity and relatively high case fatality rate of *S. dysenteriae* disease due to convulsions and coma. The cytotoxic activity leads to inhibition of protein synthesis of host cells and ultimately to cell destruction.

2. *Shigella* virulence. The virulence of *Shigella* is dependent on the presence of a **220-kDa plasmid associated with invasiveness.** A series of genes regulates secretion of specific "invasins" that localize on *Shigella* outer membranes. A 120-kDa outer-membrane protein, *vir G,* is responsible for intercellular and intracellular spread of the bacteria. Genes encoding both sets of virulence proteins are located on the plasmid. Tests for invasiveness have classically involved inoculating the rabbit or guinea pig conjunctiva with a suspension of the organisms and observing for purulent discharge and opacification (the Serény test). This procedure has been largely replaced by in vitro cell culture invasiveness assays.

Pathogenesis and Clinical Manifestations

After entry into the host during ingestion of contaminated food or water, the organisms **survive stomach acidity,** pass through the small intestine, and adhere to the mucosal epithelium of the **terminal ileum and colon.** Invasins on the bacterial surface bind to host cell surface protein receptors called "integrins." The shigellae direct host epithelial cells (nonprofessional phagocytes) to polymerize actin and accumulate myosin at the point of entry, allowing internalization of the bacteria. Once inside cells, **shigellae lyse the phagosome membrane and multiply directly in the cytoplasm.** Cell-to-cell infection is mediated by inducing host cells to create filaments of polymerized actin (F-actin) by which the bacteria invade adjacent cells.

Epithelial cells die due to **inhibition of respiratory activity.** The host responds with an acute inflammatory response and fluid exudate. After 24–48 h, continued intracellular multiplication, inflammation, and LPS release result in necrosis of mucosal surface, superficial ulceration, hemorrhage, and diarrhea. Diarrhea with blood and mucous constitutes dysentery. Patients may experience fever, severe cramping, and abdominal pain. The infectious focus remains in the epithelium of the terminal ileum and colon. The disease is usually self-limiting after 2–5 days. Fatalities due to intestinal perforation and hemorrhage occur less than 1% except for cases due to *S. dysenteriae*. The case fatality rate of 20% for disease caused by *S. dysenteriae* is due to more intensive toxin activity resulting in severe diarrhea, convulsions, coma, intestinal perforation and hemorrhage. There is a 1–3% chance that recovered patients may become chronic carriers and serve as long-term reservoirs of infection.

Immunity to Reinfection

No immunity is acquired after infection. Vaccines are in the development stages.

Laboratory Diagnosis

SPECIMENS. Stool should be collected for diagnosis of dysentery. Microbiologists will inspect the entire specimen and choose areas of blood or mucus to culture for optimal yield. Routine rectal swabs are not recommended as they may not contain sufficient material for culture and are less likely to maintain viability of shigellae. Rectal swab obtained during sigmoidoscopy is an excellent specimen. If the specimen cannot be inoculated into or onto media immediately, it must be maintained in buffered glycerol saline or Cary-Blair, a buffered thioglycolic acid semisolid agar transport medium.

PRIMARY ISOLATION AND IDENTIFICATION. Stools are inoculated to selective media. Colonies are usually detected after 24 h of incubation. These colonies are identified based on initial morphology and verification of the species by biochemical tests and serologic typing.

IMMUNOSEROLOGIC TESTS. Immunoserologic tests are of no value.

Treatment

Rehydration and restoration of electrolyte balance is essential. Oral rehydration fluids are used most often, with or without antibiotics. Ampicillin, trimethoprim-sulfamethoxazole, and trimethoprim alone have been effective for treating cases and carriers. Plasmid-mediated resistance is occurring more frequently, however. For resistant strains, nalidixic acid or newer quinolones are alternative choices.

Prevention and Control

Isolate and treat both the cases and the carriers. Emphasize proper hygiene practices, such as sewage disposal and treatment, using separate water sources for drinking and other activities. Chlorinate the water supply. Emphasize vigilance for travelers to foreign countries with endemic shigellosis.

ESCHERICHIA COLI DIARRHEA

Escherichia coli causes diarrhea by at least four mechanisms (Table 16.2). Specific serotypes are usually associated with each virulence mechanism. Because the biochemical characteristics of these strains are not distinctive and because the virulence determinants are usually plasmid mediated and can move among strains, identification of virulent *E. coli* in cultures of patient specimens is difficult.

In addition to the four well-characterized virulence mechanisms, certain serotypes of *E. coli* have been implicated in outbreaks of infant diarrhea. The virulence mechanisms have not been elucidated, but these strains can be identified by specific antisera; they are known as **enteropathogenic *E. coli* (EPEC).**

Habitat

E. coli strains are ubiquitous in the GI tracts of mammals and in the environment.

TABLE 16.2. Virulence Mechanisms of *Escherichia coli*-Associated Diarrhea

Virulence mechanism	Designation	Comments
Adherence	Enteroadherent *E. coli* (EAEC)	Newly described, not well characterized
Invasiveness	Enteroinvasive *E. coli* (EIEC)	Possess virulence plasmids similar to *Shigella*
Enterotoxin	Enterotoxigenic *E. coli* (ETEC)	Produce heat-labile toxin (LT) resembling cholera toxin and heat-stable toxin (ST)
Verotoxin	Verotoxin-producing *E. coli*	Usually serotype O157:H7; produce bloody diarrhea and hemolytic/uremic syndrome

Transmission

EXOGENOUS. Infection is usually transmitted by the fecal-oral route. For enterotoxigenic *E. coli* (ETEC), the infective dose is 10^6–10^9 organisms. In nursery outbreaks of enteropathogenic *E. coli,* transmission is thought to be by way of the hands of nurses. Verotoxic *E. coli* outbreaks have been associated with under-cooked hamburger meat served at fast-food restaurants, such as the recent serious outbreak in the Pacific Northwest.

Properties of the Organism

All *E. coli* are members of the *Enterobacteriaceae* and share the properties outlined in Chapter 15. For most strains that cause enteric disease, no definitive identifying characteristics are available. Verotoxin-producing *E. coli,* in contrast, are sorbitol negative, which distinguishes them from the majority of the indigenous intestinal strains. Extracellular products associated with pathogenicity follow:

1. Enterotoxigenic strains produce a **heat labile toxin (LT)** that is virtually identical to cholera toxin (described in this chapter) and a **heat stable toxin (ST).** The ST activates guanylate cyclase in intestinal epithelial cells, the subsequent overproduction of cyclic guanosine monophosphate (cGMP) in the cells disrupts ion exchange and results in an outpouring of fluids into the intestinal lumen.

2. Verotoxin-producing strains produce two cytotoxins that are similar to Shiga toxin. These toxins are called **Shiga-like toxins (SLTs).** The SLTs have the same three toxic activities as Shiga toxin: neurotoxic, cytotoxic, and enterotoxic. These toxins bind to the same receptors and have an identical mode of action as Shiga toxin.

3. *E. coli* that cause GI disease often possess **pili** that serve as mediators of attachment, called **colonization factor antigens (CFA).**

Pathogenesis and Clinical Manifestations

Enteroadherent strains are thought to interfere with fluid influx and eflux by **physically blocking the mucosal cell surfaces.** The pathogenic mechanism is not well understood. Enteroinvasive strains cause disease indistinguishable from that caused by *Shigella.*

Enterotoxigenic *E. coli* disease, most common in children in developing countries, is made more serious by the malnourished status of most patients. The disease is usually seen in the United States among travelers returning from foreign countries with poor sanitation. Enterotoxigenic *E. coli* diarrhea is self-limiting and not as severe as that of cholera or shigellosis. Symptoms usually begin 24–72 h after ingestion of the organisms. Disease is characterized by watery diarrhea, cramping, and vomiting.

Verotoxin-producing *E. coli* are responsible for increasingly common episodes of diarrhea in the United States. Originally thought to be important only in bloody diarrhea, the spectrum of disease syndromes is expanding. Serious secondary sequelae include hemorrhagic colitis, hemolytic uremic syndrome, and thrombotic thrombocytopenic purpura.

Immunity to Reinfection

No immunity is acquired after infection.

Laboratory Diagnosis

SPECIMENS. For most *E. coli*–associated diarrheas, special studies available only in public health laboratories are necessary to identify pathogenic strains of *E. coli*. For this reason, only specimens obtained during documented outbreaks are acceptable. Special arrangements for processing are usually required. Both DNA probes and ELISA methods are in the development stage. Stool should be collected for diagnosis of *E. coli*–associated diarrhea. The entire specimen is examined and areas of blood or mucus are chosen for culture to obtain optimal yield. A rectal swab obtained during sigmoidoscopy is an excellent specimen. If the specimen cannot be inoculated into or onto media immediately, it must be maintained in buffered glycerol saline or Cary-Blair transport medium.

PRIMARY ISOLATION AND IDENTIFICATION. Stools are inoculated onto blood agar and MacConkey agar. With the exception of some strains of verotoxin-producing *E. coli,* for which MacConkey-sorbitol agar is used, there are no selective media. Colonies are usually detected after 24 h of incubation. Colonies are identified based on initial morphology and the species is verified by biochemical tests and serologic typing. For verotoxigenic *E. coli,* particle agglutination tests for serotype O157:H7 are available.

SEROLOGIC TESTS. Serologic tests are of no value.

Treatment

As for shigellosis, rehydration and restoration of electrolyte balance is the goal of therapy. Trimethoprim-sulfamethoxazole and quinolones, such as ciprofloxacin and norfloxacin, have been used to treat serious cases.

Prevention and Control

Observe good hygienic practices. Do not eat undercooked meat products. Travelers to underdeveloped areas should eat only cooked foods or peeled fruits. Do not drink the water. Copious quantities of Pepto-Bismol[R] will prevent illness. Prophylactic norfloxacin is also effective.

YERSINIA ENTEROCOLITICA DIARRHEA

Y. enterocolitica can maintain vigor in the environment for long periods because of low nutritional requirements and ability to grow at diverse temperatures. The species is also common in domestic animals, which serve as a reservoir for human acquisition. Contaminated milk, water, and various foods have been implicated as vehicles of outbreaks.

Yersiniae possess **invasins** that mediate uptake by nonprofessional phagocytic cells (mucosal lining epithelial cells) of the GI tract. The invasive properties of these organisms are identical to those of shigellae but unlike shigellae, the disease process takes place in the **small intestine.** *Y. enterocolitica* is also able to **inhibit phagocytosis** by lipoprotein factors (V and W antigens) similar to those of *Y. pestis* (Chapter 13). Once within the cells, in a fashion similar to that of *Salmonella typhi,* the organisms are carried to the regional lymph nodes. Many strains **produce a heat-stable enterotoxin resembling the ST of *E. coli.*** The clinical syndrome can be indistinguishable from acute appendicitis, with fever, abdominal pain and guarding, and peripheral neutrophilia. Acute, watery diarrhea is the most frequent presentation.

Special media, called CIN agar, containing the antibiotics cefsulodin, irgasan, and novobiocin, can be used to isolate *Y. enterocolitica* from feces. Incubation at room temperature will enrich for yersiniae, since most fecal flora cannot multiply at that low temperature. In many parts of the United States, cultures for *Y. enterocolitica* are available only by special request.

Since this organism has only recently been recognized as an etiologic agent of diarrhea, many factors relating to pathogenesis and epidemiology remain to be elucidated. Review Chapter 13 for more details.

CHOLERA

The first major pandemic of cholera, which began in 1816, spread from India throughout the world. Since then, seven pandemics have occurred, with the seventh ongoing. India, Bangladesh, and Africa remain the areas of highest endemicity. A 1947 outbreak in Egypt involved 33,000 cases and 20,000 deaths. During the early 1960s, an epidemic emanating from Southeast Asia spread to 23 countries and resulted in 14,000 deaths. The most recent epidemic is occurring in South and Central America, where lack of chlorination of the water in some Peruvian cities has contributed to rapid spread of the organism. Small endemic U.S. foci of primarily non-O1 serogroups are present in the Gulf Coast of Louisiana, Texas, Chesapeake Bay, northern California, and the Northwest coast of the United States. Vibrios are concentrated by filter-feeding bivalve shellfish and acquired by ingestion of raw shellfish. **Two biotypes of serogroup O1 are responsible for most epidemic cholera:** the "**cholerae**" (classical) and the "**el tor**" (named after the El Tor quarantine camp where it was first isolated). Non-O1 *V. cholerae* usually cause sporadic disease, although a new epidemic serogroup (O139) has recently emerged.

Habitat

The organisms can exist in saltwater for long periods of time and are found in plankton, shellfish, and environmental samples. The organisms are harbored in the GI tracts of patients; chronic carriage is rare, occurring in 0.3–20% of patients immediately following an outbreak and usually lasting 3–4 weeks.

Transmission

EXOGENOUS. Transmission occurs after ingestion of **uncooked or undercooked contaminated seafood** or by the **fecal-oral route.** Bathing, washing clothes, and playing in water sources used for sewage are high risk activities. The infective dose is 10^{11} organisms in immunocompetent hosts.

Properties of the Organism

Resistance to environmental conditions and physical and chemical agents. Vibrios can remain viable in food and water for up to 3 weeks. Shellfish harboring

V. cholerae must be boiled for at least 10 min to kill the organisms. Chlorination of water and standard disinfectants are able to destroy the organism easily.

Microscopic morphology. V. cholerae is a **gram-negative, nonencapsulated rod** that may occasionally appear slightly curved, particularly when viewed in a saline wet preparation or under dark-field microscopy (Fig. 16.1) The organism exhibits characteristic vibratory and darting motility, mediated by a single polar flagellum. Pili act as adherence factors.

Macroscopic morphology. V. cholerae is a facultative anaerobe. The organism grows regularly on routine laboratory media, but can be enriched by incubation in alkaline broths, such as alkaline peptone water. Special selective media, such as thiosulfate-citrate-bile salts (TCBS) agar, are used for isolation of *V. cholerae* and related vibrios from clinical specimens.

Antigenic structure. Cholera vibrios are divided into six subgroups based on somatic O polysaccharide (LPS) antigens. Epidemic and most severe disease is caused by group O1; the non-O1 serogroups of *V. cholerae* (except the new O139 strain) usually cause less severe disease. All strains of *V. cholerae* share a single H flagellar antigen. **Flagellum-mediated motility is essential for attachment** and subsequent disease production; **nonmotile strains are nonvirulent.** Lipopolysaccharide has not been implicated in the pathogenesis of cholera. Pili serve as adhesins in the GI tract and are thought to mediate attachment of the bacteria to the microvilli in the epithelial cell brush border.

Biotypes. The two biotypes of serogroup O1 vibrios are based on hemolytic activity against sheep erythrocytes, biochemical reactions, susceptibility to antibiotics, and susceptibility to specific phages. The ''cholerae'' biotype and O139 serogroup are prevalent in Bangladesh and India but the current pan-American epidemic is due to the ''el tor'' biotype of *V. cholerae* O1.

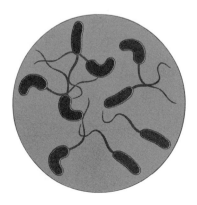

Figure 16.1.

The morphology of *V. cholerae.*

Extracellular products associated with pathogenicity

1. Cholera toxin. **Cholera toxin** (or **choleragen**) is the only virulence factor of *V. cholerae* that has been established definitively (Fig. 16.2). The genes for its production are located on the chromosome. Choleragen is made up of five polypeptide B subunits circling a central polypeptide A subunit. The B subunits bind to GM-1 ganglioside receptors on epithelial cell surfaces in the small intestine. Subunit A activates **adenyl cyclase** in the intestinal crypt cell membranes to produce cAMP. **Increased cAMP mediates hypersecretion of fluids and chloride ions and inhibition of sodium absorption.**

2. Additional extracellular properties. Additional extracellular products whose role in pathogenesis has not been elucidated include cytolysins, cytotoxins, hemolysins, enterotoxins other than cholera toxin, and proteases.

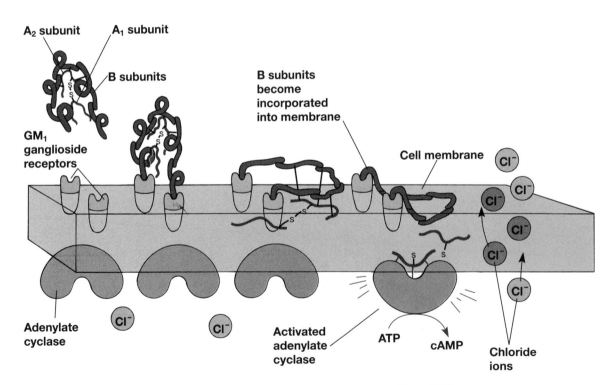

Figure 16.2.

Mechanism of the action of cholera toxin.

Pathogenesis and Clinical Manifestations

Large numbers of organisms are ingested in contaminated food or water. Those that survive the gastric acidity attach, with the aid of flagella and pili, to the brush borders of epithelial cells in the small intestine. The vibrios multiply to large numbers rapidly on the mucosal surface and produce choleragen, which binds to the ganglioside receptors on the host epithelial cells. The toxin A subunit enters through the cell membrane and activates the adenyl cyclase system. Resulting overproduction of cAMP results in release of fluids and electrolytes into the intestinal lumen. After several hours to 3-days incubation, patients experience a sudden onset of explosive, watery diarrhea with vomiting and abdominal pain. Fluid output can be voluminous, with as many as 7 L of stool per day and 20–30 evacuations. Stools do not contain polymorphonuclear leukocytes, since there is no cellular invasion and no inflammatory response. The intestinal mucosa is altered drastically and becomes eroded or ''shredded.'' Solid fecal material is depleted and stool rapidly becomes clear, containing numerous small white flecks resembling grains of rice, thought to be plugs of mucus from intestinal cells, thus the term **''rice-water stools.''** Patients rapidly become dehydrated, showing loss of skin turgor, sunken eyes, and so on.

If untreated, 60% of patients become comatose and die. With adequate fluid replacement, mortality is less than 1%. The carrier rate for untreated survivors ranges from 0.3–20% but lasts only a few weeks. Milder forms of the disease, particularly those caused by non-O1 cholera vibrios, do exist.

Immunity to Reinfection

Vaccines are available, but they are not effective in the face of a large inoculum. Recombinant vaccines are being developed. Patients experience a long-lasting and vigorous immunity to reinfection, but the total duration is unknown. Secretory or serum IgA may mediate some immunity.

Laboratory Diagnosis

SPECIMEN. Stool is the only specimen used for diagnosis of cholera. Clear rice-water stool or stool containing mucus is highly suspicious. Inasmuch as glycerol is inhibitory to *V. cholerae* and other vibrios, do not place stool into buffered glycerol saline, which is used to transport stool for isolation of other enteric pathogens. If transport is required, use Cary-Blair or alkaline peptone water.

PRIMARY ISOLATION AND IDENTIFICATION. Direct microscopic examination of a rice-water stool by dark-field microscopy may reveal characteristic motile organisms; however, only experienced technologists can rely on this technique. Stools should be inoculated into or onto standard laboratory media and TCBS selective agar. All colonies should be screened for indophenol oxidase enzyme. Oxidase-positive isolates are then identified biochemically. Most automated instruments used in clinical laboratories do not identify *V. cholerae* reliably; conventional tests are necessary. **Specific serologic typing is essential for definitive identification.**

Treatment

Fluid and electrolyte replacement is the primary treatment. Oral rehydration suspensions that promote glucose-coupled sodium and potassium ion uptake are recommended by the WHO (Table 16.3). Immediate institution of rehydration will save all but the most severely ill patients. Intravenous fluids may be necessary for such cases.

If treatment is required, tetracycline is the drug of choice.

Prevention and Control

Isolate and treat both the cases and the carriers. Emphasize proper hygiene practices, such as sewage disposal and treatment, using separate water sources for drinking and other activities, and so on. Chlorinate all potable water supplies. Boil shellfish for a minimum of 10 min before eating. Do not eat raw shellfish. If traveling to an endemic area, eat only cooked foods served hot and drink only boiled or bottled water. **Vaccines are not recommended at this time** because of their limited effectiveness. No countries currently require visitors to show evidence of cholera vaccination.

SUMMARY

1. **Bacterial diarrhea can be caused by a number of different species of organisms. The most important pathogenic mechanisms involved are (a) invasiveness (Example:** *Shigella***) and (b) enterotoxin production (Example:** *Vibrio cholerae***).**

2. **Bacterial diarrheas are transmitted by contaminated food or water (the fecal-oral route). These bacteria are primarily pathogens of humans.**

TABLE 16.3. Oral Rehydration Suspension Suitable for Undeveloped Areas (Basic Components)

Component	Units (g/L)
Sodium chloride	3.5
Potassium chloride	1.5
Rice flour	30–80
Trisodium citrate[a]	2.9

[a] The citrate component can be satisfied by adding lemon or lime juice to the solution.

3. Among the *Enterobacteriaceae*, the following genera are agents of enteric disease: (a) *Salmonella* (see Chapter 17) is an intracellular pathogen and can invade intestinal epithelium. (b) *Shigella* causes bacillary dysentery, characterized by bloody stools with pus. (c) *Escherichia coli* cause travelers' diarrhea and hemorrhagic diarrhea (the verotoxin-producing strain). (d) *Yersinia enterocolitica* causes diarrhea and pseudoappendicitis.

4. The enterotoxins produced by *Shigella* and verotoxin-producing *E. coli* act by activating guanylate cyclase in intestinal epithelial cells; the resulting production of cGMP in the cells causes ion transport dysfunction and outpouring of fluids into the intestinal lumen.

5. Cholera, caused by the gram-negative, oxidase-positive, halophilic curved bacillus *V. cholerae,* is the cause of worldwide pandemics of devastating dehydrating diarrheal disease.

6. The toxin of *V. cholerae* is the prototype two-subunit enterotoxin. The B subunits bind to the epithelial cell membrane and the A subunit activates adenylate cyclase. The resulting production of cAMP causes ion transport dysfunction and outpouring of fluids into the intestinal lumen.

REFERENCES

Anderson C (1991): Cholera epidemic traced to risk miscalculation. Nature (London) 354:255.

Brubaker RR (1991): Factors promoting acute and chronic diseases caused by Yersiniae. Clin Microbiol Rev 4:309.

Janda JM, Powers C, Bryant RG, Abbott SL (1988): Current perspectives on the epidemiology and pathogenesis of clinically significant *Vibrio* spp. Clin Microbiol Rev 1:245.

Keusch GT (1991): Workshop on invasive diarrheas, shigellosis, and dysentery. Rev Infect Dis 13S:1. (Numerous relevant papers.)

REVIEW QUESTIONS

For questions 1 to 6, a list of lettered options is followed by several numbered items. For each numbered item, select the ONE lettered option that is most closely associated with it.

A) *Shigella boydii*
B) *Shigella dysenteriae*
C) *Shigella flexneri*
D) *Shigella sonnei*

1. The species most commonly isolated from patients with diarrhea in the United States.

2. The most virulent species.

A) Thiosulfate-citrate-bile salts agar
B) Hektoen enteric agar
C) MacConkey agar with sorbitol
D) Cary-Blair transport medium
E) CIN agar (incubated at room temperature)

For each microbiological culture medium, select the associated diagnostic situation.

3. Isolation of *Vibrio cholerae* from a Californian with rice-water stools who has just returned from a trip to Peru.

4. Isolation of verotoxin-producing *Escherichia coli* from a college student with bloody diarrhea.

5. Isolation of *Shigella sonnei* in feces that must be mailed to a reference laboratory from a rural location.

6. Isolation of *Yersinia enterocolitica* from a young man admitted with a tentative diagnosis of appendicitis.

For questions 7 to 11, choose the ONE BEST answer or completion.

7. The Shiga toxin of *Shigella dysenteriae* possesses which of the following biological activities?
a) Cytotoxic
b) Neurotoxic
c) Enterotoxic
d) a and c only
e) a, b, and c

8. Loss of virulence in a laboratory-maintained strain of *S. dysenteriae* is most likely the result of
a) loss of the 220-kDa plasmid that carries genes for invasiveness

b) loss of the ability to sequester iron to use as a growth factor

c) loss of the ability to multiply at 35°C

d) mutation in the genes that produce the Shiga toxin

e) mutation in the genes that code for the 120-kDa major outer-membrane protein

9. Which statement most accurately represents the activities of shigellae in the intestinal tract early in the infectious process?

a) The organisms are phagocytized by intestinal macrophages and inhibit lysosomal fusion.

b) The organisms are engulfed by nonprofessional intestinal epithelial cells and they escape the phagosome to multiply in the cytoplasm.

c) The organisms are endocytosed by non-professional intestinal epithelial cells where they produce a potent cytotoxin that lyses the cells and allows spread of the infection.

d) The organisms adhere to the outside of intestinal epithelial cells by means of adhesins, where they multiply to large numbers.

e) The organisms adhere to integrins on the outside of intestinal epithelial cells and produce a potent enterotoxin.

10. Cholera toxin, the classical example of a subunit toxin, mediates diarrhea by

a) breaking down intestinal cell membranes and destroying absorptive capabilities

b) acting on the calcium channels in the intestinal cell membranes to induce fluid secretion

c) acting on the ganglioside receptors on intestinal cell surfaces to allow entry of the bacteria into the cells

d) acting as a classical endotoxin and mediating production of fever, cytokines, and other factors

e) acting to stimulate adenyl cyclase enzyme in intestinal cell membranes, which results in increased intracellular cAMP and hypersecretion of chloride ions and fluids

11. The main reason that cholera does not result in as many fatalities as it has in the past is that

a) an effective vaccine is available

b) sanitation is at a higher level worldwide

c) oral rehydration therapy is used effectively worldwide

d) an effective antibiotic (tetracycline) is widely available and inexpensive

e) most strains isolated today are the ''el tor'' biotype, which is less virulent than the classical ''cholerae'' biotype

ANSWERS TO REVIEW QUESTIONS

1. **D** The others are much less common; *Shigella dysenteriae* does not have a significant presence in North America but is much more common in undeveloped parts of the world.

2. **B** Bacillary dysentery, mediated in part by action of the Shiga toxin of *S. dysenteriae*, may be extremely severe.

3. **A** The TCBS agar is specific and selective for most vibrios.

4. **C** Among *Escherichia coli*, only a few strains are not able to ferment sorbitol. One of the characteristics of the verotoxic serogroups is that they are sorbitol negative, which is exploited in a selective medium, MacConkey-sorbitol. On this medium, which contains sorbitol instead of lactose, the sorbitol-negative strains appear as pink pink or colorless colonies, whereas the common, sorbitol-positive *E. coli* strains appear as dark pink colonies.

5. **D** Shigellae are so fragile in feces that they are easily destroyed by fecal enzymes once they contact the air. Transport of feces for isolation of *Shigella* must be performed in a highly buffered medium. Cary-Blair is the most commonly used transport medium for stool, since it preserves viability of many enteric pathogens.

6. **E** The CIN agar is specially formulated to inhibit most enteric pathogens and allow recognition of *Yersinia enterocolitica*. Incubation at room temperature inhibits growth of fecal coliforms, but not *Yersinia*, which are able to multiply at extremely low temperatures.

7. **e**

8. **a** Genes for invasiveness are carried on a 220-kDa plasmid. Since loss of plasmids often occurs during passage in vitro, and since invasiveness is essential for virulence, this event is the most likely cause of loss of virulence. A single mutation is less likely to completely destroy virulence since virulence is dependent on more than one component. In addition, loss of a plasmid is a more likely event than a significant mutation during standard laboratory passages.

9. **b** Once these organisms have bound to the "integrins" of host cells by means of "invasin" protein adhesins, shigellae induce their uptake into intestinal epithelial cells. Shigellae escape the phagosome

and multiply in the cytoplasm, ultimately destroying host cells and tissues and inducing an inflammatory response.

10. *e* The increased cAMP induced by activation of membrane-bound adenyl cyclase causes ion secretion and subsequent fluid secretion into the intestinal lumen. The massive outpouring of fluids is unparalleled among bacterial diarrheas.

11. *c* Cholera is still widespread and equally devastating as it has ever been, but rural health workers have been schooled in the preparation and administration of oral rehydration fluids (available to even the most undeveloped parts of the world). Recognition of the lifesaving effects of these fluids has dramatically reduced the mortality associated with cholera epidemics. Antibiotics are rarely necessary.

SALMONELLOSIS AND TYPHOID FEVER

Salmonella species are pathogenic members of the *Enterobacteriaceae* family. Classically, three species were considered: *Salmonella typhi, Salmonella choleraesuis,* and *Salmonella enteritidis* [within which fell thousands of individual serovars (serotypes), including *Salmonella typhimurium* and others]. The most recent taxonomic studies recognize two species: *Salmonella choleraesuis,* containing >2500 serovars in six subspecies groups, and *Salmonella bongori,* containing <10 very rare serovars. Most human pathogens are serovars within *S. choleraesuis.* Both classification methods are used today; the serovar is often written as if it were the species name, i.e, *S. typhimurium* and *S. enteritidis.*

S. enteritidis and related serovars are very common agents of food-borne **gastroenteritis** because of their wide distribution in animal carcasses that are mishandled during food preparation. A more serious systemic disease, **typhoid fever,** is caused by *S. typhi.* Systemic disease without a reticuloendothelial focus, caused by *Salmonella* other than *S. typhi,* is called "enteric fever" or simply **"septicemia."**

SALMONELLOSIS (GASTROENTERITIS)

Although septicemia, typhoid fever, and enteric disease caused by *Salmonella* are salmonellosis, their distinct clinical and epidemiologic features allow this differential nomenclature, in which salmonellosis refers to gastroenteritis. Approximately 50,000 cases of salmonellosis were reported in the United States in 1990, but some health experts estimate the true prevalence to be twenty times greater. The dramatic changes in food distribution, which allow products from one source to reach consumers across the entire country, and the number of people who eat away from home, serve to dilute individual cases and prevent recognition of outbreaks. Epidemiologic studies are often initiated when several isolates of an unusual serovar are identified by one laboratory.

Habitat

Salmonellae other than *S. typhi* can be found in the GI tract of many animals, including poultry, rodents, wild birds, and so on, where they either cause outright disease or are carried without apparent harmful effects on the host. A major source of human infection is commercial poultry, where overcrowding and inattention to good hygiene contribute to the colonization of the flocks. Chickens and turkey carcasses are contaminated with salmonellae from their intestinal tracts during processing. If they are not fully cooked, the poultry meat serves as a vehicle of food-borne infection. If other ready-to-serve foods are placed on unwashed areas where raw poultry was handled previously, the organisms contaminate these foods and are transmitted to the consumer. It was thought that eggs acquired the organism on the shell during laying; thus a careful washing would suffice to prevent infection. It is now known that chicken eggs can become infected in the ovaries and carry the organism internally. Consumption of raw eggs is no longer recommended. A recent outbreak in Los Angeles was traced to a bakery that used raw eggs to prepare an uncooked cake frosting for a very popular cake. Children and mothers at a number of birthday parties became ill before the common source, many miles distant, was discovered.

Chronic carriers are rare after salmonellosis (<0.1%), although many convalescent patients excrete small numbers of organisms in their feces for 3–4 weeks. Those carriers in sensitive occupations, such as food handlers, health care workers, teachers and babysitters, must practice especially good hygiene to avoid infecting others. In some cases, they are barred from returning to work by the local health authorities until their stool cultures no longer yield the offending organisms.

Transmission

EXOGENOUS. The organism is ingested with improperly prepared, previously contaminated food. Meat and dairy products are most likely, although any food containing uncooked eggs can be a vehicle. Several years ago, Easter candy from Canada caused infections across the United States. Consumption of food or water contaminated with feces of infected animals is another means of transmission. Small pet turtles were very popular in the United States during the 1950s and 1960s, until it was discovered that the turtles were infected with *Salmonella.* Young children touched the turtles and transferred the bacteria to their mouths. Such turtles are banned in most states today. Infected food handlers or other persons can transmit the infection to others. Recent outbreaks carried on cheese, icings, salads, and cold sandwiches were traced to infected workers. The infectious dose has now been down-sized. Classical studies in volunteers placed the infectious dose at greater than 10^5 organisms but recent epidemics due to very low levels of food contamination have forced recognition of previously unappreciated circumstances in which **less than 100 salmonellae can cause infection.** Whether this high infectivity is due to the organism or host factors is not yet known.

Properties of the Organism

Resistance to environmental conditions and physical and chemical agents. The organism can survive in food and water for several weeks. *Salmonella* are killed easily by proper cooking, chemical disinfection, and chlorine. Proper cooking temperature of 60°C for 15–20 min will destroy the bacteria in poultry and meats.

Microscopic morphology. Salmonella species are typical **gram-negative, nonspore-forming bacilli** that resemble all other *Enterobacteriaceae* on Gram stain. Many of them are motile and only *S. typhi* has a demonstrable capsule.

Macroscopic morphology. These facultatively anaerobic organisms grow well on most laboratory media, forming large colonies. On selective media, such as Hektoen enteric agar, xylose-lysine-deoxycholate (XLD), and Salmonella-Shigella agar, they form distinctive colonies.

Identification to species and subspecies can be accomplished biochemically (Table 17.1), but identification to serovar must be made with specific antisera.

Antigenic structure. The antigenic structure of salmonellae and its relationship to serovar is among the most well characterized in all of Bacteriology. Now that most strains fall into only a few biochemical groups, the burden of differentiating among strains for epidemiologic purposes now depends entirely on sero-

TABLE 17.1. Biochemical Characterization of Selected Subspecies of *S. choleraesuis*

Serotype	Growth on KCN	Hydrogen sulfide production	Utilization of		
			lactose	dulcitol	malonate
arizonae	−	+	−	−	+
choleraesuis	−	+	−	+	−
houtenae	+	+	−	−	−
diarizonae	−	+	+	−	+
indica	+	+	−	delayed	−
salamae	−	+	−	+	+

logic methods. Since the sophisticated serologic tests used to identify the over 2500 different serovars of *Salmonella* are beyond the scope of most clinical microbiology laboratories, these tests are performed only by public health laboratories in the event of a suspected epidemic. The serotyping scheme, called Kauffmann-White after its developers, depends on O (lipopolysaccharide) outer membrane and H (flagellar) antigens.

These methods are very powerful when they are employed. The appearance of an unusual serovar of *Salmonella, Salmonella pooni,* in episodes of diarrhea reported throughout the Midwest in 1989 pointed out the existence of a single field of cantaloupes in Mexico that was responsible for exporting contaminated fruit across the entire United States. Public health agents were able to stop shipments from this source and truncate the epidemic. Figure 17.1 illustrates the use of serotyping to solve epidemiologic questions. Antibodies developed by infected persons are not useful for diagnosis, since many people have cross-reactive antibodies or antibodies derived from previous asymptomatic infections.

Lipopolysaccharides. **The LPS of salmonellae** involved in gastroenteritis is **responsible for the associated chills and fever.** This is salmonellae's primary virulence factor.

Extracellular products associated with pathogenicity. No extracellular virulence factors are clearly implicated in pathogenesis.

Pathogenesis and Clinical Manifestations

In primary disease, after entry into the host during ingestion of contaminated food or water, the organisms **survive stomach acidity** and enzymes and **colonize the ileum and colon.** The organisms **invade** through the intestinal epithelium and

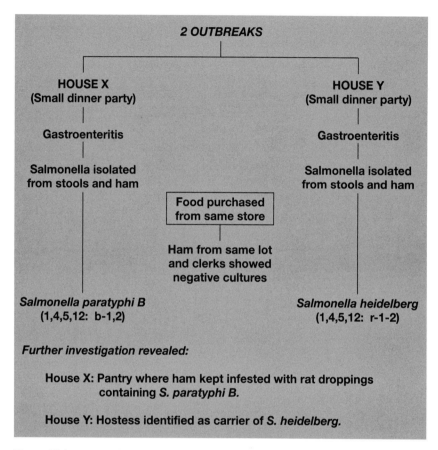

Figure 17.1.
Epidemiology of two outbreaks of salmonellosis.

are phagocytized by tissue macrophages, where they **multiply intracellularly.** The resistance of these organisms to intracellular killing may be mediated by the O antigens and other virulence factors. The host responds to the bacterial insult with an acute inflammatory infiltration of the mucous membranes of the ileum and cecum. As polymorphonuclear leukocytes destroy the bacteria, endotoxin is released, contributing to the development of chills and fever. The **incubation period** from infection to overt clinical manifestations of nausea and vomiting, diarrhea, headache, chills, and fever is usually **8–48 h, with an average of 18 h.** Patients usually recover after 2–3 days and disease is limited to the GI tract in most cases. Exceptions are patients with AIDS and those with other immunocompromising diseases, such as sickle cell anemia. The exact mechanism of the diarrheal response is not known, but cholera-like toxins, endotoxin-induced inflammation, or host response to the cellular invasion process by the salmonellae have all been proposed.

Rarely, **hematogenous dissemination,** called ''enteric fever'' or septicemia occurs. In these cases, organisms present in the GI tract invade into the GI mucosal tissue, ultimately reaching the circulatory system either directly or by lymphatic channels. A few serovars (e.g., *S. choleraesuis, S. paratyphi A, S. paratyphi B, and S. paratyphi C*) are more likely to causes systemic disease. These organisms multiply in circulating monocytes and seed any organ or tissue. The endotoxin is released during destruction, which contributes to fever, chills, and other clinical manifestations. Rarely occurring secondary processes include pneumonia and osteomyelitis. Mortality is high (25–70%) even with appropriate therapy.

Immunity to Reinfection

It is thought that no immunity is acquired after infection. Killed bacterial vaccines are available but they are of limited value.

Laboratory Diagnosis

SPECIMENS. **Stool** should be collected for diagnosis of gastroenteritis. Stool usually contains large numbers of organisms during acute disease and may continue to yield low numbers of salmonellae for several weeks. **Blood cultures** (for diagnosis of enteric fever), **sputum specimens** (for diagnosis of pneumonia), **bone biopsy** specimens (for diagnosis of osteomyelitis), and other appropriate specimens should be collected.

PRIMARY ISOLATION AND IDENTIFICATION. Stools are inoculated onto selective media; colonies are usually detected after 24 h of incubation. For identification of low level carriers, stools are inoculated into enrichment broths. All other specimens are inoculated onto supportive media and isolates are identified. Clinical laboratories identify the organisms to genus biochemically and may carry out limited serologic typing assays to place the organism into a group. For epidemiologic studies, the isolates are forwarded to a public health laboratory.

SEROLOGIC TESTS. Because the bacteria are readily isolated from clinical specimens, serologic tests are unnecessary.

Treatment

Unless patients are acutely ill with enteric fever, **antibiotic treatment is not indicated.** Such treatment may prolong the carrier state and encourage the emergence of resistant strains. Patients are given supportive therapy to prevent dehydration and electrolyte imbalance. Trimethoprim-sulfamethoxazole, amoxicillin, or chloramphenicol is used to treat septicemia, although this is a last resort.

Prevention and Control

Proper food preparation techniques and good personal hygiene practices should be used. To prevent transmission of infection by carriers; monitor their stools and ban them from sensitive occupations until they are salmonella-free.

TYPHOID FEVER

The most serious of the *Salmonella* diseases, **typhoid fever,** is an acute febrile disease with worldwide distribution caused by *S. typhi.* Around 500 cases of typhoid are reported annually in the United States, with more than one-half of these acquired by patients during overseas travel. Typhoid is endemic in many parts of the world, including developing countries in Latin America, Asia, and Africa, because of poor sanitation and the presence of chronic carriers.

Habitat

S. typhi is **restricted to the human host;** chronic carriers maintain the organism in the population. The organisms survive in the GI tract, with a predilection for the gallbladder. Approximately 3% of patients become carriers, shedding the organism for greater than 1 year after recovery. Middle-aged women are five times more likely to become carriers than similar groups of men.

Transmission

EXOGENOUS. The infectious dose seems to be quite high, with most references suggesting that greater than 10^5 organisms must be ingested. Organisms are shed into water in the **infected feces from cases** or are transmitted on the

hands of carriers who, as key links, contaminate food as they handle it. In areas with very poor sanitation, feces on the feet of flies can transmit salmonellae. Major outbreaks in developing countries are often the result of faulty water and sewage system design or maintenance. Outbreaks in the United States are often spread by fecally contaminated uncooked shellfish or by raw fruit or vegetables.

Properties of the Organism

Resistance to environmental conditions and physical and chemical agents. The organism can survive in food and water for several weeks. *Salmonella* are killed easily by proper cooking, chemical disinfection, and chlorine.

Microscopic morphology. S. typhi is a typical gram-negative bacillus that resembles all other *Enterobacteriaceae* on Gram stain. Most of them (95%) are motile. Most strains contain the **Vi capsular antigen,** which is not visible.

Macroscopic morphology. These facultatively anaerobic organisms grow well on most laboratory media, forming large colonies. On selective media, such as Hektoen enteric agar, XLD, and Salmonella-Shigella agar, they form distinctive colonies. On media containing an iron compound, colonies will show a black center due to production of hydrogen sulfide gas and subsequent precipitation of insoluble ferrous sulfide.

Antigenic structure. Both O and H antigens are similar to those of other *Salmonella* serovars. The O antigens may contribute to the ability of the organism to survive intracellularly. **The Vi capsular polysaccharide antigen is unique to** *S. typhi* and helpful for serovar identification. Human antibody response is used occasionally for diagnosis, but culture is the preferred laboratory method.

Lipopolysaccharide. Endotoxin is the primary mediator of pathology in typhoid fever.

Extracellular products associated with pathogenicity. No extracellular virulence factors are clearly implicated in pathogenesis.

Pathogenesis and Clinical Manifestations

Initially, the organisms **survive the stomach acidity** and enzymes and **penetrate the epithelial lining of the small intestine,** from which they **enter into the lymphoid tissue of the lamina propria (Peyer's patches and lymph nodes).** The salmonellae multiply in macrophages and other lymphoid tissue cells and gain access to the bloodstream. These **organisms are carried hematogenously to phagocytic reticuloendothelial cells** of the liver, spleen, bone marrow, and GI tract, as well as to the kidney and biliary tract. After phagocytosis by macrophages throughout the body, the organisms **multiply intracellularly by resisting lysosomal killing,** perhaps mediated by O and Vi antigens. The host responds with an acute endotoxin–mediated inflammatory response that produces the initial symptoms of headache, chills and fever, lethargy, generalized aches and pains, and some abdominal pain, usually **7–14 days after ingestion** of the organism. Constipation, rather than diarrhea, is common.

The organisms are again disseminated hematogenously during the second week, by reentering the circulation from the reticuloendothelial system. The resulting **bacteremia** may last for a number of days. The patient manifests high fever (up to 40°C) with occasional delirium and abdominal pain. Small petechial skin lesions called **"rose spots"** may be visible on the trunk. Diarrhea may appear at this stage due to infectious processes in the GI tract.

Systemically, the organisms at focal sites proliferate, multiplying in the GI tract, the gallbladder, the kidney, bone marrow, lungs, or CNS or any combination of sites. The host responds with an acute inflammatory infiltrate. The patient continues to display very high fever. Other clinical manifestations include hepatosplenomegaly and severe abdominal pain, renal damage, and other manifestations related to the site of salmonella proliferation. There can be serious complications from infection due to this organism. Mortality occurs in 10% of untreated patients. Necrosis of Peyer's patches and infected organs, pulmonary abscess formation, cholecystitis, and intestinal perforation and hemorrhage (0.5% of cases) are serious secondary sequelae. Approximately 3% of patients become chronic carriers. The gallbladder is often the site of carriage.

Immunity to Reinfection

Patients who survive typhoid fever retain a high level of immunity to second infections. Evidence suggests that a combination of both humoral and cellular immune mechanisms are responsible for immunity. It is postulated that opsonic antibodies directed against O and Vi antigens enhance intracellular destruction by promoting lysosomal enzyme activity within macrophages.

Laboratory Diagnosis

During the acute and early stages of typhoid, blood and urine specimens are most likely to harbor the organism. Bone marrow specimens are likely to be positive at all stages of disease. (See Table 17.2 for timing of obtaining specimens for diagnosis of typhoid fever.)

Table 17.2. Collection of Specimens for Diagnosis of Typhoid Fever

Time	Specimen
First week	Blood, bone marrow, bile
Second and third week	Blood, bone marrow, bile, stool, urine
Anytime	Abscess aspirate, tissue biopsy

During secondary stages, the infected organ should be cultured, including stool if diarrhea is present, lymph node biopsies, sputum if pneumonia is prominent, and abscess aspirates. When the patient is suffering from acute typhoid, the organism is proliferating in the gallbladder, thus culture of duodenal fluid containing bile is usually productive. The patient swallows a weighted capsule (Entero Test) attached to the patient's cheek by a string. After the appropriate time period, the capsule reaches the duodenum, is withdrawn, and the collected secretions cultured.

Of specimens obtained from carriers of typhoid fever, stool and urine specimens may be positive intermittently; gallbladder bile and bone marrow will be more productive.

Antibody assays are rarely performed due to the likelihood of false-positive results.

Treatment

Chloramphenicol has been the drug of choice historically, but resistance of greater than 15% of isolates, the rare side-effect of bone marrow suppression, and prolonged course required for effective treatment have all served to reduce its suitability. Trimethoprim-sulfamethoxazole and amoxicillin are excellent alternatives to chloramphenicol. The carrier state may not be amenable to treatment in some patients. Cholecystectomy may be required and has an 85% cure rate.

Prevention and Control

Both a phenol-inactivated injectable and a live, attenuated oral **vaccine** are available for laboratory workers and travelers. For those travelers likely to have prolonged contact with rural environments or who will eat local food, the vaccine may be used. The oral vaccine, a live avirulent mutant strain, is approximately

67% effective. The vaccine is not recommended for casual travelers or routine laboratory workers. Side effects of the vaccine may include chills and fever.

Isolation and treatment of cases and carriers is advised until clinical and bacteriologic cure is documented. Chronic carriers should be prevented from working in sensitive occupations, such as teachers of small children, nurses, and food handlers. Proper hygiene, sanitation and sewage disposal should be used. Contaminated water should be disinfected by chlorination or other means.

SUMMARY

1. Salmonellae, members of the *Enterobacteriaceae*, cause three primary diseases: gastroenteritis, septicemia, and typhoid fever.

2. Over 2500 serological types of *Salmonella* exist, identified by their O LPS antigens and their H flagellar antigens. Capsular antigens of the Vi type are found on *Salmonella typhi* and rarely on other strains; Vi is a virulence factor that acts by inhibiting nonspecific phagocytosis.

3. Salmonellae are common colonizers of domestic poultry. Chickens, eggs, and turkeys are important reservoirs involved in gastroenteritis outbreaks.

4. Salmonellae cause enteric disease by invading host epithelial cells in the ileum and colon and inducing an inflammatory response. A few serovars, notably *S. typhi* and *S. choleraesuis,* invade through the GI mucosa and enter the bloodstream to cause a systemic febrile disease, septicemia (enteric fever) or typhoid fever. Endotoxin contributes to the pathogenesis of the enteric fevers.

REFERENCES

Blaser M, Newman LS (1982): A review of human salmonellosis: I. Infective dose. Rev Infect Dis 4:1096.

Butler T, Islam A, Kabir I, Jones PK (1991): Patterns of morbidity and mortality in typhoid fever dependent on age and gender: review of 552 hospitalized patients with diarrhea. Rev Infect Dis 13:85.

Edelman R, Levine MM (1986): Summary of an international workshop on typhoid fever. Rev Infect Dis 8:329.

Ryan CA, Hargrett-Bean NT, Blake PA (1989): *Salmonella typhi* infections in the United States, 1975–1984: increasing role of foreign travel. Rev Infect Dis 11:1.

REVIEW QUESTIONS

For questions 1 to 5, choose the ONE
BEST answer or completion.

1. Which of the following practices would be
most effective in preventing an outbreak of
salmonellosis among patients in an extended
care facility?
   a) Food handlers must wash all eggs thoroughly in soap and water before cracking
   them open for cooking.
   b) Food handlers' stool must be tested for
   Salmonella, and carriers must be cured of
   their infection before they are able to begin working at the facility.
   c) Food handlers must wash their hands before beginning to work each shift.
   d) Areas where meat and poultry are prepared for cooking must be separate from
   areas where ready-to-eat foods (salads or
   sandwiches) are prepared.
   e) All tools and utensils must be washed and
   sterilized after they are used.

2. Initial recognition of the presence of salmonellae in primary cultures of feces requires
   a) use of a selective medium that allows formation of a distinctive colony morphology
   b) serologic typing of at least 10 colonies
   from the blood agar plate

   c) complete biochemical characterization of
   at least 10 colonies from the blood agar
   plate
   d) filtration of the feces sample to remove
   cross-reactive particles
   e) determination of motility of at least 10
   colonies from the blood agar plate

3. The most important factor that interferes
with the worldwide eradication of typhoid
fever is
   a) spread from country to country by migrating birds
   b) poor sanitation contributing to the maintenance of human disease
   c) the inability to eradicate the disease in
   wild animal vectors
   d) the resistance of *Salmonella typhi* to killing by cooking contaminated foods
   e) the very small infectious dose needed to
   establish infection

4. A key feature of the Vi antigen of *S. typhi* is
   a) its role as an inhibitor of intracellular killing of the bacterium within macrophages
   b) it mediates invasion of the bacterium into
   the intestinal mucosa
   c) antibody directed against Vi is measured
   to diagnose the illness in asymptomatic
   patients

d) antibody directed against Vi is used as a passive vaccine

e) its location on the bacterial cell structure

5. A young man presents to the Emergency Room with fever, chills, headache, and abdominal pain. He has just returned from a 2-week trip to Thailand and you suspect typhoid fever. What laboratory test will you order first?

a) Febrile agglutinin tests (detection of humoral antibody).

b) Culture of bone marrow.

c) Blood cultures.

d) Culture of feces.

e) Culture of urine.

For questions 6 to 8, a list of lettered options is followed by several numbered items. For each numbered item, select the ONE lettered option that is most closely associated with it. These questions concern *Salmonella*-associated gastroenteritis.

A) Lipopolysaccharide (endotoxin)
B) Major outer membrane protein (MOMP)
C) Outer membrane O antigen and virulence factor
D) Flagellar H antigens
E) Both C and D are correct

6. Serologic typing of salmonellae for epidemiologic purposes (the Kauffmann-White scheme).

7. Chills and fever associated with gastroenteritis.

8. Resistance of salmonellae to intracellular killing by macrophages.

ANSWERS TO REVIEW QUESTIONS

---

1. *d* Since uncooked poultry is the major source of *Salmonella* in this country, it must be prevented from contaminating food that is ready to be served. Cooking food destroys the organism. Hand washing is important, too, but infected food handlers pose less of a problem than the food-handling practices themselves. Regular washing will remove contaminating bacteria.

2. *a* Biochemically, all salmonellae are quite similar. Serotyping or determing motility of colonies from a blood agar plate would not be too helpful, as many other fecal bacteria would be included among the colonies selected. Colonies of salmonellae can initially be recognized only by their distinctive morphology on selective media. Usually, lactose is included in the medium, since salmonellae are unable to ferment lactose (lactose negative), whereas most other *Enterobacteriaceae* are lactose positive.

3. *b* The fact that *Salmonella typhi* is limited to humans allows the presence of infected carriers to serve as a reservoir for continuous reinfection in situations of poor hygienic practices.

4. *e* The Vi antigen is a capsular polysaccharide, unlike the other O antigens, which are outer membrane polysaccharides.

5. *c* Among those listed, blood cultures are the most productive during the first 2 weeks of illness. Bone marrow cultures are very helpful, but the invasive nature of the process precludes its use unless other methods fail to establish a diagnosis. Urine will usually become positive a bit later in the illness. Febrile agglutinin tests for anti-salmonella antibody are very nonspecific and are no longer offered by up-to-date microbiology laboratories.

6. *D* Both O and H antigens are used in identifying serovars of salmonellae.

7. *A* As with other gram-negative bacterial infections, systemic effects of endotoxin are important in salmonellosis.

8. *C* The O antigens are thought to inhibit intracellular killing of salmonellae within macrophages.

PSEUDOMONAS AND NONCHOLERA *VIBRIO* DISEASE

Unlike the *Enterobacteriaceae*, members of the genera *Pseudomonas* and *Vibrio* are free-living bacteria whose **natural habitat is soil and water.** Most species are oxidase positive, which helps microbiologists to differentiate isolates from *Enterobacteriaceae*. Pseudomonads are among the most versatile of bacterial pathogens; they can colonize and cause disease in virtually any living creature, from insects and fish to flowers and vegetables. Some of the same features that allow pseudomonads to thrive in the environment, including motility, production of a slimelike extracellular polysaccharide, elaboration of proteases, lipases, toxins, and antibiotic resistance, contribute to their pathogenicity. These organisms rarely cause disease in immunocompetent hosts, but they are powerful **opportunistic pathogens.**

As discussed in Chapter 16, *Vibrio cholerae* produces the archetype of enterotoxins. As the agent of cholera, *V. cholerae* has worldwide distribution and epidemiologic importance. Other species of *Vibrio*, however, are also important etiologic agents of disease mediated by virulence factors different from enterotoxin production. Those vibrios that produce diseases unrelated to cholera are presented in this chapter.

PSEUDOMONAS

PSEUDOMONAS AERUGINOSA AND RELATED BACTERIA

The pseudomonads are preferentially aerobic, although many of these organisms can utilize proteins anaerobically. These bacteria oxidize but do not ferment carbohydrates. Pseudomonads are important agents of nosocomial disease and **disease in certain compromised hosts,** including **burn patients** and those with **cystic fibrosis.** *Pseudomonas aeruginosa* is the most common nonfermentative bacterium isolated from clinical specimens and the fourth most prevalent agent of nosocomial disease. At least 24 species of *Pseudomonas* are known to mediate human disease, although many more species inhabit the environment and may be seen as opportunistic pathogens in immunocompromised hosts.

Habitat

Pseudomonads are found in the soil, groundwater, and on plant material in the environment. These organisms have a broad growth temperature range and are found in extremes of conditions (polar ice, hot springs, etc.). In hospitals, pseudomonads can often be isolated from sink drains, shower heads, plants in patients' rooms, and lettuce salads in the cafeteria. These bacteria are **resistant to many antibacterial substances** and have even been recovered in large numbers from disinfectant solutions! *P. aeruginosa* can be isolated from the feces of approximately 15% of normal individuals. **Hospitalized patients are at risk of becoming colonized.** As the length of stay increases, the colonization rate increases to as many as 40–70% of hospitalized patients.

Transmission

EXOGENOUS. Patient-patient spread by way of the **hands** of health care personnel is the most significant mode of transmission of *P. aeruginosa,* the most important pathogen in the group. Several outbreaks of pseudomonas-related disease have been transmitted by **contaminated instruments,** including urinary catheters, endoscopes, and respiratory therapy machines. The ability of the organism to survive and multiply in moisture containing minimal organic nutrients contributes to its pathogenic role. Ophthalmic disease has been contracted by laboratory workers who used eyewash stations containing *Pseudomonas*-contaminated disinfectant solutions to rinse out their eyes after a chemical spill. For this reason, eyewash fluids must be changed often or eyewash systems should use running tap water.

Bathing or soaking in contaminated water can transmit the organism. Incidences of skin disease related to soaking in hot tubs or whirlpool baths have been reported in both immunocompromised and nonimmunocompromised hosts. Pseudomonads and related organisms can cause serious disease when they contaminate an open wound. This condition is particularly likely for wounds acquired in or near the water, such as those resulting from fishing and boating accidents.

ENDOGENOUS. Pseudomonads can be found among the mixed flora isolated from intraabdominal disease. The organisms presumably are residents of the patient's GI tract and become agents of disease when they escape the bowel.

Properties of the Organism

Resistance to environmental, physical, and chemical agents. The organism is resistant to many chemical disinfectants, including quaternary ammonium compounds. Pseudomonads can survive in moisture without nutrients for long periods of time. These organisms are killed by boiling for 20 min and by autoclaving for a minimum of 15 min, as well as by chlorine-containing disinfectants. **Many antibiotics, including penicillins and cephalosporins, are ineffective against pseudomonads.**

Microscopic morphology. Pseudomonads are thin, straight-sided gram-negative bacilli. Some workers feel that they can differentiate them from *Enterobacteriaceae* based on Gram-stain morphology. Most species are **motile** by means of a single polar flagellum or polar flagellar tufts. Slime-producing strains of *P. aeruginosa* demonstrate a capsulelike extracellular layer.

Macroscopic morphology. Pseudomonads grow best in air, although they can use proteins to grow slowly anaerobically if necessary. Oxidation of carbohydrates is the preferred metabolic acivity. These organisms are able to grow well on most any laboratory media. *P. aeruginosa* produces a water-soluble **blue-green pigment** called pyocyanin that diffuses out into colorless media, yielding varied shades of green, blue, and purple. Other species produce other pigments. A few species of *Pseudomonas,* including *P. aeruginosa,* produce pigments that fluoresce under UV light.

A key feature of *P. aeruginosa* is its **distinctive odor,** described variously as grape-like and corn tortilla-like. *P. aeruginosa* produces a strong hemolysin that completely lyses sheep RBCs in blood agar plates. The organism is able to grow at 42°C, which differentiates it from other species that produce fluorescent pigments. Slime-producing strains yield extremely mucoid colonies with copious, gelatinous capsule-like material, also called **mucoid exopolysaccharide (MEP).** These strains are almost exclusively isolated from patients with cystic fibrosis. In addition to the macroscopic characteristics mentioned, species are identified based on biochemical and enzymatic tests.

Antigenic structure. Pseudomonads contain **LPS in their outer membrane.** Lipopolysaccharide is probably responsible for the serious manifestations of systemic disease, including septic shock, disseminated intravascular coagulation, fever, and renal failure. Surface structures, pili and flagella, mediate adherence to mucosal and injured epithelial layers. Somatic O cell wall antigens have been used for epidemiologic typing of *P. aeruginosa* isolates [the International Antigenic Typing System (IATS)]. These schemes are not used as much today, since nucleic acid fingerprinting has been used more effectively to trace the origins of strains.

Extracellular products associated with pathogenicity. Table 18.1 lists extra-

TABLE 18.1. Extracellular Products of *P. aeruginosa* That Are Important in Pathogenicity

Product	Activity
Alginate	Increases viscosity of mucous secretions in lungs of cystic fibrosis patients and thus interferes with phagocytosis and other immune responses and decreases the ability of the patient to control the infection
Cytotoxin (leukocidin)	Acts on cell membranes of eukaryotic cells; inhibits and eventually destroys polymorphonuclear leukocytes; may induce capillary endothelial cell damage
Elastase	May dissolve elastic lamina of blood vessels, leading to ecthyma gangrenosum. Also inactivates C3b and C5a complement components, inhibiting opsonization and elaboration of chemotactic factors, which serves to dampen the inflammatory response.
Exoenzyme S	Inhibits eukaryotic protein activity, contributing to tissue damage
Exotoxin A	Important toxin mediating local and systemic effects; acts in same manner as diphtheria toxin as a ribosyltransferase, inhibits EF-2 and thus protein synthesis in infected tissue, produces necrosis locally, and contributes to lethality in *Pseudomonas* sepsis
Glycolipid hemolysin	Acts synergistically with phospholipase to break down tissue lipids and lecithin; mediates local necrosis and tissue invasion
Phospholipase C	Destroys pulmonary surfactant, a lecithin-containing lipoprotein that contributes to alveolar integrity, and destroys tissue lipids, contributing to destructive lesions and spread of the disease process

cellular products of *P. aeruginosa*. The most important ones are mentioned, along with products of importance to the organism in its natural habitat:

1. The mucoid extracellular **polysaccharide slime layer,** identified in 1964 as **alginate,** seems to act as an adherence factor. It may form a protective barrier around organisms, enabling them to multiply more quickly in a sequestered environment. Some factor in the mucous secretions of cystic fibrosis patients induces production of this exopolysaccharide.

2. **Proteases,** including elastase, contribute to the **invasiveness** of the organism and to its ability to destroy tissue. One type of clinical manifestation, necrotic skin lesions called **"ecthyma gangrenosum,"** is probably mediated in part by proteases.

3. **Lipases** and **lecithinases** also destroy tissue and blood cells, enhancing invasiveness and potentiating the inflammatory response.

4. **Exotoxin A inhibits protein synthesis** by blocking the activity of elongation factor 2 (EF-2), in a manner similar to that of diphtheria toxin. This important virulence factor, exclusive to *P. aeruginosa,* contributes to the high mortality associated with septicemia involving this species.

5. **Bacteriocins** and **pyocins,** sometimes used in typing schemes, while not acting as major virulence factors in human disease, are important **colonization resistance factors in the environment.** These enzymes may act to prevent colonization of infected sites with other, less virulent bacteria.

Pathogenesis and Clinical Manifestations

Once transferred to damaged skin, the respiratory epithelium, or another vulnerable site, the organism attaches by means of its fimbriae and multiplies. In cystic fibrosis patients, abundant slime (alginate polysaccharide) allows protected growth in the lungs and urinary tract parenchyma. Extracellular toxins and enzymes break down adjacent tissue and allow spread of the infection. Tissue necrosis due to a combination of bacterial enzymes and host inflammatory response leads to local breakdown. If the organisms subsequently invade into the bloodstream, systemic clinical manifestations and shock may develop. A number of site-specific serious infectious processes can be related to pseudomonads:

1. **Corneal ulcer** and purulent conjunctivitis. *P. aeruginosa,* because of its moisture-loving character and immunity to disinfectants, can **colonize contact lens solutions.** Postcataract or other eye surgical diseases result from nosocomial acquisition. Endophthalmitis can result from hematogenous spread of the organism

after eye surgery or by direct inoculation. Enzymes break down the tissue to cause devastating and very rapidly morbid disease, usually characterized by ulcer formation. Immediate aggressive therapy is critical or the eye can be lost.

2. **External otitis** and **otitis media.** Swimmers and divers often contract ear disease with this organism. The constant moisture and excoriated epithelium due to earplugs or cotton swabs used to dry out the external ear canals provide a suitable environment for *P. aeruginosa* colonization and growth. This condition can exacerbate if the organisms invade into underlying tissue. Serious complications of this syndrome, called "malignant external otitis" include osteomyelitis, meningitis, and sinus thrombosis. *P. aeruginosa* is the most common etiologic agent of middle ear disease.

3. **Skin disease.** Debrided skin, burn wound-induced epithelial changes, and other factors allow colonization and infection of the skin. Otherwise normal individuals periodically experience episodes of **"pseudomonas folliculitis"** associated with **soaking in hot tubs** that are inadequately chlorinated.

The importance of *P. aeruginosa* in **burn wound disease** is discussed more fully in Chapter 21.

4. **Respiratory tract disease.** *P. aeruginosa* causes **pneumonia in immunocompromised and hospitalized patients.** The oropharyngeal epithelium becomes colonized and the organisms gain access to the lung by aspiration or direct inoculation by respiratory therapy manipulations or ventilating apparatus. Patients with malignancies are particularly at risk.

The most important respiratory tract manifestation, however, is the ubiquitous **colonization by mucoid strains** of *P. aeruginosa* and subsequent loss of perfusion function in the lungs of **cystic fibrosis patients.** It is postulated that the alginate layer prevents penetration of aminoglycoside antibiotics, inhibits antibody-mediated phagocytosis, and contributes to excess bronchial bulk and abnormally thick secretions in the lungs of patients with cystic fibrosis.

5. **Sepsis.** Sepsis can result from any initial infectious process, since pseudomonads can readily invade, particularly in immunocompromised hosts. Mortality is high. Bacteremia with *P. aeruginosa* may (rarely) result in skin manifestations, including **"ecthyma gangrenosum,"** bullae, or vesicular lesions. *Pseudomonas* sepsis is one of the most dreaded complications of nosocomial infections.

6. **Endocarditis.** From the bloodstream, the organism can colonize the heart valve to cause endocarditis. This complication is prevalent among **IV drug users,** who inject contaminated materials, such as nonsterile water used to dilute powdered drugs, into veins that lead to the heart. The tricuspid valve is overrepresented in such patients because of the route of injection of the organism.

Prosthetic heart valves are also at risk for *Pseudomonas*-related endocarditis, although this is rare.

7. **Urinary tract disease.** *Pseudomonas* is an important agent of UTI in hospitalized patients. In many compromised patients, infections recur or become chronic. Catheterized or otherwise compromised patients may develop *Pseudomonas* urinary tract disease. Patients with neurogenic bladders are at particular risk. The organism adheres readily to urinary tract epithelium to colonize and cause disease. In addition to the predilection of the lungs of cystic fibrosis patients to promote production of alginate by *P. aeruginosa,* alginate-producing strains are often harbored in the urinary tract, where the pathogenicity is not as pronounced. In normal hosts, especially women, the organism enters the urethral meatus by spreading across the perineum. The colonized vagina or rectum provides the reservoir.

8. Other miscellaneous diseases associated with *P. aeruginosa.* Osteochondritis following puncture wounds of the foot usually involve *P. aeruginosa.* Recent studies have shown that the lining materials used in popular tennis shoes can support low levels of viable pseudomonads. The organisms are introduced into the shoes when patients walk on damp or wet vegetation and remain indolent until a traumatic event allows them access to deep tissue. As a member of the mixed flora found in acute and complicated appendicitis, *P. aeruginosa* may contribute to lack of cure after surgery if antimicrobial agents that lack coverage for this organism are used. Occasionally, young babies, patients with malignancies, and aged patients experience a devastating necrotizing enterocolitis thought to be mediated by *P. aeruginosa.* In the bowel, toxins of pseudomonads produce ulcers, hemorrhage, and other symptoms. Although uncommon, this GI disease can be very serious. From the bowel, the organism can reach the bloodstream and cause septicemia.

Immunity to Reinfection

There is **no specific immunity to reinfection.** Several experimental vaccines have been used in attempts to prevent burn wound infection. The immunity is very short lived, but initial studies are promising.

Laboratory Diagnosis

SPECIMENS. Any infected tissue, blood, urine, sputum, or other appropriate specimen may be collected for microbiological evaluation.

PRIMARY ISOLATION AND IDENTIFICATION. Pseudomonads will grow on almost every standard laboratory medium that is incubated in the air at temperatures ranging from room temperature to 40°C. The most common species, *P. aeruginosa,* can usually be identified on macroscopic criteria alone: the colony is flat and often shows an iridescent sheen, is strongly β-hemolytic on blood agar, growth emits a characteristic sickly sweet odor described as grape-like or corn tortilla-like, and the organism is indophenol oxidase positive. Colonies on MacConkey agar are clear, reflecting the inability of *P. aeruginosa* to ferment lactose. Related pseudomonads are identified based on permissive growth temperatures, ability to oxidize carbohydrates, pigment formation, flagellar morphology, and biochemical reactions.

IMMUNOSEROLOGIC TESTS. Immunoserologic tests are not used except in a few reference laboratories. Serotyping may be used for epidemiologic studies.

Treatment

Some *Pseudomonas* diseases are so serious and rapidly progressive that surgical intervention is essential, even when antibiotics are being administered. Endophthalmitis and corneal ulcer usually require debridement or drainage. Endocarditis may require valve replacement. Osteomyelitis usually requires debridement and drainage.

Pseudomonads are notoriously **antibiotic resistant** and treatment alternatives are few. The classical treatment for serious *P. aeruginosa* disease consists of two antibiotics, namely, an **aminoglycoside,** such as tobramycin, and an **antipseudomonal β-lactam agent,** such as ticarcillin. New β-lactams, however, exhibit better activity against *P. aeruginosa,* and may be used alone for some syndromes. For example, **ceftazidime,** a third generation cephalosporin, is the treatment of choice for pseudomonal meningitis because of its excellent penetration of the blood-brain barrier.

Quinolones, primarily ofloxacin and ciprofloxacin, can be used to treat some respiratory and urinary tract diseases, and may be used as long-term oral therapy for osteomyelitis after an initial hospital course of IV therapy. Newer β-lactam antibiotics, including the monobactam aztreonam and the carbapenem imipenem-cilastatin are also effective against pseudomonads, although resistance can develop with single drug therapy.

Prevention and Control

All instruments that come into contact with patients should be disinfected and thoroughly dried. Burned skin surfaces should be treated with a topical antipseudomonal agent, such as silver sulfadiazine or mafenide acetate. Good aseptic techniques should be used when performing patient-contact health care procedures. Be certain that the water in which patients or healthy individuals are submerged, such as hydrotherapy baths and hot tubs, is properly chlorinated. Do not permit plants in the rooms of patients in intensive care settings. Do not allow disinfectants to remain in containers longer than their expiration date, which is usually only a few days. Disinfect the liners of tennis shoes periodically.

OTHER SIMILAR SPECIES OF MEDICAL IMPORTANCE

Stenotrophomonas (Xanthomonas) maltophilia

Stenotrophomonas (formerly *Xanthomonas*) *maltophilia* is an occasional agent of **nosocomial disease** and the second most common *Pseudomonas*-like agent isolated from clinical specimens. It is a common environmental contaminant. Isolates must be evaluated carefully to determine whether they are truly involved in a clinical process. This organism has an unusual antibiotic resistance pattern, susceptible only to **trimethoprim-sulfamethoxazole** and ticarcillin-clavulanic acid. One risk factor for nosocomial disease is therapy with the broad spectrum antibiotic imipenem, to which *S. maltophilia* is resistant.

Burkholderia (Pseudomonas) cepacia

This organism is an important **respiratory pathogen in cystic fibrosis patients.** Studies show that isolation of this species in association with alginate-producing *P. aeruginosa* is a poor prognostic sign. *Burkholderia* (formerly *Pseudomonas*) *cepacia* is an occasional etiologic agent of severe nosocomial disease. This species is extremely antibiotic resistant. Specific susceptibility results must be used to determine therapy, as empiric data are inconsistent.

Burkholderia (Pseudomonas) pseudomallei

This organism is the etiologic agent of **melioidosis,** a febrile disease with several manifestations, including pneumonitis, suppurative wound with regional lymph node inflammation, and sepsis. The organism is found in the environment, primarily in Southeast Asia and the Far East. It is extremely rare in the Americas. The disease itself is quite uncommon. Humans acquire the infection by walking through rice paddies or other endemic foci in bare feet, where the organism gains entrance through breaks in the skin. Humans may also become infected by inhaling aerosols. Disease in the United States is almost exclusively seen in soldiers returning from duty in endemic areas.

Burkholderia (Pseudomonas) mallei

This organism is the etiologic agent of **glanders,** a zoonotic disease of domestic animals, primarily horses. The disease is characterized by pulmonary infiltrates, ulcerative lymphoid nodules, or lymphadenopathy-like manifestations. Humans acquire glanders by close contact with infected animals. This disease is extremely rare in humans in the United States.

Numerous other species of *Pseudomonas*-like bacteria can act as opportunistic pathogens in immunocompromised and hospitalized hosts.

VIBRIO

NONCHOLERA VIBRIO DISEASE

Diseases due to vibrios are increasing due, in part, to expanded recognition of these species by microbiologists, increased consumption of raw shellfish by Americans, and to the increasing numbers of immunocompromised patients who are at risk. Like *V. cholerae,* the other pathogenic vibrios are **free-living environmental bacteria.** Most species are **saltwater** inhabitants and require increased sodium chloride concentrations for growth. These organisms are facultative anaerobes, **straight or slightly curved gram-negative bacilli,** and **motile** by means of a **single polar flagellum.** Most species are oxidase positive and able to reduce nitrate. Differentiation from *Pseudomonas* and related species depends on biochemical testing, in which the vibrios are fermentative and pseudomonads are oxidative, growth in sodium chloride, and susceptibility to specialized antibiotic-like agents. These organisms grow well on routine laboratory media and the colonies may resemble those of *Enterobacteriaceae.* Ten species of noncholera vibrios are associated with human disease (Table 18.2).

TABLE 18.2. Noncholera Vibrios

Species	Common disease process
alginolyticus	Wound infection, otitis, pneumonia
cincinnatiensis	Septicemia
damsela	Wound infection
fluvialis	Diarrheal disease
furnissii	Diarrheal disease
hollisae	Diarrheal disease
metschnikovii	Septicemia
mimicus	Otitis, diarrheal disease
parahaemolyticus	Diarrheal disease
vulnificus	Wound infection, severe septicemia

Epidemiology and Pathogenesis of Selected Species

Gastrointestinal disease due to noncholera vibrios is acquired from **raw shellfish.** Endemic pockets exist in coastal waters of Texas, Louisiana, Florida, and Maryland. *Vibrio parahaemolyticus* **is the most common agent.** Enterotoxin and hemolysin may play a role in virulence and diarrhea is usually self-limiting.

Vibrio vulnificus **is the most virulent of the noncholera vibrios,** causing a **fulminant** and often **fatal septicemia** in susceptible hosts. This organism can be differentiated from other vibrios by its ability to ferment lactose. Primary septicemia occurs in compromised individuals when the organisms, originally acquired by ingestion of contaminated raw seafood, traverse the damaged GI tract and enter the bloodstream. The other most common mode of acquisition is through a contaminated wound or abrasion that occurs near or in the water. Most patients who suffer severe consequences have a predisposing liver condition, such as cirrhosis, or cancer.

Wound infections, acquired by abrasion or trauma, can be quite serious. The organism seems to possess potent proteases that enhance invasiveness and tissue destruction. *V. vulnificus* also seems to produce a cytolysin and a cytotoxin. Once infected, major tissue destruction is possible. *V. vulnificus* possesses an antiphagocytic and antiopsonic capsule. Mortality related to *V. vulnificus* sepsis ranges from 40 to 60%.

Treatment

Tetracycline, aminoglycosides, and chloramphenicol are considered effective antimicrobial agents.

SUMMARY

1. *Pseudomonas* and *Vibrio* species are oxidase-positive, free-living water and soil dwelling gram-negative bacteria. These species produce potent exotoxins and numerous other virulence factors.

2. *Pseudomonas aeruginosa*, the most common nonfermentative gram-negative isolate in clinical microbiology laboratories, causes severe infections in immunocompromised hosts. One of the most important is pneumonia in cystic fibrosis patients due to an alginate (slime)-producing strain.

3. Pseudomonads are able to survive in under-chlorinated water and often in disinfectants. Members of this group are important agents of nosocomial disease.

4. *Pseudomonas aeruginosa* virulence factors include production of alginate (slime), exotoxin A, proteases, exoenzymes, hemolysins, and adhesins. The organisms destroy host tissue and mediate an inflammatory response.

5. Most pseudomonads and related organisms are extremely resistant to antimicrobial agents; aminoglycosides, quinolones, and some newer β-lactam agents are usually necessary.

6. *Vibrio* species other than cholera are important etiologic agents of gastroenteritis following ingestion of raw shellfish (*V. parahaemolyticus*), wound infection and primary septicemia (*V. vulnificus*), and other syndromes. Acquisition is usually associated with activities around water.

REFERENCES

Gilligan PH (1991): Microbiology of airway disease in patients with cystic fibrosis. Clin Microbiol Rev 4:35.

Janda JM, Powers C, Bryant RG, Abbott SL (1988): Current perspectives on the epidemiology and pathogenesis of clinically significant *Vibrio* spp. Clin Microbiol Rev 1:245.

Khardori N, Eltin L, Wong E, Schable B, Bodey GP (1990): Nosocomial infections due to *Xanthomonas maltophilia (Pseudomonas maltophilia)* in patients with cancer. Rev Infect Dis 12:997.

May TB et al. (1991): Alginate synthesis by *Pseudomonas aeruginosa:* a key pathogenic factor in chronic pulmonary infections of cystic fibrosis patients. Clin Microbiol Rev 4:191.

REVIEW QUESTIONS

For questions 1 to 6, a list of lettered options is followed by several numbered items. For each numbered item, select the ONE lettered option that is most closely associated with it.

A) *Pseudomonas aeruginosa*
B) *Stenotrophomonas maltophilia*
C) *Vibrio parahaemolyticus*
D) *Vibrio vulnificus*
E) *Burkholderia pseudomallei*

For each patient, select the organism most likely to have been the etiologic agent.

1. A soldier returns from Southeast Asia with fevers, sepsis, and a severe pneumonia-like disease.

2. An alcohol-abusing elderly man cuts his foot while walking on the beach and develops a fulminating, rapidly fatal septicemia.

3. A patient hospitalized for severe pneumonia was treated initially with imipenem because the etiologic agent of his pneumonia was not known. Three days into his treatment, he spikes a fever and a new infiltrate is visible on lung roentgenograph.

4. A patient who wears soft contact lenses develops excruciating pain in her right eye. On examination, the ophthalmologist sees a small ulceration.

5. A husband and wife celebrate her promotion with a fancy dinner starting with oysters on the half-shell. The next morning, both experience cramps and diarrhea.

6. Four adults spend 2 h in a hot tub on New Year's Eve. The next day, their skin displays a painful and itching rash.

For questions 7 to 10, choose the ONE BEST answer or completion.

7. The primary characteristic of *Pseudomonas* strains that colonize the lungs and other organs of cystic fibrosis patients is
   a) fimbriae that mediate adherence to mucosal epithelial cells
   b) production of elastase, which breaks down intercellular matrix to facilitate spread of the infection
   c) production of a β-hemolysin
   d) production of exotoxin A, which inhibits protein synthesis in host respiratory epithelial cells
   e) production of an extracellular slime layer made of alginate

8. A young man develops swollen and ulcerated cervical lymph nodes. Which is the most likely scenario?
   a) He has just returned from Southeast Asia, where he became infected with *Burkholderia pseudomallei* when he waded through rice fields during the filming of a documentary.
   b) He suffers from cystic fibrosis and has become colonized with alginate-producing *Pseudomonas aeruginosa.*
   c) He is hospitalized and recovering from open heart surgery. His wound has become infected with *Stenotrophomonas maltophilia.*
   d) He is a trainer's assistant at the Kentucky Derby race track. He has contracted human glanders by acquiring *Burkholderia mallei* infection from a horse.
   e) He punctured his hand while descaling a fish that he caught during a deep sea fishing cruise. His hand became infected with *Pseudomonas fluorescens.*

9. A patient with sickle cell disease presents to your Emergency Room with symptoms of sepsis. Blood cultures yield *Vibrio vulnificus.* If all modalities were available, what is the best clinical course to follow?
   a) Watch the patient to see if his condition deteriorates.
   b) Treat the patient with a third generation cephalosporin.
   c) Treat the patient with the highest dose of aminoglycoside possible.
   d) Treat the patient with anti-endotoxin monoclonal antibody and the highest dose of aminoglycoside possible.
   e) Treat the patient with an exchange transfusion.

10. An unusual strain of *P. aeruginosa* is isolated repeatedly from the catheterized urine specimens received from the patients of one urologist. This strain has not been isolated from any other source. What is the best explanation?
    a) The disinfectant in which the physician soaks his catheters between patients is contaminated with that strain of *Pseudomonas.*
    b) All of the physician's patients are from the same family and they have been eating the same contaminated food.
    c) All of the physician's patients draw their drinking water from a single well.
    d) The patients are having sexual relations with each other.
    e) The physician's nurse is a carrier of this strain.

ANSWERS TO REVIEW QUESTIONS

1. **E** Melioidosis should be suspected in any patient with a severe pneumonic process and a history of recent travel to Southeast Asia.

2. **D** Patients with nonfunctional spleens or livers are at increased risk of systemic disease by *Vibrio vulnificus* when they develop infection. The organism is found in saltwater and a primary infection at the site of a laceration wound can rapidly lead to severe disease.

3. **B** *Stenotrophomonas maltophilia* is an occasional cause of nosocomial diseases. Resistance to imipenem and susceptibility only to trimethoprim-sulfamethoxazole make its identification imperative so that the proper therapy can be given.

4. **A** *Pseudomonas aeruginosa* causes some of the most severe infections associated with contact lens wear. It can survive and even multiply in solutions containing disinfectants.

5. **C** *Vibrio parahaemolyticus* is common in seawater. The gill-feeding used by shellfish concentrates the organisms within the shellfish. Diarrhea begins 12–24 h after ingestion of the organism and is usually self-limiting.

6. **A** *Pseudomonas* folliculitis has been traced to inadequately chlorinated hot tubs and spas. *P. aeruginosa* survives hot temperatures and invades the hair follicles and other slightly excoriated skin sites to invoke a local inflammatory response.

7. **e** All of the choices are extracellular products or antigens of *P. aeruginosa,* but the polysaccharide slime (alginate) is associated strongly with cystic fibrosis patients. In fact, when a slime-producing *P. aeruginosa* is isolated from an otherwise normal host, clinicians should begin to question whether the patient may actually have an unsuspected case of relatively asymptomatic cystic fibrosis.

8. **d** Glanders, characterized by ulcerated lymphadenopathy, is a zoonosis, primarily in horses, that only occasionally is transmitted to humans during close contact. The agent of the disease is *Burkholderia mallei.* All of the other scenarios are legitimate descriptions of pseudomonad infections, but they are not consistent with this clinical presentation.

9. **d** The mortality of *V. vulnificus* sepsis ranges from 40 to 60%. Because patients with sickle cell disease are functionally asplenic, they are at even greater risk of severe consequences. Therefore, the

most aggressive therapeutic regimen possible must be instituted immediately. Vibrios, as gram-negative bacteria, possess cell wall LPS, which contributes to the symptoms of septic shock. Both anti-LPS (if commercially available at your institution) and the appropriate antibiotic, either tetracycline, chloramphenicol, or an aminoglycoside (probably the most potent) should be given.

10. *a* *P. aeruginosa* can survive in disinfectants for long periods of time. It is not transmitted sexually, and normal stomach acidity will usually destroy the organism if it is ingested. Although it is possible that the nurse is a carrier, this mode of transmission has not been documented to be important for urinary tract infections in an outpatient setting.

CAMPYLOBACTER AND *HELICOBACTER* DISEASES

These two genera of curved, nonspore-forming, **asaccharolytic,** primarily **microaerobic gram-negative bacilli** are normal flora of the GI tracts of birds and mammals. Although they cause enteric disease, they are not members of the *Enterobacteriaceae* family, but are related more closely to vibrios (curved rods). Once introduced into the environment through contaminated feces, they can survive and multiply for long periods of time. These organisms are involved in a spectrum of diseases, ranging from septic abortion and gastroenteritis to wound infection. *Campylobacter jejuni* and related species are estimated to be responsible for 12% of diarrheas worldwide. In the United States, ***Campylobacter* is the cause of diarrhea in up to 80% of patients** from whom an etiologic agent is recovered, thus outnumbering *Salmonella* and *Shigella.* As many as 2 million cases per year have been estimated.

Helicobacter pylori, a recently characterized species, has been unequivocally determined to be **a major contributor to gastritis and peptic ulcers,** diseases traditionally thought to be noninfectious in nature. The association of an etiologic agent with these common syndromes has revolutionized both diagnostic and therapeutic approaches.

CAMPYLOBACTER DISEASE

In the late 1970s, *C. jejuni* dramatically rose from obscurity to become the most common pathogen recovered from diarrheic stools in the United States, simply because new culture methods were introduced in clinical microbiology laboratories. Due to its unusual growth requirements, the organism had not been sought or recognized. This sudden recognition of a pathogen that had been present and active the entire time is a relevant illustration of the importance of microbiological technology on the ability of a laboratory to aid in diagnosis of an infectious disease.

Campylobacters are now known to be associated with **gastroenteritis,** abortion in domestic animals (cows and sheep) and humans, **wound infections, sepsis,** meningitis, periodontal disease, and **proctitis in homosexual males.** This wide disease spectrum implies several virulence factors, which are still being characterized.

There are currently 16 named species of *Campylobacter,* most of which have been implicated as agents of human disease (Table 19.1). Several species are more commonly isolated from animals (e.g., *Campylobacter cinaedi* is part of the normal GI flora of hamsters and *Campylobacter hyointestinalis* is part of the normal GI flora of pigs). It is interesting to speculate on how these species became established as etiologic agents of proctitis in homosexual men.

Habitat

Campylobacters are usually part of the normal GI flora of birds and mammals, although they sometimes cause gastroenteritis in these animals. A ubiquitous organism in commercial poultry, campylobacters have been **estimated to be pres-**

TABLE 19.1. **Important *Campylobacter* sp. Isolated From Humans**

Species	Primary host	Primary human syndrome
cinaedi	Humans	Proctitis, enteritis
coli	Swine	Gastroenteritis
concisus	Humans (oral cavity)	Periodontal disease
fennelliae	Humans	Proctitis, enteritis
fetus ss. *fetus*	Domestic animals	Abortions, sepsis, diarrhea
hyointestinalis	Swine	Diarrhea (rare)
jejuni ss. *jejuni*	Poultry	Diarrhea

ent in huge numbers (10⁹/g) in chicken carcasses found at grocery stores and supermarkets throughout the United States. Improper handling of cutting boards, knives, and utensils or insufficient cooking accounts for numerous sporadic cases of campylobacter gastroenteritis. Fecal contamination of environmental sites allows maintenance of the organisms in the environment. *Campylobacter fetus* subspecies *fetus, C. hyointestinalis,* and *C. jejuni* are important veterinary pathogens, causing abortions in cattle, sheep, and swine. Animal hosts transmit the organism as a sexually transmitted disease.

Transmission

EXOGENOUS. The campylobacters are often acquired as zoonoses through handling infected animals or through the **fecal-oral route.** Large food and water-borne outbreaks have resulted from distribution of contaminated milk, uncooked meat or fowl, and contaminated water systems.

ENDOGENOUS. Endogenous transmission of some species of campylobacters occurs in pregnant women and animals. It is postulated that in animals the organisms are present in the genitourinary tract and invade the developing fetus by direct extension, causing spontaneous abortions. In humans, the organism is thought to **reach the fetus by crossing the placenta during septic episodes.**

Properties of the Organism

Resistance to environmental, physical, and chemical agents. The organism is rapidly killed by acid at concentrations present in the empty stomach. Ingestion with food or milk or ingestion by persons with achlorhydria, however, will allow the organisms to avoid concentrated stomach acidity. The organism can survive for up to 5 weeks in milk or water at 4°C. Chlorination of water effectively kills campylobacters. These bacteria are susceptible to all chemical disinfectants. Pasteurization of milk and minimal cooking of food will destroy the organisms, which are not very resistant to heat.

Microscopic morphology. Campylobacters are **curved, spiral-shaped, or gullwing-shaped thin gram-negative bacilli** (Fig. 19.1). These organisms exhibit a rapid, darting motility mediated by **one or two polar flagella.** There is no demonstrable capsule.

Macroscopic morphology. Campylobacters are **microaerobes** that grow best in 5–10% oxygen with added carbon dioxide. Special media, supplemented with

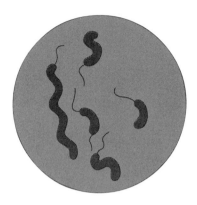

Figure 19.1.
Morphology of *Campylo-bacter* sp.

blood or other nutrients and antibiotics to inhibit normal fecal flora, are used for isolation of campylobacters from feces. Because *C. jejuni,* the most common enteric pathogen, is able to grow at 42°C, this temperature is used to inhibit other flora. Isolation of nonfecal pathogenic campylobacters should be carried out at 37°C, since these strains do not exhibit the heat tolerance of *C. jejuni.* Colonies of the enteric campylobacters are often pinkish-beige and spread along the streak line in a puddle-appearing morphology. Species are identified based on biochemical reactions and susceptibility to antibiotics.

Antigenic structure. Campylobacters contain **lipopolysaccharide (LPS)** in their outer membrane (OM), as do all other gram-negative organisms. The role of LPS in infection is not known. Although antigenic typing schemes for campylobacters have been developed, none has been universally accepted.

Extracellular products associated with pathogenicity. Strains of *C. jejuni* and *C. coli* may produce an **enterotoxin** that shares some features of cholera toxin and the labile toxin (LT) of enterotoxigenic *Escherichia coli.* The toxin is a large heat-labile protein (70,000 Da). These same species sometimes also demonstrate production of a **cytotoxin** different from the verotoxin produced by *E. coli* O157:H7. **Adhesins** on the surface of campylobacters are important for attachment to intestinal epithelium. Although the organisms do not possess pili, certain flagellar regions may serve as adhesins.

Pathogenesis and Clinical Manifestations

The infective dose can be as low as 500 organisms or as high as 10^6. Both host and organism factors probably contribute to virulence. Once past the stomach acid, the campylobacters **penetrate the mucus barrier of the small bowel** using flagellar motility and corkscrew motion facilitated by their spiral shape. The organisms colonize and **multiply in the mucus layer.** From 1 to 7 days after ingestion of the organism, patients develop one or more of several syndromes, including watery diarrhea, bloody diarrhea, and extraintestinal disease. As many as 80% of infected patients may remain asymptomatic. Diarrhea is usually self-limiting and lasts up to 1 week. **Symptoms are thought to be mediated by the enterotoxin.**

In some cases, organisms may elaborate **cytotoxin,** which may **destroy intestinal cells** and result in **bloody diarrhea.** Extraintestinal infection occurs when the campylobacters traverse the intestinal mucosa and are picked up by the tissue phagocytic cells, much like the pathogenesis of salmonella enteric fevers. Campylobacters have been shown to survive in blood monocytes for up to 7 days. Intracellular survival, therefore, seems to be a virulence factor for campylobacters as well as salmonellae. Even after recovery, patients may excrete the organism for several weeks.

Immunity to Reinfection

Once infected, patients experience long-term immunity to reinfection with serologically similar strains.

Laboratory Diagnosis

SPECIMENS. For extraintestinal disease, blood, tissue, and normally sterile body fluids are the specimens of choice. For diagnosis of gastroenteritis, feces should be collected. Feces should be placed into Cary-Blair (buffered, agar-containing thioglycolate broth) transport medium if the specimen cannot be plated immediately.

PRIMARY ISOLATION AND IDENTIFICATION. Noncontaminated specimens can be inoculated onto routine laboratory media containing blood or similar nutrients. Incubation at 37°C in a microaerobic atmosphere is necessary for optimal recovery. In the absence of other bacteria, campylobacters are easily detected. No inhibitory substances should be added to the media. Feces should be inoculated onto selective media, usually Campy blood agar or a similar medium. The addition of cefoperazone to the media has proved effective in inhibiting normal fecal flora but allowing detection of *Campylobacter* species. Incubation in a microaerobic atmosphere and at 42°C will enhance recovery.

An alternative to selective medium is the use of a 0.45-μm pore size nitro-cellulose filter overlayed on the surface of a supportive agar onto which a small amount of feces is placed. After 30 min, the filter is removed and discarded. Campylobacters, by virtue of their small size and motility, can traverse the filter and grow on the agar surface; other fecal flora will be discarded with the filter. Colonies are identified by their unique morphology; they often spread slightly on moist media. Definitive identification requires differential susceptibility to anti-biotics, enzymatic assays, and biochemical tests. Since therapy for diarrheal disease is the same for all species, laboratories usually do not pursue identification beyond the genus stage.

IMMUNOSEROLOGIC TESTS. Enzyme-linked immunoabsorbent assay methods have been used to diagnose infection and study prevalence rates for *C. jejuni*. No commercial systems are currently available.

Treatment

Except for extraintestinal infections or cases of severe dehydration, **fluid and electrolyte replacement** serve as adequate therapy. When antibiotics are necessary, **erythromycin** and **quinolones** are effective.

Prevention and Control

Milk should be pasteurized and water supplies should be chlorinated. Contact with uncooked poultry should be avoided. All surfaces and utensils that contact uncooked poultry should be washed before using with other foods that are to be eaten without cooking. Hands should be washed before and after handling food. All food should be cooked thoroughly, particularly poultry and animal products. All domestic animals and pets with diarrheal disease should be treated and ex-posure to animal feces should be avoided.

HELICOBACTER PYLORI DISEASES

The association of an infectious agent with gastritis and peptic ulcer, ubiq-uitous diseases that had been treated symptomatically for decades, was met with great skepticism. Although spiral-shaped bacteria were observed in human gastric tissue as early as the 1870s, it was not until Australian workers Marshall and

Warren announced in 1983 the isolation of an organism from a series of patients with gastritis that the topic was approached seriously. Still, it was an uphill battle until 1990, when other studies correlating cure of duodenal ulcer with eradication of *H. pylori* convinced gastroenterologists that the association was real. Today it is thought that stomach cancer may be related to the chronic presence of *H. pylori* in the GI tract.

The organism appears to be common in humans, since serologic studies show an age-related increase in prevalence. Asymptomatic patients also may harbor the organism, as indicated by biopsy studies that show microulcerations and histologic gastritis in 90% of such patients.

One significant characteristic of *H. pylori* is its ability to produce a very **strong urease enzyme.** Although the best diagnostic test is isolation of the organism from gastric biopsy tissue, this invasive procedure is being done less often. New tests are being developed rapidly, including tests of patients' breath for evidence of the urease, tests for anti-urease antibody, and specific serologic tests for antibody to bacterial antigens. Now that the organism's pathogenic potential has finally been accepted, its spectrum of disease can be determined.

Habitat

Two species of *Helicobacter* associated with gastritis are currently recognized. *H. pylori* has been recovered from the GI tract of humans and primates. A related organism, *Helicobacter mustelae,* was isolated from the gastric mucosa of ferrets and causes gastritis and peptic ulcers in those animals.

Transmission

It is unknown how the organisms are transmitted from person to person. Attempts to isolate it from feces or mucous membranes other than gastric have been unsuccessful although it has been detected in saliva.

Properties of the Organism

H. pylori is a **curved or spiral-shaped gram-negative bacillus** that displays rapid, darting motility mediated by **polar flagella.** The organism is microaerobic. A key biochemical characteristic is its ability to rapidly hydrolyze urea by means of an unusual urease enzyme. Isolates of this organism are oxidase and catalase positive.

There is speculation that the strong urease production may serve as a virulence factor by locally neutralizing gastric acidity to allow the organism to multiply more easily. This hypothesis is being studied. The ammonia produced by urease activity may contribute to necrosis of the gastric mucosal cells and act as a factor in the development of ulceration. The ability to retain motility in a viscous environment, much like *C. jejuni,* may allow *H. pylori* to penetrate the gastric mucosa and colonize epithelial cells of the gastric type.

Pathogenesis and Clinical Manifestations

The organism colonizes and multiplies in gastric mucosa directly above the epithelial cell layer (Fig. 19.2). *H. pylori* does not invade past the epithelium. The host responds with an inflammatory infiltrate, and mucin may be depleted in areas colonized by the organisms. The symptoms are apparently related to the inflammatory response. Patients develop pain, gas, dyspepsia, foul-smelling breath, and may experience nausea and vomiting. Further degradation of mucosal tissue leads to ulceration in the antrum of the stomach and duodenum.

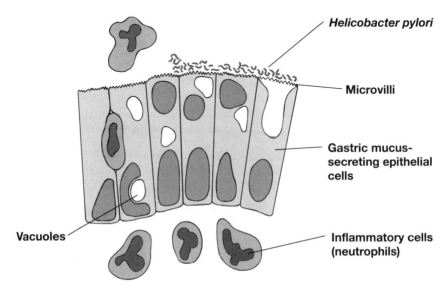

Figure 19.2.

Colonization of *H. pylori* in the mucus layer above epithelial cells of the GI tract.

Immunity to Reinfection

Although specific antibodies are present in patients with gastritis, they do not seem to be protective. Without specific antibiotic therapy, patients whose gastritis was cured by acid suppression usually relapse within a year, despite high antibody levels.

Laboratory Diagnosis

One major diagnostic method does not rely on laboratory tests, but uses a clinically derived marker. The **urea breath-test** tests the ability of patients to hydrolyze urea by measuring the amount of labeled carbon dioxide exhaled after ingestion of radioactively labeled urea. Strong hydrolysis activity implies presence of the organism.

SPECIMENS

1. Biopsy tissue. These small tissue pieces, obtained during an endoscopy procedure, can be cultured, examined microscopically for typical curved-rod morphology, or tested directly for urease production. For culture, the specimen should be transported immediately to the laboratory in a very small volume of sterile broth or buffer. Collection of biopsy material from two separate sites yields higher recovery; both antral and fundal sites are recommended.

2. Serum. Several serologic tests for antibody directed against either the organism itself or the urease enzyme have been developed. The efficacy of these tests has not yet been fully elucidated.

PRIMARY ISOLATION AND IDENTIFICATION. Direct detection of *H. pylori* in gastric biopsy touch preparations can be accomplished using a routine Gram stain with a modified counterstain using basic fuchsin instead of safranin to enhance the faint staining of these thin bacteria. The presence of typical curved rods is confirmatory. Modified silver stains (Warthin-Starry stain or Gomori methenamine silver) are used to visualize the organisms in paraffin-fixed tissue sections.

Biopsy tissue can be tested directly for the presence of urease. Several commercial systems are available; the biopsy is placed into contact with urea in a gel or broth and observed. If urease is present, the urea will be hydrolyzed to ammonia, which turns a phenol red pH indicator bright pink. Rarely would organisms other than *H. pylori* possess an enzyme active enough to yield a positive test in this system and such organisms would not normally be present in the antrum.

Culturing the specimen for *H. pylori* is the third option. Ground tissue should be inoculated onto fresh chocolate agar or modified Thayer-Martin agar, which is used routinely for isolation of *Neisseria gonorrhoeae,* and incubated under microaerophilic conditions at 35°C for up to 1 week.

IMMUNOSEROLOGIC TESTS. Several serologic tests for antibody to *H. pylori* have recently been introduced. These tests claim to test for specific antibody and to be as sensitive and specific as the invasive biopsy-dependent diagnostic tests. At least one test is based on detection of antibody directed against the high molecular weight urease enzyme. Evaluations of these tests are in progress.

Treatment

Several treatment regimens have been effective but long-term results have not been evaluated. Current therapies usually include **two agents; such as two antibiotics (metronidazole and amoxicillin)** or a **bismuth subcitrate compound and one antibiotic;** or **three agents,** including **two antibiotics** plus a **bismuth compound.**

Prevention and Control

Strategies for prevention and control cannot be defined until the epidemiology of this newly recognized infectious disease has been clarified.

SUMMARY

1. *Campylobacter* **and** *Helicobacter* **species are curved, oxidase-positive, microaerobic gram-negative bacilli whose natural habitat is the mammalian and avian GI tract.**

2. *Campylobacter* **species, especially** *C. jejuni* **and** *C. coli,* **cause gastroenteritis by colonizing the intestinal mucus layer and damaging host epithelial cell function, perhaps by means of an enterotoxin or a cytotoxin, but their exact pathogenic mechanism is unknown.**

3. Campylobacteriosis is usually acquired by ingestion of the organism on contaminated food or in contaminated water; domestic chickens and turkeys are often the source.

4. *Helicobacter pylori* has been recognized recently as the major etiologic agent of gastritis and duodenal ulcer in humans, who may be its only host.

5. *Helicobacter pylori* possesses a powerful urease enzyme, which may serve as a virulence mechanism by moderating stomach acidity in the local environment of the organism.

6. Like campylobacters, helicobacters colonize the mucus and do not penetrate into intestinal epithelial cells. The host inflammatory response results in tissue destruction and ulceration.

REFERENCES

Blaser MJ (1987): Gastric *Campylobacter*-like organisms, gastritis, and peptic ulcer disease. Gastroenterologia 93:371.

Morgan DR (ed) (1991): Symposium on *Helicobacter pylori:* a cause of gastroduodenal disease. Rev Infect Dis 13 (Suppl. 8):S655.

Rauws EAJ, Tytgat GNJ (1990): Cure of duodenal ulcer associated with eradication of *Helicobacter pylori.* Lancet 335:1233.

Walker RI, Caldwell MB, Lee EC (1986): Pathophysiology of *Campylobacter* enteritis. Microbiol Rev 50:81.

REVIEW QUESTIONS

For questions 1 to 8, choose the ONE
BEST answer or completion:

1. *Campylobacter*-associated gastroenteritis is
   transmitted primarily
   a) during handling of infected animals and
      their products
   b) person to person by the fecal-oral route
   c) by inhalation of aerosol droplets contain-
      ing viable organisms
   d) in contaminated eggs
   e) during sexual activity

2. Which set of circumstances results in best
   recovery of *Campylobacter jejuni* from stool
   specimens?
   a) Inoculate to selective media, incubate at
      37°C, and examine plate after 24 h.
   b) Inoculate to blood agar, incubate at 37°C,
      and examine plate after 48 h.
   c) Inoculate to selective blood agar, incu-
      bate at 37°C in an oxygen-depleted at-
      mosphere, and examine plate after 24 h.
   d) Inoculate to selective blood agar, incu-
      bate at 42°C, and examine plates after
      48 h.
   e) Inoculate to selective blood agar, incu-
      bate at 42°C in an oxygen-depleted at-
      mosphere, and examine plate after 48 h.

3. To cause disease in the GI tract, campylobacters
   a) adhere to mucosal epithelial cell walls by
      means of surface adhesins
   b) invade through the stomach epithelium
      using corkscrew motion and disseminate
      through the bloodstream
   c) multiply in the mucus layer above the GI
      epithelium and elaborate cytotoxins and
      inflammatory factors
   d) adhere to intestinal goblet cells by means
      of pili
   e) survive within macrophages

4. Which statement about therapy for campylobacteriosis is most correct?
   a) If one child in a day care center acquires
      campylobacter diarrhea, all other children
      should be treated prophylactically with ri-
      fampin.
   b) Treat diarrhea with erythromycin.
   c) Treat diarrhea with erythromycin plus ri-
      fampin.
   d) Treat severe disease with fluid and elec-
      trolyte replacement and a short course of
      trimethoprim-sulfamethoxazole.
   e) Treat severe disease with fluid and elec-
      trolyte replacement and a short course of
      erythromycin.

5. The association of *Helicobacter pylori* with
   gastritis and duodenal ulcer is

a) based on numerous studies, including those showing cure of gastritis associated with eradication of the organism

b) controversial, based on a study in which one volunteer developed gastritis after ingesting the organism

c) based on serological prevalence studies

d) based on noninvasive tests for *Helicobacter* antigens

e) based on subsequent development of stomach cancer following bacterial infection

6. The most striking characteristic of *H. pylori* is its
   a) curved, corkscrew shape
   b) ability to survive gastric acidity
   c) ability to survive intracellularly
   d) strongly active urease enzyme
   e) growth on selective medium

7. Diagnosis of *H. pylori* associated gastritis can be accomplished by

a) culturing the organism from antral biopsy

b) demonstrating strong urease activity in biopsied tissue

c) visualizing curved and S-shaped bacteria in stained antral biopsy material

d) measuring the presence of a strong urease by determining whether labeled carbon dioxide is exhaled by patients who have been fed labeled urea

e) all of the above

8. A common factor shared by *Helicobacter* and *Campylobacter* is that they
   a) are both members of the *Enterobacteriaceae*
   b) are both diagnosed best by a serological assay
   c) are curved, and S-shaped gram-negative bacilli
   d) both require incubation at 42°C for isolation
   e) both are found in the GI tracts of birds and mammals

ANSWERS TO REVIEW QUESTIONS

---

1. *a* Chickens and other meats contaminate food to be ingested and the organism is thus disseminated. Eggs have not been shown to harbor campylobacters. Sexual transmission occurs primarily in animals, although sexual transmission of some unusual strains does seem to occur among homosexual men. Point-source outbreaks are more common than person-person infections.

2. *e* All of these conditions will maximize recovery of *Campylobacter jejuni* and *Campylobacter coli* (the two most common

agents of diarrhea) from fecal specimens. The 42°C temperature does not inhibit growth of these campylobacters but it does inhibit growth of normal fecal flora. Because they are microaerobic, these organisms grow best at 5–10% oxygen, which is a lower concentration than that of room air. Since the organisms are somewhat slow-growing, some strains may not yield visible colonies after only 24 h.

3. *c* The organisms do not ever appear to adhere to epithelial cell surfaces, but exert their effects from within the mucus overlaying the GI epithelium. Intracellular survival in macrophages facilitates the development of extraintestinal manifestations.

4. *e* Unless disease is severe, no treatment is necessary. The organisms are susceptible to erythromycin (the drug of choice) and quinolones, but not all isolates are susceptible to sulfa drugs.

5. *a* Serologic studies, however, do show a high prevalence of antibodies, proportional to the age of the patient. Clinical evaluations of asymptomatic patients with antibodies show early changes consistent with gastritis. Until studies correlating eradication of the organism with disappearance of symptoms were published, many members of the medical community did not believe that a bacterium could cause peptic ulcer disease.

6. *d* Many organisms can survive gastric acidity in some way, but none other than *Helicobacter pylori* seem to protect themselves from the acidity by alkalinizing their immediate environment, one of the roles thought to be played by the organism's powerful urease enzyme. Most of the other selections are not unique to *Helicobacter,* and this species cannot survive intracellularly at all.

7. *e* All of the listed diagnostic methods are currently used. In addition, rapid serologic tests for antibody are also being evaluated for use as a noninvasive test system.

8. *c* Of the characteristics listed, only their cellular morphology is similar. Both genera do grow best in a carbon dioxide enriched, oxygen-depleted atmosphere.

LEGIONNAIRES' DISEASE

In 1976, the world was riveted by a medical detective story that commanded public attention for months. During the Bicentennial of the 1776 Declaration of Independence, interest was focused on Philadelphia as the historical site of the event. The story of a devastating epidemic of respiratory disease among Pennsylvania American Legion members staying at the Bellevue Stratford Hotel in downtown Philadelphia was a natural headliner for the news media. The disease struck 182 conventioneers, among whom there were 29 subsequent deaths. It was not until 6 months later that the etiologic agent, *Legionella pneumophila,* was identified and named after the American Legion. The pneumonia caused by *Legionella* species has retained the name, Legionnaires' disease.

Since that first large outbreak, there have been numerous others, caused by one of at least 40 species of *Legionella.* One of the largest occurred in the Wadsworth Veterans Administration Hospital soon after a new facility opened, a few years after the Philadelphia outbreak. A previously unused water source had been commandeered for the new hospital. It took several months of effort to control the epidemic. A 1989 outbreak in Louisiana involved 33 cases of Legionnaires' disease acquired by persons who shopped in a particular grocery store. The misting machine that kept the produce cool and moist was spewing *Legionella pneumophila* onto the vegetables and into the air. At least two persons died as a result of the disease.

In addition to pneumonia, the most common manifestation, *Legionella* is associated with several other syndromes. Before the etiologic agent was identified, a febrile, flu-like manifestation of legionellosis called Pontiac fever had struck a large number of people working in a Pontiac, Michigan Health Department. Retrospectively, this outbreak was associated with *L. pneumophila* serologically. A long standing but low incidence outbreak of prosthetic valve endocarditis caused by *Legionella dumoffii* or *L. pneumophila* in patients who received surgery at Stanford University Medical Center was reported in 1988. Pneumonia in renal transplant recipients has been traced to *Legionella micdadei*. Renal and tissue abscesses and occasional pericarditis and myocarditis have been reported. Over 100,000 cases of Legionnaires' disease occur annually in the United States, most of them sporadic.

LEGIONNAIRES' DISEASE

Habitat

The organisms are **ubiquitous in environmental fresh water,** such as ponds and streams, which they enter presumably from the soil. However, because of the many nutrients lacking in the water milieu and competition from less fastidious bacteria, it is postulated that they are not free-living. Legionellae have been shown to survive and multiply as parasites of protozoa, including the amebae *Hartmannella, Acanthamoeba,* and ciliates, such as *Tetrahymena.* It is possible that the ability to survive intracellularly in these eukaryotes contributes to the **ability of legionellae to survive in human phagocytic cells.** Patients usually acquire *Legionella* from man-made water sources, such as air-conditioning units, cooling towers, evaporative condensers, shower heads, whirlpools, mist generators, and other water outlets.

Transmission

EXOGENOUS. Airborne transmission by way of **aerosols** is the most common route. Misters, shower heads, drinking fountains, and whirlpools create aerosols that are inhaled by patients. Waterborne disease may occur, particularly in nosocomial environments. There is **no known human-human transmission** or vertical transmission from mother to fetus. Risk factors include cigarette smoking, male, more than 30 years of age, summertime, and **immunocompromised status,** such as alcohol abuse, organ transplant, malignancy, and emphysema.

Properties of the Organism

Resistance to environmental, physical, and chemical agents. Legionellae can remain viable in groundwater at 4°C for long periods and can grow at temperatures up to 50°C, but they are killed in water heated to 80°C for 30 min. **Chlorination of 2 ppm is effective** in destroying legionellae, although outbreaks often occur when chlorination of potable water sources is not adequate. Stomach acidity seems to be sufficient to kill the organisms. Sunlight and disinfectants are effective in destroying this fastidious bacterium.

Microscopic morphology. Legionellae are **gram-negative** organisms that usually appear as **short coccobacilli** when seen directly in tissue, but can exhibit **long filaments** in culture. The organisms stain poorly with standard Gram stains, but very well by silver impregnation methods. *L. micdadei* can appear partially acid-fast in tissue, and may be mistaken for a mycobacterium on direct smears and on biopsies. The organisms are usually **motile** by means of **one polar flagellum.**

Macroscopic morphology. *Legionella* species are **strict aerobes** and grow best in high humidity. Increased carbon dioxide is not necessary but does enhance growth of some species. Special media containing charcoal to remove inhibitory fatty acids and yeast extract are used for isolation. Growth requires cysteine and iron. Colonies on charcoal-yeast extract agar usually appear blue-white to gray with a pearly or ground-glass appearance. Variable colors of colony fluorescence under UV light have been used to help differentiate among species. Biochemical tests are rarely performed; strains are identified serologically. Many species of *Legionella* produce β-lactamase. The most prevalent species of *Legionella* involved in human diseases are *L. pneumophila, L. micdadei, L. bozemanii,* and *L. dumoffii.* At least 12 other species have been isolated from humans with disease, usually respiratory.

Antigenic structure. The main antigenic determinant for classification of legionellae is lipopolysaccharide (LPS). Species are derived primarily by serogroup based upon polysaccharide antigen components of LPS. *L. pneumophila,* the most prevalent species, contains at least 15 serogroups. The other species have fewer serogroups. The organisms also contain a porin protein in the outer membrane (OM).

Extracellular products associated with pathogenicity. Certain proteases may mediate tissue damage. Motility by means of flagella may help the organism invade the lung and the major outer membrane protein (MOMP) of the organism binds a complement byproduct, C3, which mediates phagocytosis.

Pathogenesis and Clinical Manifestations

The infective dose of legionellosis is thought to be as low as one colony forming unit per 50 L of air. Legionellae are inhaled into the lung, where they reach the alveoli. During the subsequent inflammatory response, C3 created by complement activation is bound to bacterial MOMP receptors. Complement receptors on alveolar macrophages and monocytes bind to the C3 on the bacterial surface and then phagocytize the organism in a ''coiling'' pseudopod-like formation (Fig. 20.1). The **organisms multiply within the phagosome vacuole and inhibit lysosomal fusion.** The vacuole becomes lined with ribosomes. The bacteria are also somehow able to maintain a rather high pH within the phagosome. Multiplying bacteria induce development of an inflammatory infiltrate in the alveoli consisting of neutrophils, macrophages, and fibrin deposits. The loss of gas exchange in the alveoli causes the clinical syndrome of **pneumonia.**

Legionnaires' disease presents as a typical pneumonia. After the initial encounter, the disease manifests after a 2–10 day incubation period. The attack rate, however, is less than 5%. In addition to the characteristic pneumonia, the disease often results in multiple system damage, such as renal failure and diarrhea. The putative nonspecific mechanism for multisystem effects is not known. Fatalities occur in older or debilitated patients.

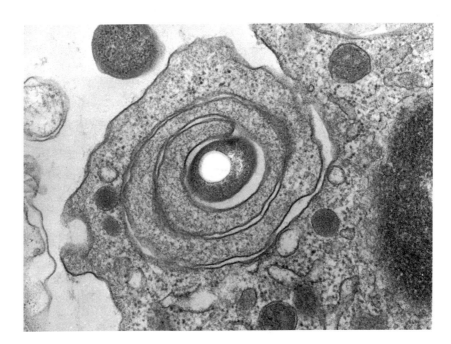

Figure 20.1.

Transmission electron micrograph of *Legionella* being engulfed by coiling pseudopod of nonprofessional phagocyte [Reproduced with permission from Horwitz MA (1984): Phagocytosis of the Legionnaire's disease bacterium (*Legionella pneumophila*) occurs by a novel mechanism: engulfment within a pseudopod coil. Cell 36:28]

Pontiac fever syndrome, a milder manifestation of *Legionella* disease, is diagnosed serologically, since the bacteria have never been isolated from patients. An aerosol inoculum is believed to be the portal of entry. The incubation period after exposure is 1–2 days . Clinical manifestations are mild and include fever, chills, headache, myalgia, and respiratory disease without pneumonia. The attack rate is greater than 90%. Fatalities are not reported.

For endocarditis and other extrapulmonary diseases the portal of entry still seems to be by the respiratory route in most cases, but dissemination occurs. Inflammatory exudates are the prominent feature. Clearing of lung lesions after resolution of clinical manifestations progresses very slowly, often requiring months.

Immunity to Reinfection

Humoral immunity is not effective, since the organism is not killed by antibody and complement. Although long-term studies are not available, cell-mediated immunity probably accounts for acquired resistance in previously infected hosts. Animal studies indicate that a vaccine prepared from either the major secretory protein of *L. pneumophila,* cell membranes, or an avirulent mutant can induce protective immunity. However, **human vaccines have not as yet been developed.**

Laboratory Diagnosis

SPECIMENS. Specimens should not be diluted or submitted in saline, as this may be inhibitory to growth of *Legionella* sp. Distilled water is an acceptable fluid for moistening specimens. Specimen samples may include sputum and respiratory secretions; transtracheal and lung biopsy tissue; blood and other body fluids, although acellular fluids, such as pleural fluid transudates, are unlikely to harbor the intracellular organisms; and urine, for direct antigen testing.

DIRECT DETECTION

Direct Fluorescent Antibody (DFA) Stain. Sputum, respiratory secretions, and lung biopsy touch preparations are the best specimens. A monoclonal antibody cocktail directed against the most common serotypes of *L. pneumophila* is used to detect organisms in the specimen. This method is about 50% sensitive but usually quite specific. Inasmuch as the pneumonia caused by other species or serotypes of *Legionella* will not be detected, cultures must also be performed.

Urine Antigen Test. Polysaccharide antigen of legionellae is concentrated in the urine and can be detected in patients with pneumonia. A radioimmunoassay (RIA) is commercially available for *L. pneumophila* and an ELISA is in development. This test is quite sensitive and highly specific. Unfortunately, patients may continue to excrete antigen for months during convalescence so the test may be falsely positive in some patients who have recovered from legionellosis and then acquired pneumonia caused by another etiologic agent.

Genetic Probe for *Legionella* RNA. Respiratory secretions and triturated tissue can be tested by the probe, which is commercially available and requires approximately 3 h to obtain results. The assay utilizes a chemiluminescent marker of hybridization and detects species of *Legionella* with a sensitivity greater than direct fluorescent antibody stain.

PRIMARY ISOLATION AND IDENTIFICATION. Culture is still the gold standard for diagnosis of Legionnaires' disease, primarily because so many serotypes and species of *Legionella* cause disease that immunologic methods may not be broad-based enough to detect them in some specimens, such as blood, and because numbers of organisms may be too low to detect visually or with a probe.

Special media are required for isolation of *Legionella*. Buffered charcoal yeast extract (BCYE) agar and selective BCYE with antibiotics are used. A biphasic BCYE agar-broth medium is available for blood cultures. Alternatively, blood collected in lysis centrifugation tubes can be plated directly to BCYE. It is important to realize that **sputum from patients with *Legionella* pneumonia may not be purulent.** The microbiologists should be notified to culture specifically for this organism.

Specimens contaminated with normal flora, such as sputum and bronchial lavages, are plated directly and plated following dilution in water and in a weak hydrochloric acid solution. Acid wash has been shown to enhance recovery. The BCYE plates are incubated in 5% CO_2 in a humidified atmosphere for at least 10 days. Colonies are ground-glass appearing, white or shades of blue, green, or purple, often fluorescing under UV light. Colonies on BCYE that fail to grow on blood agar, exhibit a typical gram-negative morphology on Gram stain, and are catalase positive, are identified presumptively as *Legionella* sp. Further identification is usually not done, but if necessary, the isolates must be sent to a reference laboratory where they are identified serologically.

IMMUNOSEROLOGIC TESTS

Legionella-Associated Pneumonia. Indirect fluorescent assay and ELISA methods employing various strains of legionellae as the substrate have been used for serologic studies. The large number of patients who have developed antibodies to these organisms makes it unlikely that a single serum specimen can be used to diagnose definitively acute infection. A fourfold rise in titer between an acute and convalescent serum specimen can verify a diagnosis, but at least 50% of patients fail to show a rise in titer for at least 2 weeks; indeed, **20% of patients never develop antibody.** A single titer of 1:256 with a compatible pneumonia is suggestive but not definitive for the diagnosis of Legionnaires' disease.

Pontiac Fever. Diagnosis of Pontiac feverlike illness must be made **retrospectively and serologically,** as the organism has not been visualized or recovered from patients.

Treatment

Erythromycin has been the drug of choice since this syndrome was first recognized. **Rifampin** has been added for **synergistic** activity, particularly since it can enter the infected macrophage and act intracellularly. Other antimicrobial agents used to treat Legionnaires' disease include tetracycline, trimethoprim-sulfamethoxazole, and ciprofloxacin.

Prevention and Control

It is important to maintain adequate chlorine levels in all potable water sources, drain cooling towers and other reservoirs of potable water when not in use, and periodically clean surface deposits thoroughly. Periodically heating indoor water systems to 80°C for 30 min, in addition to chlorination, has been used to diminish some hospital outbreaks. Use of sterilized water for washing and wound care of postsurgical patients will reduce waterborne infections.

SUMMARY

1. More than 30 species of *Legionella*, a gram-negative, aerobic bacillus, live in environmental fresh water and soil.

2. Infection is acquired by the aerosol route.

3. *Legionella pneumophila,* the most important member of the genus, produces two distinct disease syndromes. (a) Pneumonia is characterized by additional severe and systemic effects. (b) Pontiac fever is characterized as a mild respiratory disease accompanied by fever and headache.

4. Other species including *Legionella micdadei* and *Legionella dumoffii* cause pneumonia and occasionally extrapulmonary manifestations.

5. The legionellae are intracellular pathogens. These organisms possess surface receptors that bind C3, which induces phagocytosis by alveolar macrophages and monocytes. Once inside the phagosome, they inhibit lysosomal fusion and multiply intracellularly. The presence of this pathogen and the resulting inflammatory response cause the pneumonia.

6. Diagnosis depends on detection of the organism in respiratory secretions by direct fluorescent antibody stain, DNA probe for ribosomal RNA, or culture. Alternatively, antigen can be detected in the urine using an enzyme immunoassay. Serologic diagnosis is not reliable.

REFERENCES

Fang GD, Yu VL, Vickers RM (1989): Disease due to the Legionellaceae (other than *Legionella pneumophila*): historical, microbiological, clinical and epidemiological review. Medicine 68:116.

Tompkins LS, Roessler BJ, Redd SC, Markowitz LE, Cohen ML (1988): *Legionella* prosthetic-valve endocarditis. N Engl J Med 318:530.

Thornsberry C, Balows A, Feeley JC, Jakubowski W (eds) (1984): *Legionella:* proceedings of the 2nd international symposium. Washington, DC: American Society for Microbiology.

Winn WC (1988): Legionnaires' disease: historical perspective. Clin Microbiol Rev 1:60.

REVIEW QUESTIONS

> For questions 1 to 6, choose the ONE BEST answer or completion.

During the last month, three new cases of *Legionella pneumophila* pneumonia have been diagnosed in postsurgical patients at one hospital.

1. Which measure is most likely to prevent the development of similar infections in additional patients?
   a) Hyperchlorination of the water delivery system.
   b) Adding a reverse-osmosis filtration system to the water delivery system.
   c) Instituting a respiratory isolation policy for all currently infected patients.
   d) Thoroughly cleaning and disinfecting respiratory therapy equipment after use with each patient.
   e) Terminally cleaning each infected patient's room with a sporicidal disinfectant when the patient is discharged.

2. Of the following, which is the most sensitive and specific rapid method for presumptive diagnosis of *L. pneumophila* pneumonia in subsequent patients who develop a new pulmonary infiltrate?

   a) Gram stain of bronchoalveolar lavage specimens for the typical pale-staining, gram-negative bacilli.
   b) Radioimmunoassay for antigen of *L. pneumophila* being excreted in urine.
   c) Direct fluorescent antibody stain of expectorated sputum, looking for *L. pneumophila* cells.
   d) India ink preparation of sputum looking for encapsulated cells.
   e) Testing expectorated sputum for ribosomal RNA using a chemiluminescent genetic probe for legionellae.

3. The Microbiology laboratory has chosen to culture all sputum samples received for legionellae. Which medium is most likely to recover the organisms?
   a) Brucella blood agar.
   b) Cysteine-tellurite agar.
   c) Potato dextrose agar.
   d) Buffered charcoal yeast extract agar.
   e) Thiosulfate citrate bile salts agar.

4. Patients should be treated immediately and aggressively with
   a) erythromycin
   b) erythromycin and rifampin
   c) vancomycin and rifampin
   d) penicillin and an aminoglycoside
   e) an aminoglycoside

5. The primary difference between the two main disease syndromes caused by *L. pneumophila* is that
   a) the pneumonia of Pontiac fever is much milder and is manifested by a diffuse generalized infiltrate rather than a lobar presentation
   b) patients with Pontiac fever experience a much higher temperature than do those with Legionnaires' disease
   c) Pontiac fever patients do not develop pneumonia
   d) Pontiac fever patients develop headache and high fevers, whereas Legionnaires' disease patients do not
   e) the attack rate of Legionnaires' disease is

extremely high (>50%), whereas the milder disease, Pontiac fever, has a much lower attack rate (<10%).

6. The primary virulence mechanism of *L. pneumophila* is its
   a) potent cytotoxin that inhibits motility of respiratory cilia
   b) antiphagocytic capsule
   c) proteases that inflict damage to host tissue
   d) ability to induce endocytosis by nonprofessional phagocytes and survive in the cytoplasm
   e) ability to induce phagocytosis and survive in the phagosome

ANSWERS TO REVIEW QUESTIONS

1. *a* Adequate chlorination has been shown to effectively eradicate *Legionella* spp. from potable water systems. Since the bacteria are ubiquitous throughout all water in a building, filters at certain points will not prevent growth of the bacteria in distant sites. The organism is not spread from human to human, nor does it seem to colonize respiratory therapy equipment. It is a nonspore-forming bacteria.

2. *b* The RIA of urine is the most specific and sensitive. Although the probe is almost as sensitive, its specificity is for all species

of *Legionella*, not just *Legionella pneumophila*. Direct fluorescent antibody tests are not particularly sensitive, although they are rather specific. The organism is not encapsulated.

3. *d* Only BCYE will support the growth of legionellae. The other agars listed are used as follows: Brucella blood agar for isolation of anaerobic bacteria and *Brucella* spp., cysteine-tellurite agar for isolation of *Corynebacterium diphtheriae*, potato dextrose agar to enhance sporulation of fungi, and TCBS agar for isolation of *Vibrio* spp.

4. *b* The synergistic effect of erythromycin (the drug of choice for legionellae) and rifampin (which enters the macrophage, the site of bacterial multiplication) should be chosen because of the already immunocompromised state of postsurgical, hospitalized patients.

5. *c* The two syndromes, pneumonia (exemplified by Legionnaires' disease) and Pontiac fever, are quite different. Pontiac fever is milder and does not include a pneumonia component, although the attack rate is very high (90%). The attack rate for *L. pneumophila* pneumonia is less than 5%.

6. *e* Legionellae are phagocytized by macrophages in a pseudopod-like coil of cell membrane. Once inside, they prevent lysosomal fusion with the phagosomal vacuole. Toxins have not been shown to effect virulence. The organisms are not encapsulated.

NOSOCOMIAL DISEASES

Nosocomial [*Noso* (Greek, disease); *komeo* (Greek, hospital)] **diseases are acquired by patients during hospitalization.** These infections are a major concern for health care providers.

Nosocomial diseases are usually defined as those diseases in hospitalized patients for which clinical manifestations present at **least 72 h after admission.** Bacteria, viruses, and fungi are all implicated as nosocomial pathogens. Patients are at risk for developing such diseases simply by being ill enough to be hospitalized. Additional factors that contribute to the acquisition of nosocomial disease are tissue damage (trauma or surgery); manipulations as a consequence of medical care (iatrogenic), such as catheterization, antibiotic or immunosuppressive therapy, implanted devices, and respiratory care; proximity to other infected hosts; and the presence of resistant bacteria in the environment.

Numerous studies have shown that hospitalized patients are at increased risk of becoming colonized on their skin with multiply resistant *Corynebacterium* species, yeasts, methicillin-resistant *Staphylococcus aureus,* and other microorganisms unique to the hospital environment. The patient's bowels and oropharyngeal membranes become colonized with hospital-resident *Enterobacteriaceae*, pseudomonads, and other gram-negative bacilli, usually possessing a more antibiotic-resistant profile than community microorganisms of the same genus. The source of these organisms is other patients in the hospital environment. Presumably, the organisms are carried on the hands of health care providers from colonized patients to newly admitted patients, who then become colonized themselves. Therefore, **handwashing is the single most important activity** that must be performed in an effort to control nosocomial disease.

More than 2 million patients per year, representing 5–10% of all hospitalized patients, acquire an infection during their hospital stay; the economic and social consequences are staggering. It is estimated that nosocomial diseases cost $5 billion extra health care dollars annually. The main types of nosocomial diseases are shown in Table 21.1. *Enterobacteriaceae* are the most important etiologic agents of these diseases based on numbers, primarily because **urinary tract diseases comprise the largest single type of disease,** and because *Enterobacteriaceae,* mainly *Escherichia coli,* are the **principal etiologic agents of urinary tract infections.**

Many of the organisms associated with nosocomial diseases are the patient's own endogenous flora from the GI tract. However, these bacterial strains have often colonized patients after admission, carrying with them antibiotic resistance factors acquired by selective pressure of ubiquitous antibiotic usage in the facility. When they obtain access to the urinary tract through an indwelling catheter, for example, or colonize a postsurgical wound, they can multiply, destroy tissue, and promote an inflammatory response. The 10 most frequent organisms associated with nosocomial disease are *Escherichia coli, Staphylococcus aureus, Enterococcus* spp., *Pseudomonas aeruginosa,* coagulase-negative staphylococci, other *Enterobacteriaceae, Candida albicans, Klebsiella pneumoniae, Proteus mirabilis,* and anaerobic gram-positive bacteria, primarily *Propionibacterium* spp.

BLOODSTREAM DISEASE

INTRAVASCULAR ACCESS-RELATED DISEASE

The **presence of an IV catheter is the most common predisposing factor to nosocomial bacteremia and fungemia.** Intact skin is an effective barrier to infection by microorganisms; intravascular devices allow organisms direct access to the bloodstream by providing an open conduit. Almost one-half of all patients in the United States each year have an intravascular catheter inserted during hospitalization. The risk of acquiring a catheter-related bloodstream disease is less than 1%, but with 20 million patients at risk, the number of such diseases is high.

Mortality is also high; an estimated 9000 deaths per year are attributed to catheter-associated bacteremia. Nosocomial bacteremia accounts for approximately 1 week of additional hospital care with a cost of over $7000 per case. With

TABLE 21.1. Overview of the Most Common Nosocomial Diseases, In Order of Prevalence

Type of infection	Contributing factors	Primary pathogens
Urinary tract	Catheters	*Escherichia coli*
Pneumonia	Assisted ventilation	*Pseudomonas aeruginosa*
		Staphylococcus aureus
		Enterobacteriaceae
Surgical wound		Staphylococci
Bacteremia	Intravenous lines	Staphylococci (coagulase negative)

proper skin preparation, catheter care, and frequent replacement, catheter-related septicemia can be prevented in most cases. Indeed, changing uninfected catheters after 3 days has been shown to dramatically decrease infection rates.

Pathogenesis

The organisms travel along the external surface of the catheter and **colonize the interface between tissue and catheter** (Fig. 21.1). If catheter insertion has aggravated the development of a thrombus, this protected site provides nutrients and encourages microbial growth, resulting in **septic thrombophlebitis.** Organisms are seeded directly into the bloodstream from the colonized areas. The catheter material influences the ability of bacteria to adhere. Teflon and metal catheters are less hospitable than are polyvinyl chloride. The type of catheter, single lumen versus multiple lumen, is another factor. The more complex the catheter, the higher the risk that it will become contaminated. The agent being delivered will affect the type of organism likely to cause disease. Total parenteral nutrition predisposes patients to diseases due to yeasts as well as members of the normal skin flora.

Etiologic Agents

The resident skin flora are most likely to colonize the catheter surface and seed the bloodstream. The most common catheter-related microorganisms are **coagulase-negative staphylococci.** *Staphylococcus epidermidis* is the species most often identified. This species may have certain virulence factors, such as the ability to adhere to artificial surfaces mediated by lectins or other adhesins and production of **extracellular slime** protecting the colonies from host antibacterial factors and

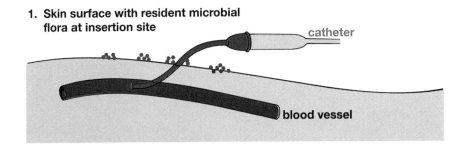

1. **Skin surface with resident microbial flora at insertion site**

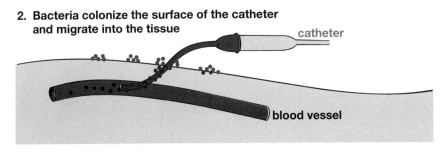

2. **Bacteria colonize the surface of the catheter and migrate into the tissue**

3. **Bacteria reach blood vessels and colonize catheter tip and lumen, from which they are sloughed into the bloodstream.**

Figure 21.1.

Schematic diagram of organisms colonizing the IV catheter.

antimicrobial agents, that contribute to its relative prominence among staphylococci as an agent of device-associated infection. Other species, however, are also involved. Coagulase-negative staphylococci are inherently quite resistant to many antibiotics, including penicillins and cephalosporins.

S. aureus is the second most common etiologic agent. Increasingly problematic are multiply antibiotic-resistant strains, particularly **methicillin-resistant S. aureus (MRSA) and Enterococcus spp. Yeast species,** particularly species of *Candida* in adults and neonates, and *Malassezia furfur,* a lipophilic fungus, in neonates receiving lipid-rich infusions, are important fungal agents of catheter-related sepsis. Other organisms that colonize the skin of hospitalized patients, such as **Corynebacterium jeikeium** and other **lipophilic corynebacteria,** *Acinetobacter* species, *Pseudomonas* species, and various *Enterobacteriaceae,* may be involved.

Laboratory Diagnosis

Diagnosis relies first upon detecting the organism in the blood. **Blood cultures** must be collected from at least **two separate venipuncture sites** to help differentiate skin contaminants from true agents of sepsis. To determine whether the catheter itself is the source of the septicemia, it can be removed and cultured. Rolling the catheter tip over the surface of a culture plate allows quantitation of colony forming units (CFU). Greater than 15 CFU per catheter has correlated with the catheter as an infectious source. Drawing simultaneous cultures through the catheter and peripherally may identify the catheter as the source.

Treatment

Removal of the catheter and empiric therapy must be instituted when clinical signs of catheter-related sepsis are present. **Vancomycin** is the drug of choice to cover coagulase-negative staphylococci and MRSA. The choice of whether to use an antifungal agent must be made based on clinical grounds. Once the etiologic agent's susceptibility pattern is known, more specific therapy can be substituted. In some cases, antibiotic therapy must be given without removing the catheter. The duration of therapy will be longer for such patients. A new treatment option for gram-negative sepsis holds much promise. Use of a molecular-engineered anti-endotoxin antibody that prevents the systemic effects of endotoxic shock is being evaluated. The treatment is currently very expensive, so its use must be justified by strong clinical or microbiological evidence of gram-negative sepsis.

Prevention

Aggressive cleansing and prophylactic treatment of skin with chlorhexidine before catheter insertion will lower the rate of subsequent disease. The antimicrobial agent mupirocin is very effective against staphylococci. Intranasal application can prevent skin colonization; mupirocin is not recommended for skin antisepsis. **Exchanging indwelling catheters every 48–72 h** will decrease the incidence of disease. If the catheter is contaminated, a new site should be chosen for the next insertion. Local insertion site care, avoidance of occlusive dressings, and application of topical antibiotics are useful preventive measures. Use of care teams to monitor catheters has been effective in reducing complications. New catheter materials, antibiotic- and heavy metal-impregnated cuffs and other technical advances are contributing to decreases in catheter-related disease.

BLOODSTREAM DISEASE FROM AN INFECTED TISSUE SITE

In compromised patients, particularly those in hospitals and skilled nursing facilities, a wound or urinary tract disease can quickly extend into the bloodstream because the host response is not strong or quick enough to prevent extension of the disease.

The most common sites from which bacteremia develops are the genitourinary tract, the respiratory tract, abscesses, surgical wound infections, and the biliary tract. Physicians can often predict the etiologic agent of a nosocomial septicemia if the causative agent in the infected source site is known.

BLOOD TRANSFUSION-RELATED DISEASE

Infusion of microbes directly into the blood from an infected donor is an uncommon type of iatrogenic infection, but it does occur. Agents acquired in this way include hepatitis B and C viruses, HIV, CMV, *Yersinia enterocolitica,* and parasites, such as *Plasmodium* spp. and *Babesia microti.*

CONTAMINATED INFUSION-RELATED DISEASES

Solutions delivered directly into the bloodstream have the potential to become contaminated with bacteria and cause sepsis in the recipient. Gram-negative bacteria are most often implicated in cases of infection due to IV fluid infection. Agents associated with reported cases include *Enterobacter cloacae, E. agglomerans, Citrobacter* spp., *Serratia marcescens,* and *Pseudomonas* spp.

Although this source of nosocomial bacteremia is rare, gram-negative sepsis is a life-threatening disease in an already debilitated patient. The presence of *Enterobacteriaceae* or any gram-negative bacteria in the bloodstream may lead to endotoxic shock and systemic disease.

RESPIRATORY DISEASE

BACTERIAL PNEUMONIA

Bacterial pneumonia is the number one cause of death among nosocomial diseases, with an overall case fatality rate of 20–50% and up to 80% in patients with *P. aeruginosa* disease.

Pathogenesis

Risk factors associated with development of nosocomial pneumonia include mechanical ventilation, loss of consciousness and subsequent aspiration, serious underlying disease or poor health, use of broad-spectrum antimicrobial therapy, and intubation.

Aspiration pneumonia is the most common form of nosocomial pneumonia. The oropharyngeal flora of hospitalized patients is different from that of healthy persons in the increased number of gram-negative bacteria and the prevalence of antibiotic-resistant strains.

Another predisposing condition to development of aspiration pneumonia is the use of **antacids and hydrogen-secretion blockers,** an extremely common measure to reduce stress-related ulcers among hospitalized patients. This therapy allows colonization of the normally sterile stomach by bacteria from the environment or the hosts oral secretions. These fluids are often aspirated by ill patients.

Aspiration of oral fluids leads to bacteria in the normally sterile lung. Normal oropharyngeal flora, such as pigmenting anaerobic gram-negative bacilli, streptococci, and actinomycetes, produce tissue-destructive enzymes and induce an inflammatory response. Hospital-acquired colonizers that reach the lung also are free to multiply and induce a host response. Encapsulated organisms such as *K. pneumoniae* are resistant to phagocytosis and their capsular polysaccharide acts to chemotactically attract macrophages, whose enzymes contribute to tissue breakdown. The resulting accumulation of cells and fluids serves to block alveolar function. Abscesses may develop after tissue destruction and necrosis.

Organisms may be introduced into a patient's respiratory tract during **assisted ventilation.** Organisms that can colonize mechanical ventilators and nebulizers, such as *P. aeruginosa, Xanthomonas maltophilia,* and *Acinetobacter* spp., are the most likely agents.

In **hematogenous spread** from other sites, staphylococci and yeast may reach the lung through the bloodstream. This acquisition mode is a rare mechanism for development of nosocomial pneumonia.

Inhalation of airborne infectious agents is another means by which bacterial pneumonia may be acquired. Tuberculosis is acquired by patients from other patients or visitors by way of aerosol droplet inhalation. A national outbreak of multiple drug-resistant *Mycobacterium tuberculosis* has recently caused major problems in urban centers in the United States. Some hospitals experienced outbreaks of Legionnaire's disease when their water or cooling systems became colonized with *Legionella* spp.

Etiologic Agents

The most common organisms associated with nosocomial pneumonia in the United States are *Pseudomonas* and *Stenotrophomonas* (*Xanthomonas*), staphylococci, *Klebsiella* spp., *E. coli*, and *Serratia* spp. **Anaerobic oral flora** as etiologic agents of aspiration pneumonia are gaining increasing recognition. Emerging but still uncommon agents include *Acinetobacter* spp., *Moraxella (Branhamella) catarrhalis*, *Haemophilus influenzae*, *Legionella* spp., *Aspergillus* spp., and influenza type A.

Laboratory Diagnosis

CLINICAL TESTS. A chest radiograph demonstrating new pulmonary infiltrates, fever, increased peripheral blood WBC count, and manifestations of pneumonia are primary criteria for diagnosis.

LABORATORY TESTS. Culture of expectorated sputum is a very poor method for diagnosis, inasmuch as this specimen is always contaminated with respiratory flora. Methods for collection of lung secretions that bypass the oral flora, such as **bronchoalveolar lavage** and collection of secretions with a **protected bronchial brush,** are more promising.

Blood cultures should always be collected, since they may reveal the etiologic agent. Culture of empyema fluid and pleural fluid should be attempted. **Transcutaneous needle aspirates** of fluid collections, if obtainable, are excellent specimens for culture.

Treatment

Empiric therapy with **broad-spectrum agents,** such as ciprofloxacin or ticarcillin plus clavulanic acid, must be instituted until the exact microbe is identified, at which time specific therapy can be targeted.

Prevention

Mechanical ventilating devices must be cleaned thoroughly to prevent colonization by organisms. Patients should be weaned of ventilators as quickly as possible. Overzealous use of broad-spectrum antibiotics should be curtailed. If possible, patients should be treated with agents such as sucralfate instead of antacids to reduce risk of stress ulcers. Sucralfate does not cause decreased gastric acidity and thus does not allow bacterial overgrowth in the stomach. Patients should be encouraged to cough, breathe deeply, and ambulate as soon as possible during their hospitalization.

VIRAL RESPIRATORY TRACT DISEASE

Nosocomially acquired **influenza** has long been a major problem among hospitalized adults, especially during community outbreaks. Either an infected patient or a visitor can transmit influenza A virus to patients. Disease is spread by way of **aerosolized virus particles.** When nosocomial outbreaks occur, high-risk patients should be treated with amantadine hydrochloride, an effective prophylactic agent.

Respiratory syncytial virus (RSV) can travel quickly through a **pediatric unit.** Inasmuch as transmission occurs primarily from hand-to-hand, thorough contact precautions are essential for prevention. For serious cases, **aerosolized ribavirin** may reduce the severity of the illness.

UNCOMMON, ENDOGENOUS ETIOLOGIC AGENTS OF NOSOCOMIAL PNEUMONIA

Pneumocystis carinii, a normal inhabitant of the lungs of healthy individuals, can multiply and cause a diffuse interstitial infiltrate in **immunocompromised hosts,** such as neonates and persons with AIDS. **Tuberculosis** may become active in patients after some aspect of their hospitalization compromises their innate immune mechanisms. Tuberculosis is an unusual etiology for nosocomial pneumonia, but is becoming more prevalent with the growing number of AIDS patients in health care facilities.

WOUND AND PROSTHESIS DISEASE

During a surgical procedure in which the internal tissues are open to the environment, some bacteria or fungal spores can enter the wound. In fact, bacteria that inhabit the crypts and hair follicles of normal skin cannot be eradicated by surface disinfection. In the **absence of adequate host immune mechanisms,** or in the **presence of an adjunct factor,** such as the foreign body of a stitch or drain, these organisms multiply and induce a host response. The subsequent inflammation and tissue destruction can be quite serious. The highest rates of nosocomial diseases are found among surgical patients who have lost the protective effect of intact skin.

Organisms are introduced either by direct physical contamination of the wound during surgery, by airborne inoculation, or by **hematogenous seeding** from a distant site. Either an infected focus such as an abscess or normal flora such as from a transient bowel spill can serve as the reservoir. The latter source of inoculum is most common in diseases involving implanted prosthetic devices, including pacemakers, heart valves, and hip joints.

Postoperative wound diseases are classified based on the extent of microbial contamination encountered during the surgical procedure (Table 21.2).

Patients likely to develop postsurgical wound disease are diabetics, elderly patients, or those with a serious underlying condition.

Bacterial Agents

RESIDENT SKIN FLORA. Bacteria already present on the skin are most likely to colonize the compromised tissue of a surgical wound site. **Coagulase negative staphylococci** are involved most, particularly if a **foreign body** is present. Because of its ability to adhere to certain plastics, *S. epidermidis* may have a slight advantage. *S. aureus,* yeast spp., and gram-negative rods are more common on the skin of hospitalized patients than on healthy patients and they are often implicated. *C. jeikeium,* a lipophilic, multiply antibiotic-resistant coryneform gram-positive rod, seems to colonize hospitalized patients preferentially. This species is occasionally involved in postsurgical wound disease.

TABLE 21.2. Types of Surgical Wounds

Classification	Characteristics
Clean	No adjacent mucous membrane flora, no break in technique, noninflamed tissue
Clean contaminated	Mucous membranes entered without break in technique, noninflamed tissue
Contaminated	Dirty wounds acquired from a contaminated source, previously infected wounds, major break in technique, such as a bowel spill, or wounds that occur through a contaminated mucous membrane.

A number of sternal wound diseases involving *Mycoplasma hominis* has recently been reported. This organism is gaining wider acceptance as a cause of postsurgical wound diseases.

ENDOGENOUS GASTROINTESTINAL FLORA. The facultative bacilli in the bowels, primarily *Enterobacteriaceae* and *Enterococcus* spp., are often found on the skin of hospitalized patients. These bacteria gain access to underlying tissue through loss of skin integrity, multiply, and induce a host inflammatory response.

Surgical procedures involving the GI tract, oropharyngeal mucous membranes, or female genital tract may permit the extremely heavy normal flora of these areas access to a previously sterile site. Anaerobic bacteria are often associated with abscesses and other infectious complications after surgery in such areas of the body.

HOSPITAL-RESIDENT BACTERIA. *P. aeruginosa, Legionella* spp., and other bacteria live in collections of moisture throughout the hospital. If allowed entry to compromised tissue, they quickly multiply and cause infection.

Fungal Agents

Fungi are increasingly involved in nosocomial disease. *Aspergillus* spp., whose **spores are ubiquitous in dust and in the air,** can be introduced into an open surgical field from the air supply during an operative procedure. One highly publicized outbreak of aspergillosis orthopedic wound disease resulted from the application of *Aspergillus*-contaminated bandage material postoperatively.

Etiologic Agents of Prosthesis-Associated Bone, Joint, and Soft Tissue Disease

1. Prosthetic heart valves and indwelling vascular prostheses. **Skin or environmental flora,** presumably **introduced at the time of surgery,** include staphylococci, corynebacteria, yeast spp., *Aspergillus,* and gram-negative bacilli. Disease due to these agents usually occurs within several weeks of surgery. Organisms that reach the site by way of **hematogenous spread** include normal oral flora, particularly **viridans streptococci,** and *Enterobacteriaceae.* When animal tissues that cannot be sterilized, such as porcine valves, are used, *Mycobacterium chelonae* and other unusual agents can be implanted along with the valve.

2. Prosthetic joints. **Normal skin flora, introduced at the time of surgery,** can multiply slowly over long time periods before they reach a critical mass and elicit a host inflammatory response. Common agents include coagulase negative staphylococci and *Propionibacterium acnes,* an anaerobic gram-positive rod that lives in hair follicles and crypts on normal skin. **Hematogenous seeding** of prostheses usually involves oral flora, particularly **streptococci,** and bowel flora.

Laboratory Diagnosis

Clinical signs and symptoms are important clues to the presence of a surgical wound infection, for example, increased peripheral WBCs, fever, pain, and exudate at the site.

Wound cultures and Gram stains are essential for diagnosis. In patients able to mount a cellular immune response, the presence of polymorphonuclear neutrophils in the Gram stain will help determine whether normal skin flora, such as staphylococci, are actually involved in an infectious process.

For laboratory diagnosis of prosthetic valve endocarditis, **blood cultures** must be obtained from **at least two separate venipunctures,** to help differentiate true pathogens from procurement contaminants.

Treatment

Empiric treatment should be based on the likely etiology of the disease and **should be narrowed once the susceptibility pattern of the actual microbe is known. Vancomycin,** as initial coverage for methicillin-resistant staphylococci, is almost always used. Other agents are added based on clinical and epidemiologic grounds.

Prevention

Prophylactic regimens are used for proscribed surgical procedures where the risk of disease is high. Antibiotics should be instituted **just prior to the procedure and continued for 1 or 2 days postoperatively,** based on the risk of contamination of the wound. Prolonged hospitalization should be avoided prior to surgery to decrease the risk of colonization of the patient with antibiotic-resistant hospital-resident flora. Prepare the incision site with antibacterial agents. Avoid shaving the skin, if possible. Some surgeons opt to irrigate the field with antibiotic solutions. **Keep the operative time as short as possible.** Operate in a room with a filtered, laminar-flow air-handling system. Change gloves and instruments when moving from a contaminated to a clean site. Remove any necrotic tissue at the time of surgery. **Remove stitch material, drains, and other foreign bodies as soon as possible** after surgery. Maintain rigorous standards of postsurgical wound care, using antibacterial ointments and **nonocclusive dressings.**

URINARY TRACT DISEASE

Nosocomial urinary tract diseases (also called UTIs for urinary tract infections) **are the most common nosocomial diseases** in the United States; the great majority are associated with urinary tract catheterization. Closed catheter systems are the standard today, but there are still opportunities for microbes to invade the system.

Pathogenesis

Irritation of the urinary tract epithelium and the presence of a favorable environment for the multiplication of bacteria (the collection bag) combine to encourage **growth of bacteria in the bladder (bacteriuria).** Microbes enter the bladder by **reflux** if the collection bag is inadvertently lifted higher than the patient's bladder, or by migration of bacteria along the catheter into the bladder. In some cases, organisms colonizing the urethra are introduced into the bladder as the catheter is inserted. **The longer the catheter is in place, the more likely it is that the patient will develop bacteriuria.** Although the historical definition of significant bacteriuria requires that urine cultures show greater than 100,000 CFU/ml of one species of bacteria, experience has shown that UTI is present in catheterized patients when CFU are much lower.

Etiologic Agents

Most UTI bacteria are **endogenous flora from the patient's GI tract.** Occasionally, organisms from one patient may be transmitted to another on the hands of health care personnel, but this is less likely now that **Universal Precautions** require caregivers to wear gloves when contacting any serum or blood containing body fluids. Bacteria likely to cause UTIs early during the course of catheterization are *E. coli, Candida* spp. and other yeasts, *P. aeruginosa,* various *Enterobacte-*

riaceae, and *Enterococcus* spp. Bacteria that are the most common agents of UTI in patients with long-term indwelling urinary tract catheters are *Providencia stuartii, Proteus vulgaris, Proteus mirabilis, E. coli, P. aeruginosa, Enterococcus* spp., and other *Enterobacteriaceae.*

It is quite **common to find multiple species in the urine of catheterized patients.** Much work remains to be done to determine which are significant pathogens and how microbiologists should interpret mixed culture results.

Laboratory Diagnosis

The **quantitative urine culture, in association with a comprehensive urinalysis,** is the primary diagnostic tool. The presence of **blood and WBCs in the urine indicates an infectious process.** Determination of the significance of a culture result depends on the type of patient, the number of species isolated, and the colony counts of bacteria isolated. A direct Gram stain can be done to detect greater than 100,000 CFU/ml on an emergency basis. Several rapid screening tests are available. The presence of leukocyte esterase correlates to polymorphonuclear neutrophil numbers, nitrite suggests the presence of nitrate-reducing bacteria, and there are several other easily measured variables. Some laboratories only perform urinalyses and cultures on urine specimens yielding positive screening test results.

Treatment

Certain antibiotics, including sulfa derivatives, nitrofurantoin, and broad-spectrum cephalosporins, concentrate in the urine and are effective against the gram-negative bacteria likely to cause nosocomial UTI. Quinolones, aminoglycosides, and aztreonam are all effective for susceptible bacteria. Choice of **treatment should be guided by the antimicrobial susceptibility pattern** of organisms common in the institution and the specific susceptibility results of the infecting bacteria.

Prevention

Avoid inserting an indwelling catheter if possible. **Intermittent catheterization** has been widely accepted as an alternative. Cleanse the insertion site thoroughly. **Maintain the closed catheter system.** Health care workers should withdraw urine only through a rubber septum port that has been thoroughly disinfected with alcohol using a sterile needle and syringe. Gloves should be worn during all phases of catheter care. Remove indwelling catheters as quickly as is medically prudent.

OTHER NOSOCOMIAL DISEASES

VIRAL DISEASE

1. **Rotavirus gastroenteritis. Rotavirus is among the most common etiologic agents of childhood diarrhea,** and can quickly spread through a nursery once introduced. Signs and symptoms include fever, vomiting, and watery diarrhea. **Spread is by the hands of caregivers.**

2. **Herpesvirus disease.** Herpes simplex and varicella-zoster viruses (VZV, the etiologic agent of chickenpox and shingles) can be transmitted nosocomially. Incidence of patients acquiring herpes skin lesions from health care workers or other patients is low; immunosuppressed patients are at greatest risk. Outbreaks of nosocomial chickenpox are not uncommon, usually occurring in pediatric populations. **Chickenpox is spread by the aerosol route.** Children and adults with chickenpox should be housed in rooms with air-handling systems separate from the rest of the hospital. Transmission of chickenpox to susceptible hosts from patients infected with shingles by the hands of personnel has occurred.

3. **Hepatitis.** Patient-patient and patient-health care worker transmission of hepatitis occurs among hospitalized patients, since occasional asymptomatic or undiagnosed cases are admitted. The mandated use of Universal Precautions for handling blood and blood and serum-containing body fluids should decrease the incidence of this type of nosocomial disease. Two safe and effective vaccines, a hepatitis B recombinant vaccine and an inactivated viral antigen vaccine, are available and their use is highly encouraged for those persons at risk who have not yet acquired antibody to HBsAg.

ANTIBIOTIC-ASSOCIATED COLITIS

Clostridium difficile **has been recognized recently as the major cause of diarrhea in hospitalized patients.** The spores can survive on environmental surfaces for long periods of time.

Pathogenesis

Patients whose **bowel flora is decimated by therapy with broad-spectrum antibiotics** are at risk for colonization by *C. difficile*. The organism is also commonly passed from patient to patient on the hands of health care providers. It gains a foothold on the colonic mucosal epithelium in the absence of colonization pressure from other bacteria. Once *C. difficile* has colonized the GI tract, the organism produces at least two toxins, an **enterotoxin** and a **cytotoxin.** The enterotoxin is thought to mediate diarrhea, although tissue damage and ulceration, perhaps caused by the cytotoxin, are hallmarks of severe disease (see discussion of pathogenicity in Chapter 10). Collections of necrotic mucosal cells and polymorphonuclear neutrophiles on the luminal surface of the colon, as visualized during endoscopy or colonoscopy, resemble a white membrane, hence the name **"pseudomembranous colitis."**

Laboratory Diagnosis

Inasmuch as many as 20% of hospitalized patients may become colonized with *C. difficile,* culture for the organism alone is not specific enough for a reliable diagnostic test. New ELISA tests for enterotoxin and cytotoxin are being evaluated, but diagnosis is still primarily a clinical decision based on clinical manifestations and a history of recent antibiotic use. A cell culture test for cytotoxin correlates most closely with *C. difficile*-associated disease.

Treatment

For mild cases, discontinuing the antibiotic therapy may be enough to ameliorate the diarrhea. For more severe cases, therapy with either **metronidazole** or **vancomycin** has been shown to effectively reduce the numbers of *C. difficile* in the gut. Relapses are not uncommon.

DIALYSIS-ASSOCIATED DISEASE

Patients undergoing hemodialysis are most at risk of acquiring **hepatitis,** especially hepatitis B and C viruses. Contact with the infected blood or serum of other patients is the most likely source, although contact with the virus on instruments and fomites in the hemodialysis unit may serve as another source of acquisition.

Patients undergoing **continuous ambulatory peritoneal dialysis (CAPD)** are at risk of acquiring several types of disease. Although not strictly considered nosocomial, these diseases are certainly iatrogenic.

Peritonitis is the greatest infectious risk for these patients; on average, patients on CAPD suffer one episode of peritonitis per year. Normal skin flora are the most common pathogens. The presence of permanently placed transcutaneous shunts in these patients allows access to bacteria from the patient's hands during manipulation of the shunt. The bacteria commonly isolated from peritonitis fluids are coagulase negative staphylococci, *S. aureus,* streptococci, coryneform gram-positive rods, *E. coli* and other *Enterobacteriaceae, P. aeruginosa, Candida* spp., and anaerobes. Other organisms are involved occasionally.

BURN WOUND DISEASE

Patients whose protective skin barrier has been compromised by burns are at risk for severe disease. Not only is the underlying tissue open for ready access by infectious agents, but the circulatory system and tissue perfusion are also disrupted. The most common etiologic agents are *Enterobacter* spp., *P. aeruginosa, S. aureus,* coagulase negative staphylococci, *Enterococcus* spp., and other *Enterobacteriaceae.* In some burn units, fungal pathogens, such as *Candida* spp. and *Aspergillus,* are important infectious agents. Herpetic diseases are also being recognized more frequently in this group of compromised patients.

Treatment of skin injury involves removal of necrotic tissue, early grafting, and maintenance of a near-sterile environment to keep levels of contamination low. If burn patients are adequately treated with topical disinfectants to reduce surface disease, they are still at increased risk of pneumonia because of injury to the lungs from inhalation of hot gases and systemic immune system degradation. **Pneumonia currently carries the highest case fatality rate** among infectious complications in burn patients.

SUMMARY

1. Nosocomial diseases, namely, those acquired after a patient is hospitalized (manifesting 72 h after admission), strike 5–10% of all hospitalized patients in the United States at an estimated cost of $5 billion annually.

2. The most important types of nosocomial disease, in order of prevalence, are urinary tract, respiratory tract, postsurgical wound, and bacteremia secondary to IV catheter.

3. The most important etiologic agents are (a) *Escherichia coli* because of its domination of UTIs; (b) coagulase negative staphylococci and *Staphyloccocus aureus* because of their tendency to colonize the nasal mucosa and skin of hospitalized patients and ability to gain access through iatrogenic breaks in the skin, including catheter insertion sites and surgical incision sites; (c) *Enterococcus* spp., which is part of the host's GI flora but flourishes when other organisms are inhibited by cephalosporin therapy; (d) *Pseudomonas aeruginosa*, which grows in sink water, colonizes burned skin, lungs of cystic fibrosis patients, urinary tract of compromised patients. Mortality of nosocomial pneumonia is extremely high.

4. Recently recognized new agents of nosocomial diseases are (a) *Legionella* species: pneumonia, surgical wound infections, and endocarditis; (b) *Clostridium difficile:* antibiotic-associated diarrhea; (c) coagulase negative staphylococci: catheter-associated sepsis; (d) *Candida albicans:* catheter- and parenteral-nutrition associated sepsis; (e) *Corynebacterium jeikeium:* catheter-related sepsis and postsurgical wound infection; (f) *Mycoplasma hominis:* postsurgical wound infections; and (g) rotavirus: nursery outbreaks of diarrhea.

5. The single most productive activity to prevent nosocomial diseases is handwashing and changing gloves between patients.

REFERENCES

Corona ML, Peters SG, Narr BJ, Thompson RL (1990): Infections related to central venous catheters. Mayo Cl Proc 65:979.

Cruse PJE, Foord R (1980): The epidemiology of wound infection. A 10-year prospective study of 62,939 wounds. Surg Clin North Am 60:27.

Gilchrist MJR, Brooks LH (1989): Nosocomial infections. In Davis BG, Bishop ML, Mass D (eds): Clinical Laboratory Science: Strategies for Practice. Philadelphia: J.B. Lippincott pp 768–780.

Kiehn TE (1989): Bacteremia and fungemia in the immunocompromised patient. Eur J Clin Microbiol Infect Dis 8:832.

Maki DG (1989): Risk factors for nosocomial infection in intensive care: 'devices vs nature' and goals for the next decade. Arch Intern Med 149:30.

Scheld WM, Mandell GL (1991): Nosocomial pneumonia: pathogenesis and recent advances in diagnosis and therapy. Rev Infect Dis 13(S9):S743.

REVIEW QUESTIONS

For questions 1 to 6, choose the ONE
BEST answer or completion.

1. Which is the most important factor accounting for the 133% increase in nosocomial
   bloodstream diseases recognized over the
   past 10 years?
   a) Increased use of broad-spectrum antibi-
      otics.
   b) More severely ill patients living longer.
   c) More respiratory therapy associated
      pneumonias.
   d) More patients requiring urinary catheters.
   e) More IV and central-venous access lines
      being placed.

2. Why is *Escherichia coli* still the most commonly recognized nosocomial pathogen?
   a) It is the most common etiologic agent of
      urinary tract diseases, the most prevalent
      type of nosocomial disease.
   b) It is inherently resistant to most com-
      monly used antimicrobial agents.
   c) It is carried in the nasal passages of many
      hospital personnel.
   d) It is so benign that most physicians do not
      treat it until the infection has become se-
      vere.
   e) It is the most important cause of neonatal
      sepsis.

3. Recently, nosocomial transmission of viral
   infections has been recognized. Which list
   contains viruses that have been shown to be
   important agents of nosocomial outbreaks?
   a) Cytomegalovirus, lymphocytic choriom-
      eningitis virus, hepatitis.
   b) Hepatitis, herpes simplex, rhinovirus.
   c) Hepatitis, respiratory syncytial virus, ro-
      tavirus.
   d) Herpes simplex, hepatitis, HIV.
   e) Cytomegalovirus, herpesvirus, Epstein-
      Barr virus

4. What activity will decrease the number of
   catheter-related gram-positive septic episodes experienced in a hospital?
   a) Removal of the colonized IV catheter
      tips.
   b) Wearing gloves when performing any pa-
      tient contact activities.
   c) Treating the catheter insertion site with
      chlorhexidine before inserting the cathe-
      ter.
   d) a and b.
   e) a, b, and c.

5. Why are methicillin-resistant *Staphylococcus aureus* considered to be such important
   agents of nosocomial infection?
   a) These agents are the most common or-
      ganism colonizing the skin of hospital-
      ized patients.

b) These agents are carried in the nasal passages of almost 50% of health care workers.

c) There is no effective vaccine for prevention of infection.

d) These agents must be treated with IV vancomycin.

e) These agents possess more virulence factors than do methicillin-susceptible strains.

6. What is the most important activity for reducing nosocomial diseases?

a) Handwashing and wearing gloves during patient contact.

b) Aggressive antibiotic therapy for all colonizations.

c) Treating health care workers with mupirocin to reduce carriage of staphylococci.

d) Changing urinary bladder catheters every 72 h.

e) Terminally cleaning all respiratory therapy equipment between patients.

> For questions 7 to 11, a list of lettered options is followed by several numbered items. For each numbered item, select the ONE lettered option that is most closely associated with it.

A) *Pseudomonas aeruginosa*
B) *Prevotella melaninogenica*
C) Coagulase-negative staphylococci
D) *Corynebacterium jeikeium*
E) *Clostridium difficile*

> For each of the cases, choose the most likely etiologic agent.

7. A young girl is burned over 40% of her body. She is in the burn unit awaiting her first skin graft.

8. A patient develops a sternotomy wound infection with an organism identified by the laboratory as a "diphtheroid."

9. A patient develops aspiration pneumonia while he is still groggy from the anesthesia.

10. A patient being treated with antibiotics and surgical debridement for a diabetic foot ulcer develops diarrhea on his sixth hospital day.

11. The site of a prosthetic hip joint placed into an elderly patient 4 months earlier becomes painful, swollen, and warm.

ANSWERS TO REVIEW QUESTIONS

1. *e* Most nosocomial bloodstream diseases are related to vascular access lines.

2. *a* Indwelling urinary tract catheters almost always become colonized with *Escherichia coli.* Under many compromising circumstances, the organism goes on to induce an inflammatory response and thus an infection. *E. coli* is not particularly antibiotic resistant, and physicians always treat symptomatic patients. Gram-negative bacilli are rarely carried in the nasal passages of health care workers, as inherent host defense mechanisms do not allow more than transient colonization by such bacteria.

3. *c* Rotavirus and respiratory syncytial virus have recently been shown to be important agents of hospital outbreaks among pediatric and neonatal patients. At least one virus in each of the other lists has not been implicated in nosocomial outbreaks. These include lymphocytic choriomeningitis virus, rhinovirus, HIV, and Epstein-Barr virus. One highly publicized case of health care-associated transmission of HIV involved a Florida dentist and several patients. The details of that case are still not entirely known, but it is possible that the dentist infected his patients with his own virus. This case is still not considered to be an ''outbreak.''

4. *e* All three activities should reduce nosocomial gram-positive line-related sepsis.

5. *d* Although these bacteria are not common in most hospital environments, methicillin-resistant *Staphylococcus aureus* cause serious infections. This infection must be treated aggressively with IV vancomycin, which usually extends the hospital stay of infected patients by as much as 10 additional days.

6. *a* Since most nosocomial diseases are transmitted by hand-hand contact, handwashing and gloves will reduce more infections than will any of the other activities listed. Some of the answers are contraindicated, such as treating patients who are colonized; this will only serve to encourage development of antibiotic resistance. Cleaning respiratory therapy equipment between patients would be prohibitively expensive. Finally, urinary tract catheters are usually left in place for extended periods unless the patient develops an infection. Changing catheters every 72 h would cause irritation of the bladder and urethral epithelium and may actually lead to infection.

7. *A Pseudomonas aeruginosa* and *S. aureus* are the two most likely agents of nosocomial burn wound infection.

8. **D** *Corynebacterium jeikeium* seems to colonize readily the skin of hospitalized patients. Although the Gram-stain morphology is diphtheroid-like, the organism is multiply resistant to antibiotics and can cause sepsis in debilitated hosts.

9. **B** The oral anaerobic flora, including pigmented gram-negative bacilli, such as *Prevotella melaninogenica,* are important agents of aspiration pneumonia in hospitalized patients due to loss of consciousness.

10. **E** Antibiotic-associated *Clostridium difficile* diarrhea is the most common cause of diarrhea in hospitalized patients.

11. **C** Staphylococci are the second most common cause of nosocomial disease (after *E. coli*). As normal skin flora, coagulase-negative staphylococci can easily contaminate a wound during surgery. The low virulence of this organism leads to an indolent course during which they multiply to a critical mass in the tissue, mediated by their ability to adhere to artificial materials used in prosthetics and catheters.

MYCOBACTERIAL DISEASES, ACTINOMYCOSIS, AND SYSTEMIC NOCARDIOSIS

Members of the *Mycobacterium, Actinomyces,* and *Nocardia* genera of bacteria are morphologically similar in that they are straight or slightly curved rods or branching filamentous organisms. *Mycobacterium* and *Nocardia* species are acid-fast and, with the exception of the noncultivatable *Mycobacterium leprae,* are aerobic in their growth requirements. In contrast, *Actinomyces* species are nonacid-fast and anaerobic or microaerophilic.

MYCOBACTERIUM

TUBERCULOSIS

Mycobacterium tuberculosis and *Mycobacterium bovis* are the etiologic agents of tuberculosis, a worldwide disease responsible for about 2,000,000 deaths annually. Greater than 99% of the cases of tuberculosis in the United States are due to *M. tuberculosis.* Effective cattle control and pasteurization of milk and milk products have essentially eradicated disease due to *M. bovis.* Iatrogenic disseminated disease occurs among patients with certain types of carcinomas that are "treated" with this organism.

From 1953 to 1984, the number of new active cases of tuberculosis in the United States declined significantly from more than 84,000 to approximately 22,000 with a case fatality rate of 8–10% and 4% among untreated and treated cases, respectively. However, from 1985 to 1991, the long-standing annual decline in cases of tuberculosis in the United States abruptly ended with approximately 39,000 more cases reported than would have been expected had this decline continued.

Much of this recent case increase is believed to be due to multidrug-resistant (MDR) tuberculosis among HIV-infected individuals and in institutional settings, such as correctional facilities and homeless shelters, where host resistance may be impaired. Approximately 10% of the 1 million HIV-infected individuals in the United States develop coexisting *M. tuberculosis* infection while 40% of those exposed develop active tuberculosis. These patients develop a rapidly progressive disease with case fatalities ranging from 72 to 89% due to MDR.

Of the approximately 10–15 million individuals in the United States with a healthy immune system and infected with *M. tuberculosis,* about 10% will develop active tuberculosis during their lifetime.

Habitat

While *M. tuberculosis* is restricted to humans and primates, *M. bovis* occurs in humans, primates, cattle, and a wide variety of other animals. Both species may be found in the respiratory tract of their respective hosts. *Mycobacterium bovis* may also be found in the udder and GI tract. Both species cause infection or disease in their animal hosts.

Transmission

EXOGENOUS. Transmission of *M. tuberculosis* occurs in children and adults by **droplet nuclei** from a case resulting in the **primary pulmonary** or **first-infection** type of tuberculosis. Crowded conditions and impaired host resistance tend to enhance the possibility of acquiring infection or disease. Certain ethnic groups, such as Asians, American Indians, Eskimos, and Blacks, are more likely to develop disease as opposed to infection. Among Black Americans, a higher incidence occurs in those with HLA-Bw 15 histocompatibility antigen.

Transmission of *M. bovis* occurs in children and adults usually as a result of the ingestion of raw milk or dairy products. When the disease involves the respiratory tract, human-human transmission can occur by droplet nuclei resulting in an infectious process similar to that seen with *M. tuberculosis.* The use of *M. bovis* for treatment of certain carcinomas may result in disseminated disease.

ENDOGENOUS. Endogenous activation of *M. tuberculosis* disease occurs due to a **waning acquired resistance and reactivation of quiescent primary foci usually within the respiratory tract** resulting in the postprimary pulmonary or reactivation type of tuberculosis. Factors thought to influence reactivation include malnutrition, alcoholism, diabetes, immunosuppression (such as patients with AIDS), and occupational respiratory hazards. The same mechanism of endogenous activation and the same influencing factors as those described for *M. tuberculosis* occur for *M. bovis* except that reactivation is usually from an extrapulmonary primary focus.

Properties of the Organism

Resistance to environmental, physical, and chemical agents. These organisms are the **most resistant of the nonspore-forming bacteria** and are resistant to drying, remain viable in dried sputum for as long as 8 months, and show a high degree of resistance to disinfecting agents. Waxes and long-chain mycolic acids in the cell wall of the organism contribute to environmental survival. The resistance of these organisms to acids and alkalis allow the latter to be used in sputum concentration techniques employed in the laboratory diagnosis of tuberculosis.

Microscopic morphology. The organisms are **acid-fast,** nonmotile, nonencapsulated, rods. Waxes and long-chain fatty acids in the cell wall also contribute to dye uptake resistance and decolorization resistance during the acid-fast staining process. The organisms are slender, straight, or slightly bent and may appear ''beaded'' or ''granular'' after staining. Both *M. tuberculosis* and *M. bovis* are **facultative intracellular parasites.**

Macroscopic morphology. These pathogens are strict aerobes that grow best on potato-egg (e.g., Lowenstein-Jensen) and serum agar base (e.g., Middlebrook 7H10) media, both of which contain malachite green dye to inhibit the growth of other bacteria. Optimal growth occurs on or in these media at 37°C in the presence of 5–10% carbon dioxide. The organisms are relatively **slow growers.** On solid media, colonies appear as dry, wrinkled, and cream colored (nonpigmented) after

10 days to 8 weeks. The **production of niacin by *M. tuberculosis*** is an important biochemical reaction in the laboratory identification of the organism, inasmuch as nonpathogenic and other pathogenic or potentially pathogenic mycobacteria do not produce niacin.

Differentiation from parasitic and free-living mycobacteria. There are several parasitic and free-living species of mycobacteria that must be differentiated from *M. tuberculosis* and *M. bovis.* Some may be responsible for "atypical" mycobacterial disease under circumstances to be described while others may be frank nonpathogens. **Differentiation is based upon their more rapid growth characteristics, yellow pigmentation, and/or biochemical reactions.**

Antigenic structure. Antigenic structural components related to virulence, have not been well defined. Inasmuch as the cell walls of both pathogens can induce a DTH and some resistance to infection, it is conceivable that wall glycolipids, lipoproteins, and/or lipids may play a role in the stimulation of delayed hypersensitivity and/or immunity. On the basis of experimental evidence, **sulfatides (cell wall glycolipids) interact with polymorphonuclear leukocytes and macrophage lysosomal membranes to prevent their fusion with phagosomes.** Antibodies to cross-reactive or pathogen-unique epitopes have not been shown to be associated with pathogenesis or resistance and are of no value in the laboratory diagnosis of tuberculosis.

Extracellular products associated with or thought to be associated with pathogenicity. No extracellular virulence factors are known.

Pathogenesis and Clinical Manifestations

THE PRIMARY PULMONARY TYPE. The primary pulmonary (first-infection) type of tuberculosis is almost invariably due to *M. tuberculosis* (Fig. 22.1). First exposure occurs mostly but not exclusively in childhood, at which time droplet nuclei containing tubercle bacilli are inhaled and lodge beneath the pleura in the area of the lung where the greatest gaseous exchange takes place. There is an **early exudative response** on the part of the host characterized by polymorphonuclear leukocytic infiltration, edema, and fluid accumulation within the alveolar spaces. The organisms are phagocytized by or "enter" the polymorphonuclear leukocytes and, possibly by a mechanism involving **sulfatide** activity, inhibit phagolysosomal fusion, multiply within the cells, and destroy them.

At some unknown period of time after polymorphonuclear leukocytic infiltration, macrophages and lymphocytes infiltrate the areas. Alveolar macrophages also phagocytize the living tubercle bacilli, which again are able to escape destruction and multiply within the cells by inhibiting lysosomal fusion by a potential

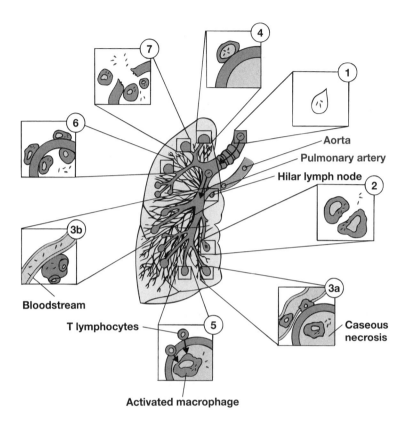

1. **Aerosol droplet containing _M. tuberculosis_ reaches alveoli. Initial event is an early exudative response with destruction of polymorphonuclear leukocytes by the organism.**

2. **Alveolar macrophages ingest _M. tuberculosis_, which multiply intracellularly.**

3a&b. **Center of lesion undergoes caseous necrosis. Some _M. tuberculosis_ are carried in phagocytic cells to hilar lymph nodes and then gain access to the bloodstream.**

4. **Small foci of infection are established in the lung apex by _M. tuberculosis_ arriving in the bloodstream.**

5. **DTH and CMI kick in; T lymphocytes release lymphokines that activate macrophages to kill _M. tuberculosis_. Some organisms within the caseous necrotic lesion remain viable.**

6. **At most sites, DTH keeps infection sequestered and under control. This "arrested" stage can last years.**

7. **When host immunity wanes, organisms can again multiply in macrophages. The lesion wall breaks down and the infection spreads.**

Figure 22.1.

Pathogenesis of primary pulmonary (first infection) TB in a normal host.

sulfatide mechanism. At this time, a **granulomatous or productive response** to the actively multiplying organisms develops characterized by microscopic granulomas referred to as **"tubercles."** Tubercles are composed of central organized aggregations of enlarged macrophages resembling epithelial cells (referred to as "epithelioid" cells), multinucleated Langhans giant cells (fused macrophage cytoplasm) containing tubercle bacilli, and peripheral lymphocytes, macrophages, and fibroblasts. The center of the tubercle undergoes a characteristic **caseous necrosis.** Some organisms gain access to the lymphatics, hilar lymph nodes, and circulation, where they are carried to and lodge in areas of high O_2 tension such as the apex of the lung. Three to four weeks after exposure to the organisms, **DTH** and **CMI** develop.

The developing immune response is entirely CMI. The great majority of individuals develop a relatively high degree of CMI by a mechanism in which alveolar macrophages, activated by the lymphokine MAF (macrophage activating factor) released from antigen-sensitized T lymphocytes, phagocytize and digest the organisms. An adequate CMI response results in healing of most infected sites by fibrosis and calcification, although calcified areas may still harbor tubercle bacilli for years or for life. The calcified primary site lesions, including those in the lymph nodes, are visible on X-ray and are referred to as the Ghon complex. The disease following calcification of the productive lesions is considered "arrested" although organisms may still be present. Inasmuch as the capability of eliciting a DTH response is still present at this time, the individual is considered to be infected or asymptomatic. Occasionally, the host fails to mount an adequate CMI response and the organisms multiply unrestricted producing numerous tubercles in the lung and/or, by hematogenous dissemination, in virtually every organ and tissue **(miliary tuberculosis).**

THE POSTPRIMARY PULMONARY TYPE. The postprimary pulmonary (reactivation) type of tuberculosis due to *M. tuberculosis* is of endogenous origin and results from a **waning CMI and reactivation of quiescent primary foci.** In more than 95% of patients, clinical disease evolves years after the original infection. The apex of the lung, where the oxygen tension is highest, is invariably the site of reactivation. The organisms initiate a chronic inflammatory response and the reactivated focus becomes caseous. The caseous tubercle liquifies and breaks into an adjacent bronchus resulting in cavity formation and aspiration into other parts of the lung where a new infectious process is initiated. Erosion of the tuberculous process into a pulmonary blood vessel leads to hemorrhage in the cavity and hemoptysis. The onset is insidious with constitutional clinical manifestations of fever, cough, malaise, and weight loss. The reactivation process may originate from an extrapulmonary focus or may result in hematogenous dissemination from the lung resulting in disease of other organs and tissues. Although there is a waning of CMI, it may still be adequate enough to account for the usual limitation of the reactivation type to the lung.

INTESTINAL TUBERCULOSIS. This form of tuberculosis results from the ingestion of raw milk and dairy products contaminated with *M. bovis.* The organisms invade the cervical lymph nodes and tonsils producing a lymphadenitis, referred to as scrofula, and tonsillitis through host-parasite interactions as described for *M. tuberculosis.* The organisms penetrate the intestinal mucosa and are carried to the mesenteric lymph nodes where they produce a mesenteric adenitis. Again, healing versus dissemination versus reactivation are determined by the extent and persistence of CMI.

CMI and the Role of DTH in Immunity

Although both CMI and humoral antibody develop during the course of first-infection tuberculosis, **only CMI is responsible for the acquired resistance** as previously indicated. The development of **DTH** during the first-infection process has evoked considerable controversy as to whether DTH is involved in acquired resistance by a mechanism similar or identical to that of CMI or whether they exhibit independent and diverse functions during host-parasite interaction. The concept of a similar or identical mechanism is supported because CMI and DTH can be adoptively transferred by lymphoid cells from individuals expressing DTH, a high incidence of reactivation tuberculosis occurs among low DTH responders, and patients with miliary tuberculosis have enhanced suppressor T-cell activity associated with a failure to show a DTH response (anergy). However, the view that DTH is responsible for severe tissue reactions, cavitation, and pulmonary spread in reactivation tuberculosis in the face of an inadequate CMI suggests that they may be mediated by two different mechanisms.

Laboratory Diagnosis

Although not a part of laboratory diagnosis, it is essential to note that combined history, clinical manifestations, tuberculin skin testing, and chest X-ray are useful adjuncts but not definitive in the differential diagnosis of tuberculosis.

SPECIMENS. The specimens obtained depend on the disease process and include sputum (the most common), gastric washings, urine, and cerebrospinal fluid. Sputum and urine **concentration** utilizing a bactericidal agent, such as 2% sodium hydroxide and a mucolytic agent, such as *N*-acetyl-L-cysteine, to liquefy and decontaminate the specimen is necessary prior to culture. The presence of acid-fast bacilli (AFB) in direct smears from untreated and/or concentrated sputum and urine specimens, as well as in other untreated applicable specimens, is strong presumptive evidence for tuberculosis if the patients exhibit referrable clinical manifestations. Culturing, however, is essential, inasmuch as specimens, such as sputum and urine, may contain saprophytic acid-fast bacilli and isolates of tubercle bacilli must be tested for antimicrobial susceptibility prior to, during, and after the completion of therapy.

PRIMARY ISOLATION AND IDENTIFICATION. These procedures require initial cultivation of concentrated sputum and urine sediment and untreated, uncontaminated specimens on media such as Lowenstein-Jensen and Middlebrook 7H10. Incubation under aerobic conditions at 37°C is required for optimal growth, which may require as long as 8 weeks. *M. tuberculosis* and *M. bovis* appear as acid-fast bacilli producing dry, wrinkled, cream-colored colonies. ***M. tuberculosis is niacin positive,*** which distinguishes it from other members of the genus. Newly developed instrumentation techniques for rapid detection of mycobacterial growth in broth medium has reduced the time for identifying culture positivity to less than 2 weeks.

Treatment

Combined chemotherapy with drugs having different modes of action is essential in order to reduce the risk of selecting out resistant mutants. The most common first-line chemotherapeutic agents used in combined therapy are isoniazid (isonicotinic acid hydrazide or INH), ethambutol, rifampin, and streptomycin, each of which have potential side effects that must be considered. Although treatment is often successful, **a relatively high percentage of patients in the United States are single-drug or multidrug resistant,** particularly, but not exclusively, those with coexisting HIV infection, AIDS, or other immunosuppression diseases.

Other agents are available for retreatment if resistance develops to the first-line drugs. Most of these second-line agents exhibit greater toxicity. Furthermore, resistance to these drugs may also develop. With successful therapy, sputum cultures become negative within 3 weeks and clinical cure is usually accomplished within 1 year. Prolonged bed rest and surgery, the mainstays of therapy for tuberculosis prior to chemotherapy, are rarely indicated.

Prevention and Control

Patients must be isolated (respiratory isolation) until negative sputum cultures are obtained.

THE TUBERCULIN SKIN TEST. This test serves as an excellent epidemiological and diagnostic aid in the prevention and control of tuberculosis when used with other armamentaria. The test is a measure of **DTH** as determined by the intradermal injection of 0.1 ml of intermediate strength purified protein derivative **(PPD),** which is a tuberculoprotein derived by fractionation of a broth culture filtrate of *M. tuberculosis.* Results are read 48–72 h after injection. **Induration of greater than or equal to 10 mm is considered positive,** 5–9 mm doubtful and probably due to a cross-reaction with "atypical" mycobacteria (see below and Table 22.1), and less than 5 mm negative. A **positive tuberculin test** indicates **infection with *M. tuberculosis* or *M. bovis*** as a result of first exposure and not necessarily disease. Occasionally, patients with leprosy give a positive reaction. A **negative tuberculin test** may indicate either **the absence of infection or "anergy"** in patients critically ill with tuberculosis or immunosuppressive diseases in which suppressor T cells are activated due to excess antigen. If recent conversion from tuberculin negative to tuberculin positive can be documented, prophylactic INH therapy for 1 year results in ridding the host of viable organisms, as evidenced by conversion back to negative. In many areas of the country, tuberculin skin testing and INH treatment of converters is required for children prior to school admission. The INH prophylaxis should also be administered to household contacts of active cases and tuberculin reactors who are immunosuppressed. As with its use in treatment, INH prophylaxis must be monitored carefully due to its potential toxicity.

CHEST X-RAY. This technique also serves as an excellent epidemiological and diagnostic aid in the prevention and control of tuberculosis. Mass X-ray programs, although no longer conducted in the United States, are useful in other countries where the disease is more difficult to control.

BACILLUS OF CALMETTE AND GUERIN. Bacillus of Calmette and Guerin (BCG) vaccine, which consists of a live, attenuated strain of *M. bovis,* is administered only to individuals who are tuberculin negative. This vaccine has been used with variable degrees of success in countries where the prevalence of tuberculosis is high. Inasmuch as BCG vaccination causes tuberculin conversion to positive and thus loss of the tuberculin skin test as an epidemiological and

TABLE 22.1. Selected Characteristics of the "Atypical" Mycobacteria and the Diseases They Produce

Organism (Runyan groups)	Habitat	Transmission	Growth properties		
			Rate of growth	Colonial pigment	Niacin production
Mycobacterium kansasii (group I) (photochromogen)			Slow (weeks)	In light: yellow-orange In dark: non-pigmented	
Mycobacterium scrofulaceum (group II) (scotochromogen)	Occur in soil, dust, water, and/or the throat of normal humans and animals	Thought to be from the enviroment *Not* transmissible from human to human	Slow (weeks)	In light: yellow-orange In dark: yellow-orange	*Not* produced
Mycobacterium avium-intracellulare complex (group III) (non-chromogen)			Slow (weeks)	In light: non-pigmented In dark: non-pigmented	
Mycobacterium fortuitum (group IV) (non-chromogen)			Rapid (2–6 days)	In light: non-pigmented In dark: non-pigmented	

diagnostic aid, its use in the United States has been limitied to those at high risk, such as personnel at hospitals specializing in chest diseases.

DISEASE DUE TO "ATYPICAL" MYCOBACTERIA

Diseases produced by these acid-fast organisms are grouped as pulmonary diseases, localized lymphadenitis, cutaneous disease, and occasionally disseminated disease. The organisms may be opportunistic or frank pathogens.

In the United States, the most common clinical manifestation is pulmonary

TABLE 22.1 (*Continued*)

Pathogenicity for experimental animals	Disease	Diagnosis	Treatment
	In the United States most common in Texas Produces a pulmonary disease similar to tuberculosis, but not as severe Dissemination is rare	Chest X-ray, history, and clinical manifestations are useful	More resistant to chemotherapy than *M. tuberculosis*
	In the United States most common in the Great Lakes area Produces cervical lymphadenitis in children Dissemination is rare	Tuberculin skin testing not used due to unavailability of most skin test antigens and cross-reactivities	Multiple drug therapy is essential, but often ineffective
Not pathogenic	Occurs throughout the United States Produces a pulmonary disease indistinguishable from tuberculosis Dissemination is rare, *except* in AIDS patients	Direct acid-fast staining of smears is unreliable due to natural ubiquitous nature of the species	Treatment of AIDS patients with MAC disease requires up to five antimycobacterial drugs, yet therapy is still inadequate
	Occurs throughout the United States Produces a pulmonary disease similar to tuberculosis Produces abscesses in wounds following open-heart surgery, renal grafting, and venous stripping	Culture of sputum and other pertinent specimens is essential	Surgical resection of diseased areas of the lung is often required

disease, although the **disseminated disease due to *Mycobacterium avium-intra-cellulare* complex (MAC) in AIDS patients is of considerable concern.** Dissemination of MAC disease is rare, *except* in AIDS patients. Treatment of AIDS patients with MAC disease requires up to five antimycobacterial drugs, yet the **case fatality rate is still high due to multidrug resistance.** Pulmonary disease due to these organisms occur mostly in elderly Caucasian males with chronic bronchitis and emphysema. It has been estimated that "atypical" mycobacteria are responsible for as much as 10% of disease caused by acid-fast bacilli. Selected characteristics of these organisms and the diseases they produce are outlined in Table 22.1.

LEPROSY

Leprosy or Hansen's disease, the etiologic agent of which is *Mycobacterium leprae,* is a disease that has been known since the time of Aristotle. Despite the availability of effective antimicrobial agents for controlling leprosy, there are still about 15,000,000 lepers throughout the world. In the United States, about 140 cases are reported each year to the CDC with most occurring among immigrants in Hawaii, Louisiana, Florida, Texas, and California.

Habitat

M. leprae is an obligate parasite of humans and nine-banded armadillos. The organisms are harbored in the nasal secretions, ulcerative lesions, and sputum of patients.

Transmission

EXOGENOUS. Transmission is not completely understood, but appears to be exclusively exogenous. The most probable portals of entry are the respiratory and cutaneous routes following intimate and prolonged contact with lepromatous leprosy patients who shed large numbers of organisms in their nasal secretions and ulcerative lesions. Children and young adults are particularly susceptible. Multiple cases occur commonly within a single family suggesting that genetic factors may predispose to disease.

Properties of the Organism

Resistance to environmental, physical, and chemical agents. M. leprae can survive for years in nasal secretions and dried sputum and are relatively resistant to disinfecting agents.

Microscopic morphology. The organisms are **acid-fast,** nonmotile, nonencapsulated rods. They are straight or curved and may appear uniformly stained or beaded after staining. *M. leprae* is an **obligate intracellular parasite.**

Macroscopic morphology. The organism **has never been cultured** in or on artificial media or in tissue culture. Mice injected through the foot pads and armadillos are susceptible to *M. leprae* disease, the latter being used to generate large numbers of organisms for experimentation.

Antigenic structure. Antigenic structural components related to virulence have not been defined. Inasmuch as the organism can induce **DTH,** it is conceivable that cell wall components may play a role in the stimulation of hypersensitivity and/or immunity. Antibodies to cross-reactive or pathogen-unique epitopes do not appear to play a role in pathogenesis, resistance, or laboratory diagnosis.

Extracellular products associated with or thought to be associated with pathogenicity. No extracellular virulence factors are known.

Pathogenesis and Clinical Manifestations

Following introduction of the organisms into the host through respiratory or cutaneous routes, the organisms slowly multiply inducing a chronic granulomatous response characterized by an influx of mononuclear cells. After an incubation of 3–5 years or longer, the disease manifests as the lepromatous or tuberculoid type with at least three intermediate stages.

LEPROMATOUS LEPROSY. The organisms **proliferate within macrophages (foam cells)** at the site of entry and in the epithelial tissues, particularly around the face and ear lobes. **Suppressor T lymphocytes are numerous but epithelioid and giant cells are rare or absent. CMI is impaired,** massive numbers of organisms appear within the macrophages, and the patient becomes **anergic to DTH reactivity** with a leprosy tissue extract referred to as ''lepromin.'' Papules and macules appear at the site of entry and coalesce with marked folding of the skin. Gradual destruction of the cutaneous nerves leads to failure of the patient to recognize trauma and secondary bacterial infection.

TUBERCULOID LEPROSY. *M. leprae* multiplies at the site of entry, usually the skin, and invades and colonizes Schwann cells. In contrast to the lepromatous type, the organism **induces helper T lymphocytes, epithelioid cell, and giant cell infiltration of the skin. DTH reactivity to lepromin and CMI develop and remain vigorous** during the course of the disease, which in all probability accounts for the **scarcity or absence of organisms within lesions.** Key clinical manifestations are the macule at cutaneous entry and anesthesia (loss of pain sensation).

INTERMEDIATE STAGES. There are at least three intermediate stages of leprosy, which represent forms of the disease with characteristics of both the lepromatous and tuberculoid types.

Immunity

The pathogenesis and clinical manifestations of lepromatous and tuberculoid leprosy correlate closely with their CMI status. The impaired CMI seen in lepromatous leprosy accounts for the severity and progressive nature of the lesions, as well as the numerous organisms seen in the macrophages within the lesions. This is in marked contrast to the vigorous CMI demonstrable in patients with tuberculoid leprosy, in which the lesions tend to be more localized and organisms are either rare or absent. Humoral antibody plays no role in acquired resistance.

Laboratory Diagnosis

History and clinical manifestations are useful adjuncts but not definitive in the diagnosis of leprosy.

SPECIMENS AND DIRECT EXAMINATION. Specimens depend on the disease process and include skin lesion biopsies (including the ear lobes) and nasal secretions. Definitive identification is based upon the demonstration of typical acid-fast bacilli within phagocytic foam cells; numerous packets of organisms or "globi" are observed in lepromatous leprosy (Fig. 22.2), but are difficult or impossible to observe in the tuberculoid type.

Treatment

Although at one time the sulfone drug dapsone (4,4'-diaminodiphenyl sulfone, DDS) was the antimicrobial of choice in the treatment of leprosy, the development of a high degree of resistance has prompted the recommendation of combined dapsone, rifampin, and clofazimine for patients with lepromatous leprosy and dapsone and rifampin for those with the tuberculoid type. Evidence indicates that combined treatment may be required for only 2 years to effect a cure or significant remission of the disease in contrast to the lifelong therapy required with dapsone alone.

Prevention and Control

The early detection and treatment of patients is essential. Family contacts of patients with the disease, especially children and young adults, must be given prophylactic therapy. BCG vaccination for the active immunization of family con-

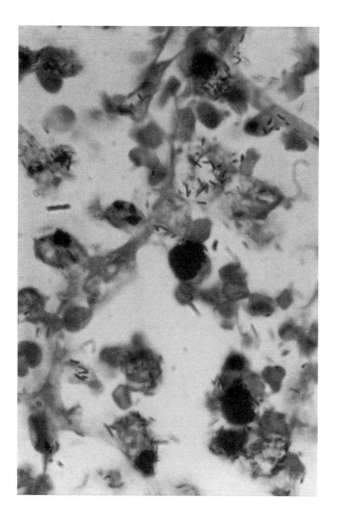

Figure 22.2.
Acid-fast stain of a skin biopsy section showing the characteristic ''packets'' of *M. leprae* within phagocytic cells. (Courtesy of Tom Rea, University of Southern California.)

tacts in highly endemic areas has been suggested, but the divergent nature of the data obtained to date has precluded a WHO recommendation.

ACTINOMYCES

ACTINOMYCOSIS

Actinomycosis is a chronic, suppurative, granulomatous disease caused most commonly by *Actinomyces israelii.* The organisms are normal inhabitants of the oral cavity predominating in and around the teeth and gum margins. The disease is the result of endogenous activation and is initiated by trauma, such as tooth extraction or pyogenic bacterial disease of the oral cavity. Human-human transmission does not occur. The organisms are gram-positive, nonacid-fast, branching, filamentous, and **strict anaerobes or microaerophiles.** From the mouth, the organisms may spread to the face and neck to produce cervicofacial disease, be aspirated into the lung with resultant thoracic disease, or be swallowed to produce abdominal disease. Multiple draining abscesses occur. The laboratory diagnosis is made by demonstrating ''sulfur granules'' in pus, sputum, or tissue biopsy material and by primary isolation and identification of the organism by strict anaerobic culture and biochemical reactions. Sulfur granules are lobulated bodies composed of delicate tangled masses of gram-positive filaments, the ends of which are club shaped. Combined drainage, debridement, and penicillin are effective in the treatment of actinomycosis.

NOCARDIA

SYSTEMIC NOCARDIOSIS

Systemic nocardiosis is a chronic granulomatous disease caused most commonly by *Nocardia asteroides.* The organisms are found in soil and water. The disease is the result of exogenous transmission and is usually initiated by inhalation. Most cases are **opportunistic,** occurring in immunosuppressed patients. Human-human transmission is possible but rare. The organisms are gram-positive, acid-fast, branching, filamentous, **strict aerobic** rods. Laboratory isolates are slow-growing, pigmented, rough-surfaced colonies that often smell ''musty.'' Following inhalation, a chronic lobar pneumonia develops with hematogenous dissemination most often to the CNS resulting in brain abscesses. The laboratory diagnosis is made by demonstrating gram-positive, acid-fast, branching, filamentous rods in sputum, cerebrospinal fluid, or tissue biopsy material, and by primary isolation and identification of the organism by strict aerobic culture and biochemical reactions. The sulfanilamides, when administered early, can reduce significantly the 80% case fatality rate that occurs in the untreated disease.

SUMMARY

1. *Mycobacterium tuberculosis* and *Mycobacterium bovis* are the etiologic agents of tuberculosis. In the United States, greater than 99% of tuberculosis cases are due to *M. tuberculosis*. Of great concern in the United States

is the growing number of multidrug resistant (MDR) cases of tuberculosis among individuals with impaired host resistance, particularly among patients with HIV infection and those with AIDS.

2. *M. tuberculosis* and *M. bovis* are acid-fast, nonmotile, nonencapsulated, facultative intracellular rods. They are strict aerobes that grow slowly on potato-egg or serum agar base media as dry, wrinkled, and nonpigmented colonies. Among the mycobacteria, niacin is produced only by *M. tuberculosis*.

3. Primary pulmonary (first-infection) tuberculosis is due almost exclusively to *M. tuberculosis* with first exposure by droplet nuclei occurring mostly in childhood. The organisms multiply within the polymorphonuclear leukocytes and destroy them, spreading to the lymphatics and hilar lymph nodes. Macrophages and lymphocytes soon infiltrate the areas, the former phagocytizing the living tubercle bacilli, which inhibit phagolysosomal fusion. The development of DTH and CMI results in a granulomatous or productive response characterized by microscopic granulomas or tubercles, the center of which undergoes caseous necrosis. An adequate CMI response results in healing of the caseous tubercle fibrosis and calcification although calcified areas may still harbor tubercle bacilli for years or life.

4. The postprimary pulmonary (reactivation) type of tuberculosis due to *M. tuberculosis* is of endogenous origin resulting from a waning CMI response and reactivation from quiescent foci. The apex of the lung is invariably the site of reactivation. The organisms initiate a chronic inflammatory response and the reactivated focus becomes caseous, liquifies, and breaks into an adjacent bronchus resulting in cavity formation and aspiration into other parts of the lung initiating a new infectious process.

5. Intestinal tuberculosis results from the ingestion of raw milk or dairy products contaminated with *M. bovis*.

6. The "atypical" mycobacteria are opportunistic or frank pathogens that may produce a wide spectrum of clinical syndromes including pulmonary diseases, localized lymphadenitis, cutaneous disease, and occasionally disseminated disease. In the United States, disseminated disease due to MAC in AIDS patients is of considerable concern.

7. *Mycobacterium leprae*, the etiologic agent of leprosy (Hansen's disease), is an obligate parasite of humans and nine-banded armadillos and is most probably transmitted following intimate and prolonged contact with lepromatous patients who shed large numbers of organisms in their nasal secretions and ulcerative lesions.

8. *M. leprae* is an acid-fast, nonmotile, nonencapsulated, obligate intracellular rod that has never been cultured in or on artificial media or in tissue culture. Mice and armadillos are susceptible to experimental disease.

9. Following introduction of *M. leprae* into the host, the organisms multiply slowly inducing a chronic granulomatous response characterized by an influx of mononuclear cells. After an incubation period of 3–5 years, the disease manifests as the lepromatous or tuberculoid type with three intermediate stages.

10. In lepromatous leprosy, the organisms proliferate within macrophages (foam cells) at the site of entry and in the epithelial tissues, particularly around the face and ear lobes. Suppressor T cells are numerous, but epithelioid and giant cells are rare or absent. CMI is impaired, massive numbers of organisms appear within macrophages, and the patient becomes anergic to DTH reactivity with lepromin. Papules and macules appear at the site of entry and coalesce with marked folding of the skin. Gradual destruction of the cutaneous nerves leads to failure of the patient to recognize trauma and secondary bacterial infection.

11. In tuberculoid leprosy, the organisms multiply at the site of entry and invade and colonize Schwann cells. In contrast to the lepromatous type, the organisms induce helper T cells, epithelioid cells, and giant cell infiltration of the skin. DTH reactivity to lepromin and CMI develop and remain vigorous during the course of the disease, which probably accounts for the scarcity or absence of organisms within lesions.

12. Actinomycosis is a chronic, suppurative disease caused most commonly by *Actinomyces israelii*, a normal inhabitant of the oral cavity predominating in and around the teeth and gum margins. Systemic nocardiosis is a chronic granulomatous disease caused most often by *Nocardia asteroides*, a soil and water inhabitant. Most cases occur as opportunistic disease in immunosuppressed patients.

REFERENCES

American Thoracic Society (1987): Mycobacteriosis and the acquired immunodeficiency syndrome. Am Rev Respir Dis 136:492.

American Thoracic Society (1990): Diagnosis and treatment of disease caused by nontuberculous mycobacteria. Am Rev Respir Dis 142:940.

Bullock WE (1985): Leprosy (Hansen's Disease). In Wyngaarden JB, Smith LH Jr (eds): Cecil Textbook of Medicine. 17th ed, Vol. 2, Philadelphia: W.B. Saunders, p 1634.

Dannenberg AM Jr (1989): Immune mechanisms in the pathogenesis of pulmonary tuberculosis. Rev Infect Dis 11 (Suppl 2):369.

Des Prez RM, Heim CR (1990): *Mycobacterium tuberculosis.* In Mandell GL, Douglas RG Jr, Bennett JE (eds): Principles and Practice of Infectious Diseases, 3rd ed. New York: Churchill Livingstone, pp 1877–1906.

Ellner JJ, Goldberger MJ, Parenti DM (1991): *Mycobacterium avium* infection and AIDS: A therapeutic dilemma in rapid evolution. J Infect Dis 163:1326.

Gangadharam PRJ, Iseman MD (1987): Antimycobacterial drugs. Antimicrob Agents Ann 2:14.

Goodfellow M, Mordarski M, Williams ST (eds) (1984): The Biology of the Actinomycetes. London, England: Academic Press.

Horsburgh CR, Mason UG, Farhi DC, Iseman MD (1985): Disseminated infection with *Mycobacterium avium-intracellulare.* Medicine 64:39.

Horsburgh CR, Selik RM (1989): The epidemiology of disseminated nontuberculous mycobacterial infection in the acquired immunodeficiency syndrome (AIDS). Am Rev Respir Dis 139:4.

Jacobson RR (1990): Hansen's disease drugs in use. Current recommendations for treatment. The Star (Carville, La.) 49:1.

Simpson GL, Stinson EB, Egger MJ, Remington JS (1981): Nocardial infections in the immunocompromised host: A detailed study in a defined population. Rev Infect Dis 3:492.

Storrs EE, Walsh GP, Burchfield HP (1974): Leprosy in the armadillo: A new model for biomedical research. Science. 183:851.

U.S. Department of Health and Human Services (1987): Diagnosis and management of mycobacterial infection and disease in persons with human immunodeficiency virus infection. Ann Intern Med 106:254.

U.S. Department of Health and Human Services (1991): Nosocomial transmission of multidrug resistant tuberculosis among HIV-infected persons-Florida and New York, 1988–1991. MMWR 40:585.

U.S. Department of Health and Human Services (1992): National action plan to combat purified protein derivative (PPD)-tuberculin anergy and HIV infection: Guidelines for anergy testing and management of anergic persons at risk of tuberculosis. MMWR 40:27. Multidrug-resistant tuberculosis. Meeting the challenge of multidrug-resistant tuberculosis: summary of a conference. Management of persons exposed to multidrug-resistant tuberculosis. MMWR 41:1 (entire issue).

Woods GL, Washington WA (1987): Mycobacteria other than *Mycobacterium tuberculosis:* Review of microbiologic and clinical aspects. Rev Infect Dis 9:275.

REVIEW QUESTIONS

For questions 1 to 12, choose the ONE
BEST answer or completion.

1. Multidrug-resistant (MDR) tuberculosis
   a) occurs only in HIV-infected patients
   b) is rarely fatal
   c) is a rapidly progressive disease
   d) is more apt to occur in children
   e) is usually caused by *Mycobacterium bovis*

2. The primary pulmonary (first-infection) type of tuberculosis
   a) is initiated by droplet nuclei from a patient
   b) is the result of endogenous activation of *Mycobacterium tuberculosis* due to a waning of acquired resistance and reactivation of quiescent primary foci within the respiratory tract
   c) has no special ethnic predilection for disease production
   d) is usually the result of drinking raw milk
   e) is the result of endogenous reactivation of quiescent primary foci from an extrapulmonary source

3. *M. tuberculosis* and *M. bovis*
   a) are highly susceptible to disinfecting agents
   b) are facultative intracellular parasites
   c) are spore-forming, acid-fast rods
   d) produce niacin
   e) have never been cultured in vitro

4. Postprimary pulmonary tuberculosis *differs* from primary pulmonary tuberculosis in that the *former*
   a) is characterized by the development of humoral mechanisms responsible for healing of caseous lesions
   b) results from a waning CMI response
   c) is of exogenous origin
   d) commonly disseminates hematogenously from the lung
   e) is characterized by a positive tuberculin test

5. Definitive identification of *M. tuberculosis* in sputum concentrates from patients with disease referrable to tuberculosis necessitates
   a) demonstration of acid-fast bacilli in direct smears, demonstration of dry, wrinkled, cream-colored colonies (acid-fast) on potato-egg medium (e.g Lowenstein-Jensen), and the production of niacin
   b) inoculation of armadillos, blood culture isolation, and acid-fast identification of the organism on suitable culture medium, and the production of niacin
   c) demonstration of acid-fast bacilli in direct smears, demonstration of dry, wrinkled, cream-colored colonies (acid-fast) on

chocolate agar, and the production of niacin
d) incubation of sputum concentrate cultures under anaerobic conditions
e) only the demonstration of acid-fast bacilli in direct smears

6. The treatment of tuberculosis
   a) is initiated with a single first-line chemotherapeutic agent
   b) usually requires prolonged bed rest and surgery
   c) in adults should be continued until the tuberculin test reverts to negative
   d) always results in negative sputum cultures and clinical cure within 3 weeks
   e) always necessitates the use of combined chemotherapy

7. A positive tuberculin test with purified protein derivative (PPD)
   a) indicates relatively high humoral antibody levels in patients with active tuberculosis
   b) never occurs following vaccination with Bacillus of Calmette and Guerin (BCG)
   c) is an indicator of active tuberculosis
   d) is a measure of DTH and indicates infection with *M. tuberculosis* or *M. bovis*
   e) indicates either the absence of tuberculous infection or "anergy" in patients critically ill with tuberculosis

8. One of the following statements relating to members of the *Mycobacterium avium-intracellulare* complex (MAC) "atypical" mycobacteria is NOT TRUE.
   a) The organisms produce disseminated disease in AIDS patients.

b) Therapy is usually inadequate despite the use of up to five antimycobacterial drugs.
c) The organisms are transmissible from human to human.
d) The organisms produce a pulmonary disease indistinguishable from tuberculosis.
e) The organisms are slow growing, acid-fast rods.

9. One of the following statements relating to *Mycobacterium leprae* is NOT TRUE.
   a) The organisms have never been cultured in or on artificial media.
   b) Armadillos and mice are susceptible to experimental infection.
   c) The organisms are obligate intracellular parasites.
   d) The organisms are acid-fast rods.
   e) The organisms can survive for years in nasal secretions due to their ability to form spores.

10. Lepromatous leprosy *differs* from tuberculoid leprosy in that the *former*
    a) is characterized by massive numbers of *M. leprae* within macrophages
    b) is characterized by the development of a strong DTH reactivity
    c) is characterized by the development of a vigorous CMI response
    d) is not transmissible from human to human
    e) cannot be treated effectively, even with combined dapsone, rifampin, and clofazimine

11. The definitive identification of *M. leprae* in skin lesions from patients with lepromatous leprosy

a) requires inoculation of the armadillo
b) requires the demonstration of acid-fast bacilli within phagocytic foam cells
c) requires cultivation on Lowenstein-Jensen medium
d) cannot be done without a corroborative positive skin test
e) requires the inoculation of mice

12. Actinomycosis and systemic nocardiosis are both

a) caused by organisms that are normal inhabitants of the oral cavity
b) caused by strict aerobes
c) the result of endogenous activation
d) characterized by the presence of "sulfur granules" in pus, sputum, or tissue
e) chronic granulomatous diseases with human-human transmission either rare or absent

---

ANSWERS TO REVIEW QUESTIONS

---

1. *c* Multidrug-resistant tuberculosis is a rapidly progressive, highly fatal disease that occurs in patients with an impaired host resistance, including HIV-infected patients. It occurs in any age group and is caused by *Mycobacterium tuberculosis.*

2. *a* Primary pulmonary (first-infection) tuberculosis is transmitted exogenously by droplet nuclei from a patient. Endogenous activation initiates postprimary (reactivation) tuberculosis. Certain ethnic groups, such as Asians, American Indians, Eskimos, and Blacks, are more likely to develop disease as opposed to infection following droplet nuclei exposure.

3. *b* *M. tuberculosis* and *M. bovis* are non-spore-forming, acid-fast, facultative intracellular parasites that are highly resistant to disinfecting agents. Both can be cultured in vitro, but only *M. tuberculosis* is niacin positive.

4. *b* Postprimary pulmonary tuberculosis is the result of the waning of an adequate CMI response in contrast to primary pulmonary tuberculosis, which occurs because the host has not as yet mounted or has failed to mount an adequate CMI response. As already indicated, postprimary tuberculosis is the result of endogenous activation. In both types, humoral mechanisms play no role in the development or persistence of acquired resis-

tance, dissemination rarely occurs from the lung after exposure or reactivation, and there is usually a positive tuberculin test.

5. *a* The definitive identification of *M. tuberculosis* in sputum concentrates from patients with potential tuberculous disease necessitates the demonstration of acid-fast bacilli in direct smears, growth of dry, wrinkled, cream-colored colonies (acid-fast) on a potato-egg (or serum agar base) medium, and the production of niacin. Armadillos are not susceptible, the organisms do not grow on chocolate agar, and culture is carried out aerobically in the presence of 5–10% carbon dioxide. The possible presence of non-pathogenic, acid-fast organisms in sputum concentrates precludes the use of direct smear staining alone for definitive identification.

6. *e* The treatment of tuberculosis always necessitates the use of combined chemotherapy with drugs having different modes of action in order to reduce the risk of selecting out resistant mutants. Prolonged bed rest and surgery are rarely required. Treatment has no effect upon a positive tuberculin test unless the disease is recognized early in its course. If therapy is effective, sputum cultures become negative in 3 weeks, but clinical cure may take up to 1 year.

7. *d* A positive tuberculin test is a measure of DTH and indicates infection with *M. tuberculosis* or *M. bovis,* not necessarily

disease. Vaccination with BCG results in a positive tuberculin test. A negative tuberculin test indicates absence of tuberculous infection or "anergy" in patients critically ill with tuberculosis.

8. *c* Members of the MAC, like all the "atypicals," are not transmissible from human to human. The organisms are slow growing, acid-fast rods capable of producing syndromes that include a pulmonary disease indistinguishable from tuberculosis and a highly fatal, disseminated disease in AIDS patients.

9. *e* *Mycobacterium leprae* does not form spores. The organisms are acid-fast, have never been cultured in or on artificial media, produce experimental infection in the mouse and armadillo, and are obligate, intracellular parasites.

10. *a* In contrast to tuberculoid leprosy, the lepromatous type is characterized by massive numbers of *M. leprae* in macrophages. The tuberculoid type is characterized by the development of strong DTH reactivity and a vigorous CMI response. Lepromatous leprosy is transmissible following intimate and prolonged contact with patients who shed large numbers of organisms in their nasal secretions and ulcerative lesions. Both types can be treated effectively with combined chemotherapy.

11. *b* The definitive identification of *M. leprae* in skin lesions from patients with lepromatous leprosy requires the demonstra-

tion of acid-fast bacilli within phagocytic foam cells. Animal inoculations are not necessary and, as indicated above, the organisms cannot be cultured in vitro. A positive skin test is indicative of infection and not necessarily disease.

12. *e* Actinomycosis and systemic nocardiosis are both chronic granulomatous diseases with human-human transmission either rare or absent. *Actinomyces israelii* is a strict anaerobe or microaerophilic and a normal inhabitant of the oral cavity, while *Nocardia asteroides* is a strict aerobe and found in soil and water. Actinomycosis is the result of endogenous activation and is characterized by the presence of "sulfur granules" in pus, sputum, or tissue. In contrast, systemic nocardiosis is the result of exogenous transmission and "sulfur granules" do not occur.

CHLAMYDIAL, RICKETTSIAL, AND MYCOPLASMAL DISEASE

The genera *Chlamydia, Rickettsia,* and *Mycoplasma* cause a number of important diseases ranging from Rocky Mountain spotted fever to sexually transmitted cervicitis. These bacteria share several characteristics: small size, an unusual or absent cell wall, and specialized growth requirements. In fact, chlamydiae and rickettsiae are not free-living, but require host cell cytoplasm for growth. Members of these genera are **obligate intracellular parasites.** Many rickettsial diseases are transmitted to humans by an insect vector.

CHLAMYDIA

The genus *Chlamydia* contains three species. The key characteristics of this genus are shown in Table 23.1.

The chlamydial cell wall is unusual among bacteria in that **peptidoglycan is virtually absent.** The organism maintains structural rigidity by means of a disulfide bond lattice arranged between outer membrane proteins. Chlamydiae are **nonmotile coccobacilli.**

The outer surface of chlamydiae presents several antigenic components to

TABLE 23.1. Characteristics of *Chlamydia*

Species	Inclusions	Major infections
trachomatis	Round, glycogen-containing, vacuolar	Trachoma (ocular infection), inclusion conjunctivitis, cervicitis, urethritis, pelvic inflammatory disease, lymphogranuloma venereum
pneumoniae	Round, dense, glycogen negative	Atypical pneumonia
psittaci	Dense, irregular, glycogen negative	Ornithosis, psittacosis

the host immune system, including a genus-specific lipopolysaccharide that resembles that of other gram-negative bacteria. The antigen may not be a virulence factor, but antibody developed against it can be exploited for serologic diagnosis of some chlamydial diseases, particularly psittacosis.

Chlamydia have developed a unique developmental cycle. Disease is spread by adherence of the **elementary body (EB),** the infectious phase of the organism, to mucosal epithelium. The mechanism of species-specific adherence is not known although a major outer membrane protein (MOMP) has been implicated. After attachment, the chlamydiae induce the host cell, a nonprofessional phagocyte, to **endocytose them in a cell membrane invagination.** Once inside the cell, they **inhibit phagolysosomal fusion** and begin their developmental cycle (Fig. 23.1). Although the EB can survive outside of a living host cell, it normally does not produce energy or synthesize adenosine triphosphate (ATP), thus requiring an intracellular existence for reproduction.

Approximately 12 h after the organism enters a host cell, the EB has reorganized to form a more metabolically active structure, the **reticulate body (RB),** which divides actively by binary fission. At 18–24 h after the initial infection, the RBs can be visualized in their cytoplasmic vacuole by special stains as a large, **intracellular inclusion** containing as many as 1000 RBs, the **inclusion body.** Glycogen-containing inclusion bodies, such as those formed only by *Chlamydia trachomatis,* stain orange-brown with iodine (Fig. 23.2). Characteristics of inclusion bodies (Table 23.1) can help to differentiate among species growing in cell culture.

As the RBs mature, they each "reorganize" into small, denser, EBs, which are released when the cell ruptures, usually 48–72 h after initial infection. The freed EBs go on to infect other cells.

Chlamydiae also possess a number of MOMP antigens. Antibodies directed against MOMPs are used as immunoreagents for differentiating among strains of

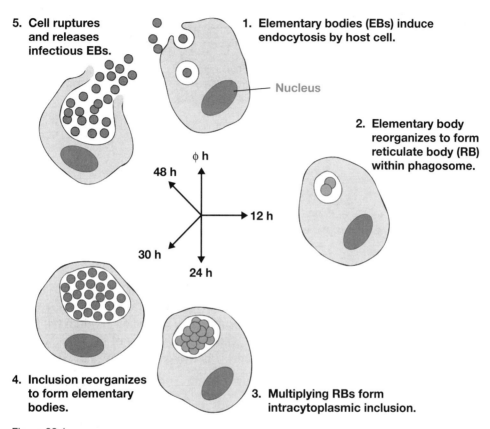

Figure 23.1.
Developmental cycle of *Chlamydia.*

C. trachomatis. Different serovars or immunotypes are usually associated with different diseases, although there is considerable overlap (Table 23.2).

The major diseases of *C. trachomatis* species (trachoma, genital tract infections, neonatal pneumonia and pneumonitis, and lymphogranuloma venereum) are discussed in the following five sections.

TRACHOMA

More than 400 million people worldwide suffer from the devastating effects of trachoma, which, when untreated, ultimately leads to blindness (the fate of at least 20 million people). In the United States, cases are sporadic, with a few endemic foci on reservations populated by Native Americans.

TABLE 23.2. Serovars of *C. trachomatis* Associated With Different Diseases

Serovar	Infection
A, B, Ba, C	Trachoma, inclusion conjunctivitis
D-M	Inclusion conjunctivitis, infant pneumonitis
L1, L2, L3	Lymphogranuloma venereum

Habitat

C. trachomatis is an **obligate intracellular parasite of humans.** Asymptomatic carriers exist, and trachoma conjunctivitis ranges from very mild early forms to serious scarring of the eye and blindness.

Transmission

EXOGENOUS. Spread from **person to person** occurs in areas where poor hygiene and crowding are rampant. **Direct contact** occurs when children rub their eyes, mothers clean their childrens' eyes with the dirty edges of their clothing or towels, or even, perhaps, spreading occurs when organisms are carried on the appendages of flying insects.

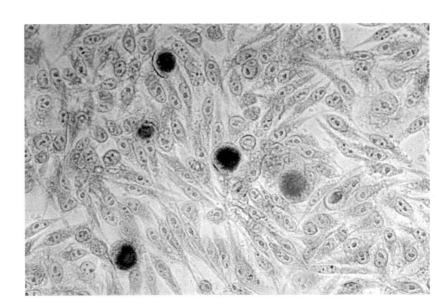

Figure 23.2.

Iodine-stained inclusion bodies in a monolayer of *Chlamydia*-infected McCoy cells. (Courtesy of Dr. Ellena Peterson, University of California, Irvine.)

ENDOGENOUS. A carrier of the organism in a latent state may develop disease if the organism becomes activated by an as yet unknown mechanism.

Pathogenesis and Clinical Manifestations

Once introduced into the secretions of the eye, the organisms attach to conjunctival cells, where they invade and proceed through the developmental cycle described previously. In most instances, the host responds with an acute inflammatory response characterized by **subepithelial infiltration of polymorphonuclear leukocytes and mononuclear cells.** The subsequent mucopurulent discharge, eyelash follicular hypertrophy, and conjunctival hyperemia (swollen, inflamed capillaries) follows within 3–10 days. The conjunctival surface becomes roughened, thus the name **trachoma,** which in Greek means ''rough.''

With repeated infections, the insult to host tissue results in corresponding **conjunctival scarring,** capillary extension into the cornea (known as **pannus**), deformation of the eyelid, and often damage to the eye surface due to **mechanical damage** inflicted by turned-in eyelashes. **Blindness** occurs as a result of repeated chlamydial infection and/or secondary bacterial infection of the eye.

Immunity to Reinfection

The human immune response is inadequate to prevent reinfection or reactivation from the latent stage.

Laboratory Diagnosis

DIRECT DETECTION IN CONJUNCTIVAL SCRAPINGS. A sterile silver spatula or other instrument should be used to **gently scrape the surface of the conjunctiva.** Since the organisms are obligate intracellular parasites, it is important to collect **infected epithelial cells,** rather than simply purulent discharge material. Monoclonal antibody-based fluorescent stains can readily detect the etiologic agent on direct smears. The advantage of fluorescent stains is that they can stain the elementary body as well as the reticulate bodies, and free elementary bodies may be the only detectable morphotype. Only experienced microscopists are able to reliably identify the tiny EB structures. Alternatively, inclusions, if present, may be visualized with Giemsa stain.

CULTURE. The conjunctival epithelial cells or the discharge should be placed in *Chlamydia*-**transport medium** immediately. The specimen is inoculated onto cycloheximide-treated McCoy cells, a mouse epithelioid cell line. The cycloheximide prevents the cells from dividing but allows continued viability, enhancing infectivity of the chlamydiae. After 24–72 h, depending on the sensitivity of the stain, the cell monolayer is stained with iodine, Giemsa, or specific monoclonal antibodies conjugated to a fluorescent or enzyme marker and examined for inclusions.

IMMUNOSEROLOIC TESTS. In areas of low prevalence, detection of antibody to chlamydiae may aid in establishing a diagnosis. Although culture or direct detection are the best methods, demonstration of serovar-specific antibody by indirect fluorescent-antibody staining can also support the diagnosis. The microimmunofluorescent test uses tiny dots of heavily infected material prepared in embryonated egg yolk cultures placed in a structured array on a slide as the substrate. Dots of antigens from all serovars of *C. trachomatis* are included. Patient antibodies bind to the specific antigen in the appropriate dot and are detected with a fluorescent antihuman antibody counterstain.

Treatment

Although the organisms are susceptible to **doxycycline, erythromycin,** second- and third-generation **cephalosporins,** and **sulfonamides,** treatment is not very effective, partly due to the occurrence of **relapse** after therapy. Either topical or systemic therapy will cause regression of clinical manifestations but the organism will remain viable in the conjunctiva. Better results are achieved with a minimum of 3 weeks of systemic therapy.

Prevention and Control

Educate people on the importance of adequate personal hygiene, and improve public sanitation facilities and access to health care.

GENITAL TRACT AND ASSOCIATED INFECTIONS

During the last decade, the scope of genital tract-associated chlamydial infections has been recognized. Today these infections are **among the most prevalent sexually transmitted disease (STD) in the United States,** estimated at over

3 million cases. There are 3–10 million new infections annually. Worldwide cases are estimated at 300 million. Numerous types of infections are caused by *C. trachomatis* (Fig. 23.3).

It is interesting that an estimated one-third to one-half of patients with gonococcal disease are also coinfected with chlamydiae. These two STD agents share several syndromes and sequelae, including Reiter's syndrome, pharyngitis, conjunctivitis, pelvic inflammatory disease (PID), and perihepatitis. Pelvic inflammatory disease due to *C. trachomatis* results in **infertility** or **ectopic pregnancy** in a significant number of infected women, with chances for these sequelae increasing dramatically with each reinfection (20% risk after the first infection and 75% risk after the third infection).

Habitat

The organism only infects and survives in humans, in whom both a symptomatic and an asymptomatic carrier state can exist.

Transmission

EXOGENOUS. **Infected secretions from the genital tract** spread the infection through **sexual activity,** including anal-genital sex, and by direct contact. Adults can transfer the organism to their eyes after touching their genital tracts. Infants usually acquire inclusion conjunctivitis or pneumonitis during **passage through the infected birth canal** of the mother, although postnatal transmission does occur by carriage of organisms on the hands.

ENDOGENOUS. Reactivation of latent infection occurs, sometimes leading to extension from the primary focus; the mechanism is not understood.

Pathogenesis and Clinical Manifestations

GENITAL TRACT DISEASE. Once introduced into the urethra, rectum, or cervix, usually by sexual activity with an infected partner, the EBs begin their developmental cycle of attachment, endocytosis, and growth. Most individuals produce little or no host response and the infection is asymptomatic (latent). Primary disease occurs when the host responds with an acute inflammatory infiltrate characterized by polymorphonuclear neutrophils. After a 2–8-day incubation pe-

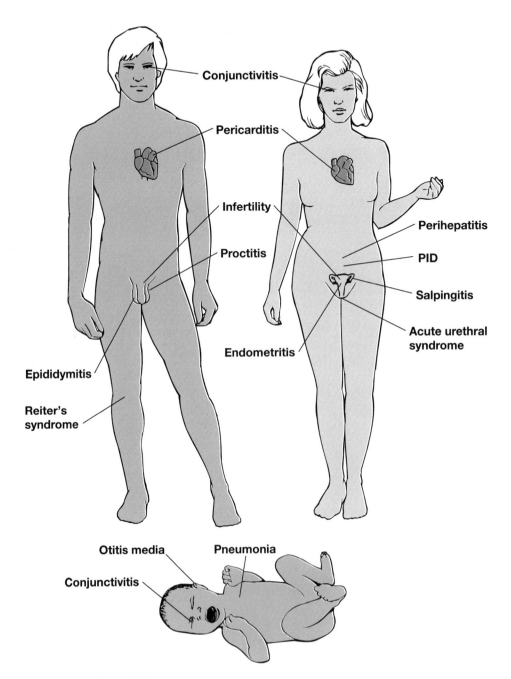

Figure 23.3.

Sites of clinical manifestation of chlamydial disease in the male, female, and baby.

riod, the disease manifests as a **mucopurulent** or "watery" discharge from the infected site. Chlamydiae are the most common etiologic agents of "nongonococcal urethritis" in males and females. This syndrome in females, often without noticable discharge but consisting of pain, frequency, and urgency surrounding urination, is called the "acute urethral syndrome" and may also occur as a result of infection with other organisms.

UPPER TRACT DISEASE. In the male, the infection can disseminate by direct extension into the epididymis to produce **epididymitis.** In the female, the organisms can travel up the fallopian tubes into the peritoneal cavity and produce **salpingitis and PID.**

NEONATAL INCLUSION CONJUNCTIVITIS

The infant becomes colonized with the organisms as it passes through the infected birth canal of the mother. Colonization may occur rarely in the vagina of infant girls or on the conjunctiva of babies of either sex. Mucopurulent conjunctivitis, with sequelae similar to that of trachoma (such as pannus and scarring), develops 1–2 weeks after delivery.

NEONATAL PNEUMONIA AND PNEUMONITIS

This syndrome is often preceded by conjunctivitis. The organisms are inhaled by the infant during passage through an infected birth canal, although disease usually does not develop until 1–6 months after birth. Infection of lung epithelial cells, with resulting cell function disruption and inflammatory infiltrate, results in pneumonitis with inflammatory cells filling airways and blocking gas exchange.

LYMPHOGRANULOMA VENEREUM (LGV)

This syndrome is caused by invasive LGV serovars. For the last 10 years, around 300 cases of domestic LGV have been reported to the CDC each year. The disease is **sexually transmitted** and often presents in conjunction with other STDs. After the organisms infect the genital epithelial cells, they invade the lymphatic systems and are carried to regional lymph nodes, often in the groin. The host responds with a cellular infiltrate of macrophages, lymphocytes, and plasma cells. The primary initial clinical manifestation, occurring 7–28 days later, is painful and swollen femoral or inguinal lymph nodes referred to as **"buboes,"** which may ultimately necrose and develop fistulae. Systemic manifestations may include fever, nausea, and vomiting. Disruption of lymphatic drainage due to swelling and necrosis may lead to elephantiasis, called "esthiomene" when it involves the vulva. Rectal complications include strictures, proctitis, and perforation.

Immunity to Reinfection

Although antibody to *C. trachomatis* is formed as a result of infection or disease, it does not seem to be protective. Relapse following a latent period is known to occur.

Laboratory Diagnosis of Genital Tract Chlamydial Diseases

DIRECT MICROSCOPIC VISUALIZATION. Direct visualization of the organism (usually EBs) is possible in genital mucosal cell scrapings, conjunctival scrapings of neonates, bubo aspirates, and other specimens.

Direct detection by **fluorescent antibody staining** is most effective with genital specimens and conjunctival scrapings. **Collection of infected cells** is critical for diagnosis of chlamydial STD, as for trachoma. Monoclonal antibodies directed against MOMP or the LPS of *C. trachomatis* are used in very sensitive and specific assays, yielding results that compare favorably with culture in some studies. These immunofluorescent reagents have largely supplanted the detection of inclusions by Giemsa stain.

DIRECT ANTIGEN DETECTION BY ELISA. These assays are used for genital swabs and scrapings and occasionally for conjunctival scrapings and may parallel direct visualization in sensitivity. These assays are particularly useful for specimens that must be transported some distance, since a positive result does not depend on viable organisms.

DIRECT DETECTION OF *CHLAMYDIA* BY GENETIC PROBE. At least two commercially available DNA probes have been evaluated extensively for detection of *Chlamydia* in genital and ocular discharge material. Chemiluminescent markers identify the double-stranded hybrids that occur when the probe binds to a homologous DNA or ribosomal RNA sequence, indicating the presence of the organism in the sample. These methods have shown sensitivity and specificity comparable to the best conventional laboratory methods. Polymerase chain reaction amplification probe tests are now available and their exquisite sensitivity may move them into the "gold standard" position. Theoretically, the DNA of even one organism may be sufficient for detection by this method.

CULTURE. As with trachoma, culture is still the "gold standard" for diagnosis of genital chlamydial disease. LGV cultures, however, are less sensitive than those involving other serovars.

IMMUNOSEROLOGIC TESTS. Microimmunofluorescence, described above for trachoma diagnosis, is still the best diagnostic modality for LGV. Complement fixation lacks sensitivity. Because of the high prevalence of sexually transmitted disease due to *Chlamydia* in the United States, immunoserology is unlikely to be helpful in establishing a diagnosis for urethritis or cervicitis. Infants with perinatal pneumonia, however, develop a rapid and specific IgM response, detection of which is the diagnostic test of choice for this disease.

Treatment

Since asymptomatic genital infection is common, all partners of infected patients should be treated. **Tetracycline or doxycycline,** followed by erythromycin and sulfasoxazole are still the therapies of choice. Combinations of cefoxitin and doxycycline may be effective when upper tract disease is present Treatment of sexually transmitted chlamydial disease includes treatment of possible coexisting gonococcal infection.

Prevention and Control

Sexually transmitted diseases, including chlamydial infections and disease, are dramatically reduced by **condom** use. Neonatal inclusion conjunctivitis (and gonococcal conjunctivitis) can be prevented by instillation of **0.5% erythromycin ointment** or **1% tetracycline ophthalmic ointment** into the eyes at birth. This topical treatment has little effect on subsequent development of pneumonitis. Unfortunately, penicillin and silver nitrate, at one time used to prevent gonococcal ophthalmia neonatorum, have no effect on chlamydiae. Except for LGV, chlamydial infections and disease are not notifiable in the United States. Thus, the public health activities of case finding and contact treatment are dependent on individual physicians. There is no effective vaccine available.

CHLAMYDIA PNEUMONIAE DISEASE

Chlamydia pneumoniae was first discovered in Taiwan as an unusual agent of sinusitis, although it was not thought to cause eye disease. The isolate, grown in the yolk sac of an embryonated hen's egg, was called TW-183. A second isolate, called AR-39, gave the species its nickname, TWAR. Serologic and culture studies of college students in Seattle, Washington, established that this strain of *Chlamydia,* first thought to be a variant of *Chlamydia psittaci,* caused **pharyngitis, bronchitis,** and an **atypical pneumonia.**

The organism received species status in 1989. It has since been associated with **respiratory disease in elderly and debilitated patients,** as well as otherwise healthy adults.

Habitat

C. pneumoniae is thought to be a human parasite, with no other environmental niche.

Transmission

The agent is thought to be spread by aerosol droplets, but the exact mode of transmission is not known.

Pathogenesis and Clinical Manifestations

Recognition of *C. pneumoniae* as an important etiologic agent of respiratory disease is too recent to allow definitive characterization of the pathogenesis or to describe all of the clinical manifestations. Presently, associated clinical manifestations include pharyngitis, fever, pleural effusion, bronchitis, and pneumonia. Evidence exists that prolonged infection after an acute episode, despite appropriate therapy, may not be uncommon.

Immunity to Reinfection

Antibody develops after infection. Preliminary studies indicate that reinfection is common. Information about the immune response to this agent is sparse.

Laboratory Diagnosis

No commercial products are universally accepted at this time. Microimmunofluorescent tests for specific antibody are available. The organism can be cultured in HeLa cell culture and inclusions stained with monoclonal antibody-conjugated fluorescent stains.

Treatment

No definitive data are available yet. Several patients treated with erythromycin were shown to suffer relapses of clinical manifestations once treatment was stopped.

CHLAMYDIA PSITTACI DISEASE

C. psittaci is a **parasite of psittacine birds,** such as parrots, parakeets, finches, and other exotic species; domestic birds, such as pigeons, turkeys, and chickens; and their close companion mammals including livestock, pets, and horses. These animals comprise the sources of this zoonosis in humans. Approximately 120 cases are reported annually in the United States. The term "ornithosis" was used originally to characterize disease of nonpsittacine birds, such as wild and domestic fowl, whereas "psittacosis" was used in reference to the disease in psittacine birds. This distinction is no longer used, since the etiologic agent and the disease are always identical. The human disease is now called **"psittacosis."** Poultry industry workers, pet owners, pigeon raisers, and others who have avian contact are at increased risk.

Habitat

The organism is mostly asymptomatic in birds, where it colonizes the mucous membranes of the respiratory and GI tracts. If birds and animals become ill, they usually develop diarrhea. The organism is shed in secretions and in the feces, but in smaller numbers from asymptomatic animals. Once shed into the environment, *C. psittaci* can survive for long periods in feces or soil.

Transmission

Transmission to humans is mostly through **inhalation of aerosols** containing viable organisms, such as from dried feces, although an ocular infection similar to trachoma has been described. Handling infected bird tissues or feathers is another source of disease. Human-human transmission is extremely rare. Even when no identifiable contact is found, the source is thought to have been pigeon feces or other environmental exposure.

Pathogenesis and Clinical Manifestations

After the organism colonizes the respiratory mucosal cells and undergoes its developmental cycle, it is carried by macrophages and other phagocytes to the spleen and liver, from which it disseminates through the bloodstream. Nausea, vomiting, fever, headache, and other constitutional symptoms accompany this stage, which occurs 7–14 days after exposure. The organism is seeded to the lungs, where it multiplies and causes a hacking, nonproductive cough and **pneumonia,** which can persist for another 7–10 days. Fatal cases usually involve infection of additional organs, including, spleen, heart, and liver. The case fatality rate of untreated disease is 20%.

Immunity to Reinfection

Patients develop antibodies directed against *C. psittaci,* although they are not protective. Recovered patients have been known to shed the organism in their sputum for as long as 10 years.

Laboratory Diagnosis

Culture is not performed by routine laboratories because of the hazardous nature of working with the etiologic agent, thus immunoserology is the mainstay of laboratory diagnosis. **Microimmunofluorescence or ELISA tests** are highly sensitive; some laboratories still perform the less-specific complement-fixation test. Cross-reactivity with other chlamydiae complicates the serologic diagnosis.

Treatment

Doxycycline is the antibiotic of choice. Effective therapy has reduced mortality to less than 2%.

Prevention and Control

Quarantine for all imported exotic birds, the use of antibiotic-containing bird feed, and a high index of suspicion when a pet bird becomes ill have all contributed to a drop in the incidence of psittacosis. When human disease is diagnosed, epidemiologic studies to identify and control the source should be conducted. There is no vaccine available.

RICKETTSIAE AND RELATED ORGANISMS

The rickettsiae are **obligate intracellular parasites.** With the exception of Q fever, which is transmitted by aerosols, these organisms are transmitted to humans by **arthropod vectors.** The most common disease in the United States, caused by *Rickettsia rickettsii*, a member of this group, is Rocky Mountain spotted fever (RMSF), which accounts for greater than 95% of rickettsial diseases reported in the United States. Approximately 600–700 cases are reported annually. Most cases of RMSF occur in the South Central and Southeast states, rather than in the Rocky Mountains. Two newly described diseases in humans, bacillary angiomatosis and ehrlichiosis, have also been associated with related bacteria. *Rochalimaea* and *Bartonella* species, fastidious gram-negative bacteria that are related to the rickettsiae, can be grown on artificial media. Key etiologic agents, their diseases, and their vectors are shown in Table 23.3. Treatment of rickettsial diseases usually involves tetracycline or doxycycline, but **not penicillins** (due to the organism's lack of cell walls).

ROCKY MOUNTAIN SPOTTED FEVER

Rocky Mountain spotted fever is a disease of individuals who work or play in endemic areas and thus can become exposed to **infected ticks.** The disease is not confined to rural areas, however. A surprising mini-epidemic occurred in New York City in 1987 when infected ticks established a focus in a local park in the

TABLE 23.3. Etiologic Agents, Their Diseases, and Vectors

Species	Disease	Vector
Rickettsia akari	Rickettsialpox	Mites
Rickettsia prowazekii	Brill-Zinsser Epidemic typhus	Lice
Rickettsia rickettsii	RMSF	Ticks
Rickettsia tsutsugamushi	Scrub typhus	Mites
Rickettsia typhi	Murine (endemic typhus)	Fleas
Rochalimaea (Bartonella) quintana	Trench fever	Lice
Rochalimaea (Bartonella) henselae	Bacillary angiomatosis	Cats (Cat fleas?)
Coxiella burnetii	Q fever	Ticks, aerosols
Ehrlichia chaffeensis	Ehrlichiosis	Ticks
Ehrlichia canis	Ehrlichiosis	Ticks

Bronx. *R. rickettsii* organisms enter the bloodstream from the tick saliva and disseminate hematogenously.

The disease is characterized by fever, headache, and an unusually distributed **rash** that often **spreads from the extremities toward the trunk.** Older patients are more vulnerable and the case fatality rate is approximately 8% in persons 30 years or older versus 1% for younger patients. As with most of the rickettsial disease, the rash is the result of organisms (*R. rickettsii*) proliferating in the endothelial cells of the circulatory system causing vasculitis.

Specific immunofluorescent stains are available at state health departments in endemic areas for use in visualizing the organism directly in biopsy specimens obtained from the skin rash. In most cases, the **diagnosis is made serologically.** Latex agglutination and microimmunofluorescence tests are useful. The Weil-Felix test, an agglutination of certain strains of *Proteus* species by patient serum, has been used historically for serologic diagnosis, but has been supplanted by newer, more specific methods.

Rickettsialpox is a milder disease caused by a similar agent, *Rickettsia akari*, and is characterized by a vesicular rash with vesicles that crust over and heal.

TYPHUS

Brill-Zinsser disease or recrudescent typhus and the primary disease, **louse-borne typhus** or **epidemic typhus,** are characterized by headache, chills, fever, and a rash that spreads from the trunk to the extremities. The *Rickettsia prowazekii* organisms infect the GI tract of lice and gain entry to the human host when the louse defecates during feeding. The louse itself is killed by the infection, in contrast to RMSF in which rickettsiae are transmitted vertically to the offspring of infected ticks.

Conditions of overcrowding and poor hygiene foster louse infestation and encourage disease acquisition. The disease is rare in the United States. Although a moderately effective vaccine exists, it is recommended only for persons at high risk, such as visitors to foreign endemic areas. Epidemic typhus has been enormously important throughout history, contributing to victories and defeats in major wars. It has added to the devastation of populations during times of plague. Thus, the disease has probably played a role in shaping the political and economic state of the world today.

Murine typhus, caused by *R. typhi,* is more common in the United States, with 50 cases reported in 1990. The oriental rat flea is the primary vector, thus persons living in contact with rats are at risk. As with epidemic typhus, feces of the arthropod vector carry the organism (*R. typhi*) into the human host. The associated rash usually remains on the trunk.

Diagnosis is made serologically. Although the organism can be cultured from blood, this is attempted only by a few specialized laboratories.

Q FEVER

Q fever usually presents as an acute febrile illness with headache and frequently hepatitis. Although tick-borne Q fever is known, most cases are acquired by **aerosols.** The etiologic agent, *Coxiella burnetii,* is shed in the feces and genital secretions (placentas or birth fluids) of infected domestic animals, such as sheep, cattle, and goats. Because of its resistance to drying, the organism remains viable in aerosols and causes disease when inhaled by humans. Slaughterhouse workers and veterinarians are at particular risk. A recent outbreak was also reported in California in which the disease was acquired by drinking unpasteurized milk. The organism grows in the phagolysosome and is an example of an acidophilic pathogen.

As with the other rickettsial diseases, laboratory diagnosis is made by immunofluorescence tests because of the danger to laboratory workers associated with attempts to isolate the agent in culture.

TRENCH FEVER AND BACILLARY ANGIOMATOSIS

Rochalimaea (Bartonella) quintana is the etiologic agent of a rare febrile disease, trench fever. Patients are infected by human body lice and exhibit fever, rash, splenomegaly, and myalgias.

The very recently discovered new member of the genus, *Rochalimaea (Bartonella) henselae*, was isolated from the blood of patients with fever. Concurrently, the same organism was identified by molecular methods to be associated with bacillary angiomatosis, a vascular proliferative disease of immunocompromised patients. Cat scratch disease is also associated with these agents. Cats and possibly cat fleas have been associated with transmission. Further studies are in progress to characterize the agent and define the spectrum of diseases with which it may be associated. Both *Rochalimaea (Bartonella)* species can be cultivated on artificial media, although the methods are laborious.

Another bacterium similar to the rickettsiae, *Bartonella bacilliformis*, produces a vascular proliferative lesion similar to that of *R. (Bartonella) henselae*. The disease caused by *B. bacilliformis,* verruga peruana or Carrion's disease, is limited to certain areas of South and Central America. Its vector is the phlebotomus sandfly. The relationships among these rare bacterial strains and emerging new diseases is a fascinating and evolving story.

EHRLICHIOSIS

Canine ehrlichiosis is transmitted by the dog tick and is characterized by an acute phase of pancytopenia and a chronic phase with fever, anemia, and occasional bleeding from the capillaries. Diseases caused by both *Ehrlichia canis* and *Ehrlichia chaffeensis* have been described only recently in humans. Thought to be transmitted by ticks, human ehrlichiosis resembles rickettsial disease, with fever, headache, hepatitis, and myalgias. Hematologic abnormalities, such as leukopenia and thrombocytopenia, are common. *Ehrlichia* species grow in leukocytes. Ehrlichiosis is distinguished from RMSF by the absence of a rash. Most cases have occurred in the Southeast or South Central United States.

MYCOPLASMA

Mycoplasmas are the **smallest prokaryotes capable of extracellular self-reproduction.** The name pleuropneumonia-like organism (PPLO) was given to early isolates because they resembled the original strain recovered from the lungs of a cow suffering from pleuropneumonia. The name is still used to refer to some mycoplasma media. There are more than 10 species of *Mycoplasma* and *Ureaplasma,* but only a few species have been associated with human disease. As laboratory tests for detection of these agents become more prevalent, mycoplasmas are being associated with an increasing number of infectious conditions.

Mycoplasmas share the same general properties. These organisms have a poorly gram-negative staining cell membrane. **Absence of a cell wall and peptidoglycan layer** explains their **resistance to penicillins** and other cell wall active antibiotics. Mycoplasmas are highly pleomorphic and flexible, which allows them to pass through filters that would retain other bacteria.

MYCOPLASMA PNEUMONIAE PNEUMONIA

Mycoplasma pneumoniae is the agent of **"primary atypical pneumonia,"** also called "walking pneumonia." It is the best characterized of the human pathogens among the mycoplasmas. The organism may be responsible for as many as 50% of all noninfluenza community-acquired pneumonias. The disease is primarily seen in children and young adults, particularly college students and military recruits.

Habitat

M. pneumoniae is a respiratory pathogen of humans, with no other known animal host. Once infected, patients continue to shed the organism in respiratory secretions for long periods of time.

Transmission

The disease is transmitted from human to human through respiratory secretions.

Pathogenesis and Clinical Manifestations

Once **inhaled,** the organisms **attach by their tips to a glycoprotein** on the host **epithelial cell surface** that is also present on the surface of erythrocytes (Fig. 23.4). The mycoplasmas remain extracellular and exert damaging effects on the

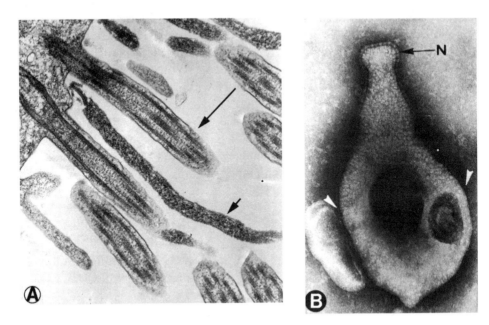

Figure 23.4.

(A) Transmission electron micrograph of *Mycoplasma* (short arrow) attached to cilia (long arrow) of respiratory epithelial cell. (Courtesy of Albert M. Collier, University of North Carolina at Chapel Hill.). (B) Negative staining of intact *Mycoplasma* cell. Note the flask like shape, the truncated tip, the nap (N) on the terminus extending distally to the area marked by the arrowhead. [Reproduced with permission from Tully JG, Taylor-Robinson D, Rose DL, Cole RM, and Bove JM (1983): *Mycoplasma genitalium*, a new species from the human urogenital tract. Int J Syst Bacteriol 33(2):387. © American Society for Microbiology.]

host ciliated respiratory epithelial cell membranes. Approximately 3 weeks after infection, the membranes begin to leak, ciliary activity is disrupted, and the host responds with a mononuclear cell infiltrate. It is postulated that most of the disease syndrome is due to subsequent epithelial cell damage inflicted by the **host immune response.** A broad range of manifestations have been documented, from asymptomatic infection to serious systemic disease involving the CNS or the heart. Serious disease is quite rare and usually occurs in older patients.

The major syndrome is **pneumonia,** characterized by nonproductive cough, fever, and chest pain. Pharyngitis and bronchitis are additional disease manifestations.

Immunity to Reinfection

Antibodies and memory T cells are produced in response to primary infection. Although reinfection does occur, the normal immune response appears to be somewhat protective.

Laboratory Diagnosis

Several tests are now available to substantiate the clinical diagnosis. Either sputum or a nasopharyngeal swab should be collected. Isolating the organism in culture is not difficult, although culture is not always available. Direct detection of *M. pneumoniae* nucleic acid by a commercially available DNA probe yields results similar to those of culture. Serologic tests, including indirect immunofluorescence, latex agglutination, and ELISA assays for both IgG and IgM have been shown to detect specific antibody during the acute stage of the disease. These newer tests have supplanted the classical complement-fixation and ''cold agglutinin'' assays.

Treatment

Erythromycin is the traditional drug of choice, although treatment is not always effective. Tetracyclines have also been used with some success.

Prevention and Control

There is no effective vaccine available.

OTHER MYCOPLASMAL DISEASES

Several other species of mycoplasmas have now been unequivocally implicated as etiologic agents of infection. *Mycoplasma hominis,* a member of the normal genitourinary flora in humans, can cause postsurgical wound infections and is one of the most common agents of postpartum septicemia in women. Intraamniotic disease and disease in neonates leading to premature labor and delivery have also been attributed to *M. hominis. Mycoplasma genitalium,* another human genital mycoplasma, has been implicated as a cause of pneumonia.

Ureaplasma urealyticum, a mycoplasma that possesses a urease enzyme, is extremely common (up to 70%) in the vaginas of sexually active young women. Although it does not seem to be pathogenic in males, it is thought to be an agent of the acute urethral syndrome in women and to contribute to neonatal morbidity as a cause of chorioamnionitis. *U. urealyticum* also causes respiratory tract infection in neonates.

A previously rarely isolated mycoplasma, *Mycoplasma fermentans* (also called *Mycoplasm incognitus*), has been isolated from AIDS patients and from a small number of immunologically competent patients that suddenly suffered massive and fatal systemic disease. This agent may be one ''cofactor'' in the multisystem degeneration seen in AIDS patients, although its role in disease is controversial.

SUMMARY

1. The chlamydiae and mycoplasmas are bacteria with unusual or absent cell walls. *Chlamydia* **and** *Rickettsia* **are obligate intracellular parasites, causing disease by damaging the host cells in which they reproduce.**

2. *Chlamydia trachomatis, Chlamydia psittaci***, and** *Chlamydia pneumoniae* **are the three species that cause human disease.** *C. trachomatis***, the agent of trachoma, is the most important cause of blindness worldwide.**

3. *C. trachomatis* **diseases are among the most common STDs in the United States. These diseases include cervicitis, which often leads to pelvic inflammatory disease and subsequent infertility, urethritis, and LGV.**

4. Infants acquire *C. trachomatis* **conjunctivitis and pneumonia after becoming colonized by organisms acquired in the birth canal of the mother.**

5. *C. pneumoniae* **(TWAR strain of** *Chlamydia***) causes an atypical pneumonia similar clinically to that of** *Mycoplasma pneumoniae***.**

6. *Chlamydia psittaci* **causes an acute, febrile pneumonia in persons who handle birds.**

7. *Rickettsia* **spp. are almost all transmitted to humans by way of arthropod vectors. For example, (a) epidemic typhus: lice; (b) Rocky Mountain spotted fever: ticks; (c) scrub typhus: mites; (d) murine typhus: fleas; and (e) trench fever: lice.**

8. *M. pneumoniae* causes atypical pneumonia, the most common pneumonic respiratory tract disease in young adults. The organism attaches to respiratory epithelial cells and interferes with their function without producing toxin or invading the cells.

9. Other mycoplasmas, including *Mycoplasma hominis* and *Ureaplasma urealyticum*, are found in human genital tracts. These organisms cause postpartum fever and may contribute to infertility. *M. hominis* can cause postsurgical wound infections.

REFERENCES

Barnes RC (1989): Laboratory diagnosis of human chlamydial infections. Clin Microbiol Rev 2:119.

Feld RD (1990): Q fever. Diagn Clin Testing 28:30.

Grayston JT, Kuo C-C, Wang S-P, Altman J (1986): A new *Chlamydia psittaci* strain, TWAR, isolated in acute respiratory tract infections. N Engl J Med 315:161.

Hammerschlag MR, Chirgwin K, Roblin PM, Gelling M, Dumornay W, Mandel L, Smith P, Schachter J (1992): Persistent infection with *Chlamydia pneumoniae* following acute respiratory illness. Clin Infect Dis 14:178.

Lo SC et al. (1989): Identification of *Mycoplasma incognitus* infection in patients with AIDS: an immunohistochemical, *in situ* hybridization and ultrastructural study. Am J Trop Med Hyg 41:601.

Maeda K, Markowitz N, Hawley RC, Ristic M, Cox D, McDade JE (1987): Human infection with *Ehrlichia canis,* a leukocytic rickettsia. N Engl J Med 316:853.

McMahon DK, Dummer JS, Pasculle AW, Cassell G (1990): Extragenital *Mycoplasma hominis* infections in adults. Am J Med 89:275.

Moulder JW (1984): Looking at chlamydiae without looking at their hosts. ASM News 50:353.

Relman DA, Loutit JS, Schmidt TM, Falkow S, Tompkins LS (1990): The agent of bacillary angiomatosis: an approach to the identification of uncultured pathogens. N Engl J Med 323:1573.

Rikihisa Y (1991): The tribe *Ehrlichieae* and ehrlichial diseases. Clin Microbiol Rev 4:286.

Salgo MP, et al. (1988): A focus of Rocky Mountain Spotted Fever within New York City. N Engl J Med 318:1345.

Slater LN, Welch DF, Hensel D, Coody DW (1990): A newly recognized fastidious gram-negative pathogen as a cause of fever and bacteremia. N Engl J Med 323:1587.

Thompson SE, Washington AE (1983): Epidemiology of sexually transmitted *Chlamydia trachomatis* infections. Epidemiol Rev 5:96.

REVIEW QUESTIONS

For questions 1 to 4, choose the ONE
BEST answer or completion.

1. Which response is true for both *Chlamydia*
   and *Rickettsia*.
   a) The primary mode of transmission is by
      way of respiratory secretions.
   b) Only those β-lactam antibiotic agents that
      penetrate into infected human cells are ef-
      fective for treating these agents, since
      they are intracellular pathogens.
   c) Both genera contain some species that are
      carried to humans by an arthropod vector.
   d) They both cause disease characterized by
      a prominent skin rash that begins on the
      extremities.
   e) Both genera consist of bacteria without
      cell walls.

2. The etiologic agents of *Chlamydia*-associ-
   ated neonatal pneumonitis (*Chlamydia trachomatis*) and adult atypical pneumonia
   (*Chlamydia pneumoniae*) can be distinguished from each other on the basis of
   a) type of inclusion seen in tissue culture
      (glycogen containing versus nonglycogen
      containing)
   b) serologic typing of isolated strains

c) biochemical reactions (urease, esculin
   hydrolysis, etc.)
d) presence or absence of elementary bodies
   on direct fluorescent antibody stained ocular secretions
e) ability to grow in yolk sac of embryonated hens' eggs

3. The primary virulence factor of chlamydiae
   is
   a) major outer membrane proteins that me-
      diate attachment to host epithelial cells
   b) production of a toxin that inhibits mu-
      cociliary action
   c) antiphagocytic capsule
   d) ability to multiply intracellularly by in-
      hibiting lysosomal fusion with the phag-
      osome
   e) ability to multiply intracellularly by es-
      caping the phagosome and carrying on
      the developmental cycle in the cytoplasm

4. Which one of the following disease-vector
   pairs is correct?
   a) Epidemic typhus: lice
   b) Scrub typhus: ticks
   c) Rocky Mountain spotted fever: mites
   d) Trench fever: ticks
   e) Ehrlichiosis: fleas

For questions 5 to 12, a list of lettered options is followed by several numbered items. For each numbered item, select the ONE lettered option that is most closely associated with it.

A) *Chlamydia trachomatis serovar* A–C
B) *Chlamydia trachomatis serovar* L1–L3
C) *Chlamydia psittaci*
D) *Chlamydia pneumoniae*
E) *Mycoplasma pneumoniae*

For each species, select the most likely associated disease characterization.

5. A young, sexually active woman presents to the Emergency Room with abdominal pain, a high WBC, and increased liver function tests. The diagnosis is pelvic inflammatory disease with Fitz-Hugh Curtis syndrome (perihepatitis).

6. A young man visited a prostitute during a recent trip to Kenya. He presents to his physician 3 weeks later with prominent swollen and painful inguinal lymph nodes.

7. A baby born to a sexually active drug abuser in New York City has respiratory distress and pneumonitis within 2 months of leaving the hospital. She had been given erythromycin eyedrops at birth, according to the hospital policy.

8. A college student feels slightly fatigued and short of breath. The doctor diagnoses "primary atypical pneumonia."

9. A young man acquires a new job handling cockatoos at Wild Animal Park in San Diego. Within 2 weeks, he develops headache and fever, and, after an additional week, he develops a hacking cough.

A) *Mycoplasma pneumoniae*
B) *Mycoplasma hominis*
C) *Mycoplasma genitalium*
D) *Mycoplasma fermentans*
E) *Ureaplasma urealyticum*

For each of the species of mycobacteria listed, select the associated clinical syndrome.

10. Post-open-heart surgery sternal wound infection

11. Postpartum fever in a gravida one, para one female

12. Asymptomatic vaginal carriage by the majority of sexually active younger women

ANSWERS TO REVIEW QUESTIONS

1. *e* These obligate intracellular parasites do not possess a typical bacterial cell wall, so β-lactam agents are never effective agents for treatment. Only rickettsiae are transmitted by arthropods; chlamydiae are primarily transmitted by contact with secretions. Chlamydial infection does not result in a rash.

2. *a* Culture results in definitive diagnosis, although serologic tests on patient sera are used more commonly in reality.

3. *d* The organisms induce endocytosis in nonprofessional phagocytes. Once inside, they prevent lysosomal fusion and multiply within the phagosome. As intracellular parasites, they inhibit host cell function and induce an inflammatory response. Antibodies directed against MOMPs are not protective, thus these proteins are probably not virulence factors. The organisms do not produce toxins.

4. *a* Epidemic typhus and Trench fever are both spread by lice. Rocky Mountain spotted fever and Ehrlichiosis are both carried by ticks. Scrub typhus is transmitted by mites.

5. *A* *Chlamydia trachomatis* serovars A–C is the most prevalent sexually transmitted

disease in the United States. Complications include pelvic inflammatory disease and perihepatitis.

6. *B* The L-lettered serovars of *C. trachomatis* cause lymphogranuloma venereum, characterized by painful inguinal "buboes," or swollen lymph glands. This is another sexually transmitted chlamydial disease.

7. *A* *Chlamydia trachomatis* serovars A–C can be acquired by the neonate during passage through an infected birth canal. The resulting diseases include inclusion conjunctivitis (prevented by erythromycin drops, whose primary function is to prevent neonatal gonococcal conjuncitivitis) and later neonatal pneumonitis.

8. *E* *Mycoplasma pneumoniae* is the classical cause of "primary atypical pneumoniae." Although *Chlamydia pneumoniae* may cause a similar disease, it is less common and seems to cause more serious disease in elderly and debilitated patients.

9. *C* Parrots, parakeets, cockatoos, and other exotic and domestic birds may harbor *Chlamydia psittaci,* which causes a systemic and pneumonia-like disease called ornithosis or psittacosis in susceptible

patients. The organism is probably transmitted by aerosols from droppings and secretions on feathers.

10. **B** Recently recognized to be an important cause of postsurgical wound infections, *Mycoplasma hominis* is often not detected on routine bacteriological cultures.

11. **B** *Mycoplasma hominis* is carried asymptomatically in the vaginas of a small percentage of women; during delivery it can enter the bloodstream and cause postpartum fever in the mother and perinatal sepsis in the fetus.

12. **E** *Ureaplasma urealyticum* is the most common mycoplasma in humans. Its role in infectious disease has not been elucidated.

SPIROCHETAL INFECTION AND DISEASE

Spirochetes are unicellular, slender, helical-shaped or corkscrewlike, flexible organisms actively motile by virtue of periplasmic flagella (syn: endoflagella, axial filaments) that lie in the periplasmic space between the cytoplasmic and outer membranes. Many occur as free living saprophytes in soil, water, and decaying matter, while others are either animal and/or human pathogens or host indigenous nonpathogens. The three genera of the order Spirochaetales that contain human pathogens are *Treponema, Borrelia,* and *Leptospira.*

TREPONEMATOSES

The treponematoses are chronic inflammatory diseases, primarily of the skin and mucous membrane surfaces, which may affect other organs and tissues usually following a latent period. The comparative etiologic agents, portals of entry, incubation periods, and basic clinical manifestations of the treponematoses are described in Table 24.1.

Although DNA homology between *Treponema pallidum* subsp. *pallidum* and *Treponema pallidum* subsp. *pertenue* is almost 100%, subspecies nomenclature is

459

based on differences described in Table 24.1 and the differences in their geographic location and pathogenicity for experimental animals. The variant status of *Treponema pallidum* subsp. *endemicum* has warranted subspecies classification for this organism. However, the inability to obtain sufficient numbers of *Treponema carateum* to conduct homology studies has precluded assignment of subspecies status to this treponeme. In addition to the similarities and differences noted in Table 24.1, each of the organisms are obligate parasites of humans and morphologically identical, but differ in their pathogenicity and degree of virulence for experimental animals. Furthermore, the diseases differ in their geographic distribution, with only syphilis occurring in the United States, but the laboratory diagnosis and treatment for each are similar.

TABLE 24.1. Some Basic Features of the Treponematoses

	Syphilis	Yaws	Endemic syphilis	Pinta
Etiologic agent	*Treponema pallidum* subsp. *pallidum*	*T. pallidum* subsp. *pertenue*	*T. pallidum* subsp. *endemicum*	*Treponema carateum*
Portal of entry	Genitalia and extragenital	Exposed skin	Oral mucosa and skin	Exposed skin
Incubation period	Usually 3 weeks (10–90 days)	Usually 3 weeks (10–90 days)	3 weeks	Usually 2–3 weeks (3 days to 2 months)
Primary lesions	Yes	Yes	Rare	Yes
Lymphadenitis	Yes	Yes	Yes	Occasional
Secondary lesions	Yes Any tissue	Yes Skin, cartilage, and bone	Yes Skin, buccal mucosa, and bone	Yes Skin
Latency	Yes	Yes	Yes	Unknown
Tertiary lesions Benign Malignant	Yes Yes	Yes No	Yes Rare	Yes No
Congenital	Yes	No	No	No

SYPHILIS

Syphilis is sometimes referred to in the vernacular as "lues" or "bad blood". In the United States, approximately 28,000–50,000 new cases of primary and secondary syphilis have been reported annually to the CDC since 1985, representing a steady increase (Fig. 24.1B). Alarmingly, early congenital syphilis has risen sharply from about 300 reported cases in 1985 to 2850 in 1990 (Fig. 24.1A); 1702 cases have already been reported through mid-1992. Although the acquired disease can occur in any sexually active individual, there has been a shift in greater prevalence from the male homosexual to the heterosexual population, presumably due to AIDS awareness and adjustment. It has been estimated that there are more than 100,000 patients with syphilis in the United States, due mostly to under reporting by physicians. Furthermore, millions of dollars are spent caring for those suffering from the debilitating tertiary manifestations of the disease.

Habitat

T. pallidum subsp. *pallidum* is an obligate parasite of humans. The organism does not occur in nature or in animals.

Transmission

EXOGENOUS. Acquired disease may be transmitted by the exogenous route. Organisms gain entrance through the abraded skin or onto mucous membrane surfaces following sexual contact, including oral and anal sex, with patients in the primary or secondary stage of the disease. Congenital syphilis is the result of exogenous transmission from the infected mother to the fetus. Although transmission of infection or disease to the fetus may result from a female in any stage of the disease, the greatest frequency (70–100%) occurs among patients with primary or secondary syphilis. Passage across the placenta prior to the eighteenth week of gestation is an **infrequent** occurrence.

ENDOGENOUS. Endogenous activation resulting in secondary disease may occur in patients with latent infection. Endogenous activation resulting in tertiary or late syphilis may also occur in patients with latent syphilis.

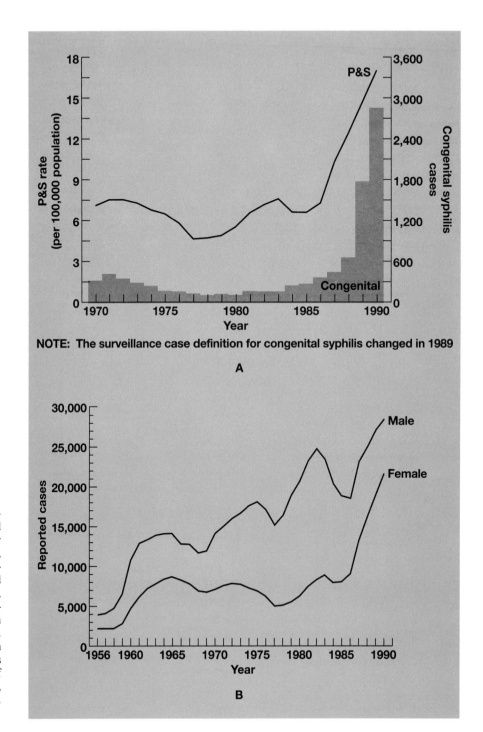

NOTE: The surveillance case definition for congenital syphilis changed in 1989

A

B

Figure 24.1.

Syphilis. (A) Congenital (under 1 year) and primary and secondary (P&S) among women, United States, 1970–1990. (B) Primary and secondary, by sex, United States, 1956–1990. [Redrawn with permission from U.S. Department of Health and Human Services (1991): Summary of notifiable diseases, United States, 1990. MMWR 39:no. 53.]

Properties of the Organism

Resistance to environmental, physical, and chemical agents. Treponemes are very sensitive to environmental conditions and to physical and chemical agents. The organisms die rapidly on fomites, such as doorknobs and toilet seats.

Microscopic morphology. T. pallidum subsp. *pallidum* is a medium coiled, thin, flexible spirochete, 5–20 μ in length and 0.2 μ in diameter. The organism is actively motile, exhibiting a "shimmering" motion in serous exudate and a directional, corkscrewlike motion in fibrinous exudate. Treponemes stain poorly or not all with the usual aniline dyes, but stain well by silver impregnation methods. The organism is best recognized and studied by **dark field microscopy** (Fig. 24.2).

Macroscopic morphology. **None of the pathogenic treponemes has been cultured in/on artificial media.** Limited growth of *T. pallidum* subsp. *pallidum* has been accomplished in a tissue culture monolayer system under microaerophilic conditions. Primary disease and latency can be induced experimentally in the **rabbit,** which serves as a source of treponemes for propagation, specific antigen preparation, and experimental studies.

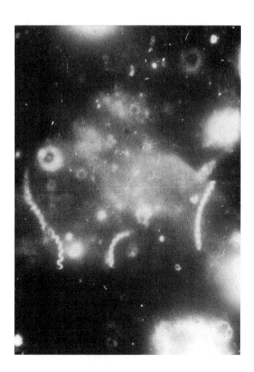

Figure 24.2.

T. pallidum subsp. *pallidum* by dark field microscopy in exudate from a human chancre. (Courtesy of the J.B. Lippincott Co.)

Nonpathogenic treponemes. There are several nonpathogenic species of *Treponema* indigenous to humans. They are harbored in the oral cavity, GI tract, and/or in and around the genitalia, and may closely resemble or be identical to the pathogen in morphology and motility. Like the pathogenic treponemes, they stain well by silver impregnation methods. Unequivocal differentiation may be difficult or impossible in early lesions.

Antigenic structure. Antigenic structural components related to virulence and diagnosis are not well understood. Recent evidence indicates that the **outer membrane of *T. pallidum* subsp. *pallidum* contains rare protein that may be essential for virulence and protective immunogenicity.** Endoflagellar, periplasmic, and/or inner-membrane proteins or lipoproteins are undoubtedly responsible for the stimulation of antibodies that develop during the course of the disease, but those responsible for the specific reactivity obtained with the standard diagnostic treponemal tests have not been isolated or identified. There is no definitive evidence that the haptene cardiolipin, an active phospholipid present in normal mammalian tissue and the antigen utilized in nontreponemal tests, is present in pathogenic treponemes. Antibody formation in these assays appears to be the result of cardiolipin release from tissues following the active disease process, and subsequent combination with treponemal or host protein to stimulate the antibody. The organism does not contain LPS.

Extracellular products associated with or thought to be associated with pathogenicity. Extracellular virulence factors have not been identified.

Pathogenesis and Clinical Manifestations

ACQUIRED SYPHILIS. In the acquired form of the uncomplicated disease, organisms gain entrance through the abraded skin or onto mucous membrane surfaces, **attach by their tips to host cells,** and colonize. Within a few hours, significant numbers of organisms leave the local site and are carried to the regional lymph nodes. Dissemination to several organs and tissues, particularly the liver, spleen, and bone marrow, occurs through the circulation, the organisms exiting through the tight junctions of the vascular endothelial cells and appearing to take up an extracellular and intracellular residence.

Establishment of the organisms in the CNS, kidneys, and bone does occur in some patients, but transient location appears to be the rule. Multiplication at the site of entry and in the regional lymph nodes, where the organisms are predominantly extracellular, induces primarily a **chronic inflammatory response** characterized by an influx of **plasma cells, lymphocytes, and macrophages,** and a leakage of fluid containing **immunoglobulin and complement.**

Primary Stage. This stage of the disease occurs after an incubation period ranging from 10 to 90 days, but usually 3 weeks, and is the end result of the local confrontation. Primary syphilis is characterized by the appearance of a painless, indurated, well-circumscribed ulcer, known as a **chancre,** accompanied by a regional lymphadenopathy that is usually bilateral. At this time, the chancre and lymph nodes contain treponemes and the disease is **communicable.** As the inflammatory cells peak, the primary lesions heal in 1–6 weeks, presumably due to **CMI** mechanisms involving macrophages activated by MAF released by antigen-specific, sensitized T cells with some contribution from relatively low levels of complement-mediated treponemicidal antibody. During this local healing process, organisms within the deeper tissues survive and undergo slow but continuous multiplication, setting up foci of infection. Survival may be the result of **intracellular establishment** by relatively few organisms following their introduction into the host and/or **few outer membrane targets for the immune response.**

Secondary Stage. This stage of the disease is initiated when organisms gain access to the circulation from these infected foci, produce a **septicemia,** and are carried to lymph nodes and previously infected and uninfected tissues, where extracellular multiplication again induces a chronic inflammatory response and some organisms presumably take up an **intracellular residence.** It occurs simultaneously with or up to 6 months after the healing of the primary lesions and is the end result of the confrontation.

Secondary syphilis is characterized by fever, headache, **generalized lymphadenopathy, a generalized rash with lesions characteristically on the palms and soles, mucous patches in the oral cavity, condylomata in the moist regions, and alopecia.** Occasionally, hepatosplenomegaly, nephritis due to immune complex formation, and periostitis may occur. At this time, secondary lesions also contain treponemes and the disease is **communicable.**

Latent Stage. This stage of the disease, representing a perfect host-parasite relationship in which there are no clinical manifestations, is ushered in when healing of the secondary lesions occurs, usually in 3 weeks to 3 months. This occurrence is presumably due to a more **pronounced and generalized CMI** and humoral response in which activated macrophages and complement-mediated treponemicidal antibody are operative on **extracellular (but not intracellular)** organisms. **At least 25% of patients develop a recurrence of the secondary stage,** usually within 1 year after healing of the initial secondary lesions, by mechanisms as yet unknown. Healing, resulting in latency, again occurs for the putative reasons described. For epidemiological tracing and the administration of appropriate treatment regimens, latency has been divided into early latent syphilis of less than 1-year duration and late latent syphilis of more than 1-year duration. Although transmission of treponemes from an infected mother to fetus can occur during latency, the absence of exposed lesions precludes communicability of the acquired disease during this stage. About two-thirds of untreated patients remain in the latent state for the rest of their lives or ''spontaneously cure,'' depending on their level of complement-dependent treponemicidal antibody, the extent of their CMI response, and the degree of access of intracellular treponemes to immune components.

Tertiary or Late Stage. This stage of the disease occurs in the remaining (approximately one-third) patients, in which there is an upset in host-parasite balance in favor of the spirochete, presumably due to a **waning of complement-dependent treponemicidal antibody and CMI.** This loss of acquired resistance may occur anywhere from months to more than 50 years after the initiation of latency. As a result, treponemes exit from the host cells and invade the CNS, cardiovascular system, eye, skin, and/or other internal organs, where they produce damage by virtue of their **invasive properties or DTH reaction** on previously sensitized tissues.

There are two types of neurosyphilis. **Symptomatic neurosyphilis** is the result of treponemal invasion and destruction of the brain parenchyma (paresis), dorsal roots of the spinal cord (tabes), or both (taboparesis); meningitis, optic atrophy, or meningovascular damage may also occur. **Asymptomatic neurosyphilis** occurs when treponemes invade the CNS without producing overt clinical manifestations.

Damage to the cardiovascular system may be the result of invasion or a DTH response, resulting in **cardiovascular syphilis**. This disease manifests as a thoracic aortic aneurysm, aortitis, and/or aortic endocarditis.

Benign gummatous syphilis manifests as destructive, granulomatous, non-progressive lesions of the skin, bone, or viscera and may occur as a result of a DTH response to treponemal antigens. Treponemes are rarely, if ever, found in the lesions, which are referred to as **benign gummas.** Transmission of the acquired disease during the tertiary stage does not occur, while congenital transmission during this stage of the disease is rare.

Acquired Syphilis in AIDS and HIV-Positive Patients. This disease usually results in a higher prevalence of recurrent secondary syphilis, and a **more rapidly progressive involvement of the CNS** during or shortly following the early course of the disease. The response is presumably due to impaired CMI.

CONGENITAL SYPHILIS. Congenital syphilis is the result of transplacental transmission from an infected mother to the fetus, **usually not until 18 weeks after gestation.** Although the mechanisms of pathogenesis are unknown, the extent of damage to the fetus depends on the stage of the disease and the number of treponemes circulating in the pregnant female at the time of transmission. Overwhelming invasion by the organisms results in a miscarriage or stillbirth.

In **early congenital syphilis,** depending on the infecting dose, the infant may present with typical clinical manifestations of early congenital syphilis either at birth or up to 2 years of age following in utero septicemic spread. These manifestations include extensive cutaneous lesions characterized as vesicular, bulbous, or papulosquamous, mucous membrane lesions that manifest as a mucoid discharge from the nose (snuffles) or rhinitis, osteochondritis of the long bones, anemia, hepatosplenomegaly, and/or CNS disease.

In **late congenital syphilis,** damage of certain tissues in utero may not appear until beyond 2 years of age. Clinical manifestations include interstitial keratitis, eighth nerve deafness, interference with second tooth development (notched and spaced incisors, ''raspberry'' molars), damage to long bones (sabre shins), perforated nasal septum (saddle nose), and/or cutaneous gummas.

Immunity to Reinfection

Little or no immunity develops to reinfection following treated or untreated primary and secondary syphilis. Immunity to reinfection in treated and untreated latency varies from partial to complete.

Laboratory Diagnosis

An accurate history of recent sexual contact or past disease is essential. Although the patient could present with no clinical manifestations referrable to syphilis, a physical examination should be conducted. It is important to bear in mind that this disease has been called ''the great imitator'' due to the great diversity of clinical manifestations that can be expressed.

SPECIMENS AND DIRECT EXAMINATION. Specimens obtained depend on the disease process. They include material from early acquired and congenital lesions, lymph node aspirates, blood for serology, and cerebrospinal fluid. The identification by **dark field microscopy** of morphologically typical treponemes with characteristic motility in genital and skin lesions of early acquired and congenital syphilis is compelling evidence that the organism is *T. pallidum* subsp.

pallidum (see Fig. 24.2). However, the potential presence of nonpathogens with similar morphology and motility precludes a definitive conclusion. The demonstration by dark field microscopy of typical treponemes in aspirated lymph nodes is definitive inasmuch as these tissues are sterile in the absence of infection.

Dark field examination of oral and anal lesions is often not attempted due to the likelihood of error that can result from the presence of nonpathogenic treponemes. In addition to the limitations of specificity, dark field microscopy may fail to reveal pathogenic treponemes due to the presence of few organisms in the lesion or lymph node.

A PCR assay has been developed for use in the diagnosis of syphilis, but is frought with problems relating to specificity.

IMMUNOSEROLOGIC BLOOD TESTS. Immunoserologic blood tests, of which there are two types, are the most commonly employed assays in the laboratory diagnosis of syphilis.

Nontreponemal tests are **screening procedures** that utilize as antigen an active phospholipid known as cardiolipin fortified with lecithin and cholesterol. The two assays performed routinely in almost all laboratories in the United States are the Venereal Disease Research Laboratory (VDRL) slide flocculation and the Rapid Plasma Reagin (RPR) circle card tests, both of which measure either IgG or IgM, and have the same qualitative sensitivity and specficity.

Although the sensitivity is excellent among patients with untreated secondary syphilis, early congenital syphilis, neurosyphilis (with the exception of tabes), and gummas, as many as 30% of syphilitics with untreated primary, latent, cardiovascular, late congenital, and tabes may exhibit false negative reactions. Of equal concern is the occurrence of **false positive reactions,** ranging from 0.1 to 10%, among patients with acute or chronic diseases other than syphilis and among pregnant, vaccinated, and drug-addicted individuals. The highest prevalence of false positive reactions occurs among patients with autoimmune diseases, particularly those with disseminated lupus erythematosis.

The nontreponemal tests are used as a **limited criterion for early syphilis cure following therapy** once syphilis has been confirmed. In early syphilis, a fourfold drop in titer indicates effective therapy, while a fourfold increase indicates relapse or reinfection. Titers that remain the same after treatment are not easily interpretable, but may indicate a coexisting nontreponemal disease. Inherent quantitative differences between the VDRL and RPR tests necessitate that the same assay be used for initial and posttherapy testing. Patients with early syphilis exhibit a significant drop in titer 2–3 months after effective treatment with conversion to nonreactivity occurring in 6 months to 2 years. Titers of patients with late latent or late syphilis usually show little or no change and, therefore, cannot be generally used as a criterion for cure.

The diagnosis of early congenital syphilis can be made on the basis of nontreponemal titers. However, inasmuch as nontreponemal antibody can cross the placenta, a distinction must be made between passive transfer of antibody from the mother and antibody manufactured by the newborn in response to the organism. Evidence for early congenital syphilis is definitive if the newborn serum titer is fourfold greater than that of the serum from the mother, or if the neonate shows a fourfold increase in titer during a 3–6 month observation period. In the absence of disease, reactivity due to passive transfer should revert to nonreactive in 3–6 months.

Treponemal tests are **confirmatory procedures** that utilize as antigen *T. pallidum* subsp. *pallidum* either killed, living, or as an ultrasonic lysate. The two assays performed routinely in almost all laboratories in the United States are the fluorescent treponemal antibody absorbed (FTA-ABS) and the microhemagglutination assay-treponema pallidum (MHA-TP) tests, both of which measure IgG or IgM. These assays are employed qualitatively to resolve diagnostic problems among patients with no history or clinical manifestations of syphilis who exhibit a reactive nontreponemal test, and those patients with clinical manifestations referrable to syphilis whose nontreponemal test is nonreactive. The sensitivities of both procedures are similar except in the primary stage, where a slightly larger number of patients exhibit FTA-ABS reactivity.

In contrast to the nontreponemal tests, 96–100% of all treated and untreated patients with congenital syphilis and acquired syphilis beyond the primary stage show FTA-ABS and MHA-TP reactivity. A reactive test indicates present or past syphilis, is therefore not necessarily an indication of active disease, and **cannot be used as a criterion for cure.** Overall, the specificity of both treponemal tests is greater than **99%.** However, false positive reactions can occur among individuals with other acute or chronic diseases and conditions, including AIDS, HIV positive and autoimmune patients, as well as pregnant females and narcotic addicts. False positive FTA-ABS tests can also occur in patients with Lyme borreliosis. Inasmuch as treponemal antibodies cross the placenta, passively transferred FTA-ABS or MHA-TP antibodies may appear in neonatal serum and persist for as long as 1 year in the absence of syphilis. Persistence beyond 1 year is suggestive of congenital syphilis.

CEREBROSPINAL FLUID ASSAYS. Cerebrospinal fluid assays are used in the diagnosis of acquired and congenital neurosyphilis.

VDRL Test. A reactive VDRL test is diagnostic for treated or untreated symptomatic or asymptomatic neurosyphilis. False positive reactions rarely, if ever, occur. A nonreactive VDRL does not rule out neurosyphilis, inasmuch as 30% of such patients exhibit false negativity.

Cell Count and Total Protein. An increased cell count (>4 lymphocytes/mm^3) and/or an elevated total protein (>40 mg/dl) may suggest neurosyphilis. However, it must be kept in mind that such abnormalitites may occur in patients with other diseases of the CNS. If the assays are abnormal, the cell count tends to revert to normal in 3–6 months following effective therapy while the VDRL and total protein may not respond or revert until 1–3 years later. The relatively high false positive and false negative FTA-ABS and MHA-TP reactions on cerebrospinal fluid render these procedures of little value in the diagnosis of neurosyphilis.

IMMUNOSEROLOGIC AND CEREBROSPINAL FLUID ASSAYS ON AIDS AND HIV-POSITIVE PATIENTS WITH PROFOUND AND PROGRESSIVE SYPHILITIC DISEASE. These patients may occasionally fail to exhibit serological reactivity. Such patients must be diagnosed by the demonstration of treponemes in biopsied skin lesions utilizing silver impregnation or specific immunofluorescent techniques. In the great majority of patients, however, the serological tests are reactive and the cell count and total protein abnormal on the appropriate serum and cerebrospinal fluid samples. Nontreponemal titers are significantly higher than in non-HIV-positive or non-AIDS patients. The response of quantitative nontreponemal tests, cell counts, and total protein to effective therapy is slow compared to the treated disease in non-HIV-positive and non-AIDS patients.

Treatment

Penicillin is the drug of choice in the treatment of all stages of acquired and congenital syphilis. **Penicillin-resistant strains of *T. pallidum* have not been reported.**

For non-HIV-positive and non-AIDS patients, 2.4 million units of benzathine penicillin G administered intramuscularly in one dose is recommended for primary, secondary, and early latent syphilis of less than 1 year duration and 7.2 million units in three equal doses at weekly intervals is recommended for late latent syphilis of more than 1-year duration and tertiary syphilis excluding neurosyphilis. Neonates with congenital syphilis should be treated with 100,000–150,000 units of aqueous crystalline penicillin G daily per kilogram of body weight or 50,000 units of procaine penicillin daily per kilogram of body weight for 10–14 days. Older children and infants with congenital syphilis should be treated with 200,000–300,000 units of aqueous crystalline penicillin G daily per kilogram of body weight for 10–14 days. Patients with neurosyphilis should be treated intravenously with 12–24 million units of aqueous crystalline penicillin G daily for 10–14 days or 2.4 million units of procaine penicillin intravenously per day together with 500 mg of probenecid orally four times daily, both for 10–14 days; each regimen should be followed by 7.2 million units of benzathine penicillin G administered intramuscularly in three equal doses at weekly intervals.

Doxycycline, tetracycline, or erythromycin has been recommended for the treatment of nonpregnant penicillin-allergic patients who are neither HIV positive nor have AIDS. However, considering the inconclusive nature of their efficacy, desensitization followed by penicillin therapy is the better choice. Desensitization and penicillin therapy is also recommended for treatment of syphilis in pregnancy.

For AIDS and HIV positive patients with syphilis the following treatments are recommended. Patients with primary, secondary, early latent, and late latent syphilis with no cerebrospinal abnormalities should be treated with 7.2 million units of benzathine penicillin G in three equal doses at weekly intervals. Patients in any stage of syphilis in which there are also cerebrospinal abnormalities, including asymptomatic neurosyphilis, should be treated with the same aggressive penicillin regimen as recommended for non-HIV-positive and non-AIDS patients with neurosyphilis. Penicillin-allergic patients should be desensitized, then treated appropriately.

Prevention and Control

Case reporting to health authorities, epidemiological tracing of contacts, adequate treatment of both cases and contacts, education of populations at high risk, and the use of condoms, are essential elements for effective prevention and control. Both VDRL or RPR screening programs are of great value in controlling syphilis.

An effective vaccine has not been developed as yet. All states require prenatal and blood bank testing, several require premarital testing, and most states recommend testing hospital admissions. A nontreponemal test is performed during routine physical examinations by most physicians.

BORRELIA

LYME BORRELIOSIS

Lyme borreliosis is a tick-borne disease first recognized as a clinical entity in 1975 in Lyme, CT. The etiologic agent, in the United States and in most other parts of the world where the disease occurs, is *Borrelia burgdorferi,* named after Dr. Willy Burgdorfer, who in 1982 was the first to isolate the organism from an *Ixodes* tick vector and relate it to the disease; two additional species have been described as causative agents in areas of Europe and Asia. The disease occurs worldwide and has been reported in 46 of the 50 states in the United States. It is highly endemic in the Northeast and Midwest, particularly in the states of Connecticut, Massachusetts, Rhode Island, New Jersey, New York, Wisconsin, Minnesota, and in northern California (Fig. 24.3). A total of 9344 cases of Lyme borreliosis was reported to the CDC during 1991, establishing it as the most common vector-borne disease in this country.

Habitat

Rodents and **birds** are the primary reservoir hosts, although the organism may be harbored for short periods of time in domestic and wild animals. *Ixodes* deer ticks are the vectors known to transmit *B. burgdorferi* to humans. *Ixodes scapularis* (formerly *I. dammini*) is the vector in the Northeast and Midwest and *Ixodes pacificus* in the West; *Ixodes ricinus* and *Ixodes persulcatus* are vectors in Europe, Asia, and Australia.

Transmission

EXOGENOUS. Transmission is exclusively by the exogenous route. Although the ticks can initiate the disease during any stage in its development, transmission occurs mainly by nymphs. Spirochetes are introduced into the human host from contaminated tick saliva and feces during a blood meal. These organisms are injected directly into the circulation and/or deposited onto epidermal surfaces. Congenital disease due to maternal-fetal transmission has been reported but is not well documented.

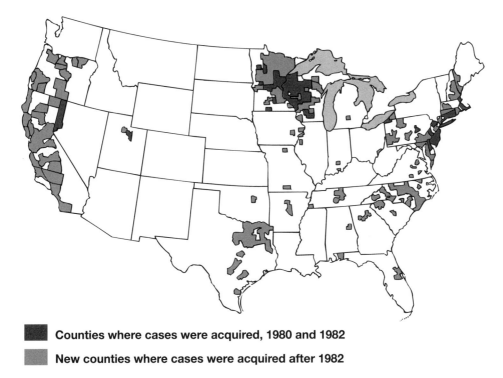

■ **Counties where cases were acquired, 1980 and 1982**

▦ **New counties where cases were acquired after 1982**

Figure 24.3.

Cases of Lyme borreliosis in the United States, by county of acquisition, 1980–1986 (excludes 1981). [Redrawn with permission from Ciesielski CA et al. (1989): Lyme disease surveillance in the United States, 1983–1986. Rev Infect Dis 2(Suppl):S1437.]

Properties of the Organism

Resistance to environmental, physical, and chemical agents. B. burgdorferi survives for relatively long periods of time in its vector and reservoir hosts. The organisms are highly sensitive to physical and chemical agents.

Microscopic morphology. The organism is a medium-to-loosely coiled, thin, flexible spirochete 4–30 μ in length and 0.18–0.25 μ in diameter (Fig. 24.4). It is actively motile, exhibiting rotational and translational movements. *B. burgdorferi* is gram-negative and stains well by Giemsa, Wright, and silver impregnation methods but, like treponemes, is best recognized and studied by **dark field microscopy**.

Macroscopic morphology. The organisms are microaerophiles that grow best at 34–35°C in Barbour-Stoenner-Kelley (BSK) broth medium, which is a complex enriched medium containing bovine serum albumin (BSA) and heat-inactivated rabbit serum. Experimental infection and/or disease has been produced and studied in rhesus monkeys, mice, hamsters, and, more recently, rabbits.

Antigenic structure. Antigenic structural components related to virulence, protective immunogenicity, diagnosis, and classification are not well defined. Two lipoproteins, designated **Osp A** and **Osp B,** once thought to be exclusively outer surface proteins, are now known to have a subsurface location. Their role in virulence, as well as the role of other subsurface molecules, such as endoflagella, are unknown. Although Osp A has been used successfully as a vaccinogen against experimental disease in the mouse, its efficacy in humans has not as yet been established. As with the pathogenic treponemes, endoflagellar, periplasmic, and/or inner membrane proteins and lipoproteins are undoubtedly responsible for the stimulation of antibodies that develop during the course of the disease, but those responsible for ''specific'' serological reactivity have not been isolated or identified. There is evidence for significant **antigenic diversity** among strains of *B. burgdorferi,* but their role in virulence and in the development of a potential classification scheme is also unknown. True LPS molecules have not been identified.

Exracellular products associated or thought to be associated with pathogenicity. Extracellular virulence factors have not been identified.

Pathogenesis and Clinical Manifestations

EARLY LYME BORRELIOSIS. *B. burgdorferi* is introduced into the host by the tick during a blood meal or following a tick bite. Tick salivary and fecal products are also introduced into the host. Organisms invade and migrate to the skin, where **attachment, colonization, and multiplication** are initiated. Some leave the local site and are carried to the regional lymph nodes. In addition, organisms enter the circulation and are carried to other organs and tissues, particularly the **joints, nervous system, and heart,** where they take up residence. Like *T. pallidum* subsp. *pallidum,* these organisms exit the circulation through the tight junctions of the vascular endothelial cells. Local multiplication and spread at the skin site and to the lymph nodes result in a **relatively minimal host response characterized by a predominantly plama cell, macrophage, and lymphocytic infiltration.**

After an incubation period of 2–32 days (usually 8–9 days), the host-parasite and host-tick product confrontation usually results in the appearance of a single lesion or multiple macular lesions at or near the bite site that become papular, then gradually expand to form an annular, erythematous circular plaque with pale-to-red intensities within the central area. This distinctive, characteristic lesion(s), which occurs in 60–80% of patients, is referred to as **erythema migrans (EM)** and ranges from 5 cm in diameter early in development to as large as 70 cm in diameter as it expands. Erythema migrans may require several months to resolve by a mechanism that appears to involve phagocytosis of the organism by macrophages. These organisms may recur as secondary annular lesions at the same or distal sites. During this early stage of the disease, some patients develop a regional or generalized lymphadenopathy. The great majority of patients with multiple EM present with fever, headache, fatigue, arthralgias, myalgias, and stiff neck.

LATE LYME BORRELIOSIS. Single or multiple late manifestations of Lyme borreliosis occur weeks to months or years following the tick bite as a result of either the slow activation and multiplication of disseminated spirochetes and/ or damage by immune complexes. **Arthritis,** more frequent in the United States than in Europe, is the **most common form of late disease in the United States,** occurring in about 50% of patients. Large joints, particularly the knee, are most often affected and recurrences occur in the same or other joints after the initial lesion wanes. Progression to a more severe, chronic, and erosive arthritis occurs in about 10% of patients and is frequently associated with the HLA-DR2 and HLA-DR4 alloantigens.

Neurologic abnormalities are more frequent in Europe than in the United States, where they occur in up to 40% of patients. Clinical manifestations include aseptic meningitis, meningoencephalitis, Bell's palsy, cranial neuritis, and radiculoneuritis. **Cardiac abnormalities** occur in about 8% of patients and may manifest as an A-V block or myopericarditis. Rarely, conjunctivitis or keratitis develop. More commonly in Europe than the United States, chronic disseminated disease may manifest as a sclerotic or atrophic skin lesion known as acrodermatitis chronica atrophicans (ACA) or a lymphocytoma with predilection for the ear lobes in children and the nipple-areola region in adults.

Immunity to Reinfection

Immunity to reinfection has been demonstrated for rabbits, but has not been investigated in humans.

Laboratory Diagnosis

An accurate history of tick bite or visitation to tick-infested and reservoir host areas is essential. A careful physical examination must be conducted for the presence of the characteristic EM lesion(s), as well as other clinical manifestations referrable to the disease, such as arthritis and/or neurological or cardiological abnormalities.

SPECIMENS AND DIRECT EXAMINATION. Specimens obtained depend on the disease process and include material from early lesions, skin biopsy, lymph node aspirates, blood for culture and serology, synovial fluid, and cerebrospinal fluid. Silver impregnation staining of skin biopsies is time consuming, difficult to interpret due to the staining of tissue artifacts, and not used on a routine basis.

At present, the false positive and false negative results obtained with the PCR assay precludes its use as a diagnostic tool.

PRIMARY ISOLATION AND IDENTIFICATION. Culture of skin, lymph node, blood, synovial fluid, and cerebrospinal fluid cultures should be attempted despite the relatively low percentage of isolation. Specimens are inoculated into BSK medium, incubated under microaerophilic conditions at 34–35°C for a minimum of 12 weeks, and examined periodically for *B. burgdorferi* by dark field microscopy and or by staining.

IMMUNOSEROLOGIC BLOOD TESTS. The two immunoserologic blood tests employed most frequently in laboratory diagnosis are the indirect fluorescent antibody (IFA) assay and ELISA that utilize as antigen killed *B. burgdorferi* and an ultrasonic lysate of the organism, respectively. A fourfold rise in titer on paired acute and convalescent sera taken at 6 to 8-week intervals is diagnostic. Individual quantitative determinations utilizing acceptable diagnostic cut-off values are only about 50% reactive in the early stages of the disease, but range from 71 to 100% reactive among patients with late manifestations.

The reliability of these procedures on a single serum specimen in the accurate diagnosis of Lyme borreliosis is subject to considerable doubt. False positive reactions occur among patients with both acute and chronic diseases, including those with treponemal disease, autoimmune disease, AIDS, and occasionally among apparently normal individuals. Antimicrobial therapy may prevent antibody formation. Lack of standardization of these assays has resulted in poor interlaboratory reproducibility. Western blot analysis is both insensitive and nonspecific during early Lyme borreliosis. Its potential usefulness in identifying specific antibodies in late disease is tempered by the lack of standardization and difficulty in interpretation of results.

CEREBROSPINAL FLUID ASSAYS. These assays are useful in the diagnosis of aseptic meningitis and meningoencephalitis. Patients usually exhibit significant levels of specific antibody, an elevated cell count with a preponderance of lymphocytes, and normal total protein and glucose levels.

Treatment

Oral doxycycline or amoxicillin plus probenecid is effective in the treatment of early Lyme borreliosis. Oral erythromycin has been recommended for treatment of penicillin-allergic children and pregnant females despite its lesser efficacy. High dose and prolonged IV ceftriaxone or penicillin G therapy is recommended for patients with late neurological Lyme borreliosis. Oral doxycycline or amoxicillin plus probenecid have proven effective in the treatment of Lyme arthritis. Patients with cardiac abnormalities do not require antibiotic therapy, inasmuch as the disease is usually self-limiting. However, a temporary pacemaker may be necessary for patients with heart block.

Prevention and Control

Vector and reservoir control, education relating to areas of tick endemicity, prevention of tick bites, and recognition of clinical manifestations referrable to the disease are important parameters in prevention and control. Inasmuch as the tick must remain in contact with the host for more than 24 h in order to transmit the organism, individuals in tick-endemic areas are urged to inspect themselves once every 24 h and to remove any ticks discovered. Although vaccines for humans have not as yet been developed, an Osp A vaccine is presently being evaluated.

RELAPSING FEVER

Relapsing fever is an acute arthropod-borne disease characterized by alternating febrile and afebrile periods. The louse-borne type, or epidemic relapsing fever, occurs worldwide with the exception of the United States, and is caused by *Borrelia recurrentis.* The tick-borne type, or endemic relapsing fever, also has a worldwide distribution that includes the United States, where the disease focus is mostly in the western and Rocky Mountain states. Speciation of the etiologic agents is based upon their vector association despite their close DNA homology. The three species of *Borrelia* responsible for human disease in the United States are *Borrelia hermsii, Borrelia parkeri,* and *Borrelia turicatae.* Relapsing fever is a classic example of how antigenic variation influences the pathogenesis of disease.

Habitat and Transmission

EXOGENOUS. Transmission is exclusively by the exogenous route.

LOUSE-BORNE TYPE. The vectors for the louse-borne type are the body and head louse **Pediculus humanus corporis** and **Pediculus humanus capitis,** respectively. **Humans are the sole host.** The louse cannot infect the host during a blood meal or transmit borreliae to another louse by transovarian passage, inasmuch as the organisms are located only in the central ganglion and lymph nodes of the vector. Thus, humans can only become infected by crushing infected lice on their skin and creating an abrasion for entrance of the organisms. Explosive outbreaks have been reported among refugees, prisoners, Armed Forces personnel, and other clusters of individuals where hygienic conditions are poor and crowded conditions exist among those wearing louse-infested clothing.

TICK-BORNE TYPE. The vectors for the tick-borne type are species of soft ticks belonging to the genus **Ornithodoros.** The major reservoir hosts in the United States are **ground squirrels, chipmunks, prairie dogs, rats, and opossums.** Ticks become infected with borreliae by feeding upon infected reservoir hosts, after which the organisms gain access to their coxal and salivary glands and gonads. Borreliae are introduced into the human host from contaminated tick saliva, coxal fluid, and feces during a blood meal. Reservoir hosts, together with the fact that the borreliae can be transmitted transovarially from tick to tick, accounts for the endemic nature of the disease. The acquisition of relapsing fever is dependent on the opportunity for contact with infected ticks in areas such as caves and mountain cabins, where people visit during hiking and camping outings.

Properties of the Organism

Resistance to environmental, physical, and chemical agents. Vector and reservoir hosts of relapsing fever borreliae remain infected for the duration of their lives. The organisms are highly sensitive to physical and chemical agents.

Microscopic morphology. Relapsing fever borreliae are identical appearing as loosely coiled, thin, flexible, actively motile spirochetes 8–40 μ in length and 0.2–0.6 μ in diameter. These organisms are gram-negative and stain well with Giemsa and Wright stains, which are used to identify the organisms in blood smears (Fig. 24.4).

Macroscopic morphology. Several species have been cultured in artificial medium, including *B. hermsii, B. parkeri,* and *B. turicatae.* The organisms are microaerophiles that grow best at 35°C in Kelley's medium, which is a complex enriched medium containing BSA and rabbit serum.

Antigenic structure. Antigenic structure, as it relates to virulence, is still not completely understood. The striking capacity of these organisms to undergo **several antigenic variations within a given host during a single infection** permits the organism to survive and accounts for the relapsing nature of the disease. The

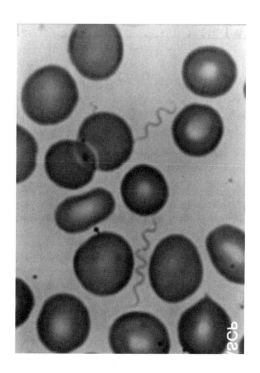

Figure 24.4.

Pathogenic *Borrelia* in Giemsa-stained blood smear or from a patient with relapsing fever. (Courtesy of the American Society of Clinical Pathology.)

mechanism has been linked putatively to an immunodominant **variable outer membrane protein (VMP)** that undergoes changes in molecular weight and protein sequences with each episode of antigenic variation. As many as 26 distinct serotypes with an epitope-unique VMP are recognizable among strains isolated from a patient or experimental animal infected with a single strain. For each antigenic serotype, VMP expression and structure is controlled by silent versus expressed genes and resultant DNA rearrangements. LPS has not as yet been identified.

Extracellular products associated or thought to be associated with pathogenicity. Extracellular virulence factors have not been identified.

Pathogenesis and Clinical Manifestations

In general, the pathogenesis of epidemic and endemic relapsing fever are similar, although the clinical manifestations of the former may at times be somewhat more severe. After entry into the host from the louse or tick vector, the organisms enter the circulation, where they multiply to produce a septicemia. Borreliae invade the spleen, liver, bone marrow, lungs, and/or the CNS where they take up **both an intracellular and extracellular residence.** Multiplication may or may not occur in these organs and is determined by as yet unknown factors. After an incubation period of 2–14 days (usually 6–7 days), the host-parasite confrontation results in a sudden onset of **fever of 38.9–40.6°C** accompanied by chills and headache that lasts for 3–7 days. At this time borrelial antibody appears and causes **destruction and elimination of the organisms by mechanisms thought to involve complement-mediated lysis and phagocytosis of agglutinated organisms by polymorphonuclear leukocytes.** Surviving organisms within the tissues **alter their antigenic structure** by means of genetic mechanisms that control VMP (?) modification and expression, enter the circulation, and **multiply in the presence of the antibody to the initial infecting strain,** thereby resulting in another febrile period and a repeat of the pathogenesis and clinical manifestations. Although the number of relapses is usually 3–4, as many as 10 have been reported. Other clinical manifestations resulting from septicemia and multiplication in the tissues may occur and include a macular rash, hepatosplenomegaly, jaundice, bronchopneumonia, and meningitis.

Immunity to Reinfection

Immunity to reinfection does not develop.

Laboratory Diagnosis

As with Lyme borreliosis, an accurate history of vector exposure and visitation to reservoir host areas is essential.

SPECIMEN AND DEFINITIVE IDENTIFICATION. A blood specimen is obtained during the febrile period and a thin film prepared and stained with either Giemsa or Wright stain. Borreliae are identified as thin, loosely wound spirochetes in the stained blood smear (Fig. 24.5).

Treatment

Early treatment of both louse-borne and tick-borne relapsing fever with doxycycline, tetracycline, erythromycin, or chloramphenicol is effective. Penicillin and streptomycin have been used but fail to prevent relapses. Therapy has reduced the case fatality rate from 5–10% to less than 1%.

Prevention and Control

Vector and reservoir host control, education relating to areas of tick endemicity, prevention of tick and louse bites, and proper personal hygiene and public health standards, are important parameters in prevention and control. Awareness of the possibility of relapsing fever is essential considering its similarity in clinical manifestations to other febrile diseases, such as malaria.

LEPTOSPIRA

LEPTOSPIROSIS

Leptospirosis is a worldwide, acute, febrile disease caused by serotypes (serovars) of *Leptospira interrogans*. Over 180 serotypes of *L. interrogans* pathogenic for animals and/or humans have been described. Of the eight associated with human disease in the United States, the most common are the serotypes *icterohaemorrhagiae, canicola,* and *pomona.* The source of most of the reported cases are **pet dogs and domestic livestock.** The disease manifests as a wide variety of clinical syndromes that vary from mild to severe and is dependent, to some extent, upon the infecting serovar and host response. Thus, leptospirosis may masquarade as a multiplicity of different entities.

Habitat

Pathogenic leptospirae are harbored in the **renal tubules** of numerous domestic and wild animals throughout the world but **in the United States, domestic animals are the major reservoir hosts.** Although organisms may reside in several different animals, many serotypes appear to have host(s) predilection. The major reservoir hosts for the three principal human pathogenic serotypes in the United States are rats, dogs, cattle, and swine for *icterohaemorrhagiae*; dogs, cattle, and swine for *canicola*; and cattle, swine, dogs, goats, and horses for *pomona*.

Transmission

EXOGENOUS. Transmission is exclusively by the exogenous route. Leptospirae enter through the abraded skin, oral or nasal mucosa, or conjunctiva following contact with urine-contaminated water by drinking, immersion of hands, or swimming. Transmission may also result from the handling of infected animals.

Properties of the Organism

Resistance to environmental, physical, and chemical agents. Leptospirae survive in untreated water for months to years. These organisms are highly sensitive to physical and chemical agents, including chlorine concentrations used in the chlorination of water.

Microscopic morphology. Leptospirae are identical appearing as tightly coiled, thin, flexible spirochetes 6–20 µ in length and 0.1 µ in diameter with their terminal ends frequently bent in the form of characteristic "hooks." The organisms are actively motile spinning on their long axis in a characteristic rotary motion. Leptospirae stain poorly or not at all with the usual aniline dyes, but stain well by silver impregnation methods. Like treponemes and *B. burgdorferi,* these organisms are best recognized and studied by **dark field microscopy.**

Macroscopic morphology. The organisms are strict aerobes and grow best at 29°C in either Fletcher's semisolid medium, which contains inactivated rabbit serum, or Ellinghausen's semsolid medium, which contains Tween 80 and BSA.

Antigenic structure. Antigenic structural components related to virulence are not well understood. Surface or subsurface structures associated with virulence have not as yet been identified. However, limited knowledge of the antigenic structure has allowed the formulation of a classification scheme useful in diagnosis and epidemiological tracing of outbreaks. The more than 180 pathogenic serotypes (serovars) of *L. interrogans* have been differentiated and identified on the basis of agglutination and cross-absorption agglutination studies, which strongly imply the presence of outer membrane molecules with serotype-unique epitopes. For the purpose of serodiagnostic screening, the serotypes have been placed into 19 serogroups on the basis of common agglutinogens. Some serotypes contain LPS-like molecules, but their role in pathogenesis is unknown.

Extracellular products associated or thought to be associated with pathogenicity. Extracellular virulence factors have not as yet been clearly defined. The role of a demonstrable but not as yet isolated soluble hemolysin is still uncertain.

Pathogenesis and Clinical Manifestations

FIRST-PHASE LEPTOSPIROSIS. After entry of the leptospirae into the host, they enter the circulation and multiply to produce a **septicemia.** The organisms invade the spleen, liver, kidneys, GI tract, and/or the CNS, where they are thought to take up **both an extracellular and intracellular residence.** Multiplication may or may not occur in these organs and is determined by as yet unknown factors. After an incubation period of 7–12 days, the first phase of the disease manifests as fever, chills, headache, GI disturbance, and conjunctival redness. In 2–7 days, the clinical manifestations diminish and the patient becomes afebrile. Organisms are still present in the eyes and kidneys and remain there during the disease, but are rarely found in other tissues, including the blood and cerebrospinal fluid, presumably as a result of their **destruction and elimination by complement-dependent lysis and by phagocytosis by mononuclear cells following opsonization.**

SECOND-PHASE LEPTOSPIROSIS. After a 1–3 day afebrile period, a **recurrence of fever,** which persists for only 1–2 days, ushers in the second phase of the disease despite the presence of relatively high levels of leptospiricidal and opsonizing antibodies and the rarity of organisms in the circulation and most tissues. If other more serious clinical manifestations develop, they tend to persist for up to 30 days. The infecting serovar and the host response to the organism influence the pathogenesis and resulting severity of the disease.

During either phase of the disease, jaundice, rash, hepatosplenomegaly, petechial hemorrhage, meningitis, and/or renal damage may occur, but the exact role of virulence factors versus immune damage is not known. Several serovars produce mild disease characterized by a single phase of fever of short duration.

Immunity to Reinfection

Immunity to reinfection is serovar-specific and permanent, presumably due to protective antibodies that lyse the organisms in the presence of complement and enhance mononuclear cell phagocytosis of the leptospirae by opsonization.

Laboratory Diagnosis

In addition to pertinent clinical manifestations, an accurate history relating to occupation (e.g., dog breeding, veterinarian, farmer, miner, or sewer worker) and pet dog ownership, assists in the determination of whether leptospirosis should be considered in the differential diagnosis.

SPECIMENS. Specimens obtained depend on the disease process and include blood for culture and serology, urine obtained by clean-catch or catheterization, and cerebrospinal fluid.

PRIMARY ISOLATION AND IDENTIFICATION. This requires cultivation of blood, cerebrospinal fluid, and/or urine in Fletcher's or Ellinghausen's semisolid medium. Incubation aerobically in the dark at 29°C is optimal for isolation of the organism. Cultures should be examined by **dark field microscopy** for at least 10 weeks for the presence of tightly coiled, ''spinning'' spirochetes with hooked ends. Positive blood and cerebrospinal fluid cultures should be obtained during the first-phase febrile period. Urine cultures are most often positive during the second phase of the disease.

IMMUNOSEROLOGIC BLOOD TESTS. These tests rather than culture methods are the assays used most frequently to diagnose leptospirosis due to the failure to consider the disease in the differential diagnosis during the early febrile period and the need for specialized media not generally available in the routine clinical laboratory.

A macroscopic slide agglutination test employing formalinized serogroup-specific organisms as antigen is a useful rapid screening procedure for detecting broad, cross-reacting leptospiral antibody. Antibody appears 1–2 weeks after the appearance of first-phase clinical manifestations, reaches a maximum during convalescence, and may persist for years thereafter. A fourfold increase on paired acute and convalescent sera taken at 4-week intervals, and a titer of greater than or equal to 1:100 on a single specimen in the presence of referrable clinical manifestations, provide definitive evidence for active leptospirosis.

The demonstration of serovar-specific antibodies requires the use of living or formalinized individual serovars as antigen in a microscopic agglutination test read by dark field microscopy and is performed only by special reference laboratories.

Treatment

Penicillin and tetracycline are effective if administered within the first 2–4 days after the initial onset of clinical manifestations. Later administration has no effect upon the course of the disease. Because the uncomplicated, febrile disease is usually self-limiting and treatment is usually begun relatively late in the disease, the case fatality rate is 1–2% in both the treated and untreated disease. However, mortality may reach as high as 50% among treated and untreated patients with jaundice and renal failure.

Prevention and Control

Rodent-control methods, such as rat-proofing, and education of those in hazardous occupations (e.g., miners, sewer workers, and veterinarians) as to proper attire and hygienic conditions are essential. Swimming in stagnant waters must be avoided. **An effective vaccine required for dogs and one recommended for cattle** is available in the United States. A **heat-killed vaccine** is being used effectively for coal miners in Japan and Poland.

SUMMARY

1. *Treponema pallidum* **subsp.** *pallidum,* **the etiologic agent of syphilis, is the major pathogen of the four treponemes that cause human disease. It is transmitted either by sexual contact or transplacentally from an infected mother to the fetus.**

2. The pathogenic treponemes are actively motile spirochetes that stain

poorly or not at all with the usual aniline dyes. They are best recognized by dark field microscopy.

3. In uncomplicated acquired syphilis, organisms gain entrance to the host as described, and within a few hours are carried to the regional lymph nodes and disseminated mainly to the liver, spleen, and bone marrow. The end result of local multiplication is the communicable primary stage. As the inflammatory cells peak, the primary lesion heals. During this local healing process, organisms within the deeper tissues undergo slow but continous multiplication, setting up foci of infection. The communicable secondary stage is initiated when treponemes gain access to the circulation from infected foci, produce a septicemia, and are carried to lymph nodes and other tissues. Lesions heal but at least 25% of patients develop recurrent secondary syphilis. Latency is the result of the healing of secondary lesions and the survival of some treponemes. The tertiary stage occurs in approximately one-third of patients with latent infection. Treponemes exit cells and invade the CNS system, cardiovascular system, eye, skin, and/or other internal organs. In congenital syphilis, overwhelming invasion of the fetus may lead to a miscarriage or stillbirth.

4. Lyme borreliosis, the etiologic agent of which is *Borrelia burgdorferi*, is a worldwide tick-borne disease. The primary reservoir hosts of *B. burgdorferi* are rodents and birds. Transmission occurs from infected *Ixodes* deer ticks.

5. *B. burgdorferi* is a gram-negative, actively motile spirochete that is best recognized by dark field microscopy. The organism is microaerophilic and can be cultured in vitro.

6. In early Lyme borreliosis, organisms invade and migrate to the skin, where they produce distinctive single or multiple lesions referred to as erythema migrans (EM). Organisms are also carried to other organs and tissues, particularly the joints, nervous system, and heart. In late Lyme borreliosis, manifestations may occur months or years following the tick bite. They usually manifest as arthritis, neurological abnormalities, and/or carditis.

7. Relapsing fever, caused by members of the genus *Borrelia*, is an acute arthropod-borne disease characterized by alternating febrile and afebrile periods. The tick-borne (endemic) type occurs in the United States with a disease focus in the western and Rocky Mountain states. The vectors are soft ticks (*Ornithodoros*), and the major reservoir hosts are ground squirrels, chipmunks, prairie dogs, rats, and opossums.

8. Relapsing fever borreliae are actively motile, gram-negative spiro-chetes that stain well with Giemsa and Wright stains, which are used to iden-tify the organisms in blood smears.

9. The pathogenesis of the relapsing fevers begins with the entrance of the spirochetes into the circulation after entry of the organisms into the host. Host-parasite confrontation results in a sudden onset of high fever accom-panied by chills and headache. Antibody appears and causes destruction of the organisms by mechanisms thought to involve complement-mediated lysis and phagocytosis of organisms. Surviving spirochetes within the tissues alter their antigenic structure, enter the circulation, and multiply in the presence of antibody to the initial infecting strain, resulting in another febrile period. The number of relapses is usually 3–4.

10. Leptospirosis, caused by serotypes of *Leptospira interrogans,* is a worldwide, acute, febrile disease that may manifest as a multiplicity of dif-ferent clinical entities. In the United States, the most common are the sero-types *icterohaemorrhagiae, canicola,* and *pomona.* The spirochetes are har-bored in the renal tubules of their hosts, and are transmitted following contact with urine-contaminated water.

11. Leptospirae are actively motile spirochetes with their terminal ends frequently bent in the form of characteristic ''hooks.'' They are best recog-nized by dark field microscopy and are strict aerobes that grow best in serum-enriched, semisolid media.

12. The pathogenesis of leptospirosis begins with the entrance of the spirochetes directly into the circulation from the portal of entry; the organ-isms multiply and produce a septicemia. Invasion of the spleen, liver, kidneys, GI tract, and/or the CNS occurs. In 2–7 days, the clinical manifestations diminish and the patient becomes afebrile. Recurrence of fever occurs after the short afebrile period. The severity of the disease depends upon the in-fecting serotype and the host reponse.

REFERENCES

Barbour AG (1988): Plasmid analysis of *Borrelia burgdorferi,* the Lyme disease agent. J Clin Mi-crobiol 26:475.

Barbour AG (1990): Antigenic variation of a relapsing fever *Borrelia* species. Annu Rev Microbiol 44:155.

Barbour AG, Fish D (1993): The biological and social phenomena of Lyme disease. Science 260:1610.

Crissey JT, Denenholz DA (1984): Syphilis. Clin Dermatol 2:1.

Erdile LF, Brandt MA, Warakomski DJ, Westrack GJ, Sadziene A, Barbour AG, Mays JP (1993): Role of attached lipid in immunogenicity of *Borrelia burgdorferi* Osp A. Infect Immun 61:81.

Faine S (1990): Leptospirosis. In Evans AE, Brachman PS (eds): Bacterial Infections of Humans. 2nd ed. New York: Plenum Press.

Fikrig E, Barthold SW, Kantor FS, Flavell RA (1992): Long-term protection of mice with Lyme disease by vaccination with Osp A. Infect Immun 60:773.

Fiumara NJ, Lessell S (1970): Manifestations of late congenital syphilis. Arch Dermatol 102:78.

Hook EW III (1989): Syphilis and HIV infection. J Infect Dis 160:530.

Johns DR, Tierney M, Felsenstein D (1987): Alteration in the natural history of neurosyphilis by concurrent infection with the human immunodeficiency virus. N Eng J Med 316:1569.

Larson SA, Hunter EF, Kraus SJ (eds) (1990): A Manual of Tests for Syphilis. Washington, DC: American Public Health Association.

Malison MD (1979): Relapsing fever. JAMA 241:2819.

Miller JN (1975): The value and limitations of non-treponemal and treponemal tests in the laboratory diagnosis of syphilis. Clin Obstet Gynecol 18:191.

Miller JN, Beachler CW (1992): Nonvenereal treponematoses. In Feigin RD, Cherry JD (eds): Textbook of Pediatric Infectious Diseases. Chap 117, 3rd ed. Vol. 1, Philadelphia: W. B. Saunders, pp 1197–1204.

Rahn DW, Malawista SE (1991): Lyme disease: Recommendations for diagnosis and treatment. Ann Intern Med 114:472.

Ricci JM, Fojaco RM, O'Sullivan MJ (1989): Congenital syphilis: the University of Miami/Jackson Memorial Medical Center experience, 1986–1988. Obstet Gynecol 74:687.

Steere AC (1989): Lyme Disease. N Eng J Med 321:586.

U.S. Department of Health, Education, and Welfare (1968): Syphilis: A synopsis. Publication No. 1660.

U.S. Department of Health and Human Services (1989): Sexually transmitted diseases. Treatment guidelines. MMWR 38:S8.

Walker EM, Zampighi GA, Blanco DR, Miller JN, Lovett MA (1989): Demonstration of rare protein in the outer membrane of *Treponema pallidum* subsp. *pallidum* by freeze-fracture analysis. J Bacteriol 171:5005.

REVIEW QUESTIONS

For questions 1 to 14, choose the ONE
BEST answer or completion.

1. Primary and secondary syphilis
   a) are usually the result of endogenous activation
   b) are communicable
   c) occur only in hot and humid climates
   d) can be diagnosed by culturing lesion exudates on serum-enriched media
   e) occur only in AIDS and HIV-positive patients

2. *Treponema pallidum* subsp. *pallidum* and *Borrelia burgdorferi differ* in that the *former*
   a) is gram-negative
   b) is best recognized by dark field microscopy
   c) contain endoflagella
   d) stains well by silver impregnation methods
   e) is usually transmitted to humans by sexual contact

3. The pathogenesis of primary syphilis is best described as
   a) extracellular multiplication of treponemes at the site of entry and in the regional lymph nodes with the induction of a chronic inflammatory response characterized by an influx of plasma cells, lymphocytes, and macrophages, and a leakage of fluid containing immunoglobulin and complement
   b) a perfect host-parasite relationship in which treponemes reside intracellularly without producing clinical manifestations
   c) predominantly the result of LPS release and damage to genital tissue resulting in chancre formation
   d) extracellular multiplication at the site of entry and in the regional lymph nodes with the release of a powerful exotoxin responsible for the characteristic chancre and regional lymphadenopathy
   e) extracellular multiplication of treponemes at the site of entry and in the regional lymph nodes with the release of cardiolipin from the host tissues and the formation of cardiolipin-antibody immune complexes responsible for the tissue damage

4. Patients with coexisting untreated latent syphilis and AIDS
   a) usually exhibit a serum nonreactive nontreponemal blood test
   b) usually exhibit a serum nonreactive treponemal blood test
   c) usually undergo rapid nontreponemal serological conversion to nonreactivity after therapy compared to the response in non-AIDS patients

d) should be treated aggressively with erythromycin

e) may develop a rapid, progressive involvement of the CNS

5. One of the following statements relating to congenital syphilis is NOT TRUE:
   a) The fetus usually becomes infected early in the first trimester.
   b) Penicillin therapy can be instituted without considering desensitization, inasmuch as neonates are not allergic to penicillin.
   c) Transplacental transmission occurs most often when the pregnant female has primary or secondary syphilis.
   d) The clinical manifestations of late congenital syphilis may not manifest in the infant until after the age of 2 years.
   e) Both nontreponemal and treponemal antibody cross the placenta during the development of the disease in utero.

6. One of the following statements relating to tertiary or late syphilis is NOT TRUE. These diseases
   a) may manifest as benign gummatous lesions that are usually a source of transmission by sexual contact
   b) are the result of an upset in host-treponeme balance in favor of the treponeme during latency, presumably due to a waning of treponemicidal antibody and CMI
   c) may manifest as either symptomatic or asymptomatic neurosyphilis
   d) are treated with higher doses of penicillin than other stages of the acquired disease
   e) may result in nontreponemal antibody titers that usually fail to change with effective therapy

7. During a routine physical examination, an adult male with no history, clinical manifestations, or treatment referrable to syphilis was shown to have a quantitative VDRL titer of 1:4 (4 dils) on his serum.
   a) A definitive diagnosis of syphilis can be made by demonstrating the presence of treponemes in the blood by dark-field microscopy.
   b) The VDRL, cell count, and total protein determinations should be conducted on cerebrospinal fluid immediately.
   c) Treatment for syphilis should be instituted and the VDRL response to therapy monitored.
   d) An FTA-ABS or MHA-TP test should be done in order to establish or rule out present or past syphilis.
   e) A definitive diagnosis should be made by injecting a rabbit intradermally with a blood sample and observing the animal for the development of a primary lesion.

8. The transmission of *B. burgdorferi* to humans
   a) usually occurs from handling infected reservoir hosts, such as mice and deer
   b) is often by sexual contact
   c) occurs from contaminated *Ixodes* tick saliva and feces during a blood meal
   d) is often the result of drinking contaminated water
   e) commonly occurs by the maternal-fetal route

9. Early Lyme borreliosis *differs* from late Lyme borreliosis in that the *former*
   a) commonly manifests as an arthritis
   b) is characterized by an extensive acute inflammatory response

c) requires high dose and prolonged IV therapy
d) commonly manifests as a carditis
e) often manifests with an annular lesion referred to as erythema migrans

10. One of the following statements relating to the unreliability of the IFA and ELISA tests on sera in the diagnosis of Lyme borreliosis is NOT TRUE:
    a) False positive tests occur in patients with other diseases.
    b) Lack of standardization of the tests has resulted in poor interlaboratory reproducibility.
    c) A high proportion of false negatives occur during the early stage of the disease.
    d) A fourfold rise in titer on paired acute and convalescent sera taken at 6-8-week intervals provides a presumptive diagnosis.
    e) False positive tests may occasionally occur among normal individuals.

11. Louse-borne and tick-borne relapsing fevers are *similar* in that
    a) both are characterized by alternating febrile and afebrile periods resulting from borreliae antigenic variation
    b) both have animal reservoir hosts
    c) both result from infection during a blood meal taken by their arthropod vector
    d) their spirochetes can be transmitted from vector to vector by transovarian passage
    e) both occur in the United States

12. The best approach to the definitive diagnosis of relapsing fever is

a) assaying for specific antibody in serum during the febrile period utilizing an ELISA test
b) culturing a blood specimen in Kelley's enriched medium
c) the observation of a Giemsa- or Wright-stained thin blood smear prepared from a specimen obtained during the febrile phase for thin, loosely wound spirochetes
d) obtaining an accurate history of vector exposure
e) Western blot analysis of serum for specific antibody

13. The pathogenic leptospirae
    a) are harbored in the renal tubules of reservoir hosts
    b) are usually transmitted from human to human by droplet infection
    c) have never been cultured in or on artificial media
    d) can be identified in blood smears as gram-negative, tightly coiled spirochetes
    e) contain LPS responsible for most of the clinical manifestations observed in leptospirosis

14. One of the following statements relating to leptospirosis is NOT TRUE.
    a) The disease may masquerade as a multiplicity of different clinical entities which depend on the infecting serovar and the host response.
    b) An ulcerative lesion develops at the site of entry of the leptospirae.
    c) The first phase afebrile stage of the disease is the result of the destruction and

elimination of leptospirae by complement-dependent lysis and by phagocytosis by mononuclear cells following
opsonization.

d) The disease can be diagnosed by the
demonstration of a fourfold rise in titer
on paired acute and convalescent sera

taken at 4-week intervals or by the demonstration of greater than or equal to
1:100 titer on a single serum specimen.

e) The disease can be effectively treated
only when therapy is instituted within
the first 2–4 days after the initial onset
of clinical manifestations.

ANSWERS TO REVIEW QUESTIONS

---

1. *b* Primary and secondary syphilis are communicable through their exposed lesions.
These syndromes are the result of exogenous transmission and occur in all climates and in uncomplicated acquired
syphilis. None of the pathogenic treponemes can be cultured in or on artificial
media.

2. *e* *Treponema pallidum* subsp. *pallidum*,
the etiologic agent of syphilis, is usually
transmitted by sexual contact in contrast
to *Borrelia burgdorferi*, the etiologic
agent of Lyme borreliosis, which is
transmitted to humans by infected *Ixodes*
ticks. Treponemes stain poorly or not at
all with the usual aniline dyes, while *B.
burgdorferi* is gram-negative. Both spirochetes are best recognized by dark field
microscopy, contain endoflagella (the organelles of locomotion), and stain well
by silver impregnation methods.

3. *a* The pathogenesis of primary syphilis is

best described as extracellular multiplication of treponemes at the site of entry
and in the regional lymph nodes with the
induction of a chronic granulomatous response characterized by an influx of
plasma cells, lymphocytes, and macrophages, and a leakage of fluid containing
immunoglobulin and complement. Latency is characterized as a perfect host-
parasite relationship in which treponemes reside intracellularly without
producing clinical manifestations. There
is no definitive evidence that cardiolipin-
antibody immune complexes are responsible for the tissue damage observed in
primary and secondary syphilis. The organism does not contain LPS and does
not produce exotoxin.

4. *e* Patients with coexisting untreated latent
syphilis and AIDS may develop a rapid,
progressive involvement of the CNS. In
the great majority of such patients, both
nontreponemal and treponemal tests on

serum are reactive. The response of quantitative nontreponemal tests to effective therapy is much slower compared to the treated uncomplicated disease. High dose therapy with penicillin is essential for these patients.

5. *a* The fetus usually does not become infected until 18 weeks (during the second trimester) after gestation. Neonates are not allergic to penicillin, transplacental transmission is highest when the pregnant female has primary or secondary syphilis, late congenital syphilis may not manifest in the child until after the age of 2 years, and both nontreponemal and treponemal IgG antibody can cross the placenta in utero during the development of the disease.

6. *a* Gummatous lesions may occur during tertiary syphilis, but the rarity or absence of organisms precludes them as a source of transmission during sexual contact. Tertiary syphilis is the result of an upset in host-treponeme balance in favor of the treponeme during latency, presumably due to a waning of treponemicidal antibody and CMI, may manifest as asymptomatic or symptomatic neurosyphilis. This disease is treated with higher doses of penicillin than other stages of the acquired disease and may result in nontreponemal antibody titers that usually fail to change with effective therapy.

7. *d* Patients with no history, clinical manifestations, or treatment referrable to syphilis and exhibiting a reactive VDRL slide flocculation or RPR circle card test may have had or may have syphilis, or may be false positive reactors due to the presence of an acute or chronic disease or a condition, such as pregnancy. An FTA-ABS or MHA-TP test will determine whether the patient is a false positive reactor or whether he has or has had syphilis. Lumbar puncture should not be done and treatment for syphilis and VDRL monitoring should not be initiated until the diagnosis of syphilis has been established definitively. If the treponemal test is reactive, treatment will depend on the reliability of a history of adequate therapy for past syphilis, if available. Rabbit inoculation with blood or other tissues to establish the presence of treponemes is unreliable, expensive, and cumbersome.

8. *c* *B. burgdorferi* is transmitted to humans by contaminated *Ixodes* tick saliva and feces during a blood meal. Transmission rarely occurs as a result of handling infected reservoir hosts or by the maternal-fetal route and never occurs as a result of sexual contact or drinking contaminated water.

9. *e* Early Lyme borreliosis often manifests with a characteristic annular lesion (erythema migrans) and requires standard dose oral doxycycline or amoxicillin plus probenecid therapy. The relatively minimal host response is predominantly plasma cells, macrophages, and lymphocytes. Arthritis and carditis are manifestations of late Lyme borreliosis.

10. *d* A fourfold rise in IFA or ELISA titers on paired acute and convalescent sera taken at 6–8-week intervals provides a *definitive* not a presumptive diagnosis. The remaining statements are valid reasons for the unreliability of these tests, namely, that false positives occur in patients with other diseases and in some normal individuals, they lack standardization, and false negatives occur in early disease.

11. *a* Louse-borne and tick-borne relapsing fevers are similar in that both are characterized by alternating febrile and afebrile periods resulting from borreliae antigenic variation. The louse-borne type has only a human host and can infect the host only through an abrasion caused by crushing of the louse; taking a blood meal does not result in infection, inasmuch as the organisms are located only in the central ganglion and lymph nodes of the louse. The louse-borne type does not occur in the United States and *Borrelia recurrentis* cannot be transovarially passaged.

12. *c* The diagnosis of relapsing fever is best accomplished by demonstrating thin, loosely wound spirochetes in a Giemsa- or Wright-stained thin blood smear prepared from a specimen obtained during the febrile phase of the disease. A specific and sensitive ELISA and Western blot test have not been developed and culturing is insensitive and impractical. An accurate history of vector exposure provides essential information but does not by itself enable a definitive diagnosis to be made.

13. *a* The pathogenic leptospirae are harbored in the renal tubules of reservoir hosts. These organisms are usually transmitted to humans through the abraded skin, oral or nasal mucosa, or conjunctiva following contact with urine-contaminated water by drinking, immersion of hands, or swimming. The spirochetes can be isolated by culturing appropriate specimens in Fletcher's or Ellinghausen's semisolid medium. The organisms stain poorly or not at all with the usual aniline dyes and therefore a Gram stain on a blood smear would be of no value. Although the leptospirae contain an LPS-like substance, its role as a virulence factor is unknown.

14. *b* Leptospirae enter the circulation directly after entry into the host without local multiplication and lesion development. Leptospirosis may masquarade as a multiplicity of different clinical entities that depend on the infecting serovar and the host response. The first-phase afebrile stage is the result of leptospirae destruction and elimination by lysis and phagocytosis. A definitive diagnosis can be made on the basis of a fourfold rise titer on paired sera taken at 4-week intervals or by the demonstration of a greater than or equal to 1:100 titer on a single specimen. The disease can be effectively treated only when therapy is instituted within the first 2–4 days after the initial onset of clinical manifestations.

INDIGENOUS MICROBIOTA

The human body is host to an almost inconceivable number of microorganisms. More microorganisms live in 1 cubic inch of human mucosal tissue than there are people on the earth. Most of the flora that we harbor are harmless parasites (gaining benefit but returning none to the host), living with us in harmony. Some of our resident microflora provide critical functions that allow our survival (symbiotic relationship). If some members of the normal flora gain access to a normally sterile site, however, and natural defenses are somehow compromised, these previously harmless organisms can cause disease. Another group of microorganisms initiates association with a human host by ingestion or inhalation, or by deposition on intact skin. In most cases, these associations are transitory, as innate defense mechanisms eliminate the interlopers without incident.

The concept of a ''pathogenic'' organism has been altered dramatically by the advances in medical science that prolong the lives of seriously ill individuals; by virtue of the medical treatment that has altered the host state, such patients are at risk of infection from microorganisms previously considered harmless. As Dr. Michael Rinaldi (University of Texas, San Antonio) has stated, the ''human petri dish,'' those patients whose immune systems have been compromised by medical treatment, will support the destructive growth of many microbes, both normal environmental inhabitants and normal human flora, that would have been destroyed easily by an intact immune system.

Knowledge of the normal flora, then, can be useful for predicting the agents likely to be involved in an infection that involves loss of integrity of the adjacent mucous membrane. For example, certain oral flora are involved in endodontal abscesses and chronic sinusitis, and normal bowel flora possessing some virulence factors are involved in intraabdominal abscess formation. The most common etiologic agents of IV catheter-related sepsis are commensal inhabitants of normal skin, the coagulase-negative staphylococci.

INDIGENOUS MICROBIOTA BY BODY SITE

Each separate environment on the external and mucosal surfaces of the body provides a unique niche that supports a diverse and interactive microbiota. The state of the host with respect to nutritional status, age, immunological functions, external physical environment, internal physical condition, and emotional status are all important determinants of what constitutes "normal flora." For example, hospitalized individuals become colonized with hospital-resident fungi and bacteria soon after admission. Once they are discharged, these organisms disappear. Patients with anatomical defects of the urinary tract, either permanent or transitory (e.g., during pregnancy) may harbor a low level of bacterial colonizers in the urinary tract. It is well known that human herpesvirus 1, which resides in a latent state in the trigeminal nerve of infected individuals, can exacerbate to cause symptomatic disease when the host undergoes emotional stress.

An overview of the flora of a healthy human host is presented in Figure 25.1. Viruses are not considered as normal flora, although certain latent viruses, such as cytomegaloviruses (CMV) and other herpesviruses, may be present within the host without producing symptoms.

Skin, Including External Ear Canal

Examples of normal microbiota:

1. *Staphylococcus* spp., primarily coagulase negative.
2. Streptococci, including group A streptococci.
3. *Propionibacterium acnes,* found in **sweat glands** and in **hair follicles.**
4. Aerobic coryneform bacteria, including *Corynebacterium* spp. and others.
5. *Micrococcus* spp., almost never involved in infection.
6. *Bacillus* spp.

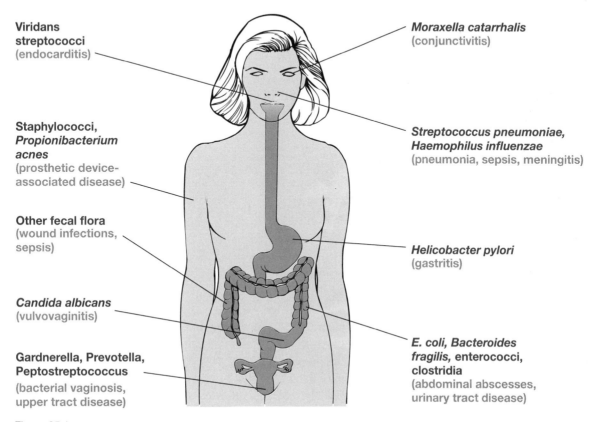

Viridans streptococci
(endocarditis)

Staphylococci, Propionibacterium acnes
(prosthetic device-associated disease)

Other fecal flora
(wound infections, sepsis)

Candida albicans
(vulvovaginitis)

Gardnerella, Prevotella, Peptostreptococcus
(bacterial vaginosis, upper tract disease)

Moraxella catarrhalis
(conjunctivitis)

Streptococcus pneumoniae, Haemophilus influenzae
(pneumonia, sepsis, meningitis)

Helicobacter pylori
(gastritis)

E. coli, Bacteroides fragilis, **enterococci, clostridia**
(abdominal abscesses, urinary tract disease)

Figure 25.1.

Figure of human showing indigenous microbiota that are most involved in infectious processes and naming key examples of such infections.

    7. *Candida* spp.

    8. *Pityrosporum ovale* (a yeast that causes seborrheic dermatitis, pityriasis versicolor, or folliculitis in some individuals but is harbored without reaction by most people; a slight T-cell defect may predispose affected individuals)

    9. *Malasezzia furfur,* a lipid-loving yeast.

    10. Mycelial fungi.

    11. Tiny mites, *Demodex folliculorum* (hair follicles) and *Demodex brevis* (sebaceous gland) colonize over one-half of all adults, primarily in the eyebrows and around the nose.

Conjunctiva

Examples of organisms found in normal conjunctiva:

1. Coagulase-negative staphylococci.
2. Micrococci.
3. *Neisseria* spp.
4. *Moraxella catarrhalis.*
5. Corynebacteria.
6. *Propionibacterium acnes* and other propionibacteria.
7. Anaerobic bacteria.
8. *Candida albicans.*

Upper Respiratory Tract

Because organisms are rapidly cleared by innate defense mechanisms in the lower respiratory tract, **areas below the larynx and trachea are usually sterile.** The upper respiratory tract (nose and throat) of normal humans, however, harbors numerous microorganisms, many of which are agents of infectious disease under appropriate circumstances. These organisms are listed below:

1. Viridans streptococci.
2. Anaerobic streptococci.
3. Staphylococci, both coagulase negative and *Staphylococcus aureus.*
4. *Neisseria* spp., such as *Neisseria sicca, Neisseria lactamica,* and the potential pathogen *Neisseria meningitidis.*
5. *Stomatococcus mucilaginosus,* common oral flora that acts as an opportunistic pathogen on occasion.
6. *Veillonella* spp.
7. Corynebacteria.
8. *Haemophilus influenzae* and *Haemophilus parainfluenzae.*
9. *Streptococcus pneumoniae.*
10. *Candida* spp.
11. *Enterobacteriaceae.*
12. *Enterococcus* spp.

Oral Cavity and Saliva

The mouth is the gateway to the entire GI tract. All flora that eventually colonize the lumen of this pipeline snaking through the body enter through the mouth. A list of some of these flora follows:

1. Viridans streptococci.
2. Staphylococci, coagulase negative and *S. aureus.*
3. *Neisseria* spp.
4. Anaerobic streptococci and anaerobic gram-negative bacilli.
5. Beta-hemolytic streptococci of various species.
6. *Streptococcus pneumoniae.*
7. *Enterobacteriaceae.*
8. *Haemophilus* spp.
9. *Capnocytophaga* spp.
10. Lactobacilli.
11. Several species of spirochetes.
12. *Eikenella corrodens.*
13. *Candida* spp.
14. The protozoans *Trichomonas tenax* and *Entamoeba gingivalis.*

Gingival Crevices

The gingival crevices provide a specialized environmental niche, with a very **low oxidation-reduction potential** and the surface of teeth as attachment sites. Certain organisms are found exclusively in this area; others are sloughed from this site and continue to survive and multiply in other areas of the oral cavity. The agents of periodontal and endodontal disease are normal flora in the healthy host. Certain host factors, not yet fully characterized, predispose the patient to dental caries and gingival disease. A list of organisms commonly found in gingival crevices follows:

1. Spirochetes.
2. Anaerobic gram-negative rods, such as *Wolinella* spp. and the black-pigmenting *Porphyromonas* and *Prevotella* spp.
3. Viridans streptococci, including *Streptococcus mutans* (the **etiologic agent of caries**).

4. *Actinomyces* spp.

5. *Actinobacillus actinomycetemcomitans* (a facultative gram-negative rod that may be associated with periodontal disease).

6. Lactobacilli.

7. Fusobacteria.

8. *Peptostreptococcus* spp. (anaerobic streptococci).

Gastrointestinal Tract

STOMACH. The stomach, because of its very low pH, usually sterilizes the bacteria that enter by ingestion. The normal stomach should be bacteria-free.

DUODENUM. *Helicobacter pylori* appears to be carried by some individuals. It is possible that a great majority of such carriers develop gastritis, but the epidemiology is not well understood.

ILEUM. The upper small intestine is sterile in normal individuals. Small numbers of organisms carried in on ingested food may be present soon after meals, but these do not persist.

The terminal ileum, however, contains as many as 10^6 bacteria per milliliter of fluid. These flora are similar to the flora of the colon, where anaerobes outnumber aerobes 1000:1. Some of the more common species are listed here, but all of the types found in the colon may be present in lesser numbers in the terminal ileum. Organisms include:

1. *Bifidobacterium* spp. (bifurcated anaerobic gram-positive rods) are numerically most prevalent.

2. *Bacteroides fragilis* group (possesses virulence factors that mediate abscess formation).

3. Other anaerobic gram-negative rods.

4. Anaerobic cocci.

5. *Enterobacteriaceae* (*Escherichia coli, Enterobacter* spp., *Proteus* spp., and others).

6. *Enterococcus* spp.

COLON. Some of the more common colon microbes:

1. *Eubacterium* spp.

2. *Bifidobacterium* spp.

3. *Bacteroides* spp., including the *B. fragilis* group and other anaerobic gram-negative rods.

4. *Peptostreptococcus* spp. and other anaerobic cocci.

5. *Clostridium* spp.

6. *Enterobacteriaceae.*

7. Enterococci.

8. Staphylococci.

9. Viridans and β-hemolytic streptococci.

10. *Pseudomonas* spp. and other nonfermentative aerobic and facultative gram-negative bacilli.

11. Protozoan parasites, such as *Trichomonas hominis, Endolimax nana, Iodamoeba bütschlii, Chilomastix mesnili, Retortamonas intestinalis,* and *Entamoeba coli.*

12. A number of patients harbor the protozoan *Blastocystis hominis* in the feces, but its role as a pathogen is still controversial. It may be normal flora in some hosts.

13. Enteric viruses, such as caliciviruses, coronaviruses, various enteroviruses, and rotaviruses may be present in the stool of asymptomatic patients, but they are not thought to be normal flora.

Anterior Urethra

These organisms are flushed into urine during normal voiding; they are present in numbers ranging from 10^2 to 10^4/ml of urine:

1. Anaerobic gram-negative rods, including *Bacteroides* spp., *Fusobacterium,* and *Prevotella* spp.

2. *Peptostreptococcus* spp.

3. *Clostridium* spp. and nonspore-forming anaerobic gram-positive rods.

4. Coagulase-negative staphylococci.

5. Coryneform facultative and aerobic gram-positive rods.

6. *Mycobacterium smegmatis, Mycobacterium gordonae.*

7. *Acinetobacter calcoaceticus.*

8. *Gardnerella vaginalis* (a gram-positive bacillus that stains as a gram-variable coccobacillus and is associated with bacterial vaginosis).

9. *Mycoplasma hominis* and *Mycoplasma genitalium.*

10. Yeasts, particularly *Candida* spp.

11. *Trichomonas vaginalis,* rare.

Genital Tract

EXTERNAL GENITALIA. Microbiota of the external genitalia are similar to skin flora, but enteric flora are more prevalent because of the proximity of the anus and the warm, moist nature of the site. A list of the flora found commonly follows:

1. Coagulase-negative staphylococci.
2. Viridans streptococci.
3. *Peptostreptococcus* spp.
4. Coryneform facultative and aerobic gram-positive rods.
5. *Enterococcus* spp.
6. *Enterobacteriaceae.*
7. *Mycobacterium smegmatis.*
8. *Bacteroides fragilis* group and other anaerobic gram-negative rods, including *Fusobacterium* spp.
9. *Mycoplasma genitalium, M. hominis.*
10. Yeasts, primarily *Candida* spp.

VAGINA. The vagina is sterile at birth, but within a few hours acquires a gram-positive flora consisting of streptococci, micrococci, and coryneforms. Estrogen in the blood (from the maternal circulation) induces vaginal epithelial cells to secrete glycogen, which encourages the growth of lactobacilli, but these are lost after several weeks and the original gram-positive flora remains until puberty. At puberty, redeposition of endogenously produced glycogen stimulates development of the adult flora, consisting primarily of anaerobes. It is thought that at least some of the microbial flora of the vagina originate in the feces and migrate along the moist perineal surface to the vagina. A list of microbial flora found in the vagina follows:

1. Lactobacilli, predominantly.
2. Anaerobic gram-negative bacilli, including *Prevotella bivia, Prevotella disiens, Porphyromonas* spp., *Bacteroides fragilis* group, and fusobacteria.
3. *Peptostreptococcus* spp.
4. *Veillonella* spp.
5. Anaerobic gram-positive bacilli, including *Propionibacterium* spp., *Actinomyces* spp., *Eubacterium* spp., *Bifidobacterium* spp., and others.
6. *Clostridium* spp.

7. Transient aerobic flora, such as *Enterobacteriaceae* and other gram-negative bacilli.

8. β-hemolytic streptococci, especially Lancefield group B *(Streptococcus agalactiae)*.

9. Staphylococci, including *S. aureus* and micrococci.

10. Coryneforms.

11. *Gardnerella vaginalis*.

12. *Mycoplasma* spp.

13. *Ureaplasma ureolyticum* is present in up to 70% of sexually active asymptomatic adults but is probably acquired during sexual activity and is not a part of normal vaginal flora.

14. Yeast spp., predominantly *Candida albicans*.

15. Filamentous fungi occasionally colonize the vagina for short periods of time.

16. Some viruses, notably CMV, are shed in vaginal secretions of asymptomatic women, but they are probably not ''normal.'' Adenoviruses are found occasionally in healthy vaginas. The role of adenoviruses as pathogens in this site is not clear.

ROLE OF NORMAL FLORA IN PROTECTION FROM INFECTION

Secretion of fatty acids by some skin-dwelling normal flora may help inhibit the ability of infectious agents to gain a foothold. The **lactobacilli in the vagina secrete peroxidase enzymes** that inhibit growth of infectious agents, and the presence of lactobacilli maintains a **low pH** by producing acid metabolic end products. Normal bacteria colonizing the lumen of the colon secrete inhibitory factors against foreign bacteria. By occupying the space on the mucosa epithelial wall, they **prevent the adherence and multiplication of enteric pathogens.** Normal viridans streptococci in the oropharynx help to **prevent colonization** by pathogenic streptococci.

"INFECTIONS" THOUGHT TO OCCUR AFTER INDIGENOUS MICROBIOTA OVERGROWTH

Infections that occur when the normal flora grows out of control are bacterial vaginosis, small bowel bacterial overgrowth, periodontal disease, and appendicitis.

SUMMARY

1. The human body is host to a large number and assortment of microorganisms, most of which are harmless.

2. A number of etiologic agents of serious diseases, such as group A beta streptococci, *Neisseria meningitidis*, *Streptococcus pneumoniae*, and *Haemophilus influenzae* on respiratory mucosal epithelium and *Streptococcus agalactiae*, *Staphylococcus aureus*, and *Candida albicans* in the vaginal tract, are carried as part of the normal flora by the majority of individuals. A predisposing event or a temporary loss of immunocompetence often allows these colonizers to become pathogens.

3. Some normal inhabitants of the epithelium may serve as deterrents to colonization by exogenous pathogenic species by elaborating inhibitory products, physically preventing adherence of pathogens, and maintaining a local environment incompatible with growth of pathogenic microorganisms.

REFERENCES

Isenberg HD, D'Amato RF (1991): Indigenous and pathogenic microorganisms of humans. In Balows A, Hausler WJ Jr., Herrmann KL, Isenberg HD, Shadomy HJ (eds): Manual of Clinical Microbiology, 5th ed. Washington DC: American Society for Microbiology.

Marples MJ (1969): Life on the human skin. Sci Am 220:108.

Rosebury T (1961): Microorganisms Indigenous to Man. New York: McGraw-Hill Book Co.

Skinner FA, Carr JG (1974): The Normal Microflora of Man. London: Academic Press.

REVIEW QUESTIONS

For questions 1 to 4, choose the ONE BEST answer or completion.

1. A patient with a several week history of low-level fever of unknown origin has three blood cultures drawn, only one of which yields a bacterial isolate. Which is the most likely organism and what is its clinical significance?
   a) *Acinetobacter anitratus,* a skin contaminant with no clinical significance.
   b) *Escherichia coli,* originating from a urinary tract infection.
   c) *Pseudomonas aeruginosa,* originating from a burn wound.
   d) Viridans streptococcus species, indicative of endocarditis.
   e) *Propionibacterium acnes,* a skin contaminant with no clinical significance.

2. Bacterial vaginosis is a syndrome characterized by a foul-smelling, thin, homogeneous vaginal discharge and vaginal pH greater than 4.5. Organisms that are isolated from vaginal discharge in this case include *Prevotella bivia, Peptostreptococcus* spp., and *Mobiluncus* spp. What would be most likely visualized in a Gram stain of vaginal discharge from a patient with bacterial vaginosis?

   a) Numerous gram-variable coccobacilli and cocci indicative of the anaerobic flora overgrowth.
   b) Numerous long, gram-positive rods characteristic of *Lactobacillus* spp.
   c) Numerous large, budding yeast cells.
   d) Numerous large, gram-negative bacilli characteristic of *Enterobacteriaceae.*
   e) Numerous gram-positive cocci characteristic of staphylococci.

3. A premature infant has been receiving lipid-enriched parenteral IV nutrition since birth. She began to appear septic and the neonatologist ordered blood cultures. What special procedure should the laboratory use to maximize the chance of recovering the pathogen?
   a) Supplement the blood culture medium with olive oil or some other lipid to allow growth of *Malassezia furfur,* a yeast that requires lipids.
   b) Draw two separate blood cultures from two separate sites to help rule out skin contaminants.
   c) Use povidone-iodine to disinfect the skin site prior to drawing the blood.
   d) Incubate the blood culture at room temperature to enhance recovery of cold-loving organisms.
   e) Use cycloserine-cefoxitin-fructose agar to maximize recovery of *Clostridium difficile.*

4. Which list of members of the normal flora contains only organisms that have been shown to be pathogens under appropriate conditions?

a) *Mycobacterium smegmatis, Streptococcus pneumoniae, Demodex folliculorum.*

b) *Staphylococcus epidermidis, Haemophilus influenzae, Bacteroides fragilis.*

c) *Trichomonas tenax, Fusobacterium nucleatum, Entamoeba coli.*

d) *Escherichia coli, Proteus vulgaris, Entamoeba gingivalis.*

e) *Neisseria sicca, Micrococcus luteus, Demodex brevis.*

For questions 5 to 7, a list of lettered options is followed by several numbered items. For each numbered item, select the ONE lettered option that is most closely associated with it.

A) Coagulase-negative staphylococci.
B) *Candida albicans.*
C) *Bacteroides* spp.
D) *Neisseria* spp.
E) *Actinomyces* spp.

For each ecological niche on immunocompetent human hosts, select the member of the normal flora that is most likely to cause a local infection following a breakdown of innate host defenses.

5. Human gingival crevices

6. Feces

7. Skin on back of hand

ANSWERS TO REVIEW QUESTIONS

---

1. *e* The only organism among those listed that inhabits normal skin is *Propionibacterium acnes*. Because only one of three blood cultures yielded the organism suggests that it is a procurement contaminant, rather than a true pathogen. When viridans streptococci are isolated from blood, the patient usually has endocarditis and the organisms are shedding into the bloodstream continuously. In that case, the blood cultures would all have yielded the organism. If the patient's isolate originated from a burn wound or urinary tract derived sepsis, he would be acutely ill.

2. *a* Enterobacteriaceae, staphylococci, and yeast are not normal vaginal flora, nor are they anaerobic bacteria as characterizes

bacterial vaginosis. The normal vaginal lactobacilli create a very acidic local environment (pH often <3.0) that helps maintain homeostasis. The increased pH would rule out lactobacilli.

3. *a* A common cause of sepsis in lipid-fed neonates and occasionally adults is *Malasezzia furfur,* a member of the normal skin flora that requires lipid for growth. The organism survives on the lipids present on the skin of normal individuals, but growth is enriched in the area surrounding the catheter insertion site where lipid content is high. The yeast colonizes the catheter and goes on to cause fungemia. Answers *b* and *c* are appropriate strategies useful for decreasing the chance of a procurement contaminant and for determining the presence of a contaminant in the culture. Cold-loving organisms may cause blood transfusion reactions, but rarely cause sepsis in nontransfused patients. *Clostridium difficile* has not been shown to be an agent of bacteremia or sepsis.

4. *b* All three species cause serious infections in hosts compromised by trauma or immune defect. Other organisms listed: *Trichomonas tenax, Entamoeba gingivalis, Mycobacterium smegmatis, Mycobacterium gordonae, Micrococcus luteus, Demodex folliculorom, Demodex brevis,* and many others have not yet been implicated in disease.

5. *E* The other genus present in most normal mouths, *Neisseria* spp., is found in the saliva and on the squamous epithelium, but not in the gingival crevices, where the oxygen concentration is very low.

6. *C* Anaerobes outnumber aerobes 1000:1 in the bowel; *Bacteroides* spp. and *Bifidobacterium* are predominant among the anaerobes.

7. *A* Normal skin staphylococci gain entrance to subcutaneous tissues through an intravenous catheter insertion site. Local infection can lead to septicemia; coagulase-negative staphylococci are the most common agents of nosocomial bacteremia.

MYCOLOGY

MYCOLOGY

Mycology is the scientific study of a unique group of microorganisms called **Fungi** (sing., Fungus). Medical mycology is a specialized branch of the discipline which is concerned with those fungi that produce disease in humans and other animals. The word zoopathogenic is used to indicate such medically important fungi.

CHARACTERISTICS

The fungi are **eukaryotes.** A eukaryotic cell is one in which the nucleus is separated from the cytoplasm by a membrane. The DNA of the eukaryotic nucleus is divided into individual packets known as chromosomes. Eukaryotic cells have other membrane-bound structures, such as mitochondria (sing., mitochondrion), in their cytoplasm. By way of contrast, the bacteria (sing., bacterium) are **prokaryotes,** a word that signifies the organisms do not have a membrane-bound nucleus. The genetic information of prokaryotes is instead carried by a single, highly convoluted filament of double-stranded DNA that lies unbounded by a membrane in the cytoplasm of the cell. The DNA of prokaryotes is not divided into chromosomes and the cytoplasm of the cell does not contain mitochondria or other membrane-bound structures. The separation of the fungi from the bacteria is based on the fundamental difference in the nuclear structure of eukaryotes and prokaryotes. The biology of prokaryotic and eukaryotic cells is distinctive, and because of this difference antibacterial substances do not ordinarily affect eukaryotic cells.

The fungi are typically surrounded by cell walls that contain complex polysaccharides (e.g., chitin, chitosan, glucans, and mannans). These structural elements of the fungi can be specifically stained, and this characteristic is used to recognize fungi in tissues or exudates of an infected host. Three such cell wall stains are the **periodic acid-Schiff (PAS) stain,** the **Gomori methenamine silver (GMS) stain,** and the **calcifluor (CFL) stain.** The GMS stain is also used to reveal some bacteria, most notably, the spirochaetes and the actinomycetes.

The plasma membrane (plasmalemma) of a fungus contains sterols, principally ergosterol. This sterol or the synthetic pathways leading to its production are frequently the site of action of antifungal drugs, and changes in the ergosterol composition of the membrane can lead to drug resistance.

The fungi lack chlorophyll and are accordingly heterotrophic in their nutrition. Such nutritional constraints mean that the fungi need an organic source of energy in order to grow and multiply. Fungi may satisfy their energy needs as saprobes in nature or as parasites of other organisms. Among the latter are those that cause disease in humans and other animals, but most of the zoopathogenic fungi are also saprobes and are acquired by susceptible hosts from environmental locations.

GROWTH

The fungi are divided into two groups on the basis of their growth pattern: **yeasts** and **moulds.** The yeasts are unicellular fungi that reproduce by budding or, in a few species, by fission. Macroscopically, in culture on solid media, the yeasts produce colonies that are soft in consistency and similar in form to those of bacteria. The cell cycle of a budding yeast is similar to the growth cycle in other eukaryotes, but the method of reproduction (budding) is unique. The moulds (also spelled molds) are multicellular fungi. The growth cycle may be pictured as beginning with the germination of a reproductive propagule (Fig. 26.1). The germ tube produced by germination grows from the tip (apex) and the growth process is therefore called apical extension. The continued extension of the germ tube with ramifications (side branching) results in a network of filaments called **hyphae** (sing., hypha). The collection of hyphae so generated gives rise to a cottony colony that is also called a **mycelium** (pl., mycelia) or a **thallus** (pl., thalli).

The cytoplasm of one type of hypha is uninterrupted by any cross walls or

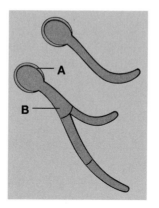

Figure 26.1.

Germination of a fungal reproductive propagule. (A) Reproductive conidium or spore. (B) Germ tube.

septa (sing., septum) throughout the entire mycelium. Such hyphae are coenocytic and are termed **nonseptate.** In contrast, the cytoplasm of another type of hypha is regularly interrupted by septa and such hyphae are accordingly called **septate** hyphae. The two types of hyphae, nonseptate and septate, are illustrated in Figure 26.2.

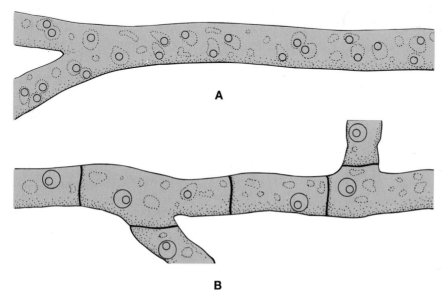

Figure 26.2.

Types of hyphae. (A) Non-septate. (B) Septate.

REPRODUCTION

The two major ways in which fungi reproduce are asexual and sexual. The processes are not exclusive and a given fungus may reproduce in one or the other way or in both ways.

Asexual Reproduction

VEGETATIVE REPRODUCTION. The hyphae that comprise the mycelium of a mould may grow vegetatively and initiate a new mycelium if a small portion of them is transferred to a fresh medium. Special propagules (reproductive units) are not required for this sort of reproduction. One group of fungi, the Mycelia Sterilia, reproduce exclusively in this manner, but most fungi also form reproductive propagules.

REPRODUCTION BY PROPAGULES. The asexual growth form of a fungus is called its anamorphic state and is accomplished by reproductive propagules called **conidia** or **sporangiospores,** depending on their mode of production.

Conidia (sing., Conidium). The conidium is usually deciduous (released) at maturity and is not developed by cytoplasmic cleavage or free cell formation. The ontogeny (development) of conidia is one basis for delineation of form species among those fungi that produce only the anamorphic form of growth. A comprehensive consideration of conidium ontogeny is beyond the scope of this chapter. Some definitions need to be given so that the terms can be used in the description of zoopathogenic fungi developed in the subsequent chapters.

Conidia develop from fertile hyphae by one or the other of two fundamental processes termed: (1) the **blastic** process or (2) the **thallic** process (Fig. 26.3). In the blastic sort of conidium formation a recognizable portion of the fertile hyphae (Fig. 26.3) markedly enlarges (blows-out) before being separated by a septum. When both the inner and outer walls are involved in the formation of the blastic conidium, the process is termed holoblastic (entire) (Fig. 26.3A and B). When only the inner wall is involved in the formation of the blastic conidium and the outer wall breaks away when the conidium is released, the process is called enteroblastic (internal) (Fig. 26.3C and D). Thallic development involves the conversion of an entire segment of the fertile hypha into a conidium. When the process involves the entire wall of the hypha, the event is called holothallic. Such conidia may occur at the end of a hypha (Fig. 26.3E) or in an internal (intercalary) segment (Fig. 26.3F). Thallic conidia that are produced in succession along the entire length

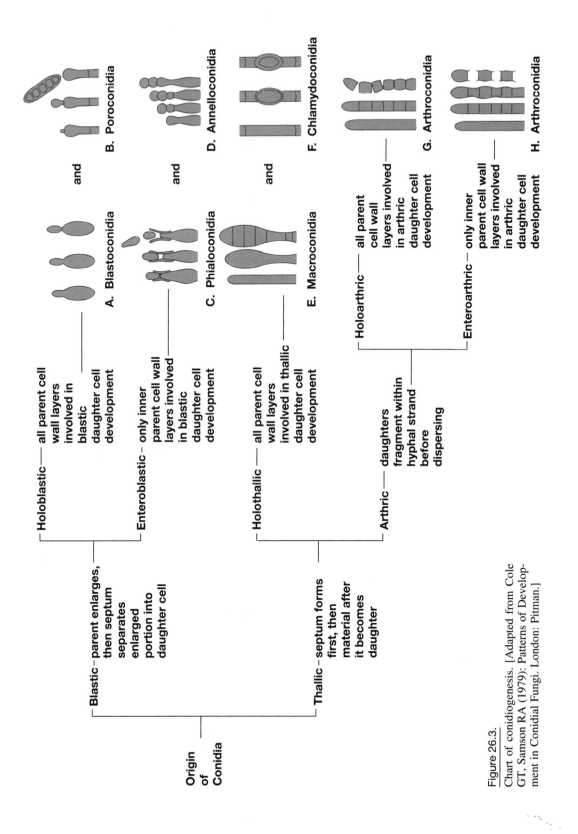

Figure 26.3.

Chart of conidiogenesis. [Adapted from Cole GT, Samson RA (1979): Patterns of Development in Conidial Fungi. London: Pitman.]

of a hyphal strand are termed arthric and may be holoarthric (Fig. 26.3G) or enteroarthric (Fig. 26.3H) depending on the method of their release.

The portion of the fertile hypha that produces a blastic or thallic conidium is called the conidiogenous cell (conidium-producing cell). This cell may be formed on a morphologically modified unit that is itself borne on a specialized branch of hyphae called the conidiophore (conidium bearer). Conidia are often given special names that more concisely define the nature of a morphologically distinctive conidiogenous cell.

A complete delineation of the nomenclature of such conidia will not be given in this chapter, but those conidial names used in subsequent chapters are defined as follows:

Arthroconidium (pl., Arthroconidia). Arthroconidia are thallic conidia characterized by the conversion of a preexisting, entire hyphal element (Fig. 26.3G and H). At maturity these conidia break loose from each other and initiate another cycle of growth by germination and apical extension as described on page xx under Growth. The method of release (i.e., holoarthric or enteroarthric) is not indicated in common usage but is shown in Figure 26.3G and H. Some texts refer to these conidia as arthrospores, but the term arthroconidium is widely accepted.

Blastoconidium (pl., Blastoconidia). Most of the yeasts reproduce by a blastic process (budding) and the whole cell may be thought of as a blastic conidium even though it does not usually initiate a new cycle of growth by germ tube formation.

The yeast cell itself, then, is referred to as a blastoconidium (Fig. 26.3A). Sometimes the blastoconidia do not separate at maturity but continue to grow and thus elongate into sausage-shaped filaments termed pseudohyphae. Species of zoopathogenic yeasts that form pseudohyphae and the condition under which they do so are described in Chapter 28.

An older term, blastospore, for the budding yeast cell continues to be used by some, but blastoconidium is more widely accepted. The reproductive element of the fission yeasts is considered an arthroconidium.

Moulds may also produce conidia holoblastically. The process is the same regardless of whether the conidiogenous cell is formed by a unicellular fungus (yeast) or a multicellular fungus (mould).

Chlamydoconidium (pl., Chlamydoconidia). This asexual unit arises by a holothallic process (Fig. 26.3F). The conidium is thick-walled and is usually thought of as fostering survival but not dissemination or multiplication of a fungus. The proper name for this type of conidium is not commonly agreed upon. Some refer to it as a chlamydospore because it is unlike a conidium in that it is not deciduous and because its function does not appear to be involved in reproduction. Nevertheless, the more consistent designation is given here.

Macroconidium (pl., Macroconidia). Some fungi produce conidia of two separate sizes: large ones (macroconidia) and small ones (microconidia). The terms are useful with those fungi that produce both sizes, but the names do not indicate anything about conidiogenesis, and both large and small may be produced either blastically or thallically. A representative macroconidium is depicted in Fig. 26.3E.

Phialoconidium (pl., Phialoconidia). This asexual propagule arises by an enteroblastic process (see Fig. 26.3C). The conidiogenous cell is called a phialide (Fig. 26.3C). Sometimes the lips of the phialide are very much reduced, and the structure is not apparent in light microscopy.

Poroconidium (pl., Poroconidia). These holoblastic conidia are formed by the emergence of the newly formed conidium through a pore in the conidiogenous cell (Fig. 26.3B).

Annelloconidium (pl., Annelloconidia). The first annelloconidium to arise is formed holoblastically, but all of the successive ones are enteroblastic. As each conidium emerges it leaves a ring of parental outer-cell wall. These remnants are called annellations (rings), and the conidiogenous cell is termed an annellide (Fig. 26.3D).

These are the sorts of conidia seen among the zoopathogenic fungi. The microscopic appearance is the major basis for identification in the laboratory and will be an important part of the following descriptions.

Sporangiospore (pl., Sporangiospores). This spore is produced by cytoplasmic cleavage (Fig. 26.4) within a structure called a **sporangium** (pl., sporangia). The hyphae of sporangiospore producers are nonseptate, for the most part, though septum formation can occur to isolate the sporangium from the hyphal element from which it was produced and to contain the cytoplasm of the cell involved in sexual reproduction.

Sexual Reproduction

Most fungi engage in sexual reproduction and the form of growth that it encompasses is called the teleomorphic state of the fungus. The mode of sexual reproduction is the basis of taxonomy of the fungi. The process of sexual reproduction in fungi involves the same basic process as in all other eukaryotes. Each of the products of meiosis that result from sexual reproduction is housed in a

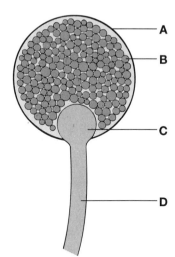

Figure 26.4.

Diagrammatic representation of the asexual spores of a zygomycete. (A) Sporangium. (B) Sporangiospores. (C) Columella (structural element of the sporangium. (D) Sporangiophore (sporangiospore-bearing structure).

specialized structure, the sexual spore. There are three types of sexual spores: **zygospores, ascospores,** and **basidiospores.** The morphology and development of these spores are the basic criteria for distinguishing among the five phyla in the kingdom Fungi. The events of sexual reproduction involve complicated morphological transformations that will not be described here.

It should be noted that while some of the zoopathogenic fungi do engage in sexual reproduction, the consequences of that interaction are not known to play a role in pathogenesis and are not routinely used in laboratory identification.

DIMORPHISM

Dimorphic zoopathogenic fungi express one distinct form in tissue, and may also grow in that form at body temperature on artificial medium, and a second distinct form in nature or on artificial medium under appropriate incubation conditions. The tissue form may be referred to as the parasitic form, and the form found in nature as the saprobic form.

CLASSIFICATION

The fungi are contained in a separate biological kingdom called **Fungi.** There are five phyla in the kingdom. The divisions are based on the type of sexual reproduction, or lack thereof, within the division. The phyla and the type of sexual spores produced are: (1) **Zygomycota** (zygospores), (2) **Ascomycota** (ascospores), (3) **Basidiomycota** (basidiospores), (4) **Deuteromycota** (sexual reproduction unknown), and (5) **Mycophycophyta** (ascospores or, more rarely, basidiospores). Zoopathogens are found in the first four phyla but the majority occur in the Ascomycota and Deuteromycota. Members of the different phyla are commonly indicated by appending the suffix -etes to the stem of the word for the phylum. Thus, Zygomycetes are members of the Zygomycota, Ascomycetes are members of the Ascomycota, and so on. Many taxonomists feel the Deuteromycetes or **Fungi Imperfecti** should not be given phylum status since they represent only the anamorphic states of the Ascomycota and the Basidiomycota for which a teleomorphic state has not been discovered and perhaps has been lost during the evolution of the species. But the more traditional approach is used here. The Mycophycophyta, which contains the **lichens,** is a distinct group each of whose members is a symbiotic association of a fungus (an ascomycete or, more rarely, a basidiomycete) and an alga. There are no zoopathogens in this group. The detailed classification of the fungi or consideration of phylogeny cannot be given here but reference texts are provided.

SUMMARY

1. **The fungi are eukaryotes.**

2. **There are two growth forms of fungi: yeasts (unicellular) and moulds (multicellular).**

3. **The filaments of multicellular fungi are called hyphae and may be nonseptate (coenocytic) or septate.**

4. **The mycelium of a mould is the collection of hyphae that form a colony of growth.**

5. **There are two sorts of reproductive elements among the fungi: asexual propagules, which are called either conidia or sporangiospores depending on how they are formed, and sexual spores.**

6. **Conidia develop from fertile hyphae by two processes: blastic, in which a portion of the wall of the fertile hyphae blows out to form a conidium, and thallic, which involves the conversion of an entire segment of the fertile hyphae into a conidium.**

7. **Blastic conidia are termed holoblastic, when both the inner and outer**

walls of the hypha are involved, and enteroblastic, when only the inner wall is involved and the outer wall breaks away.

8. Thallic conidia are called holothallic when the entire wall is involved in formation of the conidium. Thallic conidia produced along the entire length of the hyphal strand are termed arthric and may be called holoarthric or enteroarthric depending on the method of their release.

9. Most fungi engage in sexual reproduction and the form of growth that it encompasses is called the teleomorphic state of the fungus.

10. Many zoopathogenic fungi exhibit dimorphism that consists of a saprobic growth form found in nature and a parasitic growth form found in the tissues and exudates of an infected host.

11. The fungi are classified in the kingdom Fungi, which is comprised of five phyla: (1) Zygomycota, (2) Ascomycota, (3) Basidiomycota, (4) Deuteromycota, and (5) Mycophycophyta. Zoopathogenic fungi are found among members of phyla numbers 1–4 but not among those in phylum number 5.

REFERENCES

Cole GT, Samson RA (1979): Patterns of Development in Conidial Fungi. London: Pitman.

Hawksworth DL, Sutton BC, Ainsworth GC (1983): Ainsworth and Bisby's Dictionary of the Fungi. Kew, Surrey: Commonwealth Mycological Institute.

Howard DH (1983–1985): Fungi Pathogenic to Humans and Animals (in three parts). New York: Marcel Dekker.

Kwon-Chung KJ, Bennett JE (1992): Medical Mycology. Philadelphia: Lea & Febiger.

Margulis L, Schwartz KV (1988): Five Kingdoms. New York: W.H. Freeman.

REVIEW QUESTIONS

For questions 1 to 6, choose the ONE BEST answer or completion.

1. Fungi are considered to be eukaryotic microbes because
   a) they grow by apical extension
   b) they form spores
   c) they possess both types of nucleic acids
   d) they possess membrane-bound nuclei

2. Dimorphism of zoopathogenic moulds is exemplified by
   a) the symbiotic association of a mould with an alga among the Lichens
   b) the existence of both macro- and microconidia
   c) the expression of two distinct morphologic forms: one in the tissues of the host, the other in nature
   d) the expression of both sexual and asexual propagules by a mould

3. Conidium formation that involves conversion of an entire segment of a fertile hypha is called

   a) thallic
   b) enteroblastic
   c) holoblastic
   d) sporangiosporogenesis

4. When both the inner and outer walls of a fertile hypha expand rapidly (blow out), the resulting conidium is called
   a) holoblastic
   b) enteroblastic
   c) holothallic
   d) holoarthric

5. A very useful staining procedure for revealing fungi in tissue is
   a) the Gram stain
   b) the periodic acid-Schiff's stain
   c) lactophenol cotton blue stain
   d) the hematoxylin and eosin stain

6. The major sterol in the membranes of fungi is
   a) lanosterol
   b) cholesterol
   c) ergosterol
   d) estradiol
   e) testosterone

ANSWERS TO REVIEW QUESTIONS

1. *d* The fungi are eukaryotes, which means they have a membrane-bound nucleus. The other answers are true of fungi but not uniquely so.

2. *c* The term dimorphism simply means two forms but is reserved, in medical mycology, for that common expression of two growth forms displayed by zoopathogens: one in nature, and the other in the tissues or exudates of a host.

3. *a* Thallic conidia are those produced by the conversion of an entire length of a fertile hypha.

4. *a* The word holo means entire. Thus holoblastic indicates all layers of the cell wall engage in the blow out or blastic process.

5. *b* The PAS stain interacts with polysaccharides of the fungal cell walls.

6. *c* Ergosterol is the prominent component of the plasma membrane of fungi. Cholesterol is the major sterol component of mammalian cells.

DERMATOMYCOSES

The term **dermatomycoses** signifies any infectious disease of the skin caused by a fungus. Such afflictions include (1) the dermatophytoses (ringworms), (2) certain skin infections caused by *Candida* spp., and (3) a number of miscellaneous, superficial diseases of the skin, hair, and nails. In this chapter dermatophytoses and miscellaneous superficial infections will be considered. *Candida* infections of the skin are presented in Chapter 28.

DERMATOPHYTOSES

Dermatophytoses are fungous infections of humans and other animals confined almost exclusively to the cutaneous layers of the body including the hair and nails. The infections are also known colloquially as **ringworm** and medically as *tinea*. A large number of closely related fungi known collectively as the **dermatophytes** are the causative agents.

Epidemiology

SOURCE. The dermatophytes are worldwide in distribution; however, some species are strictly limited to certain geographical areas. **Anthropophilic** species

523

are those found solely on humans and commonly show reduced conidiation in culture. **Zoophilic** species occasionally infect humans, but are predominantly found on other animals (cattle, cats, dogs, etc.). **Geophilic** species are those found in soil. The source of certain representative dermatophytes is given in Table 27.1.

TRANSMISSION. The ringworm infections are transmitted by direct contact with infected humans or other animals, by contact with skin scales or hair shed from lesions, or through contaminated fomites (inanimate objects used by humans). Such infected materials have been shown to remain infectious for periods

TABLE 27.1. Some Representative Dermatophytes

Genus	Prominent clinical feature[a]	Type of hair involvement[b]	Wood's light fluorescence	Epidemiology[c]
Microsporum				
audouinii	T. cap.	Ecto	+	A
canis	T. cap.	Ecto	+	Z
gypseum	T. corp.			G
	T. cap.	Ecto	−	
Trichophyton				
mentagrophytes	T. cap.	Ecto	−	A,Z
	T. corp.			
	T. ped.			
rubrum	T. cap.	Ecto	−	A
	T. corp.			
	T. ped.			
	T. cru.			
	T. ung.			
schoenleinii	T. cap.	Endo	+	A
concentricum	T. corp.		−	A
violaceum	T. cap.	Endo	−	A
verrucosum	T. cap.	Ecto	−	Z
	T. corp.			
tonsurans	T. cap.	Endo	−	A
	T. corp.			
Epidermophyton				
floccosum	T. cru.	NA[d]	−	A
	T. ped.			
	T. corp.			

[a] Abbreviations: T. cap. is tinea capitis; T. corp. is tinea corporis; T. ped. is tinea pedis; T. cru. is tinea cruris; and T. ung. is tinea unquium. The indicated clinical features are the most prominent but not exclusive ones.
[b] Abbreviation: ecto is ectothrix and endo is endothrix. In some instances hair involvement may be rare, but the type is indicated.
[c] Abbreviations: A is anthropophilic; Z is zoophilic; G is geophilic.
[d] NA, hair not involved by *Epidermophyton* spp.

greater than 1 year. The dermatophytoses are contagious, whereas almost all other mycoses are not (an uncommon exception and will be noted in Chapter 28).

Pathogenesis and Virulence Factors

The infectious element of the dermatophytes is an arthroconidium or undifferentiated fragment of hyphae. The macroconidia and microconidia commonly seen in cultures in vitro are not produced in vivo and are not the agents of natural infections but may occasionally initiate infection in laboratory personnel engaged in handling cultures.

In a susceptible host the infectious arthroconidium germinates and grows in the stratum corneum. Fragments of hyphae may also initiate growth directly in the skin. Living tissue is only rarely invaded (see Immunology, p. 529). On the skin, the infection spreads centrifugally.

Hair invasion proceeds as follows: An infectious arthroconidium germinates proximal to the hair shaft (pilus). The emergent germ tube descends the hair follicle. The external root sheath is penetrated, but this external colonization is transient, and the hair shaft is invaded about midway down the follicle. The intrapilary hyphae grow downward toward the upper limits of the zone of active keratinization. Living cells are not invaded. The hyphae are carried upward by the hair growth and, in the case of those fungi that produce the **ectothrix type** of hair involvement, break out of the hair shafts and back onto the surface at about the level of the follicle orifice. These secondary extrapilary hyphae form a dense mycelium that produces arthroconidia. Thus, the arthroconidia are outside the hair shaft (ectothrix) while some hyphae remain within the hair shaft. Hairs may fall out or break off leaving the areas of alopecia characteristic of the disease. In the **endothrix type** of involvement the initial invasion steps are the same, but the intrapilary hyphae remain within the hair shaft and form arthroconidia therein. In the **favus type of endothrix involvement** the stages are the same, but intrapilary growth is not so abundant and thus hairs are not usually weakened and do not break off.

The sensory signals and their transduction, which account for the patterns of skin, nail, and hair involvement in the dermatophytoses, are unknown. Some of the enzymes required for keratin utilization have been identified, and a few other enzymes, such as elastases, collagenases, and proteases, have been described. Generally, such virulence factors are useful in explaining the ability of dermatophytes to colonize the skin and its appendages, but the major manifestations of disease appear related to the host response to fungous antigens.

Clinical Manifestations

In general, dermatophytoses involve the nonviable keratinized layer of skin. The diseases are called tinea, a word to which is appended an adjective that defines the area of involvement.

1. **Tinea capitis:** Ringworm of the scalp and hair.
2. **Tinea barbae:** Chronic dermatophytic infection of the bearded area of the face and neck.
3. **Tinea corporis:** Ringworm of the glabrous (smooth) skin. Lesions vary from superficial scaling to deep granulomata (rare). The superficial lesions spread centrifugally and have an erythematous border containing actively growing organisms and a central clear area where few living organisms exist.
4. **Tinea cruris** (jock strap itch): Ringworm of the groin, perineum, and perianal regions.
5. **Tinea pedis** (athlete's foot): Ringworm of the feet, particularly the toe webs and soles.
6. **Tinea unguium:** Dermatophytic involvement of the nails.
7. **Tinea favosa** (also called favus): This is a chronic dermatophytic infection of the scalp where cup-shaped crusts called scutula are formed around the hair shafts.
8. **Tinea imbricata:** A superficial dermatophytosis with a bizarre pattern of concentric lesions caused by a single species of dermatophyte, *Trichophyton concentricum.*

Mycology and Laboratory Diagnosis

The appearance of lesions is typical for tinea, but other organisms can cause similar symptoms and a number of noninfectious dermatitides may resemble dermatophytoses. A definitive diagnosis depends on the demonstration of a dermatophyte by one or another of the following techniques.

DIRECT MOUNT. A simple scraping with a scalpel blade at the erythematous border of the lesion will often verify the diagnosis upon microscopic examination. A drop of 10–20% potassium hydroxide (KOH) solution is used as a mounting fluid that will dissolve the keratin of the skin. Scales from the lesion are placed in the drop of potassium hydroxide and a coverslip applied. Demonstration of branching hyphae that form arthroconidia (Fig. 27.1A) are diagnostic. Hair samples from tinea capitis and tinea barbae will reveal one or another of two

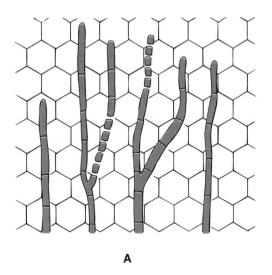
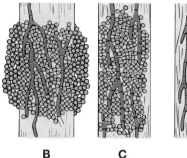
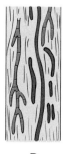

Figure 27.1.

Appearance of dermatophytes in potassium hydroxide preparations of skin and hair. (A) Hyphal elements and arthroconidia. (B) Ectothrix involvement of hair. (C) Endothrix involvement of hair. (D) Favic hair.

patterns of arthroconidial arrangement: either the conidia will surround the outside of the hair shaft (ectothrix) or they will be located within the hair shaft (endothrix) (Fig. 27.1B and C). The hair from cases of tinea favosa are quite characteristic in that shaft invasion does occur but arthroconidia are rarely seen. Thus, strands of hyphae or air spaces formerly occupied by hyphae are seen (Fig. 27.1D).

WOOD'S LIGHT. Some species of *Microsporum* cause hairs to fluoresce a greenish-yellow color when exposed to a UV light of long wavelength (365 nm, called Wood's light after Robert William Wood, an American physicist who designed the lamp that generates this wavelength). This result is useful for veterinarians, since tinea of cats and dogs is often caused by those *Microsporum* spp. that cause hair fluorescence (Table 27.1), but only 10% of tinea capitis cases in humans involve *Microsporum* spp. that evoke fluorescent hairs. Thus the value of Wood's light is limited in human disease. Hairs involved in tinea favosa also fluoresce but the color is silvery instead of the greenish-yellow seen with *Microsporum*-infected hairs. Fluorescence in the hairs is generated by intermediate products (pteridines) of fungal metabolism.

CULTURE. The dermatophytes are commonly grown on **Sabouraud dex-**

trose agar or some similar recipe of dextrose (1–4%) and peptone (2%) with agar (2%), which usually contains substances that inhibit bacteria and saprobic fungi. Originally, the medium as designed by R. Sabouraud (a nineteenth century dermatologist) was adjusted to pH 5.2. Such acidity inhibits bacterial growth but does not affect the growth of fungi. The medium thus had selective qualities useful in culturing skin, hair, and nail specimens likely to be contaminated with bacteria and noninfectious moulds. Such selectivity is achieved today by addition of chloramphenicol (to inhibit bacteria) and cycloheximide (to inhibit common saprobic moulds). Material for cultivation is obtained by scraping the lesion with a scalpel blade.

ETIOLOGIC AGENTS. The dermatophytes utilize the protein keratin in their metabolism (keratinophiles) and are placed in three genera on the basis of the elements of asexual reproduction (Fig. 27.2). The Genera *Trichophyton, Microsporum,* and *Epidermophyton* are differentiated from each other by their large, multiseptate, elongate **macroconidia** (holothallic conidia) (Fig. 27.2). A second type of conidium, which is called a **microconidium** (holoblastic conidium), is a small, unicellular, spherical, oval, or pyriform structure. These conidia are helpful in differentiation among species. The macroconidia of *Microsporum* spp. are echinulate (spiky), mostly spindle-shaped, thick-walled, and borne singly (Fig. 27.2). *Trichophyton* spp. produce macroconidia that are cylindrical, smooth, thin walled, and borne singly (Fig. 27.2). The macroconidia of *Epidermophyton* spp. are smooth, club-shaped, moderately thick-walled, and borne in clusters of two or three; microconidia are absent in this genus (Fig. 27.2). The salient features of some of the more representative dermatophytes are given in Tables 27.1 and 27.2. Nearly 30 species of dermatophytes have been associated with clinical disease.

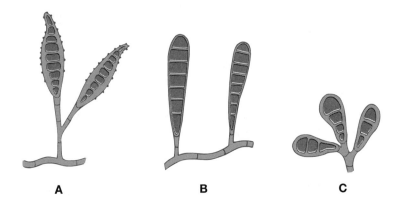

Figure 27.2.

Macroconidia of the dermatophytes. (A) *Microsporum.* (B) *Trichophyton.* (C) *Epidermophyton.*

A   B   C

However, there are only 6 species commonly encountered in urban areas of the United States (Table 27.2).

Immunology

HOST-PARASITE INTERACTIONS. The dermatophytic infections that evoke the most vigorous inflammatory responses are generally cleared rapidly and are often self-healing. Such infections are most often caused by zoophilic species of dermatophytes. By way of contrast, minimally inflammatory disease is often caused by anthropophilic species and may be associated with defective cell-mediated forms of immunity toward antigens of the dermatophytes. There is a high degree of hypersensitivity that develops in ringworm. Sometimes specific lesions that represent this aspect of the host response develop. Such lesions are called **dermatophytids** or simply **ids** and are vesicular cutaneous eruptions at sites separate from the primary lesions. The ids are sterile and represent strong delayed-type hypersensitivity (DTH). Cutaneous defenses against dermatophytoses involve the physical characteristics of the skin surface, the continual sloughing of the upper stratum corneum, the relative resistance to infection during parts of the hair growth cycle, the fungistatic lipids in sebum, and the iron-transporting protein, transferrin, in plasma that competes with the organisms for iron and may thereby limit the infection to nonliving (keratinized) tissues. An early neutrophilic leukocyte infiltrate in the epidermis and a later dermal mononuclear cell infiltrate are the inflammatory responses to dermatophytic infection. Dermatophyte infections in humans or animals are accompanied by a partial immunity to reinfection, and the second infections have a shortened, milder course. Experimental dermatophyte infections in animals appear to sensitize the animals so that they develop immediate and delayed hypersensitivity to the antigens of the infecting organisms.

SKIN TEST. Delayed-type hypersensitivity, which develops in patients with dermatophyte infection, can be displayed with the antigen **trichophytin,** a filtrate antigen prepared from the liquid medium in which special species of dermatophytes have been grown. The product is not used diagnostically because of the widespread occurrence of dermatomycoses ($> 90\%$ of adults are positive). Thus, a positive test need not relate to a current dermatosis.

Treatment

Treatment of the dermatophytoses is administered either by prescription or nonprescription drugs. Among prescription drugs, the most commonly used is griseofulvin, an antibiotic that concentrates in keratinized areas of the body. This

TABLE 27.2. Characteristics of Six Common Dermatophytes[a]

Microsporum

> *Microsporum canis:* Colonies are cottony or wooly, white to buff in color. The reverse is yellow to orange-brown. Macroconidia are numerous, large, thick-walled, spindle-shaped, echinulate, 8–20 × 40–150 μm, with 6–15 septa. Microconidia are usually scarce, clavate to elongate.
>
> *Microspum gypseum:* Colonies are downy to granular, pale buff to rosy buff. The reverse is rosy buff to amber. Macroconidia are predominantly cylindrical, slightly tapering toward both ends, 25–28 × 5–12 μm, with up to 5 septa and moderately thick, verrucose walls. Microconidia are 1.7–3.3 × 3.3–8.3 μm, clavate, smooth-walled or slightly rough-walled, borne laterally along the hyphae.

Trichophyton

> *Trichophyton mentagrophytes:* Colonies are white, floccose to granular, yellowish to peach colored. Reverse pale yellow to brown to reddish brown. Microconidia are clavate, borne laterally on undifferentiated hyphae in floccose strains or nearly spherical on conidiophores, forming clusters in granular strains. Macroconidia are rare or abundant in granular forms, clavate, 20–50 × 6–8 μm, with 3–5 septa. Spiral hyphae may be seen.
>
> *Trichophyton rubrum:* Colonies are cottony and white, later becoming velvety. The reverse side is reddish to rose purple. Macroconidia are elongate, cylindrical, thin and smooth-walled, with 3–8 septa. Generally, these are scarce. Microconidia are numerous, clavate, 2–3 × 3–5 μm, borne in clusters or singly along the hyphae. A wide variety of colonial types has been described.
>
> *Trichophyton tonsurans:* Colonies grow fairly slowly on glucose peptone agar, and are flat, somewhat powdery, with a yellowish surface. The reverse is mahogany red. Macroconidia are not frequently seen, but when found are somewhat thick-walled, club-shaped with 3–5 septa. Microconidia are numerous, clavate, 2–5 × 3–7 μm, and are borne laterally along the hyphae on pedicels of various lengths.

Epidermophyton

> *Epidermophyton floccosum:* Colonies have a velvety to powdery surface that is gently folded in a number of radiating furrows and is khaki-yellow in color. The reverse is yellow to tan. Usually, isolates mutate early and almost invariably, with the production tufts of white, sterile hyphae that soon overgrows the entire colony. Macroconidia are clavate, smooth, fairly thick-walled, with 0–4 (usually 2–3) septa; the macroconidia are borne in characteristic clusters of twos and threes. Microconidia are not produced.

[a] It should be noted that some dermatophytes reproduce sexually. The name provided for this teleomorphic form is *Arthroderma* (phylum Ascomycota). The name of the anamorphic form of growth is used in clinical reports. Among the species in this table, *M. canis, M. gypseum,* and *T. mentagrophytes* are known to have a teleomorphic form of growth.

drug has virtually eradicated classical tinea capitis in children. Another prescription drug is ketoconazole. It is used both systemically and topically. Nonprescription drugs are applied topically and are usually effective if the area of involvement is small, though recurrences are common. Among the active ingredients of such substances are undecylenic acid, tolnaftate, and miconazole. Miconazole and ketoconazole are members of a chemically distinct group of compounds called azoles.

MISCELLANEOUS SUPERFICIAL SKIN DISEASES

In addition to the dermatophytoses and certain infections caused by *Candida* spp. there are a number of afflictions of the skin and its appendages (hair and nails) that are caused by fungi. A few of the more notable ones will be briefly considered here.

Superficial Dermatomycoses

Pityriasis versicolor (also called tinea versicolor). This dermatomycosis is a chronic, mild, usually asymptomatic infection of the superficial layer of the skin (stratum corneum). The disease is caused by *Malassezia furfur*, a yeast that produces abundant blastoconidia and pseudohyphal elements in the skin scales. Diagnosis of pityriasis versicolor is based on the clinical picture and the demonstration of typical fungal elements in a KOH scraping from infected skin. The yeast requires oleic acid for growth, which has to be accommodated in cultures in vitro (cultures are rarely performed in diagnostic efforts). The yeast may also produce a folliculitis of the hair follicles called **pityriasis folliculitis** and is considered by some to be important in **seborrheic dermatitis** (dandruff). The organism is a commensal of the normal skin but the factors that cause it to precipitate, pityriasis versicolor and pityriasis folliculitis, or to be involved in seborrheic dermatitis are unknown. Ketoconazole and selenium sulfide are useful therapeutic agents, but recurrences are common.

Tinea nigra palmaris. This affliction is an asymptomatic, superficial fungous infection of the skin. Usually the palmar surface of the hands is the site of involvement and so the designation, palmaris. The lesions are brown-to-black macules (flat areas of pigmentation). There is no obvious host inflammatory response. The etiologic agent, *Phaeoannellomyces (Exophiala) werneckii,* appears in potassium hydroxide treated scrapings as pigmented (brown to black), septate, ramifying hyphae. Cultures produce black, yeast-like colonies that later become hyphal. The blastoconidia may replicate independently of the hyphae (the early yeast-like colony) but are formed on the hyphae (holoblastic annelloconidia) when these appear. Common topical fungicides are generally effective in treatment.

Piedra. The hair shaft is involved in this disease. Two forms of the infection are recognized: (1) **black piedra** in which hard, black nodules form along the hair shaft and are caused by *Piedraia hortai* (not seen in the United States) and (2) **white piedra** in which the nodules are white and are caused by *Trichosporon beigelii.* The diseases are generally diagnosed by direct examination of hair shafts emersed in potassium hydroxide. The appearance of the nodules and their contents are quite distinctive. Cultures are not often performed to establish the diagnosis. The appearance both in direct mounts and cultures is described in standard texts.

A number of other species of fungi have been associated with cutaneous diseases, but these are beyond the scope of this chapter. Standard textbooks can be consulted for further information.

SUMMARY

1. The dermatophytoses are a collection of cutaneous diseases in which the site of attack is limited to the skin, hair, and nails. The afflictions are caused by a group of related keratinophilic fungi known as the dermatophytes.

2. The dermatophytoses are known colloquially as ringworm and medically as tinea. When the term tinea is used, the area of involvement is indicated by a modifying adjective, for example, tinea capitis, ringworm of the scalp; tinea pedis, ringworm of the feet, and so on.

3. The diagnosis of a tinea infection rests on: (a) the clinical picture displayed, (b) demonstration of fungal elements in scrapings from lesions suspected of being ringworm, (c) irradiation of suspected lesions with a Wood's light (restricted to certain species of *Microsporum* and *Trichophyton schoenleinii*), and (d) culture of materials from lesions on selective media (Sabouraud dextrose agar with inhibitors).

4. The dermatophytes are divided into three genera on the basis of the morphology of an asexually produced macroconidium. Other structural elements, such as microconidia, can be helpful in species identification. A sexual form of reproduction occurs in some species of dermatophytes but this manifestation plays no role in pathogenesis of the dermatophytoses and is not commonly a part of the identification procedures in the clinical laboratory.

5. Some species of dermatophytes are worldwide in distribution (for example, *Trichophyton rubrum*), others occur in very restricted geographic areas (for example, *Trichophyton concentricum*).

6. Dermatophytes are characteristically found in defined locations: anthropophilic forms are those associated with humans though rarely they may infect animals where opportunities for contact occur; zoophilic forms are those characteristically associated with animals and may be acquired from

that source by humans. Occasionally, varieties of a particular species will be found to associate either with humans or animals (e.g., *Trichophyton mentagrophytes*); geophilic forms are those that occur in the soil and are acquired by humans and animals from that location.

7. A high degree of sensitivity (DTH) to fungal products is common with dermatophytoses. Individuals sometimes develop sterile vesicles called "dermatophytids" as a manifestation of this sensitivity.

8. Treatment may be systemic (griseofulvin and ketoconazole) or topical. Useful topical agents commonly contain undecylenic acid, tolnaftate, or one of the azoles.

9. Dermatomycosis is a broad term that includes dermatophytoses (ringworm), *Candida* infections, and a number of very superficial afflictions including pityriasis versicolor, tinea nigra palmaris, and white and black piedra.

REFERENCES

Fitzpatrick TB, Eisen AZ, Wolff K, Freedberg IM, Austin KF (eds) (1987): Dermatology in General Medicine, 2 vols. 3rd ed. New York: McGraw-Hill Book Co.

Howard DH (1983): Ascomycetes: the dermatophytes, In Howard DH (ed): Fungi Pathogenic for Humans and Animals (in three parts), Part A–Biology. New York: Marcel Dekker, p 113.

Matsumoto T, Ajello L (1987): Current taxonomic concepts pertaining to the dermatophytes and related fungi. Int J Dermatol 26:491.

Rebell G, Taplin D (1970): Dermatophytes: Their Recognition and Identification. Coral Gables, FL: University of Miami Press.

REVIEW QUESTIONS

For questions 1 to 6, choose the ONE
BEST answer or completion.

1. Ectothrix type hair involvement refers to
   a) broken hairs
   b) ingrown hairs
   c) fungous conidia within a hair shaft
   d) fungous conidia around a hair shaft

2. Sterile vesicular lesions, indistinguishable
   from a primary lesion, which arise in other
   parts of the body of an allergic individual
   infected with a dermatophyte are called
   a) dermatomycosis
   b) dermatophytes
   c) dermatophytids
   d) furuncles
   e) zits

3. A selective medium for isolating dermatophytes
   a) is impossible to design
   b) will often contain antibacterial antibiotics
      and cycloheximide

c) is useless in dealing with dermatophytes
d) ought to contain blood or serum

4. An inexpensive substance useful in direct examination of material from patients suspected of having ringworm is
   a) saline
   b) lactophenol cotton blue
   c) Sabouraud broth
   d) potassium hydroxide

5. A major feature that distinguishes among the
   three major genera of dermatophytes is
   a) growth on media containing cyclohexi-
      mide
   b) morphology of the macroconidium pro-
      duced in culture
   c) arrangement of conidia in or on infected
      hairs
   d) animal species infected naturally

6. The selection of infected hairs for fungus
   culture may be aided by the use of a
   a) high intensity light
   b) laser beam
   c) fluorescent light
   d) Wood's light

ANSWERS TO REVIEW QUESTIONS

1. *d* Ectothrix conidia surrounding the hair shaft.

2. *c* The allergic manifestation of a dermatophyte infection is called a dermatophytid or commonly simply an id.

3. *b* Media for the cultivation of dermatophytes are often various recipes of simple glucose-peptone agars. One recipe is called Sabouraud dextrose agar. The medium may be made selective by the addition of chloramphenicol (antibacterial) and cycloheximide (antifungal for certain common saprobes).

4. *d* Potassium hydroxide is used as a clarifying agent for keratin-containing skin, hair, and nails. The presence of fungal elements may be revealed after such clarification.

5. *b* The morphology of the asexually produced macroconidium is the basis for distinguishing the three genera of dermatophytes.

6. *d* The Wood's light (365 nm) causes hairs infected with certain species of *Microsporum* (greenish-yellow) and with *Trichophyton schoenleinii* (silver-blue) to fluoresce.

YEAST INFECTIONS

The yeasts are unicellular fungi. The predominant asexual reproductive unit of the majority of yeasts is a blastoconidium. A number of such fungi are pathogenic, but the two genera that contain the most important zoopathogens are *Candida* and *Cryptococcus*. In addition, there are a number of other yeasts that have been, more rarely, implicated in disease. Such organisms will be considered under the separate heading of Miscellaneous Yeast Infections at the end of this chapter.

CANDIDIASIS

Candidiasis, also known as candidosis, is an acute or subacute infection in which the causative agent commonly produces superficial disease of the skin, nails, and mucous membranes or may, more rarely, involve other deep-seated areas of the body.

Epidemiology

Zoopathogenic species in the genus *Candida* are **commensals** of the GI tract, and of the vaginal and oral mucosae. The source of infection is, therefore, most commonly **endogenous.** *Candida* spp. take advantage of certain predisposing events to cause disease. Among such events are (1) physiological situations (e.g., infancy and pregnancy); (2) traumatic changes, including maceration (softening of the skin by moisture) and postoperative contaminations; (3) endocrine dystrophies (e.g., diabetes); (4) malnutrition; (5) malignancy; (6) anemia; and (7) changes induced by antibacterial and immunosuppressive drugs. *Candida* infections are very common and may occasionally be contagious, usually by sexual contact or by contaminated hands such as nurse-to-baby transmission in newborn nurseries.

Pathogenesis and Virulence Factors

Candida spp. are commensals and disease by them is initiated after receiving sensory signals. The nature of these signals and their operation in the fungous cell are unknown. Those aspects of the host-parasite interaction that have been explored include the following:

1. **Genetics.** *Candida albicans* is a **diploid organism** and efforts to bring about haploidization have been unsuccessful. Attempts to get yeast cells to mate have failed. Thus, *C. albicans* is amyctic (does not mix, i.e., does not engage in sexual reproduction). Genetic analyses are, nevertheless, possible. The first successful genetic approach involved heterokaryon formation and parasexual genetics. These early efforts were followed by the development of plasmid genetic systems. Explanation of these are beyond the scope of this short course, but it is to be noted that approaches to an understanding of pathogenesis of *Candida* spp. will depend on the use of genetic tools such as these.

2. **Adherence.** Successful colonization of the GI tract and the mucous membranes by *Candida* spp. involves adherence of the yeast cells to the epithelial surfaces. There is a good deal of information on the role of fungal proteins and mannoproteins in adherence. Receptors have been characterized.

3. **Filament Formation.** Tissue invasion by *C. albicans* is often associated with **germ tube formation,** and the appearance of *Candida* spp. in vivo is customarily one of yeast cells and hyphal filaments. Thus, both true hyphae and pseudohyphae would appear to be involved in the disease process by different species of *Candida.* The exact signals that foster germ tube formation or sponsor pseudohyphae in vivo are unknown. Of course, filament formation plays no role in the pathogenesis of *Candida glabrata,* which does not form hyphae.

4. **Proteases.** A number of protein degrading enzymes have been described as produced by *Candida* spp. These proteases could be involved in virulence (e.g.,

by degradation of immunoglobulins, etc.), but although genetic studies show proteases are involved in candidiasis, the exact pathogenetic role is yet to be described.

Clinical Manifestations

Candida infections involve the skin, the mucous membranes or, more rarely, disseminate to other organ systems (e.g., lungs, heart, spleen, and kidneys).

CUTANEOUS LESIONS. *Candida* spp. invade the skin and nails, and such involvement produces lesions that resemble those produced by dermatophytes. Nail infection almost always includes involvement of the area around the nail leading to club-shaped fingers. The skin areas with closely opposing surfaces, such as those between the fingers, in the groin, and other sites of accumulated moisture, are often infected by *Candida* spp. For example, the most common incitant of diaper rash is *C. albicans.*

MUCOUS MEMBRANES. The yeast may infect the mucous membranes and lead to a condition known as **thrush,** which may be recurrent. Infection at the corners of the mouth, called **perlèche,** is occasioned by saliva accumulation. The mucosal surface of the vagina is a frequent site of *Candida* infection (**vulvovaginitis).** The problem is recurrent in some women and the reasons for repeated attacks are not known.

A form of candidiasis known as **chronic mucocutaneous candidiasis (CMC)** affects individuals with immunological defects in cell-mediated immunity (CMI). There are several defects of CMI known to predispose to CMC. The disease consists of repeated attacks over long periods of time of various mucocutaneous types of candidiasis. Although the infection is recurrent, the site of involvement remains localized and a spread to deeper tissues and organ systems does not occur. Thrush is frequently seen in AIDS patients but although the esophagus is often involved, systemic dissemination rarely occurs.

SYSTEMIC DISSEMINATED DISEASE. Cases of **disseminated candidiasis** are seen in advanced malignancies, such as bladder or bowel cancer. It can also be associated with Hodgkin's disease and is commonly observed in bone marrow transplant patients. Neutropenia from whatever cause often heralds deep-seated, disseminated candidiasis.

Mycology and Laboratory Diagnosis

APPEARANCE IN TISSUE AND EXUDATES. *Candida* spp. appear in tissues and exudates as **yeast cells** (blastoconidia) and **hyphal elements.** The blastoconidia or the hyphae may predominate, but both are usually present. The hyphal components are most often **pseudohyphae** but true hyphae may occur in infections caused by *C. albicans* (Table 28.1). Exceptions to this generalization are *C. glabrata*, which does not form hyphae of either sort and *Candida guilliermondii* in which pseudohyphal formation is much reduced.

APPEARANCE IN CULTURE. Cultures of the fungus grown on most laboratory media produce soft, cream-colored colonies comprised of unicellular organisms, that is, yeast cells (Fig. 28.1A). These blastoconidia sometimes do not separate at maturity but rather remain attached and elongate to form pseudophyphae (Fig. 28.1B). The yeast cells of *C. albicans* can form germ tubes when incubated at 37°C in serum or on certain other substrates. Such germ tubes give rise to a true mycelium comprised of apically growing hyphae. However, the true mycelium is customarily short lived and is soon accompanied by both blastoconidia and pseudohyphae (Fig. 28.1).

IDENTIFICATION OF CANDIDA spp. IN THE LABORATORY. The identification of *Candida* spp. relies on morphological and physiological attributes.

TABLE 28.1. *Candida* **Species Involved in Human Disease**

Species[a]	Germ tube formation	Chlamydoconidia (vesicles)	Pseudohyphae
Candida albicans	+	+	+
Candida glabrata[b]	−	−	−
Candida guilliermondii	−	−	±
Candida kefyr[c]	−	−	+
Candida krusei	−	−	+
Candida lusitaniae	−	−	+[d]
Candida parapsilosis	−	−	+
Candida rugosa	−	−	+
Candida tropicalis	−[e]	−[e]	+
Candida viswanathii	−	−	+

[a] The general order of species identification is germ tube formation, pseudohyphal formation, and finally, assimilation of certain carbon sources of energy.
[b] Formerly, *Torulopsis glabrata.*
[c] Formerly, *Candida pseudotropicalis.*
[d] An interesting additional characteristic of this species is its resistance to the drug amphotericin B.
[e] Rare isolates of *C. tropicalis* have been reported to form germ tubes and chlamydoconidia (vesicles).

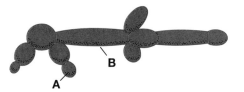

Figure 28.1.

Yeast cell and hyphal element of *C. albicans*. (A) Blastoconidia. (B) Pseudohyphae.

Germ Tube Test. The germ tube test is a rapid identification procedure of the most common incitant of candidiasis, *C. albicans* (75% of isolates of yeasts in a clinical laboratory). The test involves immersing a small portion of an isolated colony in serum (commercial animal sera; the kind of animal is probably not important). Mixtures are incubated at 37°C (mandatory), and after 3 h a sample is examined microscopically for germ tubes (Fig. 28.2). A positive test is a specific identification of *C. albicans*.

Formation of Pseudohyphae. The genus *Candida* contains a large number of species other than *C. albicans* that reproduce asexually by means of blastoconidia. In most of these species pseudohyphae are a prominent aspect of growth under certain circumstances (e.g., tissue invasion or cultivation on special media). Those species of *Candida* that have been associated with human diseases are listed in Table 28.1. The production of pseudohyphae by these species is revealed by cultivation of an isolate on some variation of **corn meal agar (CMA)** with Tween-80, or a comparable substitute for that medium, incubated at room temperature. Most *Candida* spp. produce pseudohyphae under these circumstances, and the pattern of development is useful in species delineation. A description of such patterns is, however, beyond the coverage here. It should be noted that *C. glabrata* does not form pseudohyphae and that *C. guilliermondii* forms them sparingly (Table 28.1).

Chlamydoconidia are formed on CMA by *C. albicans* (Table 28.3; Fig. 28.3C). This event is helpful because about 5% of the isolates of *C. albicans* fail to germinate in the routine germ tube test, and these false negatives are then recognized by their morphology on CMA. It should be noted that the structural element called a chlamydoconidium, or a chlamydospore by some, is neither a conidium nor a spore because it does not germinate at maturity. Most investigators

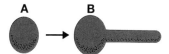

Figure 28.2.

Germination or blastoconidia of *C. albicans*. (A) Blastoconidium. (B) Germ tube.

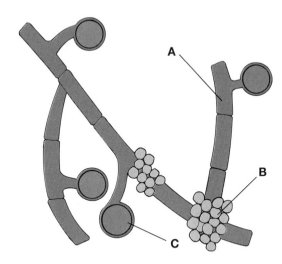

Figure 28.3.

C. albicans cultivated on corn meal agar. (A) Pseudohyphae. (B) Blastoconidia. (C) Chlamydoconidium.

consider it to be a special structural element of *C. albicans* for which a nonspecific term, such as vesicle, is more appropriate.

Substrate Assimilation. Species identification within the genus *Candida* is made on the basis of morphology on CMA and carbon source assimilation patterns. *Candida* spp. assimilate various carbon sources, and this fact can be used to separate them. Several commercial preparations have been developed to facilitate these determinations. The tests used to identify *Candida* spp. are listed in Table 28.1.

Sexual Reproduction. Some of the *Candida* spp. express a teleomorphic form (not *C. albicans*) but this expression is not related to pathogenesis of diseases for which they are responsible and is not customarily used in identification in a clinical laboratory.

Immunology

HOST-PARASITE INTERACTION. In a normal host there are a number of innate and immunological defense mechanisms, both humoral and cellular, that protect the host from infection by *Candida* spp. Among these innate mechanisms, complement and polymorphonuclear leukocyte mediated phagocytosis are of primary importance. A common predisposing factor in disseminated candidiasis is

neutropenia (a decrease in the number of neutrophilic leukocytes). The neutropenic individual often develops candidiasis. Immune responses to *Candida* have been documented in clinical as well as experimental studies, but the role of individual components of the immune system is unresolved. The immune responses to *Candida* infections that are currently being investigated are (1) the immunoregulatory effect of circulating antigens and immune complexes or both; (2) the diagnostic and prognostic value of antigenic determinants; (3) the importance of the antigenic differences between yeast and hyphal forms of the fungus; (4) the influence of hormones on the immune response; (5) the clinical significance of cell-mediated immunity and humoral immunity, including the role of IgA and IgE; (6) the development of serologic tests that will distinguish colonized, healthy individuals from those with infection; and (7) the basis of the immunosuppression in those who are infected with *Candida* spp.

SEROLOGIC AND IMMUNOLOGIC TESTS. There are a number of tests designed to detect antibodies to or antigens of *Candida* spp., but none is widely adopted as both specific and sensitive enough to assist reliably in the diagnosis of candidiasis. There is a good deal of activity in the area of development of such serologic tests, but none are widely recognized as definitive. Another approach to the problem of identifying patients with disseminated candidiasis involves the detection of specific products of fungal metabolism (e.g., D-arabinatol).

Treatment

Mucocutaneous candidiasis is treated with various topical medicaments (e.g., nystatin, clotrimazole, and ketoconazole). Ketoconazole is especially useful in CMC. At present amphotericin B is the only useful antimicrobial for systemic, widespread candidiasis but some of the newer azoles may prove useful as experience develops.

CRYPTOCOCCOSIS

In its most frequently recognized form, cryptococcosis is a chronic, wasting, frequently fatal disease (in untreated or severely immunocompromised individuals) characterized by a pronounced predilection for the CNS and caused by the basidiomycetous (phylum Basidiomycota) yeast *Cryptococcus neoformans*. The characteristics of the primary pulmonary form of the disease are not well known. Cryptococcosis most often occurs in immunocompromised hosts. In AIDS, cryptococcosis is the fourth most important cause of death due to infectious disease and occurs in 6–7% of all AIDS patients in the United States.

Epidemiology

C. neoformans is worldwide in distribution. However, there are two biotypes of the fungus, named *C. neoformans* var. *neoformans* and *C. neoformans* var. *gattii* (see p. 545). The biotypes have different geographic distributions. *C. neoformans* var. *gattii* is most often found in tropical or subtropical locations. Moreover, the two biotypes have different ecological associations: *C. neoformans* var. *neoformans* is found in association with avian habitats, especially pigeons, while the only natural source of *C. neoformans* var. *gattii* so far identified is debris from the tree *Eucalyptus camaldulensis.*

Pathogenesis and Virulence Factors

C. neoformans is primarily an **opportunistic pathogen.** Therefore, the pathogenesis of disease does not depend as much on the virulence attributes of the fungus as it does on the impaired immune response of the host. Nevertheless, several features of the biology of *C. neoformans* are clearly related to its ability to cause disease. Among those features are:

1. **Growth at 37°C.** There are several species in the genus *Cryptococcus,* but only four can grow at 37°C. Thus, the ability to survive and grow at 37°C is one of the attributes of *C. neoformans* that contributes to pathogenicity. Mutants of the pathogenic species selected for inability to grow at 37°C are avirulent.

2. **Capsule.** The capsule of *C. neoformans* is a characteristic feature that is clearly associated with virulence. Acapsular mutants are avirulent. Capsulated strains resist phagocytosis, and opsonization by specific antibody or complement or both leads to more easily resolved experimental infections. Therefore, the capsule is an important virulence attribute of *C. neoformans.*

3. **Phenoloxidase Production.** *C. neoformans* does not utilize the catecholamines of the CNS as sources of carbon and nitrogen, nor are such substances exclusively found in brain tissue. Thus, the presence of these amines in the CNS is not a trophic signal to *C. neoformans.* But the fungus does produce melanin in vivo, and that substance can scavenge oxidative intermediates, such as superoxide anion and hydroxyl radicals. Such activity could provide a mechanism of survival to *C. neoformans* confronted by reactive oxidative intermediates formed by phagocytic cells, that is, polymorphonuclear leukocytes and mononuclear phagocytes.

Clinical Manifestations

The fungus is acquired by inhalation of infectious conidia from an exogenous source. Pulmonary cases of cryptococcosis are frequently subclinical and often overlooked, but the primary infection may disseminate. The meninges and brain parenchyma are the characteristic sites involved in disseminated disease. Other tissues may be involved and skin lesions occur in about 20% of cases of disseminated disease.

Mycology and Laboratory Diagnosis

Cryptococcosis is caused by a single species of a basidiomycetous yeast that has both an anamorphic and a teleomorphic form of growth. The anamorphic form is an encapsulated yeast that has two biotypes, each of which in turn has two serotypes discerned on the basis of the antigenic epitopes within the capsule. The two biotypes are named *C. neoformans* var. *neoformans* (serotypes A and D) and *C. neoformans* var. *gattii* (serotypes B and C). These biotypes are distinguished on the basis of physiological attributes that can be identified on certain selective media. One such medium is **canavanine-glycine-bromthymol blue (CGB medium).**

The teleomorphic state of this basidiomycetous yeast is named *Filobasidiella neoformans*. Once again, there are two varieties, based on the shape of the basidiospores (sexual spores). The two varieties are *F. neoformans* var. *neoformans* (anamorph, *C. neoformans* var. *neoformans*) and *F. neoformans* var. *bacillispora* (anamorph, *C. neoformans* var. *gattii*). The teleomorphic state plays no known role in pathogenesis and is not a part of the laboratory identification in a clinical microbiological laboratory. However, the existence of the teleomorphic state provides a resource of potential value in the study of the fundamental question on the biology of *C. neoformans* including its ability to cause disease.

APPEARANCE IN TISSUE. In the tissues of an infected host, *C. neoformans* of either biotype occurs as a **blastoconidium with a capsule.** The capsule can be demonstrated in tissue sections by special stains. The encapsulated yeast cells can be visualized in fluids from patients (e.g., spinal fluid) with either India ink (Fig. 28.4) or with the CFL stain.

APPEARANCE IN CULTURE. In culture, the fungus produces mucoid colonies that contain encapsulated yeast cells customarily revealed with India ink preparations. *C. neoformans* deposits **melanin** when grown in media containing certain catecholamines. The enzyme responsible for the initial step in the produc-

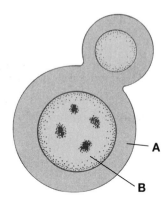

Figure 28.4.

Appearance of an India ink preparation of *C. neoformans*. (A) Capsule. (B) Blastoconidium.

tion of melanin is a **phenoloxidase,** which is relatively unique among zoopathogenic yeast that grow at 37°C and are commonly encountered in the clinical laboratory. A medium used to reveal this phenomenon is **bird seed agar,** so called because it contains an extract of the thistle seed *(Guzotia abysinica),* which is one of several types of seeds used to feed birds. The seeds are rich in di- or polyphenolic compounds that are substrates for the cryptococcal phenoloxidase.

Immunology

HOST RESPONSE AND RECOVERY FROM DISEASE. The host response to infection by *C. neoformans* is complex. The majority of individuals are protected from an infection with *C. neoformans* by three natural effector cells: polymorphonuclear leukocytes, natural killer cells, and macrophages. When an individual is exposed to large numbers of cryptococci, innate cellular mechanisms are overwhelmed and acquired resistance mechanisms must come into play. Both humoral and CMI are stimulated by *C. neoformans,* but CMI responses are more effective in eliminating the fungus. The host response is reflected by the histopathological picture observed. When the immune response is poor, a form of the disease occurs in which infiltration by granular cells is largely absent. In contrast, when the host response is adequate, a cellular infiltration by neutrophils and macrophages, in a pattern typical of other granulomatous diseases, is seen. When the fungous burden is large and not effectively controlled by innate resistance mechanisms, soluble cryptococcal antigens induce suppressor cells. These cells inhibit induction of sensitized T cells that ordinarily clear tissues of cryptococci. Certain populations of suppressor cells interfere with anticryptococcal T cells and keep them from eliminating the fungus from the tissues. While cryptococcal antigens stimulate the suppressor cell pathway, the host's acquired protective mechanisms are down regulated to an ineffective level. Long-lived suppressor memory cells may be generated during the induction of suppressor cells. Such memory cells can be transformed to suppressor cells when restimulated with cryptococcal antigen. The outcome of the exchange between the protective immune responses and the down regulatory responses determine the fate of the host. If a host's innate and acquired resistance mechanisms and antifungal drugs or both can limit the numbers of cryptococci so that the suppressor cell circuit is eliminated, then the disease will be arrested; if not, then the disease becomes progressive and fatal.

SEROLOGIC TESTS IN CRYPTOCOCCOSIS. The presence of capsular material can be detected in body fluids by the **latex agglutination (LA) test.** Specific antibody (or the derived globulin) attached to latex beads is reacted with body fluids (spinal, urine, or serum) of patients. Agglutination of latex beads indicates the presence of specific (i.e., cryptococcal) antigen in the fluid. The test is very useful (93% positive in culturally proven cryptococcosis) and is more regularly positive than is the detection of encapsulated yeast by India ink smears in spinal fluid. There is also a commercially available DNA probe for use in identification of cultures.

Therapy

Amphotericin B is currently the most effective therapy in cryptococcal meningitis. The drug is sometimes supplemented with 5-fluorocytosine. Fluconazole has been recommended for treatment of cryptococcal meningitis in AIDS patients and some of the other azoles may provide alternate therapeutic approaches in the future.

MISCELLANEOUS YEAST INFECTIONS

Many yeasts have been implicated in human infections. These yeasts are usually uncommon and almost invariably involve immunocompromised hosts. It is impossible to consider them all, but a few of the more important are included:

Torulopsosis. The yeast called *C. glabrata* was formerly known as *Torulopsis glabrata*. This name is still widely used. The phenotypes of *C. albicans* and *C. glabrata* are quite different from one another. The fungus characteristically produces infections of the genitourinary system.

Pityriasis versicolor. The etiologic agent of this skin affliction has been described in Chapter 27. *Malassezia furfur* has occasionally been implicated in systemic disease. It probably gains access to deeper tissues from its location on the skin through nosocomial (hospital) manipulations. Involvement of the heart, lung, and liver have been noted. No special medical terms have been developed to characterize these events.

Trichosporosis. Several species in the genus *Trichosporon* have been implicated in opportunistic diseases. The yeasts commonly form both arthroconidia and blastoconidia in cultures. In one species, *Blastoschizomyces capitatus* (formerly, *T. capitatum*), annelloconidia and blastoconidia are formed. Species of *Trichosporon* are separated on the basis of the assimilation of carbon and nitrogen sources.

Geotrichosis. Most yeast reproduce asexually as blastoconidia but a few of them reproduce by arthroconidia or annelloconidia. *Geotrichum candidum* reproduces by arthroconidia. This yeast is a very rare incitant of infection but lesions of the mouth, intestinal tract, bronchi, and lungs have been described. The fungus is identified morphologically on the bases of colony texture and the microscopic appearance of the arthroconidia produced.

SUMMARY

1. **Yeast infections are those caused by fungi whose predominate asexual reproductive propagule is a blastoconidium, though a few reproduce by arthroconidial formation, and some reproduce by both conidial forms.**

2. **There are two genera of yeasts that contain the largest number of zoopathogens: *Candida* and *Cryptococcus*.**

3. **Candidiasis is an infection in which the causative agents, *Candida* spp., produce superficial disease of the skin, nails, and mucous membranes or may, more rarely, disseminate to involve other areas of the body. *Candida* spp. are commensals and are customarily acquired endogenously though examples of contagious acquisition, often by sexual contact, are known.**

4. ***Candida* spp. usually appear as blastoconidia and pseudohyphae in tissues but the hyphal appearance is reduced in *Candida guilliermondii* and absent in *Candida glabrata*.**

5. ***Candida* spp. are identified by their morphological appearance and by their various assimilation of carbon compounds.**

6. Cryptococcosis in its most common clinical form involves the CNS. The disease is acquired by inhalation of infectious conidia from natural sources.

7. The zoopathogen *Cryptococcus neoformans* is a basidiomycetous yeast comprised of two varieties in its anamorphic state: *C. neoformans* var. *neoformans* and *C. neoformans* var. *gattii*. There are four serotypes of *C. neoformans* labeled A,B,C, and D. Serotypes A and D are contained in var. *neoformans* and serotypes B and C are contained in var. *gattii*. The fungus can reproduce sexually and the teleomorphic state also has two varieties: *Filobasidiella neoformans* var. *neoformans* (anamorph, *C. neoformans* var. *neoformans*) and *F. bacillispora* (anamorph, *C. neoformans* var. *gattii*).

8. *C. neoformans* is an encapsulated blastoconidium that often incites no obvious host cellular response, but more rarely evokes a granulomatous response.

9. The encapsulated yeast *C. neoformans* forms melanin on media containing di- or polyphenolic compounds. The enzyme involved in the primary step of the reaction is a phenoloxidase.

10. Polysaccharides comprising the capsules of *C. neoformans* can be discovered in body fluids. Commercial reagents are available for their detection.

11. There are a number of yeasts other than *Candida* spp. and *C. neoformans* that may cause disease. A few of these are *Torulopsis glabrata* (now named *Candida glabrata*), *Malassezia furfur* (see Chapter 27), *Trichosporon* spp., and *Geotrichum candidum*. The infections caused by yeasts are almost invariably opportunistic.

REFERENCES

Calderone RA, Braun PC (1991): Adherence and receptor relationships of *Candida albicans*. Microbiol Rev 55:1.

Koneman EW, Roberts GD (1985): Practical Laboratory Mycology. Baltimore: Williams & Wilkins.

Kregar-van Rij NJW (ed) (1984): The Yeasts. A Taxonomic Study. Amsterdam: Elsevier Science Publishers BV.

Kwon-Chung KJ, Varma A, Howard DH (1990): *Cryptococcus neoformans*—ecology and epidemiology. In 3rd Symposium Topic in Mycology. New York: Plenum Press.

Littman ML, Zimmerman LE (1956): Cryptococcosis. New York: Grune & Stratton.

Odds FC (1988): *Candida* and Candidosis. London: Baillière Tindall.

REVIEW QUESTIONS

> For questions 1 to 6, choose the ONE BEST answer or completion.

1. Chlamydoconidia (vesicles) are a *determinative* morphological feature in the identification of
   a) *Cryptococcus neoformans*
   b) *Candida albicans*
   c) *Epidermophyton floccosum*
   d) *Coccidioides immitis*

2. Involvement of tissues around the nail plate is characteristic of nail disease caused by
   a) *Trichophyton rubrum*
   b) *Candida albicans*
   c) *Trichosporon cutaneum*
   d) *Scopulariopsis brevicaulis*

3. *C. albicans* is noteworthy as the etiologic agent in
   a) valley fever
   b) thrush
   c) mycetoma
   d) pneumonia

4. An endogenously acquired fungus is one that
   a) is found only in sick people
   b) is found only inside hospitals
   c) is never found in animals other than humans
   d) is found frequently as a commensal in normal healthy individuals

5. The fungus *C. neoformans*
   a) grows as yeast cells and pseudohyphae in human tissue
   b) produces polysaccharides that can be detected in body fluids by serological techniques
   c) produces lesions that may show a remarkably high number of infiltrating inflammatory cells
   d) is a common resident of the GI tract of mammals

6. *C. albicans*
   a) may appear as blastoconidia and hyphal elements in the tissues of a host
   b) is a member of the GI biota of humans
   c) produces chlamydoconidia (vesicles) in vitro on suitable media
   d) possesses a polysaccharide capsule
   e) letters *a, b,* and *c* are correct
   f) all are correct

ANSWERS TO REVIEW QUESTIONS

1. *b* Chlamydoconidia (vesicles) are formed on special media by *Candida albicans*.

2. *b* Paronychial involvement is characteristic of nail infections by *Candida albicans*.

3. *b* Thrush is the name for the oral or vaginal forms of candidiasis.

4. *d* Commensal microorganisms, such as *C. albicans,* are acquired endogenously by immunosuppressed hosts.

5. *b* The latex agglutination test for the polysaccharide of *Cryptococcus neoformans* is a very useful test for cryptococcosis.

6. *e* Items *a, b,* and *c* are attributes of *C. albicans.*

PULMONARY MYCOSES

The pulmonary mycoses considered in this chapter have the following features in common: (1) each is acquired by inhalation of conidia produced by fungi that occur as saprobes in nature; (2) the primary infection is frequently asymptomatic or subclinical; (3) none is contagious, that is, human-human transmission has rarely been observed; (4) all may disseminate from the primary pulmonary site to involve other organ systems; and (5) each of the etiologic agents is dimorphic, that is, the saprobic form of growth in nature is different from the parasitic form of growth that occurs in the tissues of the host. There are four pulmonary mycoses with the five attributes just outlined.

COCCIDIOIDOMYCOSIS

Coccidioidomycosis (valley fever) is an infection caused by *Coccidioides immitis*. The primary infection may be asymptomatic, subclinical, or a self-limited, pulmonary disease of varying degrees of severity. In a small percentage of clinically ill individuals the fungus disseminates from the lungs to produce a chronic or acute malignant disease that may involve nearly any tissue of the body.

Epidemiology

The fungus is a **New World organism** and occurs only in the soil of North, Central, and South America. In the southwestern United States the disease occurs predominantly in the Kern, Tulare, King, and Fresno counties of California and in the Maricopa and Pima counties of Arizona. Although the major morbidity of the disease is in the southwestern portion of the United States, a few cases present outside the endemic area because an infected person may move out of the endemic area after infection or because the fungus can contaminate materials shipped out of the endemic region and infect a person in a nonendemic place. About 10–15% of the cases of coccidioidomycosis occur outside the endemic area.

C. immitis is a soil-inhabiting fungus adapted to life in semiarid regions. The conditions that favor the fungus are an arid or semiarid climate, alkaline soil, relative freedom from severe frosts, and a very hot, dry season of several months followed by some rain (an annual rainfall of $\sim$ 5–20 in.).

There is a significant difference among **ethnic groups** with regard to likelihood of disseminated disease. For example, in Kern county, California, Caucasians constitute 87% of the population, but account for only 41% of the cases of disseminated coccidioidomycosis, while the 13% non-Caucasians account for 59% of disseminated disease. In fact, over 22% of disseminated coccidioidomycosis cases occur in Filipinos, though they comprise but 0.23% of the population. This striking discrepancy is not solely a question of economic or health status; apparently, it is due to a genetic difference (this assumption is still not proven).

Pathogenesis and Virulence Factors

C. immitis is a highly infectious fungus but not a highly virulent one. Nearly all infections are self-healing and more than 60% are asymptomatic or subclinical. The malignant forms of coccidioidomycosis occur rarely, indicating that the host-parasite interaction depends heavily on the host response and only slightly on the invasive capacity of the fungus. Nevertheless, in the case of an inadequate host response *C. immitis* becomes a malignant pathogen.

Those factors of the fungus responsible for tissue invasion are largely unknown. A few isolated observations regarding unique cell wall components, chemotactic substances, and proteases have been recorded, but no suitable genetic system is available to explore them.

Clinical Manifestations

The disease is not contagious. The infectious arthroconidia are acquired by inhalation and 60% of infected individuals are asymptomatic or subclinical while 40% develop symptoms. People with or without signs after exposure convert to a positive skin test.

The clinical symptoms are influenza-like, ranging from mild to severe. These patients are rarely seen in the hospital since it is a self-limiting disease in a large portion of cases. Fifteen percent of cases cavitate. A small percent of patients disseminate the disease, which then may involve almost any organ system.

Mycology and Laboratory Diagnosis

DIMORPHISM OF *C. IMMITIS.* In vivo *C. immitis* consists of large **spherules** averaging 30–60 μm (up to 150–200 μm) in diameter, containing many small (2–5 μm) **endospores** (Fig. 29.1A,B). In vitro at room temperature, *C. immitis* grows as a mycelium comprised of hyphae which form arthroconidia (enteroarthric) that are **highly infectious.**

APPEARANCE IN TISSUE. The infectious arthroconidia enter the tissue of an infected host by the pulmonary route. The conidia grow by enlargement and the nuclei replicate (Fig. 29.1). The cytoplasm of the enlarging spherule is filled with nuclei (a syncytium). Septa divide up the cytoplasm and separate individual nuclei. The walls of these packets thicken and structures called endospores are formed. The overall picture is an endospore-filled spherule (Fig. 29.1). The spherules rupture to release the endospores that repeat the cycle of enlargement and nuclear division. This endospore-spherule cycle is the tissue (parasitic) form of growth of *C. immitis.* The spherules can be found in tissue or exudates (sputum, spinal fluid, or pus) of infected hosts.

APPEARANCE IN CULTURE. The spherules, that constitute the parasitic form of *C. immitis,* can sometimes be cultured at 37°C, but the efforts to do so have often failed in the past and are no longer customarily attempted in the clinical laboratory. The tissue form can be evoked in experimental animals injected with arthroconidia but this is not a routine diagnostic procedure. Cultures are incubated at room temperature. At this temperature the endospores germinate, and the mycelium so generated is comprised of hyphae which form arthroconidia at maturity

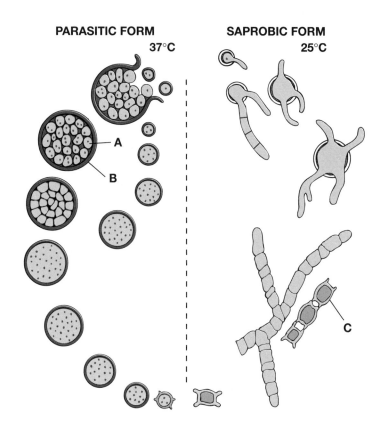

PARASITIC FORM 37°C

SAPROBIC FORM 25°C

Figure 29.1.

The dimorphism of *C. immitis.* (A) Endospores. (B) Spherule. (C) Arthroconidia.

(Fig. 29.1C). These arthroconidia are the infectious form of the fungus. Thus, cultures must be handled with **strict biosafety precautions.**

EXOANTIGEN TEST. This test is a serological procedure currently available for the definitive identification of the saprobic (mould) form of *C. immitis, Blastomyces dermatitidis, Histoplasma capsulatum,* and *Paracoccidioides brasiliensis.* The principle is the same for all four systemic pathogens, but the reagents are specific for each. The overall procedure will be given for *C. immitis* and not repeated for each of the others. Antigens are extracted from the mycelium in saline (with merthiolate) and tested against a standardized antibody in an immunodiffusion system. Positive controls are included in each test. Commercial reagents of a high degree of reliability are available. The exoantigen test provides a rapid, reliable identification method that does not depend on macroscopic or microscopic morphology of an isolate (both subject to some variation). A commercially available DNA probe can also be used for identification of cultures.

Immunology

HOST-PARASITE INTERACTION. The spectrum of disease ranges from a benign, self-limited infection to a progressive, disseminated process. The host factors that govern the course of the disease have not been fully defined. Polymorphonuclear leukocytes and mononuclear phagocytes effectively phagocytize arthroconidia and endospores, but the fungus inhibits phagolysosomal fusion (PL-F) and survives in the phagosome. Survival and propagation of the fungus in host tissues is accompanied by the activity of both T and B lymphocytes. Primary coccidioidal infection involves cellular immune reactivity and low levels of circulating antibody, whereas, chronic or progressive coccidioidomycosis is characterized by depressed or absent T-cell reactivity and proliferative B-cell responses. T-cell anergy seen in disseminated coccidioidal disease is associated with a high ratio of suppressor to helper cells. Low doses of coccidioidal antigen engender a high level of immunity to challenge accompanied by the induction of T cells that arm macrophages to restrict fungal growth. Conversely, high doses of antigen or administration of antigen through the IV route result in suppression of T-cell reactivity to the fungus.

SEROLOGIC AND IMMUNOLOGIC TESTS. The antigens used are culture filtrates. The fungus is cultivated on a specified medium and after the growth of the fungus, the broth is filtered. The filtrate is standardized for use in skin tests of DTH and in serologic tests. Both the saprobic (mycelial) and parasitic (spherule; certain laboratory strains can be grown in the parasitic form) form of growth may be used to generate the antigens. The saprobic growth filtrate (**coccidioidin**) is most commonly used, but the parasitic growth filtrate (**spherulin**) has also been used.

Skin Test. The skin test is performed by injecting the filtrate antigen coccidioidin or spherulin intradermally. The reaction measures DTH to antigens of *C. immitis*. It takes about 3 weeks after exposure to develop a positive skin test. A negative skin test may mean: (a) test performed too early in disease process, (b) the current illness is not the disease tested for, or (c) disseminated coccidioidal disease (anergy). Thus, the skin test is not a useful diagnostic procedure. A positive skin test indicates previous exposure to the fungus. Individuals with a positive skin test are immune to a second attack of the disease.

Antibody Tests. Antibodies against *C. immitis* antigens are found in IgM, IgG, IgA, and IgE classes. Two antibody responses are of particular value in serodiagnosis. These are detected by the tube preciptin (TP) and complement fixation (CF) assays and by immunodiffusion (ID) that corresponds to the TP and CF antibody (i.e., IDTP and IDCF). There are no data to support a role for antibody in recovery from disease or in acquired immunity.

   1. **TP Test.** The **TP antibody** is predominantly the IgM isotype, and is seen early in symptomatic illness ($\sim$ 53% of persons in first week, 91% during second and third weeks, and 86% during fourth week). Thereafter the response decreases rapidly.
   2. **CF Test.** The **CF antibody** is produced later in the course of coccidioidomycosis and generally persists throughout the course of infection. The CF antibody is mostly the IgG isotype. The titer of CF antibody is correlated with the severity of disease. Low titers ($<$1:16–1:32) are associated with primary pulmonary disease or with limited dissemination. High titers ($>$1:32) are associated with extensive dissemination. The prognosis of the disease is often predictably associated with the titer of CF antibodies. One notable exception is CNS involvement. When that area is the sole site of involvement, humoral CF titers are frequently less than 1:16.

Treatment

   In its common form, coccidioidomycosis is an acute self-limited infection that does not customarily require therapy. In some cavitary forms therapy is recommended and disseminated disease requires therapy. Amphotericin B is the most effective agent available, but some of the newer azoles may prove useful as experience with them develops.

HISTOPLASMOSIS

   Histoplasmosis, caused by *Histoplasma capsulatum* var. *capsulatum,* presents a variety of clinical manifestations. The primary disease may be asymptomatic, subclinical, or a self-limited pulmonary disease of varying degrees of severity that leaves multiple areas of calcification. Chronic cavitary disease occurs in 10–15% of the primary pulmonary cases. Progressive, disseminated histoplasmosis, a rare sequela, is characterized by emaciation leukopenia, hepatosplenomegaly, and irregular fevers.
   There are three varieties of *H. capsulatum: H. capsulatum* var. *capsulatum,*

H. capsulatum var. *duboisii,* and *H. capsulatum* var. *farciminosum,* each responsible for a distinctive syndrome. Only var. *capsulatum* will be considered here.

Epidemiology

The geographic distribution is worldwide with a notable intensity in the United States, especially in the areas around the major river valleys of the Missouri, Mississippi, and Ohio rivers. As with coccidioidomycosis, a few cases may occur outside the endemic area because the infected individual moves out of the area after infection or because materials shipped to nonendemic areas are contaminated with infectious conidia.

It has been clearly demonstrated that this organism can most frequently be isolated from soils contaminated with bird droppings, especially the excreta of chickens and starlings (a variety of black bird); it is also associated with bats. The fungus does not cause disease in birds, but it does in bats and the fungus is found in bat feces. On the basis of numerous small epidemics of histoplasmosis, it appears that there are focal origins of infection. There is no relation to the dry or wet seasons. Animals other than humans can become infected (e.g., dogs, cats, mice, rats, skunks, opossums, bears, raccoons, etc.).

Pathogenesis and Virulence Factors

As with *C. immitis,* the factors that account for disease causation by *H. capsulatum* are not well known. In general, the adequacy of the host response seems to be of primary importance in controlling disease. The majority of individuals recover from *H. capsulatum* infection. Defects in CMI seem more important in expression of disseminated disease than do virulence attributes of the fungus. A few observations have been made but an adequate genetic system for exploring them is only in a primitive stage of development.

Clinical Manifestations

The disease is not contagious. The clinical manifestations of histoplasmosis are similar to those of coccidioidomycosis. Of those who inhale conidia of *H. capsulatum,* 95% are asymptomatic or subclinical. The only evidence of the encounter is a positive skin test. The 5% of exposed individuals who do become ill manifest a pulmonary infection similar in clinical manifestations to coccidioidomycosis. The symptoms are influenza-like with fever and pulmonary congestion. Cavitation of the lung may occur in 10–15% of the clinically manifest primary infections. Calcifications in the lung and sometimes in the spleen (indicating extrapulmonary involvement) are common. Progressive dissemination occurs in a small percentage of cases of primary disease. Disseminated disease involves reticuloendothelial cells, such as those found in the liver, spleen, and lymph nodes. Hepatosplenomegaly is a common feature of disseminated disease.

Mycology and Laboratory Diagnosis

DIMORPHISM OF *H. CAPSULATUM*. In vivo and in vitro at 37°C, *H. capsulatum* is an ovoid budding yeast cell (blastoconidium) about 4–5 µm in diameter. In vitro at room temperature and in nature, the fungus forms a mycelium comprised of hyphae that produce characteristic tuberculate macroconidia (8–14 µm in diameter), and small spherical microconidia (2–4 µm in diameter) that are the infectious elements of the fungus (Fig. 29.2D). A teleomorphic form of growth is known. The name given it is *Ajellomyces capsulatus* (phylum Ascomycota). The teleomorphic form of growth is not used in laboratory identification of *H. capsulatum.*

APPEARANCE IN TISSUE. The microconidia are inhaled and undergo a sequence of morphologic changes that in some strains include direct budding to generate the blastoconidia of the tissue form of growth (Fig. 29.2A). The yeast cells of *H. capsulatum* are found in macrophages in tissue. It can also occur extracellularly but the fungus is primarily a facultative intracellular parasite (Fig. 29.2B).

APPEARANCE IN CULTURE. The yeast cells of the parasitic form of growth germinate in vitro at room temperature and initiate a mycelium comprised of hyphae upon which are borne both microconidia and macroconidia (Fig. 29.2C, D). The microconidia (holoblastic) may have fingerlike projections (tubercles) on their cell walls. The large macroconidia (holoblastic) characteristically have tubercles on their walls. The microconidia are infectious and cultures must be handled with **strict biosafety precautions.** The hyphal form of growth can be converted to the yeast form by cultivation at 37°C, but conversion occurs in vitro with only about 10–12% of isolates. Conversion will occur in experimental animals, but this is not commonly done as a diagnostic procedure.

EXOANTIGEN TEST. There is an exoantigen test. It is performed on cultures like the one for *C. immitis* antigens, but the reagents are specific for *H.*

PARASITIC FORM   **SAPROBIC FORM**

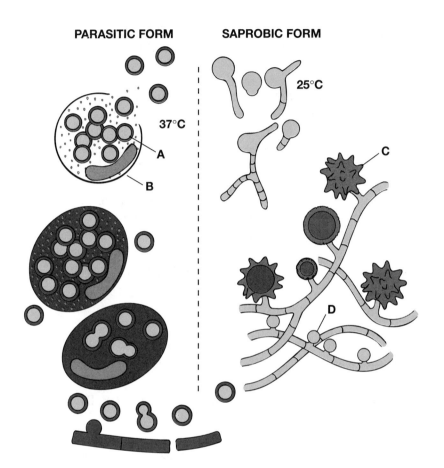

Figure 29.2.
The dimorphism of *H. capsulatum*. (A) Blastoconidia (yeast cells). (B) Macrophage. (C) Macroconidium. (D) Microconidium.

capsulatum. A commercially available DNA probe can also be used for identification of cultures.

Immunology

HOST-PARASITE INTERACTION. Infection by *H. capsulatum* frequently results in inapparent, subclinical, or completely benign disease. Reinfection after recovery from disease is extremely rare, and enhanced resistance can be established experimentally in a variety of animals. Thus, both natural and acquired resistance are prominent features of histoplasmosis.

Antibodies do not appear to play a role in resistance to *H. capsulatum,* but some plasma components (transferrin) do affect the fungous growth in vitro. In addition, antibodies and complement may play an ancillary role in phagocytosis of the fungus and in antibody-dependent cellular cytotoxicity by natural killer cells.

Cellular events are crucial to both natural and acquired resistance to *H. capsulatum*. Yeast cells of *H. capsulatum* survive in polymorphonuclear leukocytes and grow in circulating mononuclear phagocytes. Monocyte-derived macrophages, alveolar macrophages, and peritoneal exudate cells require stimulation by lymphokines, such as interferon-γ, in order to inhibit the intracellular growth of the fungus.

Experimental animals are protected against challenge by prior vaccination with viable or killed cells and fractions derived from killed cells. The protection engendered by vaccination is cell-mediated and can be adoptively transferred with immune T cells. Suppression of T-cell responses by macrophages and suppressor T cells has been documented in natural and experimental histoplasmosis.

SEROLOGIC AND IMMUNOLOGIC TESTS

Skin Test. A skin test is done with a mycelial phase filtrate antigen called histoplasmin. The uses and limitations are similar to those with coccidioidin.

Antibody Tests. Serologic tests for histoplasmosis include CF, ID, and LA. Antibodies are found in the IgM, IgG, IgA, and IgE classes.

1. **CF Test.** The CF test is performed with whole yeast cells and with a mycelial-phase culture filtrate antigen, designated histoplasmin. Demonstrable CF titers to the yeast-cell antigen are usually detected within the first 3–4 weeks of infection. Complement fixation antibodies to histoplasmin develop later, are generally of a lower titer than those obtained with yeast cells, and may occur in the absence of CF-antibody reactivity to yeast cells, particularly in patients with chronic histoplasmosis. In some studies, as many as one-third to one-half of patients with chronic pulmonary or progressive disseminated histoplasmosis are negative for CF antibodies. Although the magnitude of CF titers does not assist in distinguishing the pulmonary from extrapulmonary forms of the disease or establish the extent of disease severity, increasing titers (fourfold or greater) denote an unfavorable clinical response and, conversely, decreasing titers denote a favorable prognosis for recovery.

2. **ID Test.** The specificity of antibody responses to *H. capsulatum* can be established by use of the ID test in which reference *Histoplasma* antigen and

antiserum reagents are used. Of the multiple antigens present in histoplasmin, the two that have been designated **H** and **M** are specific for *H. capsulatum*. The occurrence of precipitin antibody to the H antigen, either alone or in combination with antibody to the M antigen, provides strong, if not definitive evidence of histoplasmosis. Reactivity to the M antigen is demonstrable in approximately 75% of patients with histoplasmosis, but does not differentiate between active or inactive disease.

3. **LA Test.** The LA test detects antibodies that are produced within 2 or 3 weeks after primary infection. Titers of greater than or equal to 1:32 are usually considered positive, but there are a number of clinical situations that give false-positive reactions (e.g., rheumatoid arthritis, tuberculosis, bronchogenic carcinoma, mycoplasmal pneumonia, and a series of other diseases unrelated to histoplasmosis).

Treatment

In its common form, histoplasmosis is an acute self-limited infection that does not customarily require therapy. In some cavitary forms therapy is recommended and disseminated disease requires therapy. Amphotericin B is the most effective agent available, but some of the newer azoles may prove useful as experience with them develops.

BLASTOMYCOSIS

Blastomycosis is a chronic infection caused by *Blastomyces dermatitidis*. The primary disease is a pulmonary infection acquired by inhalation of infectious conidia of the fungus. The disease may disseminate and may involve any part of the body but with a marked predilection for lungs, skin, and bone.

Epidemiology

Blastomycosis was once thought to be limited solely to the United States and Canada. The majority of cases occur in the south eastern United States and along the Mississippi, Missouri, and Ohio river valleys. The endemic area overlaps that of histoplasmosis to a considerable extent. Scattered cases are also found in those regions of Canada contiguous to endemic areas of the United States. However, autochthonous cases have been reported from South America, Africa, Europe, and the Middle East. Therefore, the disease is worldwide.

Cases in males outnumber those in females by about 10:1, and there is some correlation with occupation or presumptive opportunity to come into contact with the organism. Age and race are of no importance. The ecological niche of the fungus is not clear. The fungus has only been isolated a few times from natural sources. Moreover, there is no reagent available for skin testing. Thus, the geographical distribution of the disease can only be surmised from cases in humans and animals (notably dogs) and not from the distribution of skin test reactivity or soil isolates.

Pathogenesis and Virulence Factors

Only limited studies have been made on the pathogenesis of blastomycosis. As with other pulmonary mycoses, progressive disease appears to depend largely on the immune response of the host rather than aggressive attributes of the fungus.

Blastomycosis is a notably suppurative infection and a granulocyte chemotactic factor has been described. In addition, an alkali-soluble fraction of cell walls of the fungus produces, upon injection into experimental animals, a pyogranulomatous response indistinguishable from the response induced by whole cells. The active fraction could be a phospholipid because virulent strains contain many-fold more phospholipids than do avirulent strains.

Clinical Manifestations

The disease is not contagious. Clinically, this disease often presents as a chronic infection of the skin. Common sites for lesions include face, leg, and foot. The lesions are suppurative granulomas that heal spontaneously or by therapy with pronounced scar formation. In its indolent form the disease is a chronic, recurrent disease of many years' duration.

The first stage in infection is pulmonary; the number of pulmonary infections that result in skin lesions is impossible to determine because no skin test reagent is available. Therefore, there is no estimate of the number of asymptomatic or subclinical cases. Primary pulmonary blastomycosis can apparently resolve spontaneously but does so far less frequently than do pulmonary coccidioidomycosis and histoplasmosis.

Mycology and Laboratory Diagnosis

DIMORPHISM OF *B. DERMATITIDIS*. In vivo and in vitro at 37°C, the organism multiplies as blastoconidia, which are 8–15 μm in diameter, with thick cell walls, and a wide base at the juncture of budding daughter cells (Fig. 29.3A). In vitro at room temperature, the organism grows as a mycelium, with hyphae upon which are produced ovoid (3–5 μm) conidia (holoblastic), which are the infectious elements of the fungus (Fig. 29.3B). There is a teleomorphic form of growth. It is called *Ajellomyces dermatitidis* (phylum Ascomycota). The teleomorphic form of growth is not used in the laboratory identification of *B. dermatitidis*.

APPEARANCE IN TISSUE. The infectious conidia are inhaled and convert to large, solitary yeast cells (12–15 μm) embedded in abscesses (characteristically)

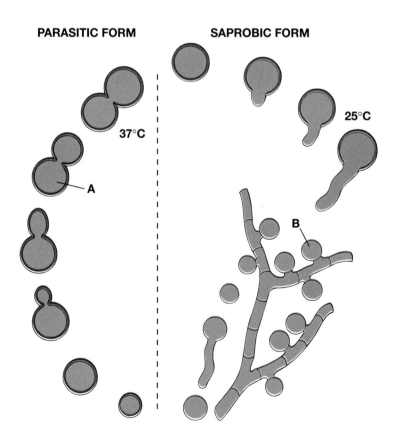

PARASITIC FORM   **SAPROBIC FORM**

37°C

A

25°C

B

Figure 29.3.

The dimorphism of *B. dermatitidis.* (A) Blastoconidia (yeast cells). (B) Conidia.

with single buds that have a broad basal attachment to the mother cell. The cells (blastoconidia) have thick cell walls and are generally not intracellular though occasionally seen in large giant cells.

APPEARANCE IN CULTURE. The yeast cells of the tissue form of growth germinate in cultures at room temperature and a white mycelium is formed that is comprised of hyphae upon which are formed single, lateral conidia (holoblastic) (Fig. 29.3B). The conidia are the infectious elements of the fungus and cultures must be handled with **proper biosafety precautions.** The tissue form of growth (i.e., large single budding yeast cells is relatively easy to generate in vitro by incubating cultures at 37°C).

EXOANTIGEN TEST. There is an exoantigen test available for *B. dermatitidis* and it is performed with specific reagents. A commercially available DNA probe can also be used for identification of cultures.

Immunology

HOST-PARASITE INTERACTION. *B. dermatitidis* evokes an inflammatory response consisting of both suppuration and granulomas. The mechanisms of killing of yeast cells remain unknown. Both polymorphonuclear leukocytes and mononuclear phagocytes do not kill the yeast cells efficiently even when they are stimulated with lymphokines. Survival of the organism within host tissues is related to its large size and to its resistance to oxidative and nonoxidative products of phagocytes. Cell-mediated immunity is critical in recovery from disease, but the process by which CMI limits the growth of the fungus is not understood.

SEROLOGIC AND IMMUNOLOGIC TESTS

Skin Test. There is no satisfactory antigen to test for DTH in blastomycosis. This lack has led to ignorance regarding asymptomatic or subclinical infections and to an inability to describe the relative occurrence of progressive, disseminated infections.

Antibody Tests. One of the impediments to serodiagnosis has been the lack of useful antigens. Early work on CF and ID has proven unsatisfactory. More recent work has revealed the presence of an antigen called the **A antigen** in culture filtrates of *B. dermatitidis* yeast cells. This antigen has been used in several serologic tests.

1. **ID Test.** In one study usc of the A antigen in an ID procedure detected 80% of proven cases.

2. **CF Test.** The A antigen has also been used in a CF procedure and was positive (titer >1:8) in 57% of proven cases. The use of both ID and CF procedures gave positive results in 88% of proven cases.

3. **Indirect Enzyme Immunoassay.** The A antigen has been used in an indirect enzyme immunoassay. Reports of positive results range from 77–100% of proven cases.

Treatment

The primary pulmonary form of the disease does not ordinarily require therapy. Prolonged progressive pulmonary disease or disseminated infections are treated with amphotericin B though the newer azoles may prove useful as experience with them develops.

PARACOCCIDIOIDOMYCOSIS

Paracoccidioidomycosis is a chronic granulomatous disease characterized by a primary pulmonary infection and by dissemination to the skin, mucous membranes, lymph nodes, and internal organs caused by *Paracoccidioides brasiliensis.*

Epidemiology

So far as is known the disease is limited to South and Central America. The natural habitat is thought to be soil and a few isolates have been recovered from that location. However, the ecology of *P. brasiliensis* is largely unknown. No animal hosts are known. There is a marked predominance of male-female patients (12:1) even though DTH reactivity is the same in both sexes.

Pathogenesis and Virulence Factors

The virulence of isolates of *P. brasiliensis* has been associated with the presence of **α-1,3-glucan** in the walls of the fungus. The yeast phase of the organism is inhibited by estrogens and this fact may account for the preponderance of severe infection in males. Very little is known of pathogenetic factors and as with the other pulmonary mycoses host response is probably the important criterion governing the appearance of progressive, disseminated disease.

Clinical Manifestations

The disease is not contagious. The infectious conidia are acquired by inhalation. Many of these encounters are asymptomatic or subclinical. People with or without signs after exposure convert to a positive skin test. The primary disease is influenza-like and may vary from mild to acute. The pulmonary disease is usually self-limiting. The disseminated forms of the disease often involve the skin and mucous membranes.

Mycology and Laboratory Diagnosis

DIMORPHISM OF *P. BRASILIENSIS.* In vivo and in vitro at 37°C *P. brasiliensis* occurs as blastoconidia that develop multiple buds. The parental yeast cell is customarily 10–12 μm (larger forms may occur). Both single and multiple buds may appear but multiple budding is the characteristic appearance. In vitro at room temperature, *P. brasiliensis* grows as a mycelium comprised of hyphae that form arthroconidia and lateral holoblastic conidia (Fig. 29.4B,C).

APPEARANCE IN TISSUE. Infectious holoblastic conidia are inhaled and convert to the parasitic form of growth (Fig. 29.4A). In the tissues of the host *P. brasiliensis* appears as multiple budding yeast cells with narrow basal attachment of the buds to the parent cell.

APPEARANCE IN CULTURE. The yeast cells of the parasitic form germinate when cultured at room temperature. The colonial form is variable. Generally, brownish flat colonies to white velvety colonies are seen. The mycelium may remain sterile for a long time in culture with only chlamydoconidia formed. Both arthroconidia and lateral holoblastic microconidia may be formed. These conidia are the infectious elements of the fungus and cultures of *P. brasiliensis* should be handled with **due regard to biosafety.** The yeast cells of the tissue phase are often easily obtained by growing the fungus at 37°C.

EXOANTIGEN TEST. There is an exoantigen test for *P. brasiliensis* and it is performed with specific reagents.

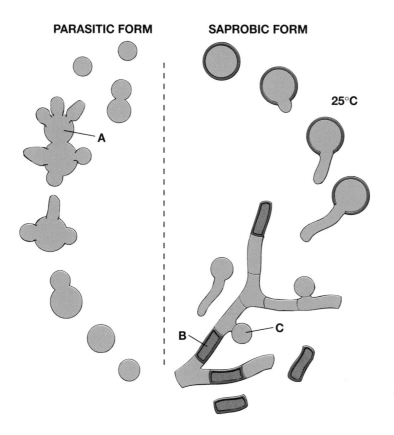

PARASITIC FORM   **SAPROBIC FORM**

25°C

A

B   C

Figure 29.4.

The dimorphism of *P. bras-iliensis.* (A) Blastoconidia (multiple budding). (B) Arthroconidia. (C) Conidia.

Immune Response

HOST-PARASITE INTERACTIONS. The spectrum of disease ranges from a benign, self-limited infection, to a progressive, disseminated process. The host factors that govern the course of the disease have not been fully defined. Polymorphonuclear leukocytes ingest yeast cells of *P. brasiliensis* and the process is augmented by specific antibodies. The yeast cells survive better in polymorphonuclear leukocytes from patients than they do in polymorphonuclear leukocytes from healthy controls. Animal mononuclear phagocytes ingest *P. brasiliensis.* The process is augmented by heat labile serum components and PL-F does not occur. Evidence exists for a role of natural killer cells in limiting the growth of *P. bras-iliensis.* Antibodies occur during the course of infection, but there is no evidence for their role in recovery from disease or in acquired resistance. To the contrary, as with the other pulmonary mycoses, there is an abundant production of antibodies that often correlates with the more malignant forms of the disease. Studies involving skin testing, lymphoblastogenic assays, lymphokine production, and cell-mediated cytotoxicity have affirmed the fundamental importance of CMI in paracoccidioidomycosis.

SEROLOGIC AND IMMUNOLOGIC TESTS

Skin Test. Delayed-type hypersensitivity is revealed by the application of a skin test with a filtrate antigen called paracoccidioidin.

Antibody Tests

1. **TP Test.** These antibodies appear early in the course of disease and disappear quickly.

2. **ID Test.** When **precipitins** are evaluated by immunodiffusion in agar, a diversity of reactivities emerges. With a culture filtrate of yeasts, three precipitin bands are found: band 1 is specific for the disease, band 2 is also specific but is not as often detected as band 1, band 3 cross-reacts with the M antigen of *H. capsulatum.*

3. **CF Test.** Complement fixing antibodies appear later in the course of illness. High titers may be found in disseminated disease.

Treatment

Primary pulmonary disease usually resolves spontaneously. Amphotericin B is used in the disseminated forms of the disease. As with the other pulmonary mycoses, azoles are beginning to be evaluated.

SUMMARY

1. The pulmonary mycoses described in this chapter: (1) are acquired by inhalation of infectious conidia produced by fungi that are saprobes, (2) consist of a primary infection that is often asymptomatic, (3) are not contagious, (4) rarely disseminate to other organ systems, and (5) are caused by dimorphic zoopathogens.

2. Recovery from the pulmonary mycoses and the basis of acquired resistance in those diseases involves CMI.

3. Useful serologic procedures are available to assist in the diagnosis of all of the pulmonary mycoses.

4. Coccidioidomycosis is found only in North, Central, and South America. In the United States it occurs in the Southwest. Histoplasmosis is worldwide with a notably large occurrence in the United States where the major endemic areas are those bordering the major river valleys of the Ohio, Missouri, and Mississippi rivers. Blastomycosis occurs in endemic areas overlapping those of histoplasmosis. The exact geographic distribution of *Blastomyces dermatitidis*, the causative agent of blastomycosis, is unknown because there is no skin test reagent available and because the fungus is rarely isolated from nature. Paracoccidioidomycosis is found only in Central and South America.

5. Amphotericin B remains the single most effective antifungal for the disseminated forms of the pulmonary mycoses but one or another of the newer azoles may prove useful as experience develops.

6. All of the agents of pulmonary mycoses produce their infectious propagules in cultures in the clinical laboratory. Strict biosafety precautions must be used in handling those cultures.

7. *Coccidioides immitis*, the causative agent of coccidioidomycosis, occurs in the tissues of an infected host as an endospore-filled spherule. In nature and in cultures in the laboratory the fungus grows as a cottony mycelium comprised of hyphae that form arthroconidia. The arthroconidia are the infectious elements of the fungus.

8. *Histoplasma capsulatum* var. *capsulatum*, the causative agent of the classical form of histoplasmosis, occurs in the tissues of a host as a budding yeast in mononuclear phagocytes. The fungus is a facultative intracellular parasite. In nature and in cultures in the laboratory the fungus grows as a mycelium comprised of hyphae upon which both holoblastic microconidia and holoblastic macroconidia are formed. Both sizes of conidia may be smooth or sculptured with fingerlike projections called tubercles. The microconidia are the infectious elements of the fungus.

9. *B. dermatitidis*, the causative agent of blastomycosis, occurs in the tissues of a host as a large yeast cell with a single bud and a thick cell wall. In nature and in cultures in the laboratory the fungus grows as a mycelium comprised of hyphae that form holoblastic, smooth-walled, lateral conidia. These conidia are the infectious elements of the fungus.

10. *Paracoccidioides brasiliensis*, the causative agent of paracoccidioi-

domycosis, occurs in the tissues of a host as multiple budding yeast cells. In nature and in cultures in the laboratory the fungus grows as a mycelium upon which are formed both arthroconidia and lateral holoblastic conidia. Both conidial forms are potential infectious elements of the fungus.

REFERENCES

Chandler FW, Kaplan N, Ajello L (1980): A Colour Atlas and Textbook of the Histopathology of Mycotic Diseases. London: Wolfe Medical Publications Ltd.

Cox RA (ed) (1989): Immunology of the Fungal Diseases. Boca Raton, FL: CRC Press.

Howard DH (1984): The epidemiology and ecology of blastomycosis, coccidioidomycosis, and histoplasmosis. Zbl Bakt Hyg A 257:219.

Schwarz J (1981): Histoplasmosis. New York: Praeger.

Stevens DA (1980): Coccidioidomycosis. New York: Plenum Press.

Szaniszlo PJ (ed) (1985): Fungal Dimorphism. New York: Plenum Press.

REVIEW QUESTIONS

> For questions 1 to 8, choose the ONE BEST answer or completion.

A 35-year-old resident of St. Louis, MO recently visited his brother in Tucson, AZ. He lived in St. Louis all of his life and this was his first visit to Arizona. He returned home after 2 weeks, and 3 days later he presented at the outpatient clinic of Barnes hospital complaining of a mild cough, a slight fever, and some difficulty in breathing. The X-ray showed multiple infiltrations in both lung fields. The hilar lymph nodes were enlarged.

1. The most likely mycosis suggested by the history and symptoms is
   a) pulmonary candidiasis
   b) pulmonary cryptococcosis
   c) coccidioidomycosis
   d) histoplasmosis
   e) blastomycosis

2. The cause of the mycosis selected in question 1 appears in exudates and body fluids as
   a) encapsulated yeast cells
   b) an intracellular parasite of macrophages
   c) endospore-filled spherules
   d) thick-walled singly budded yeast cells

3. The specimen you would choose to collect to culture for the etiologic agent is
   a) blood
   b) urine
   c) sputum
   d) saliva

4. Each of the following fungi is dimorphic *except*
   a) *Coccidioides immitis*
   b) *Blastomyces dermatitidis*
   c) *Cryptococcus neoformans*
   d) *Histoplasma capsulatum*

5. Each of the following mycoses is worldwide in distribution *except*
   a) coccidioidomycosis
   b) histoplasmosis
   c) cryptococcosis
   d) dermatomycosis

6. Each of the following mycoses is noncontagious *except*

   a) coccidioidomycosis
   b) dermatomycoses
   c) blastomycosis
   d) cryptococcosis

7. Each of the following fungi may multiply in tissue by means of blastoconidia *except*
   a) *Candida albicans*
   b) *Cryptococcus neoformans*
   c) *Coccidioides immitis*
   d) *Blastomyces dermatitidis*

8. Macroconidia that are covered with finger-like projections (tubercules) are characteristic for
   a) *Coccidioides immitis*
   b) *Blastomyces dermatitidis*
   c) *Histoplasma capsulatum*
   d) *Microsporum canis*
   e) *Aspergillus fumigatus*

ANSWERS TO REVIEW QUESTIONS

1. *c* The individual would be expected to be immune to histoplasmosis because of his long term residence in an endemic area of that disease. Therefore, his current illness is more likely to be due to his recent visit to the endemic area of coccidioidomycosis.

2. *c* *Coccidioides immitis* appears in the tissues of an infected host as endospore-filled spherules.

3. *c* Sputum is cultured for the agent of coccidioidomycosis.

4. *c* *Cryptococcus neoformans* is not dimorphic. It occurs as an encapsulated blastoconidium in the tissues of a host (parasitic form) and in culture in the laboratory (saprobic form).

5. *a* Coccidioidomycosis is restricted in geographic distribution, occurring only in the New World (i.e., North, Central and South America).

6. *b* The dermatophytoses (ringworm) are contagious. The other mycoses are usually noncontagious.

7. *c* The tissue form of *C. immitis* is a spherule with endospores. No blastoconidial reproduction is involved.

8. *c* *Histoplasma capsulatum* produces, in its saprobic form of growth, macroconidia with tuberculate projections on its cell wall surface.

INOCULATION MYCOSES

Inoculation mycoses are those in which the infectious elements of a fungus are traumatically introduced into the tissues. One might expect that such an event would result in a nondistinctive foreign body reaction in the tissues of the host and that the clinical presentation would be one of a nonspecific wound infection. This occurrence is often the case. Not infrequently, however, a very specific, clinically recognizable syndrome results from the implantation of certain fungi. The reasons for such pathogenetic distinctiveness are unknown. None of the inoculation mycoses is contagious.

The following inoculation mycoses will be described: (1) sporotrichosis; (2) chromoblastomycosis; (3) mycetoma; and (4) miscellaneous inoculation mycoses without specific clinical appearance

SPOROTRICHOSIS

In its commonly encountered form sporotrichosis is a chronic suppurative, granulomatous disease caused by *Sporothrix schenckii* and is characterized by subcutaneous nodules that develop into abscesses or indolent ulcers; the disease is usually localized but with lymphatic spread. The infection rarely disseminates to organ systems beyond the primary cutaneous and lymphocutaneous sites. Rarely seen systemic forms of disease are acquired by inhalation.

Epidemiology

Sporotrichosis is worldwide though there are endemic foci. The organism grows commonly in soil or on decaying vegetation in association with materials used for mulching (e.g., sphagnum moss). Its occurrence on thorny plants provides a mechanism for traumatic introduction into a susceptible host. Farmers, nurserymen, gardeners, and florists are most often afflicted.

Pathogenesis and Virulence Factors

Little is known about the pathogenetic factors associated with tissue invasion by *S. schenckii*. Both the dematiaceous and hyaline conidia may function as the infectious elements. After penetration of tissue the conidia undergo a series of morphologically complicated changes that result in the blastoconidia comprising the parasitic form of growth.

Clinical Manifestations

The disease is not contagious by contact with lesions; trauma is required. Sporotrichosis in its most commonly encountered form is a chronic infection characterized by nodular lesions of the skin or subcutaneous tissues and proximal lymphatics. The primary lesions are acquired by the traumatic introduction of infectious conidia of *S. schenckii*. The nodules that develop frequently suppurate, ulcerate, and drain. Secondary dissemination to other sites is uncommon. Primary infections of the lung, acquired by inhalation, have been described. Such primary pulmonary infection may disseminate, rarely, to other anatomic sites.

Mycology and Laboratory Diagnosis

DIMORPHISM OF *SPOROTHRIX SCHENCKII.* A single species of fungus, *S. schenckii,* is the etiologic agent of sporotrichosis. The fungus is dimorphic producing a mycelium with conidia (2–3 × 3–6 μm) in culture at room temperature, and blastoconidia (1–3 × 3–10 μm) in vivo and in vitro at 37°C. *S. schenckii* produces brown-to-black colonies at 25–30°C and thus presents as a dematiaceous **(i.e., darkly pigmented) fungus** (Fig. 30.1).

PARASITIC FORM   **SAPROBIC FORM**

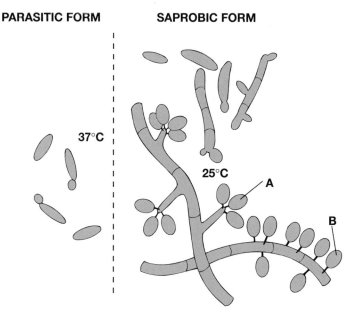

Figure 30.1.

The dimorphism of *S. schenckii*. (A) Petilate hyaline conidia borne on denticles. (B) Dematiaceous conidia borne in a sleevelike pattern.

APPEARANCE IN TISSUE. *S. schenckii* is characteristically difficult to detect in skin lesions. When observed, the fungus appears as a polymorphic yeast. The blastoconidia are round, oval, or elongate. Budding is polar or occasionally lateral and may be multiple. Round and oval forms are usually 2–6 μm in diameter but the uncommon elongate forms may be 10–15 μm in length. Even though the yeast cells are scant in tissue, the chances of isolating *S. schenckii* from cases of sporotrichosis are very good.

APPEARANCE IN CULTURE. The yeast cells germinate in cultures at room temperature and the colonies formed are moist in appearance and generally waxy in texture. The pigment is often brown to black (dematiaceous). The mycelium is comprised of hyphae that form two sorts of conidia: dark, thick-walled, holoblastic conidia borne along the hyphae in sleeves and hyaline holoblastic conidia, typically borne in a **petaline arrangement** at the tips of tapering conidiophores. The conidia are connected to the conidiophores by threadlike structures called **denticles.** At 37°C the fungus converts to the yeast cell form of growth.

Immunology

Although both a serologic test (agglutination test with patient's serum and specific yeast cell antigen) and a skin test (DTH) exist, they are rarely used, since the clinical picture is so characteristic that a strong presumptive diagnosis can be made on this basis alone, and the organism can be readily cultured. Factors involved in recovery from disease or acquired immunity have not been studied in sufficient detail to be summarized here.

Treatment

Potassium iodide (KI) administered orally is very successful in cutaneous and lymphocutaneous sporotrichosis. Amphotericin B is employed in those sensitive to iodides or in treating systemic forms of disease. No doubt, some of the azoles will be found effective.

CHROMOBLASTOMYCOSIS

Chromoblastomycosis is a chronic, slowly progressing, granulomatous disease of cutaneous and subcutaneous tissues, characterized by marked **hyperplasia** and **hyperkeratosis** of the epithelium, and caused by certain species of dematiaceous fungi.

Epidemiology

Chromoblastomycosis is found primarily in the tropics and subtropics (80% of cases), rather than in the temperate zones. The majority of cases has been reported from Cuba, Puerto Rico, and Brazil.

Pathogenesis and Virulence Factors

Virtually nothing is known about the pathogenesis of the five agents of chromoblastomycosis (Table 30.1). Experimental disease has been produced in mice and frogs.

Clinical Manifestations

The disease is not contagious by direct contact with the lesions; trauma is required. Lesions almost always appear on an exposed part of the body, most frequently on the foot or lower leg. The incubation period is unknown. The lesions usually begin as small papules or pustules, which ultimately ulcerate, then crust over, producing a dry, verrucous, raised lesion. Satellite lesions occur often and are usually more elevated than the initial lesion. The course of the disease may be extraordinarily slow; most cases are not seen until 10–15 years from the outset, probably because there is little effect on the general health of the patient. Metastasis to other organ systems are rare.

Mycology and Laboratory Diagnosis

DIMORPHISM OF THE ETIOLOGIC AGENTS OF CHROMOBLASTOMYCOSIS. In the tissues of a host the five etiologic agents of chromoblastomycosis (Table 30.1) appear the same. The form is that of dark-brown, thick-walled, more or less isolated cells that reproduce by fission. This tissue form is called a **sclerotic cell** (Fig. 30.2A). In cultures at 25°C the agents of chromoblastomycosis grow as dark olive-brown to black colonies.

APPEARANCE IN TISSUE. In tissue biopsies or in skin scrapings all of the dematiaceous agents of chromoblastomycosis appear as sclerotic cells. The sclerotic cells of the five species of dematiaceous fungi that cause chromoblas-

TABLE 30.1. Conidiation Patterns Among Species of Agents of Chromoblastomycosis

Species	Type of conidiation[a]
Cladosporium carionii	*Cladosporium* (holoblastic conidia)
Phialophora verrucosa	*Phialophora* (enteroblastic phialaconidia)
Rhinocladiella aquaspersa	*Rhinocladiella* (holoblastic poroconidia)
Fonsecaea pedrosoi	Mixed: *Cladosporium, Rhinocladiella, Phialophora*
Fonsecaea compactum	Mixed: same

[a] See Figure 30.2.

PARASITIC FORM   **SAPROBIC FORM**

37°C | 25°C

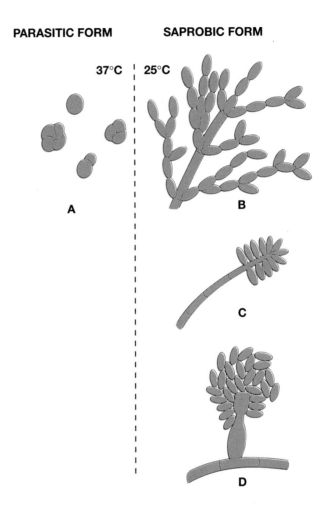

Figure 30.2.

The dimorphism of the agents of chromoblastomycosis and patterns of conidiation in room temperature cultures. (A) Sclerotic cells. (B) *Cladosporium*-type conidiation (holoblastic conidia). (C) *Rhinocladiella*-type conidiation (poroconidia). (D) *Phialophora*-type conidiation (phialoconidia).

tomycosis are indistinguishable. Occasionally, dematiaceous hyphae are also seen. There is little information on the morphologic events that accompany conversion of infectious conidia to sclerotic cells.

APPEARANCE IN CULTURE. There are five species of dematiaceous fungi that cause chromoblastomycosis. These five species are delineated on the basis of their conidiation pattern (Table 30.1; Fig. 30.2B,C,D). Although there are some reports of in vitro sclerotic cell production, usually the organisms do not convert to the parasitic form of growth when cultivated at 37°C.

Immunology

Natural resistance is high but there is little information on the mechanisms of resistance. Serodiagnostic techniques have been little explored and none is used routinely.

Treatment

Surgical excision is useful in early lesions. Antifungals include 5-fluorocytosine, amphotericin B, and one of the azoles (itraconazole) have been used successfully.

MYCETOMA

The microorganisms responsible for this affliction produce a localized, swollen lesion, generally on the hand or foot, involving cutaneous and subcutaneous tissues, fasciae, and bone. The lesions are abscesses that suppurate and drain through sinus tracts to the outside. The pus contains granules of varying size and color, dependent on the species of microbe involved.

Epidemiology

Mycetomas are worldwide in distribution, much more common in tropical and subtropical areas (India, Mexico, and Central America; more than 1200 cases per year in the Sudan). Mere presence of known etiologic agents in soil is not sufficient to insure cases of disease because trauma is required.

Pathogenesis and Virulence Factors

Experimental infections by some of the etiologic agents have been induced. Because of the diversity of etiologic agents general statements are not possible but very little is known about pathogenesis of the **eumycotic** and **actinomycotic agents** of mycetoma. Several of the true bacteria have been studied extensively, but such information is not considered in this chapter.

Clinical Manifestations

The disease is not contagious by direct contact with the lesion; trauma is required. Mycetomas are swollen deep-seated lesions most often of the hand or foot. The disease results from the traumatic introduction of any one of a large number of etiologic agents. The skin and subcutaneous tissues are initially involved. The lesions often progress to involve fascia and bone. The lesions become suppurative and sinus tracts are formed from which pus containing grains is released. The grains are the collected growth of the etiologic agent accompanied by structural elements that derive from the host response. Generally, there is no hematogenous or lymphatic spread. Some of the agents of mycetoma do produce systemic disease but these are most often acquired by inhalation of the infectious element rather than spread from a primary cutaneous site.

Mycology and Laboratory Diagnosis

These infections are caused by a large number of different microorganisms classified among the fungi, the actinomycetes, and the eubacteria. For convenience the agents are divided into three categories as follows (descriptions of individual members of the categories is not possible in this brief consideration):

1. **Eumycetoma** (true mycetoma, mycetoma vera, and maduromycosis): caused by true fungi, the Eumycetes. Some of those involved include: *Madurella mycetomatis, Madurella grisea, Pseudallescheria boydii, Acremonium* spp., *Exophiala jeanselmei, Pyrenocheata romeroi, Leptosphaeria senegalensis, Curvularia geniculata, Neotestudinata rosatii,* and *Fusarium* spp.

2. **Actinomycetoma** (actinomycotic mycetoma): caused by filamentous bacteria in the order Actinomycetales. Some of these are: *Nocardia brasiliensis, Nocardia asteroides, Nocardia caviae, Actinomyces israelii* (human bites), *Actinomadura madurae, Actinomadura pelletieri,* and *Streptomyces somaliensis.*

3. **Botryomycosis** (granuloma pyogenicum and bacterial pseudomycosis): caused by true bacteria (Eubacteriales). A few examples are: *Staphylococcus aureus, Escherichia coli, Bacteroides* spp., *Proteus* spp., and *Pseudomonas aeruginosa.*

Immunology

No serodiagnostic tests are used and little is known about immune response in general. Some information is available on host-parasite interaction with the actinomycotic agents (notably *N. asteroides*) but these data are beyond the scope of this chapter.

Treatment

It is essential to distinguish which of three categories of agents is involved: eumycotic, actinomycotic, or eubacteria because the therapy will obviously be different. The diversity of agents precludes consideration of therapy of mycetomas.

MISCELLANEOUS INOCULATION DISEASES WITHOUT EXACT CLINICAL PICTURE

Many inoculation mycoses do not display a characteristic clinical picture. These diseases manifest as deep abscesses. The etiologic agents are many and a standard text needs to be consulted to cover the salient features of each of the dozens of species involved. It should also be noted that several of the agents of inoculation mycoses may also become agents of deep-seated systemic disease. In addition to the examples noted under sporotrichosis and chromoblastomycosis, there are reports of systemic disease due to *P. boydii, Exophiala* spp., *Wangiella (Exophiala) dermatitidis, Phialophora* spp. and *N. asteroides,* among many others.

SUMMARY

1. Inoculation mycoses are those infections that occur after the traumatic introduction (inoculation) of infectious fungi into the subcutaneous tissues of a susceptible host.

2. Several of the inoculation mycoses are clinically typical: (1) sporotrichosis, (2) chromoblastomycosis, and (3) mycetoma. But many of the inoculation mycoses are not clinically distinctive.

3. Sporotrichosis is caused by *Sporothrix schenckii* a dimorphic fungus that occurs in the tissues of an infected host as a polymorphic blastoconidium and in cultures as a mycelium comprised of hyphae upon which are borne conidia arranged in a typical fashion on the conidiophore.

4. Chromoblastomycosis is caused by five species of dematiaceous fungi. All of the species of etiologic agents appear the same in the tissues of a host: dark-brown, thick-walled cells that reproduce by fission (sclerotic cells). In culture the fungi display different patterns of conidiation upon which is based their identification. These types of conidiation are characteristic of the genera *Cladosporium*, *Phialophora*, *Fonsecaea*, and *Rhinocladiella*.

5. Mycetoma is a tumefaction of the hand or foot. The lesion may be caused by a fungus (eumycetoma), a filamentous bacterium (actinomyce-toma), or a nonfilamentous bacterium (botryomycosis).

6. There are many inoculation mycoses that are not clinically distinctive. Some of the agents of inoculation mycoses may also produce deep-seated, systemic disease. Some of the fungi reported to do so are *Pseudallescheria boydii*, *Exophiala* spp., and *Wangiella (Exophiala) dermatitidis*.

REFERENCES

deHoog GS (1983): On the potentially pathogenic dematiaceous hyphomycetes. In Howard DH (ed): Fungi Pathogenic for Humans and Animals, Part A. New York: Marcel Dekker, pp 149–217.

McGinnis MR (1985): Dematiaceous fungi, In Lennette EH, Ballows A, Hausler WJ Jr, Shadomy HJ (eds): Manual of Clinical Microbiology. 4th ed. Washington, DC: American Society for Microbiology, pp 561–574.

McGinnis MR, Rinald MG, Winn RE (1986): Emerging agents of phaeohyphomycosis: pathogenic species of *Bipolaris* and *Exserohilum*. J Clin Microbiol 24:250.

REVIEW QUESTIONS

For questions 1 to 5, choose the ONE BEST answer or completion.

1. Which of the following attributes is NOT associated with the condition known clinically as mycetoma. Mycetoma
   a) is a localized infection, generally on the hand or foot
   b) produces pus containing granules of varying size and color
   c) may be caused by true fungi as well as by actinomycetes
   d) is commonly acquired by inhalation of etiologic agent with dissemination into the subcutaneous tissues

2. Fungi causing chromoblastomycosis show conidiation of the
   a) *Cladosporium* type
   b) *Phialophora* type
   c) *Rhinocladiella* type
   d) all three types listed

3. *Sporothrix schenckii*
   a) is dimorphic
   b) commonly produces acute pulmonary disease
   c) is readily observed in the tissues of an infected host
   d) is commonly acquired from bee stings

4. Which of the following is NOT generally associated with the inoculation mycoses?
   a) dark-spored fungi
   b) granules in tissue or pus from sinus tracts
   c) exogenous acquisition
   d) hematogenous dissemination
   e) dimorphism of the etiologic agent

5. Brown, spherical, septate, sclerotic bodies from pus are diagnostic of
   a) mucormycosis
   b) aspergillosis
   c) chromoblastomycosis
   d) mycetoma
   e) sporotrichosis

ANSWERS TO REVIEW QUESTIONS

1. *d* Mycetomas are acquired by direct inoculation of the etiologic agents.

2. *d* All three types of conidiation are displayed by one or another of the agents of chromoblastomycosis.

3. *a* *Sporothrix schenckii* is a dimorphic fungus.

4. *d* Hematogenous dissemination is rare in any of the inoculation mycoses.

5. *c* Sclerotic bodies is the name for the in vivo growth form of any of the agents of chromoblastomycosis.

OPPORTUNISTIC FUNGOUS DISEASES

Fungi may become particularly active incitants of disease when an individual's defense mechanisms are deficient. Such diseases are termed **opportunistic** because the fungus takes advantage of the immunosuppressed host. The factors that predispose individuals to opportunistic diseases include diabetes, lymphomas, broad-spectrum antibiotics, and immunosuppressive therapy including corticosteroids, X-irradiation, and cytotoxic drugs.

The decade of the 1950s witnessed a dramatic increase in opportunistic infections and the reason for this is probably related to three major events that took place during those years: (1) antibacterial antibiotics became established as therapeutic agents and were widely used, (2) corticosteroids became both available and commonly affordable, and (3) effective cytotoxic agents for cancer chemotherapy began to be used on a widespread basis. Antibiotics, steroids, and cytotoxic agents can alter the immune status of an individual and lead to opportunistic infection.

The spectrum of fungi involved in opportunistic infections ranges from well-known zoopathogens (e.g., *Coccidioides immitis*) to customarily nonpathogenic saprobic forms (e.g., *Aspergillus fumigatus* or *Rhizopus oryzae*).

The opportunistic behavior of *Candida* spp., of *Cryptococcus neoformans*, and of the agents of the pulmonary mycoses, has been noted in Chapters 28 and 29. Herein the important features of *Aspergillus* spp., the Zygomycetes, and miscellaneous opportunistic zoopathogens will be considered.

ASPERGILLOSIS

The members of the genus *Aspergillus* produce enteroblastic conidia (phialoconidia) arranged on a specialized conidiophore as shown in Figure 31.1. *Aspergillus* spp. may interact with animals in a variety of ways. Members of the genus may cause pulmonary infections of a localized or invasive type (rarely disseminated), allergy, or toxemias due to ingestion of secondary metabolites.

Aspergillus spp. are also important causes of pulmonary disease in wild and domesticated birds and a cause of mycotic abortion in cattle.

Epidemiology

Aspergillosis is worldwide in distribution and can affect all ages and sexes. *Aspergillus* spp. are becoming increasingly important as pathogens of immunocompromised hosts.

Pathogenesis and Virulence Factors

These comments are restricted to the infectious forms of aspergillosis. In such forms *Aspergillus* spp. are almost always opportunistic (e.g., cavity colonization and invasion of immunocompromised hosts). Thermotolerant species are potentially pathogenic. A number of toxic substances and potentially destructive enzymes including **endotoxins, mycotoxins,** and **elastases,** have been described. Some immunomodulating materials in culture supernatants have been described. One such substance interferes with complement-dependent and complement-independent phagocytosis of conidia by macrophages. In vivo production of such materials could compromise immune function.

Clinical Manifestations

Aspergillus spp. interact with animal hosts in three fundamentally different ways: (1) by inducing allergies, (2) by infectious invasion of tissues, and (3) by forming toxins that contaminate feed or food and induce toxemias in those who ingest the food products. Only the infectious forms of disease will be outlined.

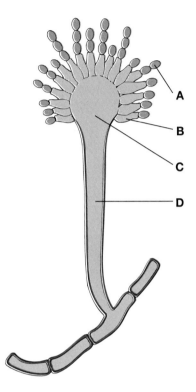

Figure 31.1.

Typical head of a member of the genus *Aspergillus*. (A) Enteroblastic conidia (phialoconidia). (B) Primary phialide. (C) Vesicle (element of conidia-bearing structure). (D) Conidiophore (conidia-bearing structure).

There are three general forms of infectious disease induced by *Aspergillus* spp:

1. **Pulmonary Aspergillosis.** Primary pulmonary aspergillosis is rare in immunocompetent humans but is an extraordinarily common disease in birds (e.g., chickens, turkeys, and penguins).

2. **Cavitary Colonization.** *Aspergillus* spp. not uncommonly colonize pulmonary cavities caused by other disease processes such as cavitary tuberculosis. The results are referred to as **fungous balls** or **aspergillomas.**

3. **Disseminated Aspergillosis.** Disseminated disease by *Aspergillus* spp. occurs in immunocompromised hosts. The route of acquisition is pulmonary and may involve several areas (e.g., skin, CNS, heart, lung, and nasal-orbital areas). The ubiquity of aspergilli allows them to precipitate infections in many ways (e.g., surgical contamination or inoculation). Traumatic implantation into the cornea results in particularly troublesome lesions.

Mycology and Laboratory Diagnosis

Aspergillus fumigatus is the most common cause of infectious aspergillosis. However, several other species including *Aspergillus flavus, Aspergillus terreus,* and *Aspergillus niger* have also been implicated in disease. The single species *A. fumigatus* is chosen as an example of the methods of identification.

APPEARANCE IN TISSUE. Septate hyphae that branch at acute angles comprise the tissue appearance of the fungus.

APPEARANCE IN CULTURE. *A. fumigatus* produces a moderately fast growing, flat, velvety, bluish-green colony, becoming brown on aging. The typical *Aspergillus* type of conidiation is produced (Fig. 31.1), with chains of enteroblastic phialoconidia produced by one row of phialides pointing upward from the upper part of the vesicle.

Immunology

Once again, only tissue invasive forms of aspergillosis are considered. In the normal host, defense against *Aspergillus* spp. depends on the ability of pulmonary macrophages to kill fungal conidia. Those individuals whose macrophage function is compromised are confronted with tissue invasion by hyphae from the germinated conidium. These fungal forms are too large for phagocytosis but are sensitive to oxidative and nonoxidative substances released by polymorphonuclear leukocytes or mononuclear phagocytes. Antibodies are produced against *Aspergillus* spp. but their presence has not been developed into a useful adjunct to diagnosis. Current efforts at serologic diagnosis are directed toward finding circulating antigens as is done in cryptococcosis or detection of unique fungal metabolites. Antibodies could be important in vivo by augmenting attachment of phagocytic cells to hyphae. The importance of CMI in aspergillosis is not yet understood.

Treatment

Treatment will depend on the form of aspergillosis involved (i.e., allergic, toxemic, or infectious). Invasive aspergillosis is difficult to treat. Amphotericin B is most often employed. The azoles may prove useful.

ZYGOMYCOSES

The zygomycoses are those diseases caused by members of the phylum Zygomycota. There is a broad range of afflictions caused by these fungi including both inoculation mycoses and deep-seated, systemic disease. All are relatively rare infections and the systemic diseases are invariably opportunistic. Only the latter will be considered here.

Epidemiology

The systemic zygomycoses are more commonly reported from North America and Europe but are worldwide in distribution. Factors that predispose to the systemic zygomycoses include: diabetes mellitus, burns, leukemia, lymphomas, chronic illnesses, and immunosuppression. Occasionally, an underlying immunosuppressive condition is not recognized.

Pathogenesis and Virulence Factors

Little is known but some useful animal models have been developed. The rapidity with which mucoraceous fungi can penetrate the tissues of an immunocompromised host indicates an armamentarium of tissue-destructive enzymes.

Clinical Disease Manifestations

The systemic zygomycoses (also known as **mucormycoses** because all of the agents are in the order Mucorales of the phylum Zygomycota) present a spectrum of clinical disease types, a complete description of which is not possible here. One of the most characteristic clinical forms is acute **rhinocerebral zygomycosis.** The infection usually begins in the turbinates or paranasal sinus. The signs first involve the nose and spread to the eye and brain.

Mycology and Laboratory Diagnosis

The Zygomycetes produce sexual spores called zygospores and asexual spores called sporangiospores (see Fig. 26.4). The mycelium is comprised of nonseptate hyphae. The zygomycetes that produce deep-seated systemic diseases are in the order Mucorales. One genus commonly encountered is *Rhizopus.*

APPEARANCE IN TISSUE. The Zygomycetes appear rather similar in tissue: broad, nonseptate hyphae that branch at right angles.

APPEARANCE IN CULTURE. The five families in the order Mucorales are Mucoraceae, Cunninghamellaceae, Syncephalastraceae, Saksenaeaceae, Mortierellaceae. Each of the families is distinguished by the morphology of its sporangium. The most common incitants of mucormycosis are contained in the family Mucoraceae. All of the species in the family Mucoraceae have similar sporangia. The species are distinguished on the basis of various morphologic features.

Immunology

The rarity of the disease indicates a high natural resistance. Bronchoalveolar macrophages are unable to kill the sporangiospores of mucoraceous fungi but do control germination of the spores. Substances that reduce the natural resistance of a host (e.g., steroids) allow spore germination and tissue penetration by hyphal elements. The hyphae of mucoraceous fungi are sensitive to oxidative and non-oxidative substances released by phagocytes. Serologic adjuncts to diagnosis are not widely used. The role of CMI is largely unknown.

Treatment

There is usually a very poor response to antifungals. Amphotericin B has been used.

MISCELLANEOUS OPPORTUNISTS

There is a very large number of fungi, both **dematiaceous** (dark-colored conidia) and **moniliaceous** (light-colored conidia) fungi that can be involved in opportunistic fungous infections. Identification of this diverse group of fungi cannot be considered in this chapter.

SUMMARY

1. Opportunistic fungous diseases are those whose incitants take advantage of an immunosuppressed host.

2. Factors that predispose individuals to opportunistic diseases include

diabetes, lymphomas, broad-spectrum antibiotics, and immunosuppressive therapy including corticosteroids, X-irradiation, and cytotoxic drugs.

3. The spectrum of fungi involved in opportunistic infections ranges from well-known zoopathogens, such as *Coccidioides immitis*, to customarily nonpathogenic saprobes, such as *Aspergillus* spp. or *Rhizopus* spp.

4. *Aspergillus* spp. interact with animal hosts in three ways: (1) induction of allergies, (2) infectious invasion of tissues, and (3) formation of secondary metabolites that are toxic upon ingestion by animals.

5. *Aspergillus* spp. produce pigmented colonies in culture. The conidia produced are enteroblastic phialoconidia arranged in a characteristic fashion on the conidiophore. In infectious invasion of tissue *Aspergillus* spp. appear as septate hyphae with branches occurring at acute angles.

6. The zygomycoses are diseases caused by members of the phylum Zygomycota. Both deep-seated, systemic diseases and inoculation mycoses may be produced. Rhinocerebral zygomycosis is one of the more characteristic clinical forms.

7. The Zygomycetes produce sexual spores called zygospores and asexual spores called sporangiospores. The mycelium is comprised of nonseptate hyphae.

8. All of the agents of deep-seated, systemic disease are in the order Mucorales. This order contains five families distinguished on the basis of the morphology of their sporangia (i.e., Mucoraceae, Cunninghamellaceae, Syncephalastraceae, Mortierellaceae, and Saksenaeceae). The family Mucoraceae contains the most frequently encountered incitants of systemic mucormycosis. These species are distinguished on the basis of morphologic features. In the tissue of a host the zygomycetes appear as broad, nonseptate hyphae with right angle branches.

9. There are a large number of fungi other than species of *Aspergillus* and the Zygomycetes that can initiate infection in an immunosuppressed host.

REFERENCES

Raper KB, Fennell DI (1965): The Genus Aspergillus. Baltimore: Williams & Wilkins.

Scholer HJ, Muller E, Schipper MAA (1983): Mucorales. In Howard DH (ed): Fungi Pathogenic for Humans and Animals (in three parts), Part A-Biology. New York: Marcel Dekker, pp 9–59.

REVIEW QUESTIONS

> For questions 1 to 3, choose the ONE
> BEST answer or completion.

Ms. J. R. is a white female 15 years of age who was in good health until about 1 year prior to admission to UCLA when she began to lose weight despite a good appetite. During the past year she has lost between 30 and 40 lb and for the past 3 months she has been tired and listless in addition to having dryness of the mouth, excess urine output, and extreme thirst. Laboratory results established that the patient was severely diabetic and in ketoacidosis. On the fourth hospital day, the patient developed cellulitis of the left orbit with slight protrusion of the eye, facial paralysis, and a stiff neck.

1. Which of the following fungi is most likely involved in the sequence of events described in the case presentation?
   a) *Aspergillus*
   b) *Candida*
   c) *Rhizopus*
   d) *Cryptococcus*
   e) *Blastomyces*

2. The possibility would be strengthened by finding which of the following structural elements is an aspirate from the afflicted area.
   a) septate hyphae whose branches form at acute angles
   b) nonseptate hyphae, quite wide in diameter with side branches at right angles
   c) budding yeasts with some hyphal strands
   d) large (15 μm) thick-walled blastoconidia with cytoplasmic retraction
   e) Encapsulated blastoconidia

3. The diagnosis would be confirmed by the isolation of a fungus showing which of the following microscopic characteristics.
   a) encapsulated blastoconidia
   b) blastoconidia, pseudohyphae, and chlamydoconidia
   c) sporangiospores within a sporangium, nonseptate hyphae with rhizoids
   d) septate hyphae with laterally borne conidia of varying sizes (4–12 μm)
   e) septate hyphae, conidiophores with vesicles from which conidia arise from phialides

ANSWERS TO REVIEW QUESTIONS

1. *c* This answer is the best choice.

2. *b* This description is that of the mucoraceous fungi in tissue.

3. *c* This answer covers the general appearance of one of the common agents of mucormycosis.

VIROLOGY

MORPHOLOGY AND TAXONOMY OF VIRUS

Conceptually, viruses are genetic elements packaged in protein coats. This packaged genetic element can penetrate a susceptible cell and replicate within the cell. Descriptively, viruses are a heterogeneous group of infectious agents that vary in sizes from 20 to about 200 nm in average diameter. The genetic element may be DNA or RNA. The essential structure of viruses consists of a central core of nucleic acid inside a shell of protein that may in turn be wrapped in a membranous envelope. There are literally hundreds of ''species'' of viruses capable of infecting humans.

MORPHOLOGY

Viral morphology is best studied by the **negative staining technique** and in an electron micrograph. This technique involves the mixing of a suspension of virus with a solution of electron dense metallic compound, such as phosphotungstic acid. The metallic compound stains the background leaving the viral structures relatively colorless in the electron micrograph (Fig. 32.1). Complementary data, especially for the larger virus, can be obtained with an electron micrograph of thin sections of infected cells (Fig. 32.2).

There are four basic morphologic types of human viruses. They are (1) viruses with an icosahedral capsid symmetry, (2) viruses with an icosahedral capsid symmetry and an outer envelope, (3) viruses with a helical capsid symmetry and an outer envelope, and (4) viruses with a complex capsid. Morphology is an important criterion in the classification of viruses.

Virus With an Icosahedral Capsid Symmetry

A virus with icosahedral capsid symmetry has two key components: a central core (the genome) and an outer shell of protein known as the **capsid** (Fig. 32.3). The capsid of each virus is an aggregation of morphologic units, known as **capsomeres.** The number of capsomeres per virus particle is constant for each species

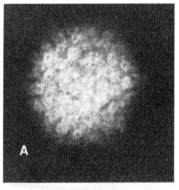

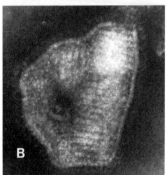

Figure 32.1.

(A) A negatively stained nucleocapsid of the herpes simplex virus. Note the individual capsomere. (B) A negatively stained influenza virion. Note the helical nucleocapsid surrounded by the envelope with surface projection. [Reproduced with permission from Madley CR (1972): Virus Morphology. Baltimore: Williams & Wilkins.]

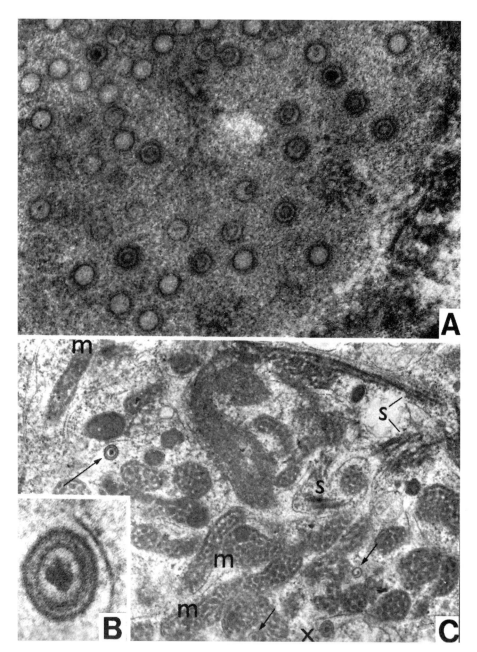

Figure 32.2.
Thin section of a cell infected by the Epstein-Barr virus. (A) Numerous nucleocapsids and empty capsids in the nucleus. (B) A mature virion (long arrow) within a membrane-bound space. (C) A mature virion. [Reproduced with permission from Epstein MA, Henle G, Achong BG, Barr Y (1965): Morphological and biological studies on a virus in cultured lymphoblasts from Burkitt's lymphoma. J Exp Med 121:761.]

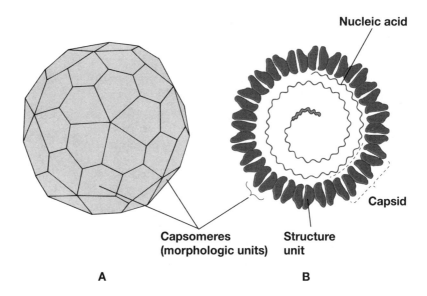

Figure 32.3.

A nonenveloped icosahedral virus (A) and its cross-section (B). [Modified from Casper DLD (1965): Cold Spring Harb Symp Quant Biol 27:4.]

of virus but usually varies between families of viruses. The core and capsid are known as the **nucleocapsid.** A virus particle with all its morphologic components is known as a **virion.** For viruses with this type of morphology, nucleocapsids are synonymous with virions (e.g., the papillomavirus).

Virus With an Icosahedral Capsid Symmetry and an Envelope

A virus with icosahedral **capsid symmetry** and an envelope is morphologically identical to the preceding group except that the nucleocapsid is wrapped in an outer **envelope** (Fig. 32.4). Between the nucleocapsid and envelope is the **matrix protein.** This viral envelope is derived from the membrane of the host cell except that membrane proteins of the host are largely replaced by viral proteins. The envelope proteins generally appear as spikes known as **peplomers.** For viruses with this type of morphology, the virion consists of the nucleocapsid and the envelope (e.g., the rubellavirus).

Virus With a Helical Capsid Symmetry and an Envelope

Here the capsid proteins are aggregated around the viral genome as a flexible hollow tube. (Fig. 32.5). The coiled nucleocapsid is wrapped in an envelope to form a virion (e.g., the influenzavirus).

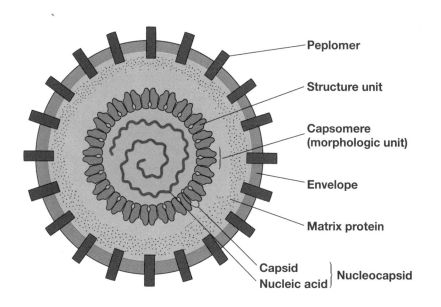

Peplomer

Structure unit

Capsomere
(morphologic unit)

Envelope

Matrix protein

Capsid
Nucleic acid } Nucleocapsid

Figure 32.4.

An enveloped icosahedral virus (cross-section). [Modified from Casper DLD (1965): Cold Spring Harb Symp Quant Biol 27:8.]

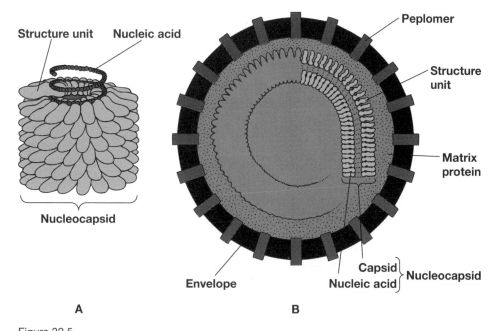

Structure unit   Nucleic acid

Nucleocapsid

A

Peplomer

Structure unit

Matrix protein

Envelope

Capsid
Nucleic acid } Nucleocapsid

B

Figure 32.5.

An enveloped helical virus. (A) A segment of its nucleocapsid and (B) its cross-section. [Modified from Casper DLD (1965): Cold Spring Harb Symp Quant Biol 27:50.]

Virus With a Complex Symmetry

Here the structure is much more complex (Fig. 32.6). The virion consists of an external envelope, a complex layer of tubular structure, and an internal structure made up of a DNA-containing core and lateral bodies. Viruses with this morphology are among the largest of all viruses (e.g., the smallpoxvirus).

FUNCTIONS OF MORPHOLOGIC COMPONENTS

Nucleic Acid Core

The nucleic acid core contains all the necessary information for virus replication in susceptible cells. For some species of virus, notably those with a single positive-sense RNA and those with small DNA genome, introduction of the nucleic acid into a susceptible cell results in viral replication and release of progeny virions.

Capsid

The capsid is necessary for morphogenesis of the virion. In the group of virus without an envelope, the capsid also determines host specificity, protects the viral genome from degradation by nucleases in body fluid, enhances the efficiency of infection, and induces the formation of neutralizing antibody.

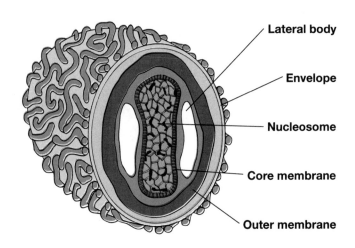

Figure 32.6.

Cross-section of a poxvirus. [Modified from Lennette EH, Halonen P, Murphy EA (eds) (1988): Laboratory diagnosis of infectious diseases. New York: Springer-Verlag.]

Envelope

The envelope is essential for infectivity of all enveloped viruses. Stripped off the envelope, the nucleocapsid of an enveloped virion is incapable of attaching to a susceptible cell. The peplomers play a key role in viral attachment to a susceptible cell and in the induction of neutralizing antibodies against the enveloped virus.

Matrix Protein

This protein is necessary for the maturation and release of enveloped virions.

TAXONOMY

Taxonomy is a system for **classification** and **nomenclature.** In dealing with a large number of viruses with varying characteristics, a system of taxonomy is a practical necessity. The orderly grouping of viruses into a small number of families facilitates learning. The identification of viral isolates from clinical materials is made easier by first identifying the family to which an isolate belongs. Standardized nomenclature is essential in communication. Viral taxonomy is based on the recommendations of the International Committee on Taxonomy of Viruses.

Classification

Viruses are grouped according to relatedness. The grouping is set arbitrarily at the hierarchial levels of family, genus, and species. A family of viruses consists of a cluster of viruses that share common characteristics and that are distinct from other major clusters (families) of viruses. Viruses within a family may be organized into genera; members of a genus share certain common characteristics that are distinct from other genera of the same family. Viruses belonging to a genus may be further separated into species. There is at this time no formal agreement on specific characteristics that distinguish species within a genus.

Grouping of viruses into families are generally based on **morphology** (size, shape, the presence or absence of an envelope, capsid symmetry, and others) and **genomic characteristics** (RNA or DNA, single or double stranded, positive or negative sense, number of segments, size of genome, etc.).

Nomenclature

Families are designated by terms with the suffix ''viridae''; and, genera with the suffix ''virus.'' For species, one simply uses the English vernacular name. For example, the full formal taxonomic terminology of type 1 poliovirus is *Picornaviridae, Enterovirus,* polio 1. In informal usage, one describes poliovirus 1 as a species of the enterovirus genus that belongs to the picornavirus family. Linnaen

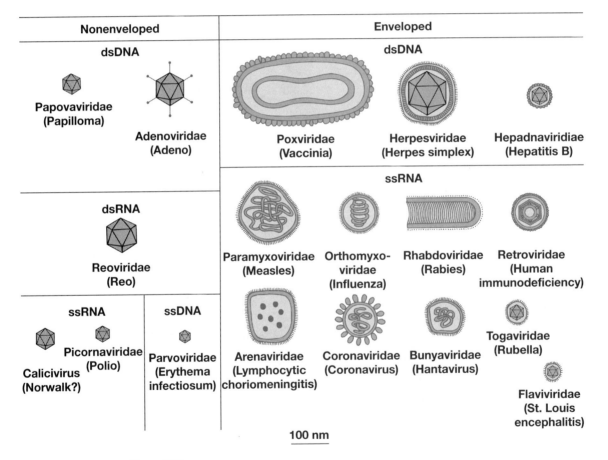

Nonenveloped	Enveloped

dsDNA

Papovaviridae
(Papilloma)

Adenoviridae
(Adeno)

dsDNA

Poxviridae
(Vaccinia)

Herpesviridae
(Herpes simplex)

Hepadnaviridiae
(Hepatitis B)

ssRNA

Paramyxoviridae
(Measles)

Orthomyxo-
viridae
(Influenza)

Rhabdoviridae
(Rabies)

Retroviridae
(Human
immunodeficiency)

dsRNA

Reoviridae
(Reo)

ssRNA

Calicivirus
(Norwalk?)

Picornaviridae
(Polio)

ssDNA

Parvoviridae
(Erythema
infectiosum)

Arenaviridae
(Lymphocytic
choriomeningitis)

Coronaviridae
(Coronavirus)

Bunyaviridae
(Hantavirus)

Togaviridae
(Rubella)

Flaviviridae
(St. Louis
encephalitis)

100 nm

Figure 32.7.

The 18 families of animal viruses pathogenic for human. *Filoviridae* is not included because human infection by this family of viruses has not been documented in the United States. [Redrawn with permission from Matthews REF (1982): Classification and nomenclature of viruses. Intervirology 17:36.]

binomials, such as *Picornavirus poliomyelitis* or *Orthomyxovirus influenzae,* are not used.

Families of Viruses Pathogenic for Humans

Virtually all viruses pathogenic for humans in the United States have been placed in **19 families,** although a few are still unclassified. The names and key characteristics of the 18 families are shown in Figure 32.7. It is recommended that students attempt at this time to memorize the names of these 18 families, their key characteristics (RNA or DNA and enveloped or not enveloped) and the name of a medically important species for each family.

Other Classification Schemes

Human viruses have also been classified by the mode of transmission and by the predominant pathology induced in the human host. For example, arboviruses (*ar*thropod-*bo*rne viruses) include all viruses that are transmitted between vertebrates by the bite of arthropods; and hepatitis viruses denote viruses that inflict hepatocellular damages. There is no relationship among the three schemes of classification. Arboviruses include many species of the togavirus, flavivirus, reovirus, and bunyavirus families. Hepatitis viruses are comprised of the hepadnavirus family, a species of the picornavirus family, and several other unclassified ones.

SUMMARY

1. A virus is essentially one or several molecules of nucleic acid enclosed in a layer of viral proteins. A virus can enter and replicate within a susceptible cell.

2. The protein layer (capsid) is comprised of many morphologic units (capsomeres) and may be shelllike (icosahedral symmetry) or tubelike (helical symmetry). The nucleic acid enclosed in the capsid is known as the nucleocapsid. For some species of viruses, the nucleocapsid is surrounded by an external membranous envelope.

3. Viral genes may be DNA or RNA and single or double stranded. For RNA viruses, the RNA may be segmented (more than one molecule) or non-

segmented (one molecule) and positive (can serve as mRNA) or negative sense. Nucleic acids of many but not all viral species, if appropriately introduced into a susceptible cell can replicate and form progeny viruses (see Chapter 33).

4. The capsid is important in the packaging of viral nucleic acids. For nonenveloped viruses; the capsid determines host specificity, increases the efficiency of infection, protects viral nucleic acids from degradation by nucleases in body fluid, and induces the formation of virus-neutralizing antibodies. For enveloped viruses, stripping off the envelope results in the loss of infectivity. It is the peplomers (spike of viral proteins on the envelope) that determine host specificity and induce neutralizing antibody.

5. Human viruses are grouped into 19 families. This grouping is based primarily on morphology and the nature of viral genes.

REFERENCES

Murphy FA (1988): Virus taxonomy and nomenclature. In Lennette EH, Halonen P, Murphy FA (eds): Laboratory Diagnosis of Infectious Diseases Principles and Practice. New York: Springer-Verlag pp 153–176.

Van Regenmortel MHV (1990): Virus species, a much overlooked but essential concept in virus classification. Intervirology 31:241.

REVIEW QUESTIONS

For questions 1 to 4, choose the ONE BEST answer or completion.

1. About the basic structure of viruses:
   a) The basic structure of all viruses consists of a molecule of nucleic acid wrapped in a layer of viral proteins.
   b) The basic structure of all viruses consists of one or several molecules of nucleic acids wrapped in a layer of proteins surrounded by an external envelope.
   c) The basic structure of all viruses is also known as the nucleocapsid.
   d) Genera of a single virus family may have icosahedral or helical nucleocapsid.
   e) A typical virion must have a nucleocapsid.

2. About functions of viral components:
   a) Capsid proteins of all viruses determine host specificity and induce neutralizing antibodies.
   b) Peplomers of all viruses including nonenveloped viruses determine host specificity and induce neutralizing antibodies.
   c) Mixing a suspension of viruses with ether (ether destroys the envelope) renders the suspension noninfectious.
   d) Mixing a suspension of herpes simplex viruses with specific antibodies against the viral capsid renders the virus noninfectious.
   e) The capsid is essential in the formation of virions.

3. Identify the incorrect statement regarding the genomic chemistry of virus families.
   a) *Herpesviridae*—DNA
   b) *Retroviridae*—DNA
   c) *Orthomyxoviridae*—segmented RNA
   d) *Reoviridae*—double-stranded RNA
   e) *Parvoviridae*—single-stranded DNA

4. Which one of the following families of viruses is nonenveloped?
   a) *Retroviridae*
   b) *Herpesviridae*
   c) *Paramyxoviridae*
   d) *Papovaviridae*
   e) *Togaviridae*

ANSWERS TO REVIEW QUESTIONS

1. *e*   3. *b*

2. *e*   4. *d*

Question Nos. 1 and 2 are essentially a reemphasis of the most important aspects of viral structure and of functions of structural components. Note that there is no question on viruses with complex symmetry. There is only one family of virus that has complex symmetry: *Poxviridae*. This family of virus is not only unique in its complex symmetry but also unique in other characteristics, such as its large size and its replication cycle. Some virologists question if poxviruses are true viruses. Because of its complexity, it is difficult to study or deduce the function of each structure component.

Question Nos. 3 and 4 are reminders that, for communication purposes, students are required to memorize names of the more important families and their medically relevant characteristics. The most important ones are *Herpesviridae, Retroviridae, Orthomyxoviridae, Picornaviridae, Hepadnaviridae, Paramyxoviridae,* and *Papovaviridae.* The more important morphologic and chemical characteristics of a virus family are the possession of an external membranous envelope and the genomic chemistry.

VIRUS REPLICATION

Viruses are **obligatory intracellular parasites.** As such, it replicates only within susceptible cells. However, its mode of replication is markedly different from prokaryotic or eukaryotic intracellular parasites. In virus replication there is intimate **mingling of viral components with the protoplasm of the host cell.** Also, the virus depends on the host cell for energy and low molecular weight precursors for the synthesis of viral components. Translation of viral mRNA into proteins depends on the host's protein synthetic machinery. Knowledge of how viruses replicate are important in the comprehension of viral pathogenesis, virus interaction, and the mode of action of antiviral chemicals.

VIRUS REPLICATION CYCLE

The cycle is generally described as consisting of six steps: attachment, penetration, uncoating, the synthetic phase, maturation, and release.

Attachment

A virus has **attachment sites** and a cell has **specific viral receptors.** The two are configuratively complementary, much like the relation between antigen and antibody. When the two sites collide, the virus is attached to the cell and the virus replication cycle is initiated. Attachment is a random physical phenomenon that follows the law of mass action. It does not require the expenditure of energy. Virus attachment sites are on the surface of each virion (e.g., capsid of nonenveloped virus and peplomer of enveloped virus). Virus receptors are usually glycoproteins embedded in the cell membrane. The receptors are virus specific and have physiologic functions. For example: the CR2 molecule on the B lymphocyte is a C3 receptor and also serves as the receptor for the Epstein-Barr virus; and, the CD4 molecules on T helper lymphocytes have immune functions and also serve as receptors for HIV. Virus attachment sites must be on the periphery of a virion and can be blocked by specific neutralizing antibodies.

Penetration

After attachment, the nucleocapsid enters the cell by **pinocytosis** or by the **fusion** of the cell membrane with the viral envelope. This fusion is usually mediated by a viral envelope protein.

Uncoating

This step involves the **disassembly** of the nucleocapsid into capsid proteins and viral nucleic acid. The disassembly is achieved by **unidentified host enzymes.** An exception is the poxvirus family. The uncoating of the genome of poxviruses requires first a host enzyme and then a virus-specified uncoating enzyme. Apparently, the host uncoating enzyme partially exposes the viral gene, a virion-associated DNA dependent RNA polymerase then transcribes the exposed viral gene and the host ribosome translates the newly formed transcript. Among the polypeptide formed is the viral uncoating enzyme that completes the uncoating of viral genes.

Synthetic Phase

This phase includes three overlapping steps: the **synthesis of virus-specific mRNA,** the **synthesis of viral genes,** and the **translation of viral mRNA** into polypeptides. The viral mRNA is often subjected to the same types of modifications found in cell mRNA (e.g., splicing, polyadenylation, and capping). Some viral polypeptides are cleaved by proteases at specific sites into two or more functional units. Pathways for the synthesis of viral nucleic acids vary considerably among the different viral families but are dependent on the chemical nature

of viral genes. The translation of viral mRNA into polypeptides depends on the
host's protein-synthesizing apparatus and is the same for all viruses. The synthetic phase, also known as virus gene expression, is often subjected to **temporal regulation.** (Students are advised to review gene replication and gene expression in a biochemistry text.)

Maturation

Maturation is the formation of infectious virions. Nucleocapsids are formed by **self-assemblage.** When the capsid proteins reach a sufficiently high concentration, they will self-assemble into capsids. This process is expedited by nucleic acids of the right sizes. Most of the capsids contain viral genomes (nucleocapsids), some are empty and a few may contain host genes (pseudovirions). For enveloped viruses, the nucleocapsid acquires an envelope by "**budding**" through cell membrane at the site where host proteins are largely or completely replaced by viral proteins. This budding process requires the participation of the matrix protein that is deposited on the portion of the cell membrane destined to become the viral envelope.

Release

The release of nonenveloped viruses occurs through **cell disintegration.** Thousands of progeny viruses are generally released from each replication cycle. For enveloped viruses, virus release from the infected cell occurs through the budding process. Cells releasing viruses through **budding** may remain viable.

Figure 33.1 depicts the replication cycle as exemplified by that of the poliovirus.

VARIATIONS IN THE SYNTHETIC PHASE

The key viral product in the synthetic phase is the **viral mRNA.** The pathway through which multiple copies of viral mRNA are formed varies with the **chemistry of the viral genome;** but the pathway through which viral mRNA is translated into viral polypeptides is the same for all viruses. All mRNA are translated into polypeptides by the host cell's protein-synthesizing machinery. The pathways leading from viral genomes to multiple copies of viral mRNA can best be described under the following three categories: RNA viruses other than retroviruses, DNA viruses, and retroviruses.

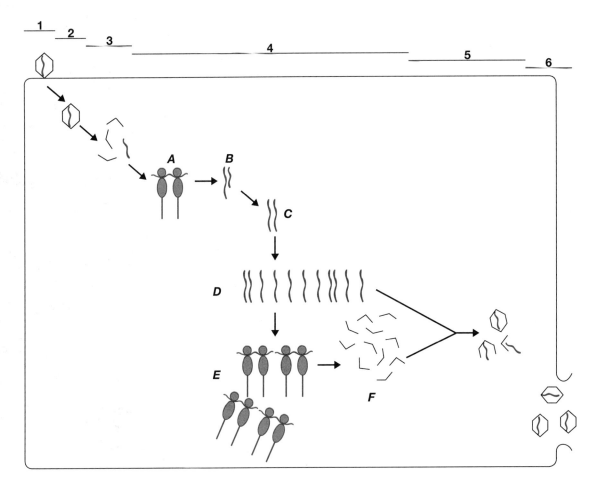

Figure 33.1.
Replication cycle of the poliovirus. (1) Attachment. (2) Penetration. (3) Uncoating. (4) Synthetic phase: (A) translation of viral RNA into RNA-dependent RNA polymerase; (B) synthesis of the negative-strand RNA; (C) formation of double-strand RNA; (D) synthesis of multiple copies of mRNA (viral genome); (E) translation of mRNA into polyproteins; (F) cleavage of polyproteins into capsid proteins. (5) Maturation. (6) Release.

RNA Viruses Other Than Retroviruses

It is important to remember that the host cell does not have an **RNA dependent RNA polymerase;** therefore, this polymerase must be encoded in the viral genome. The initial step in the synthetic phase depends on whether the viral genome is single or double stranded; and, if single stranded, whether it is positive or negative sense. In the following description, the terms ''positive-sense RNA'' and ''mRNA'' are used interchangeably.

Viruses with single-stranded positive-sense RNA (e.g., *Picornaviridae*). The viral genome is the same as viral mRNA. The uncoated viral genome is translated, yielding a RNA dependent RNA polymerase. Using the viral genome as template, this polymerase synthesizes a complimentary strand of RNA. Together, the original viral genome (positive sense) and the newly synthesized complimentary strand (negative sense) form a double-stranded RNA known as the replicative form. Using this replicative form as the template, the viral polymerase synthesizes from the negative-sense strand many copies of positive-sense RNA. These positive-sense RNAs serve as viral mRNA as well as viral genomes for progeny virions.

Viruses with single-stranded negative-sense RNA (e.g., *Orthomyxoviridae*). The uncoated negative-sense RNA cannot be translated. It must be transcribed into positive-sense RNA. This initial step is performed by an RNA dependent RNA polymerase found in the capsid. Once positive-sense RNA are formed, the synthetic phase proceeds as described for *Picornaviridae*. Both positive- and negative-sense RNA are formed. The negative-sense RNA serves as viral genomes for progeny virions; the positive-sense RNA as viral mRNA.

Viruses with double-stranded RNA (e.g., *Reoviridae*). The capsid also contains an RNA dependent RNA polymerase that transcribes the negative-strand of the uncoated viral genome into positive-sense RNA. The synthetic phase then proceeds as described for *Picornaviridae*. The double-stranded RNA serves as genomes for progeny virions.

DNA Viruses

The synthetic phase of DNA viruses differs from that of the RNA viruses in three important aspects. (1) The transcription of viral DNA depends, at least in part, on the host cell's DNA dependent RNA polymerase. (2) The viral DNA can be integrated into cell DNA and, thereby, subjected to the same regulatory mechanism of the cell. (3) Viral DNAs are **transcribed in blocks** instead of all at once. Transcription of some blocks of genes depends on the transcriptional products of other blocks. Some blocks of genes are transcribed by the host enzyme DNA dependent DNA polymerase right after uncoating, and these are known as **early genes.** Other blocks are transcribed only after a sufficient amount of early gene products are formed, and they are known as **late genes.** In general, the early genes code for products with regulatory functions while the late genes code for structural components of the virion.

Early genes are transcribed by host cell's DNA dependent RNA polymerase, while late genes require early gene products for transcription. What are these early gene products? Studies of gene regulation of DNA viruses of bacteria have shown that early gene products include repressor substances and factors that modify the host cell's DNA dependent RNA polymerase. In one bacterial virus, the promoter of the early but not the late genes is recognized by the host's DNA dependent RNA polymerase. Therefore, only the early genes are transcribed by the host's polymerase. In another bacterial virus, one product of the early genes is a substance that modifies the host's polymerase. After the modification, the host polymerase is capable of recognizing the promoter of late genes and transcribing the late genes. In still another bacterial virus (the lambda phage), the early gene product is a repressor that directly or indirectly shut off the expression of all late genes. When all the late genes are shut off by the repressor, the bacterial virus is said to be in a state of **lysogeny** (see Chapter 35). Lysogeny-like events have also been described for human viruses. For example, after the uncoating of the genome of Epstein-Barr virus in a human B lymphocyte, only the early genes are expressed and all late genes are shut off. The late genes are not shut off by any repressor but by an unknown mechanism probably related to the host cell. This relationship between the Epstein-Barr virus and the human B lymphocyte is known as a **nonproductive infection.** It should be emphasized here that, in a nonproductive infection, the cell has acquired a package of foreign genes some of which are expressed.

For the smaller DNA viruses (papova- and parvoviruses) the synthesis of viral DNA depends on the host's DNA dependent DNA polymerase. The larger DNA viruses code for their own DNA polymerases.

Retroviridae

The genome of retroviruses consists of a dimer of positive-sense single-stranded RNA. Unlike other RNA viruses, its genome codes for a RNA dependent DNA polymerase (reverse transcriptase) instead of the RNA dependent RNA polymerase. The reverse transcriptase transcribes viral RNA into viral DNA some of which may be integrated into host cell DNA. The integrated viral DNA is known as **provirus** and the nonintegrated as **episomal DNA.** The host's DNA dependent RNA polymerase then transcribes the episomal and proviral DNA into viral mRNA. Some of the mRNA serve as genomes of progeny virions.

TRANSFECTION WITH VIRAL GENOMES

Transfection is the experimental infection of host cells with naked viral genomes (viral nucleic acid completely devoid of associated proteins). If the transfection is successful and, thereby, results in the release of progeny virions, the viral nucleic acid is said to be infectious. The **infectiousness of viral nucleic acid** depends on the nature of the initial step of the synthetic pathway, which in turn depends on the genomic chemistry. The genome of all viruses, which contain polymerases in the virion, is noninfectious, because the virion-associated polymerase is essential in initiating the synthetic phase after the uncoating of viral genome.

All single-stranded negative-sense RNA viruses, the reovirus (double-stranded RNA), the retrovirus, and the poxvirus have a noninfectious naked genome. The retrovirus has a single-stranded positive-sense RNA genome; but its naked genome is noninfectious because the first step of the synthetic phase is the reverse transcription of viral RNA into viral DNA by the virion associated reverse transcriptase. This reverse transcription presumably requires the viral RNA to exist as a dimer. As expected, naked retroviral DNA isolated from infected cells are infectious. The poxvirus has a double-stranded DNA genome; but, its naked genome is noninfectious because the poxvirus is a large and complex virus with an unique and complex replication cycle. While it is theoretically possible to transfect the naked genome of large DNA viruses, such as the herpesvirus, such efforts seldom yield progeny virions. This occurs because, due to its large size, it is difficult to prepare intact herpes viral DNA genome. What is used in transfection experiments are fragments of herpesviral DNA. Some herpesviral DNA fragments are expressed after introduction into susceptible cells.

The experimental introduction of foreign nucleic acid into a mammalian cell is known as transfection if the foreign nucleic acid is expressed in the transfected cell. The foreign nucleic acid need not be a viral genome.

SUMMARY

1. The virus replication cycle consists of the following six sequential steps: attachment, penetration, uncoating, synthetic phase, maturation, and release.

2. Attachment depends on the physical complementarity of two epitopes, one on the virion and the other on the cell membrane. The viral and cell epitopes bind onto each other much like the binding of antigen to its specific antibody.

3. Penetration is the internalization of the nucleocapsid and occurs through pinocytosis or the fusion of the viral envelope with the cell membrane.

4. Uncoating requires the participation of host enzymes.

5. In the synthetic phase, viral genome, viral mRNA, and viral proteins are formed usually in abundance. The pathway through which viral genomes and viral mRNA are formed varies according to the chemistry of viral genome.

6. Maturation of nonenveloped viruses is primarily the formation of nucleocapsids. This occurs through self-assembly. In the maturation of enveloped virions, the nucleocapsid acquires an external envelope consisting of a cell membrane whose membrane proteins are largely replaced by viral proteins. The envelope is acquired at the cell membrane by ''budding.'' The matrix protein plays a role in the acquisition of the envelope.

7. For nonenveloped viruses, thousands of progeny virions are released through cell death and disintegration. For enveloped viruses, the progeny virions are released by budding out from the cell. This budding process need not result in cell death.

8. The transcription of DNA and RNA viral genome depends on host's DNA dependent RNA and virus RNA dependent RNA polymerase, respectively. For the retrovirus (an RNA virus), the viral genome is reverse transcribed to viral DNA by the viral reverse transcriptase and the viral DNA is then transcribed to viral mRNA and genomes by the host's DNA dependent RNA polymerase.

9. The naked genome of all DNA viruses except the poxvirus, which may not be a true virus, has been successfully transfected. Successful transfection of naked RNA virus genome depends on whether the viral genome can or cannot serve as viral mRNA. Those RNA viruses whose naked genomes are noninfectious are also the viruses whose virions contain the polymerase.

10. The DNA viral genes are transcribed in blocks. The early genes are those transcribed right after uncoating and the late genes, after transcription of early genes. Transcription of the late genes may be repressed.

REFERENCES

Greene WC (1991): The molecular biology of human immunodeficiency virus type 1 infection. N Engl J Med 324:308.

Joklik WK (1992): The virus multiplication cycle. In Joklik WK, Willet HP, Amos DB, Wilfert CM (eds): Zinsser Microbiology, Chap 55, 20th edition. Norwalk, CT: Appleton & Lange, pp 789–835.

Stephens EB (1988): Assembly of animal viruses at cellular membranes. Annu Rev Microbiol 42:489.

REVIEW QUESTIONS

For questions 1 to 4, choose the ONE BEST answer or completion. (Disregard poxviruses in answering the questions.)

1. About virus replication:
   a) Without exception, virus release requires cell death.
   b) Unidentified host enzymes are required in the uncoating of nucleocapsids.
   c) Without exception a virion becomes internalized (penetration step) through pinocytosis of the cell.
   d) The binding site (attachment site) of a herpesvirus locates on the surface of its nucleocapsid.
   e) The virus replication cycle consists of the following sequential steps: attachment, uncoating, penetration, synthesis (synthetic phase), maturation and release.

2. About binding of a virion to a susceptible cell:
   a) This is achieved through the binding of two molecules having epitopes that are physically complementary to each other.
   b) Virus receptors are glycoproteins on cell membrane without function other than to serve as receptors for viruses.
   c) Viruses do not bind to susceptible cells at 0°C.
   d) Virus receptor molecules for different species of viruses (e.g., HSV and HIV) are the same protein.
   e) The rate of virion-cell binding is not governed by the law of mass action; instead, it depends on the principle of chemotaxis.

3. One of the following statements regarding viral gene expression (the synthetic phase) is incorrect:

a) The transcription of viral DNA and viral RNA genomes depends on host cell DNA dependent RNA polymerase and on virus-coded polymerase, respectively.

b) The pathway for the formation of multiple copies of viral mRNA from RNA viruses varies according to the chemistry of viral genome.

c) For certain DNA viruses, it is common for certain blocks of genes to be expressed and other blocks of genes to be repressed.

d) Viral mRNA are processed and translated in much the same way as host cell mRNA.

e) Posttranslation modification of polypeptides has been described only for the poliovirus

4. One of the following statements about transfection of naked viral genome (disregarding the poxvirus) is incorrect:

a) All viral genomes that depend on cell polymerase for transcription can be transfected (at least in theory).

b) The genome of retroviruses cannot be transfected, yet its provirus has been successfully transfected.

c) The genome of any species of viruses that contain polymerase in the virion cannot be transfected.

d) All viral genomes that depend on virus-coded polymerase for transcription cannot be transfected.

e) Transfection bypasses attachment, penetration, and uncoating steps of the virus replication cycles.

ANSWERS TO REVIEW QUESTIONS

---

1. *b*

2. *a*

3. *e*

4. *d*

This chapter is very important. It is basic to all subsequent chapters in medical virology, especially the chapters on antivirals, virus mutation and interaction, and virus pathogenesis (Chapters 34, 35, and 36). The questions are essentially a reemphasis of the more important areas of the virus replication cycle.

ANTIVIRALS AND VIRAL VACCINES

ANTIVIRALS

Antivirals are substances capable of intercepting the virus replication cycle. There are literally hundreds of antivirals; but only a few have been approved by the FDA for the prophylaxis or treatment of specific virus infections or diseases in humans. Only those antivirals approved by the FDA for clinical use are described here. The antivirals are grouped according to their modes of antiviral actions.

SUBSTANCES INTERFERING WITH VIRUS ATTACHMENT

Human Serum Immune Globulin

Human serum immune globulin (IG) is a sterile concentrated solution containing about 16% of immunoglobulin. It is extracted from large pools of human plasma from a large number of adult blood donors. It contains antibodies against a wide variety of common infectious agents. Antibodies against viral proteins on the external surface of a virion can interfere with attachment of the virion to specific virus receptors on the cell surface. Given during incubation, IG reduce the severity of measles, hepatitis A, and hepatitis B. This type of protection is known as **passive immunization.**

Human Virus-Specific Immune Globulin

This globulin is essentially the same as human IG except that the IG is extracted from plasma known to have high levels of antibodies against a specific virus. Postexposure administration of virus-specific IG has been found effective in modifying or preventing varicella, hepatitis B, and rabies.

INTERFERENCE WITH PENETRATION OR UNCOATING

Amantadine and Rimantadine

Amantadine inhibits the replication of several enveloped RNA viruses; but, it is effective clinically only against influenza A. Amantadine-resistant mutants of influenza A virus have been encountered in an occasional patient suffering from influenza. Resistance is associated with mutation of the gene coding for the matrix protein. Rimantadine is an analog of amantadine and is about equally effective against influenza A virus. Amantadine-resistant mutants are also resistant to rimantadine. The exact mode of action is not known. The attachment and endocytosis of influenzavirus occurs normally in the presence of amantadine but the uncoating of viral genome is inhibited.

INTERFERENCE WITH THE SYNTHETIC PHASE

Interferons

Interferons (IFNs) are **glycoproteins** coded for and synthesized by host cells. The IFNs have antiviral, immune modulating, and anticell proliferation activities. There are three types of IFNs: **IFN-α, IFN-β,** and **IFN-τ.** These types are distinguishable by specific antibodies. The principal source of IFN-α is the leukocyte; of IFN-β is the fibroblast, and of IFN-τ is the T lymphocyte. Recombinant IFNs are now available for all three types.

In the human cell, there are 13α, 1β, and 1τ genes that are **normally repressed.** The most important inducer for α and β genes are virus infections but for the τ gene it is the activators of T lymphocytes. Many nonviral intracellular parasites are weak inducers. Double-stranded RNAs (synthetic or virus derived) are also powerful inducers of the α and β genes. Both IFN-α and IFN-β genes are more active than IFN-τ as antivirals and IFN-τ is more active as the immune modulator and antiproliferative agent.

The more important antiviral attributes of IFN are it is **active in nanogram** concentrations, it is active against **all species of viruses,** and it has **no IFN resistant** mutant. (Isolates of HIV that are naturally resistant to IFN-α have been reported recently.) The antiviral activity is, in general, **host species specific.** Therefore, IFN for treatment of human infections must be IFN produced by cultured human cells. Producing a sufficient amount of IFN from cultured human cells for clinical use is expensive and tedious. With the availability of human IFN produced by the recombinant DNA technique, the high cost of IFN has been reduced.

The principal antiviral action of IFN is interference with the translation of viral mRNA through the following sequence of events. The IFN binds onto IFN receptors on the cell surface. This binding causes the derepression of several genes, which code for **virus inhibitory proteins,** and the virus inhibitory proteins block the translation of viral but not host mRNA. The virus inhibitory proteins consist of at least two enzymes; **elF$_2$ kinase** and **oligoadenylate synthetase.** The initiation factor elF$_2$ is necessary for the binding of mRNA to ribosome; elF$_2$ kinase phosphorylate elF$_2$, and, thereby, inactivates elF$_2$. Oligoadenylate is an activator of RNA endonuclease that degrades single-stranded RNA. What is difficult to explain is why the translation of host mRNA is not or only minimally suppressed in cells exposed to IFN? One hypothesis is that viral inhibitory proteins require double-stranded RNA as cofactor. Double-stranded RNAs are intermediary products in the synthetic phase of RNA viruses (except the retrovirus) but not DNA viruses. If this hypothesis is correct, how does IFN interfere with replication of DNA viruses?

The **toxicity of IFN is minimal.** Large doses (10^6 units/kg) given intravenously may induce symptoms similar to a mild acute virus infection (fever, chill, myalgia, and leukopenia). Toxic symptoms disappear with discontinuation of treatment.

So far, IFN-α has been approved by the FDA for the treatment of venereal warts (a papovavirus infection), of Kaposi sarcoma in patients infected by the HIV, and of chronic hepatitis due to hepatitis B and C viruses. It is not clear why IFN has not been found effective in acute virus diseases. One possible reason is that IFN is released by virus-infected cells within hours of exposure to an infecting virus and that the injection of exogenous IFN would not significantly affect the disease process. Another possible explanation is that damage to host tissue is primarily due to immune response and exogenous IFN would not significantly reduce this immunologic injury.

Nucleoside Analogs

With the exception of small DNA viruses (papova- and parvoviruses), all viruses code for their own polymerases for the synthesis of viral genomes. These **virus-coded polymerases** are ideal targets for antiviral drugs of the **nucleoside analog** category. In general, the nucleoside antiviral drugs are phosphorylated into nucleoside triphosphate by the host cell or virus-coded kinases. The triphosphate will then act as a **competitive inhibitor** of a nucleoside triphosphate normally found in the cell and used by the cell as a precursor for nucleic acid synthesis. For a nucleoside analog to be an effective antiviral, it must have the following three characteristics: it can be phosphorylated into the triphosphate, it has a higher affinity for virus-coded than host cell polymerase and can be **incorporated into the elongating chain of nucleic acid** in place of its competitive analog. Two of the most widely used antiviral drugs in clinical practice are the nucleoside analogs **acyclovir** and **zidovudine** (Fig. 34.1).

Acyclovir is an analog of deoxyguanosine. It is effective in the treatment of infections due to herpes simplex and varicella viruses. Acyclovir is phosphorylated into monophosphate by a **virus-coded kinase** and then into triphosphate by host enzymes. Acyclovir triphosphate has a much higher affinity for virus-coded DNA polymerase than cell DNA polymerase; therefore, it inhibits the function of viral DNA polymerase at concentrations that are minimally inhibitory to cell DNA polymerase. Acyclovir triphosphate is also used as a precursor for DNA synthesis. When incorporated into an elongating chain of DNA in the place of deoxyguanosine triphosphate, the **DNA chain elongation is interrupted.** The mode of action of acyclovir is the inhibition of viral DNA synthesis. Acyclovir at the therapeutic concentration is virtually nontoxic because phosphorylation requires a virus-coded kinase; therefore, there is no acyclovir triphosphate in cells not infected by the herpes simplex or varicella viruses. Acyclovir-resistant mutants of herpes simplex virus have been demonstrated in clinical materials and are important primarily in immunodeficient subjects. The mutation may affect the kinase gene or the DNA polymerase gene.

Zidovudine (azidothymidine) is an analog of thymidine. It is effective in inhibiting the growth of HIV by targeting on the virus reverse transcriptase. Zidovudine is phosphorylated to the triphosphate derivative by host cell kinases. The triphosphate has higher affinity for viral reverse transcriptase than cell DNA polymerase. It is also incorporated into elongating chains of DNA substituting for thymidylic acid. Once incorporated, elongation of the DNA chain is no longer possible. Thus, zidovudine interferes with the synthesis of viral DNA from viral RNA genome. Zidovudine-resistant HIV has also been demonstrated.

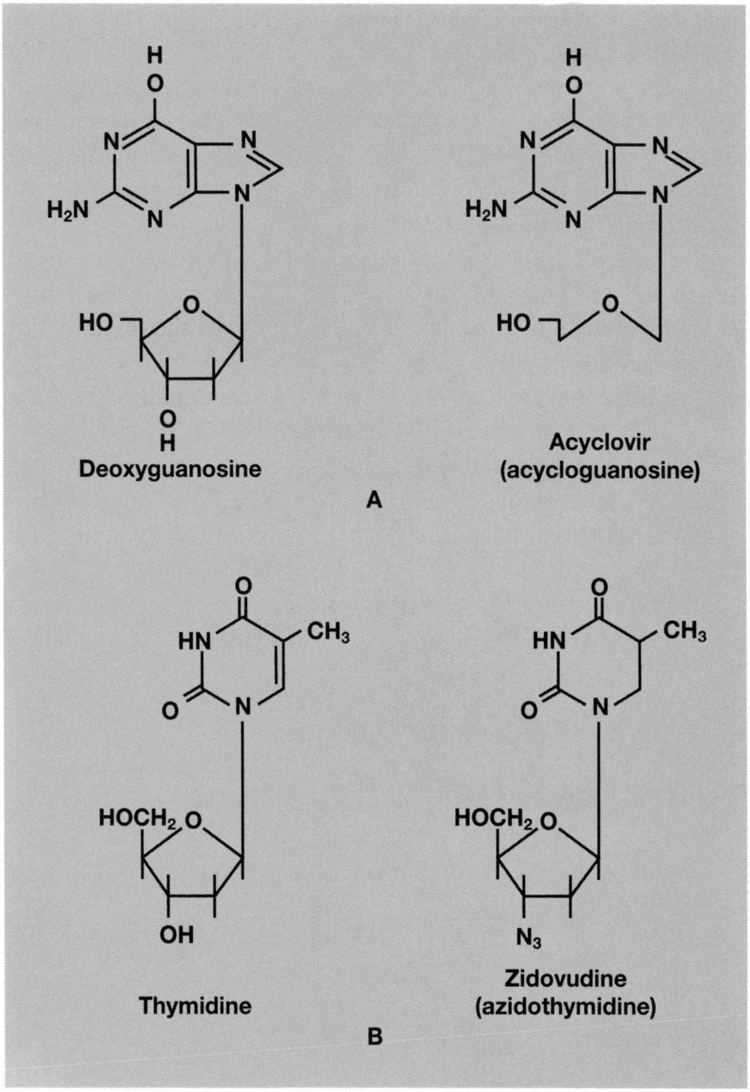

Figure 34.1.

(A) Structure of deoxyguanosine and its anti-herpes analog, acyclovir. (B) Structure of thymidine and its anti-AIDS analog, zidovudine.

Two dideoxynucleosides, **zalcitidine** (dideoxycytidine or ddC) and **didanosine** (dideoxyinosine or ddI), have been approved recently by the FDA for the treatment of AIDS. Like zidovudine, both ddC and ddI act as chain terminators and inhibitors of reverse transcriptase. Both ddC and ddI are analogs of deoxycytidine and deoxyinosine, respectively.

Ribavirin, a guanosine analog, is effective in inhibiting the in vitro growth of many RNA and DNA viruses. It is quite toxic to the host. It is approved for the treatment of respiratory syncytial virus in infants and must be administered as an aerosol. Ribavirin has also been found effective in postexposure chemoprophylaxis and treatment of Lassa fever (a highly fatal disease occurring chiefly in West Africa and caused by a bunyavirus). Despite the lack of approval by the FDA, ribavirin should be used in treating Lassa fever infection.

Other less important nucleoside analogs approved by the FDA for human use include vidarabine, ganciclovir, idoxuridine, and trifluridine. These compounds are quite toxic. **Ganciclovir** is approved by the FDA for the treatment of retinitis caused by the cytomegalovirus in patients with the immunodeficiency syndrome. The others are for the topical application in the treatment of herpetic keratitis.

Foscarnet (trisodium phosphonoformate) inactivates the DNA polymerase of the herpes virus as well as that of the hepatitis B virus and the reverse transcriptase of HIV. It is approved for the treatment of CMV retinitis in patients with AIDS. Its toxic effects can be very severe (renal impairment and electrolyte imbalance). It must be administered by IV drip. The structure of foscarnet shows some similarity with that of pyrophosphate. Some consider foscarnet as an analog of nucleotides.

INTERFERENCE WITH MATURATION OR RELEASE

There are no antivirals, approved for human use, that interfere with viral maturation or release.

VIRAL VACCINES

The administration of vaccine prior to exposure (**preexposure immunoprophylaxis**) is a major mode of reducing the morbidity and mortality of virus infections. The successful development of a vaccine generally requires that the virus in question has one or only a **few stable antigenic types** and that the virus (or its components) can be obtained in **abundance.** Virus vaccines approved by the FDA for use in the United States may contain **live attenuated virus, inactivated virus,** or **viral components.** Viral components may be produced by recombinant DNA technology or obtained from the virion.

LIVE ATTENUATED VACCINE

This type of vaccine contains **mutant virus** that has lost much of its virulence for humans. The vaccine virus induces immunity but not disease in the human host through its **limited multiplication** in the vaccinated person. In general, this is the vaccine of choice because a single administration usually induces a lifelong immunity. Live attenuated vaccine should be used with caution among the immunodefectives and during pregnancy because of the potential of disease induction. Live attenuated vaccines approved for use in the United States are those against the polio, measles, mumps, rubella, varicella, and yellow fever viruses.

INACTIVATED VACCINE

This type of vaccine contains purified and **killed virions** in sufficiently **high concentrations** to induce immunity. In general, several doses given parenterally are necessary to induce full immunity. The immunity so induced is transient and requires a booster dose to maintain immunity. It can be safely given to the immunodefectives and pregnant women. Inactivated vaccines approved for use in the United States are those against the influenza-, rabies-, Japanese B encephalitis-, and polioviruses. **Subunit (subvirion) vaccine** is a variety of inactivated vaccine; it contains primarily the immunity-inducing component of the virion. Subunit vaccines approved for use in the United States are those against the influenza and hepatitis B viruses.

RECOMBINANT VACCINE

One type of recombination vaccine contains viral components produced by DNA recombinant technology; it generally has the same attributes as the subunit vaccine. The only one approved for use is the recombinant hepatitis B vaccine. Another type of recombinant vaccine contains the modified vacciniavirus. The modification consists of the insertion into the vaccinia genome of a gene that codes for the immunity-inducing component of a virus in question. The insert is achieved by DNA recombinant technology. As the vacciniavirus grows in the host, the "foreign" gene product is also formed and immunity against both the vacciniavirus and the virus in question are induced. This type of recombinant vaccines against hepatitis B and immunodeficincy viruses are being evaluated for efficacy and safety.

SUMMARY

1. Relatively few antivirals have been approved by the FDA for the prevention modification and treatment of viral infections. The approved antivirals are immune globulins, interferon-α, nucleoside analogs, amantadine, and rimantadine.

2. Immune globulins contain neutralizing antibodies that prevent the attachment of specific viruses to susceptible cells. In clinical practice, immune globulins are generally given before exposure or during incubation to modify the infection (passive immunoprophylaxis).

3. Interferons are glycoproteins synthesized by the host cell. Normally, the host cell does not synthesize interferons. The host cell synthesizes and releases interferons only when it is stimulated. Important stimulants include some products formed during virus replication and certain chemicals, such as synthetic double-stranded RNA. In vitro studies show that interferons are powerful viral inhibitors and have broad antiviral spectrum.

4. Interferon interferes with viral replication by the following mechanism. It binds onto an interferon receptor on the cell surface. This binding incites an intracellular signal that leads to the derepression of at least two genes. The genes code for virus inhibitory proteins, an elf_2 kinase and an oligoadenylate synthetase. The elF_2 kinase phosphorylates and inactivates elF_2, which is an essential factor for the binding of mRNA to ribosome. Oligoadenylate activates an endonuclease that degrades mRNA. The end result of the derepression of these two genes is interference with the translation of viral mRNA. It is not clear why the translation of cell mRNA is only minimally inhibited.

5. Nucleoside analogs, after phosphorylation into the triphosphate derivative, serve as competitive inhibitors of nucleoside triphosphates during the synthesis of RNA and DNA. The two most important nucleoside analog antivirals are acyclovir and zidovudine. Acyclovir is an analog of guanosine. It is effective in the treatment of infections by the herpes simplex and varicella viruses and is virtually nontoxic to the host. Its phosphorylation requires a virus-coded kinase; hence, it is active only in virus-infected cells. Acyclovir triphosphates have higher affinity for viral than for cell DNA polymerase and also terminate elongation of DNA chains. Zidovudine is an analog of thymidine. It is effective against the HIV. Its phosphorylation depends on the host enzyme. It has a high affinity for the virus-coded reverse transcriptase and

inhibits the reverse transcription of viral genome into viral DNA. Didanosine (dideoxyinosine) and zalcitidine (dideoxycytidine) are effective anti-HIV agents.

6. Amantadine and rimantadine interfere with the penetration and/or uncoating of many enveloped viruses, but is effective only against influenza A infections in humans.

7. Vaccines are effective in preventing virus infections.

8. Generally, effective vaccines are available for those viruses that have one or a few stable antigenic types and that can be obtained in sufficient quantity for vaccine preparation.

9. Live attenuated vaccines generally confer lifelong immunity but may induce diseases among the immunodefectives and the fetuses.

10. Inactivated vaccines generally require multiple doses to induce immunity and booster doses to maintain immunity. They do not induce diseases among the immunodefectives or fetuses. Subunit vaccine is a variety of inactivated vaccine; its chief content is the immunity inducing component of the virion. A recombinant vaccine is essentially the same as a subunit vaccine except that the immunity-inducing virion component is produced by recombinant DNA technology.

REFERENCES

Bart KJ, Hinman AR, Jordan WS (1989): International Symposium on vaccine development and utilization. Rev Inf Dis 11:5491.

Centers for Disease Control (1994): General recommendations on immunization. MMWR 43(RR1):1.

Centers for Disease Control (1993): Use of vaccines and immune globulins in persons with altered immunocompetence. MMWR 42(RR4):1.

Cooney EL, Collier AC, Greenberg PD, Coombs RW, Zarling J, Arditti DE (1991): Safety & immunological response to a recombinant vaccinia virus vaccine expressing HIV envelope glycoprotein. Lancet 337:567.

Douglas RG (1990): Prophylaxis and treatment of influenza. N Engl J Med 322:443.

Edlin BR, St. Clair MH, Pitha PM et al. (1992): In vitro resistance to zidovudine and alpha-interferon in HIV-1 isolates from patients: correlations with treatment duration and response. Ann Int Med 117:451.

Gardner P, Schaffner W (1993): Current concept: immunization of adults. N Engl J Med 328: 1252.

Hirsh MS, D'Aquilal RT (1993): Therapy for human immunodeficiency virus infections. N Engl J Med 328:1686.

McCormick JB, King IJ, Webb PA (1986): Lassa fever: effective therapy with ribavirin. N Engl J Med 314:20.

Merigan TC (1988): Human interferon as a therapeutic agent. A decade passes. N Engl J Med 318:1458.

Peter G (1992): Current concepts: childhood immunization. N Engl J Med 327:1794.

Pfeiffer N (1991): The oral alpha-interferon craze. AIDS Patient Care 5:34.

Russell AD, Hugo WB, Ayliffe GAJ (1992): Principles and practice of disinfection, preservation and sterilization. Oxford, England: Blackwell Scientific Publications.

Whitley RG, Gnann JW (1993): Drug therapy: Acyclovir: A decade later. N Engl J Med 327:782.

Yarchoan R, Mitsuya H, Myers CE, Broder S (1989): Clinical pharmacology of 3-azido-2',3'-deoxythymidine (zidovudine) and related dideoxynucleosides. N Engl J Med 321:726.

REVIEW QUESTIONS

For questions 1 to 9, choose the ONE BEST answer or completion.

1. Which one of the following viral inhibitions intercepts virus replication by preventing attachment?
   a) Interferons
   b) Amantadine
   c) Nucleoside analogs
   d) Antibodies against virus polymerase
   e) Antibodies against virus attachment site

2. Which one of the following antiviral drugs intercepts virus replication by preventing penetration or uncoating?
   a) Amantadine
   b) Zidovudine
   c) Didanosine (ddI)
   d) Acyclovir
   e) Foscarnet

3. All but one of the following antivirals interfere with virus replication by targeting virus polymerases:
   a) Zidovudine
   b) Acyclovir
   c) Ganciclovir
   d) Interferon-α
   e) Didanosine

4. Which one of the following antiviral agents interferes with translation of virus-specific mRNA?
   a) Dideoxycytidine
   b) Ribavirin
   c) Amantadine
   d) Acyclovir
   e) Interferons

5. Acyclovir in therapeutic doses is essentially nontoxic because
   a) it targets exclusively virus-specific polymerase
   b) it causes premature chain termination during DNA synthesis

c) it is rapidly degraded by a host enzyme

d) it is phosphorylated into acyclovir monophosphate almost exclusively by virus-specific kinase

e) uninfected cells contain an inhibitor that prevents the conversion of acyclovir monophosphate into acyclovir triphosphate.

6. One of the following statements about interferons is incorrect:

a) There are, in a human cell, at least 10 genes that code for interferons.

b) Interferons partially or completely inhibit replication of all viruses in cell culture.

c) Human and rabbit interferons are equally effective in inhibiting replication of poliovirus in human cell culture.

d) Interferons are not effective in the treatment of acute virus diseases.

e) Interferons are effective in the treatment of several chronic virus diseases.

7. One of the following statements about the mechanism of antiviral action of interferons is incorrect:

a) Double-stranded RNAs (viral or synthetic) are believed to be the more effective inducers of interferon-α and interferon-β.

b) Interferons are inducers of virus inhibitory proteins.

c) Both elF$_2$ kinase and oligoadenylate synthetase are among the better characterized virus inhibitory proteins.

d) The virus inhibitory proteins interfere with translation of viral mRNA.

e) The absence of binding sites for virus inhibitory proteins on host mRNA explains the failure of virus inhibitory proteins to degrade host mRNA.

8. All but one of the following characteristics are required in the successful development of a vaccine against a newly discovered enveloped virus:

a) It must be possible to obtain a large quantity of virions or viral peplomers.

b) The virus must have no more than several serotypes.

c) The peplomer must remain antigenically stable.

d) The virus must have the capability of inducing disease in animals.

9. One of the following statements about viral vaccines is incorrect:

a) The choice of live-attenuated or inactivated vaccines is available only for the prevention of poliomyelitis.

b) Generally, immunity induced by live vaccines last longer than immunity induced by inactivated vaccines.

c) Postexposure chemoprophylaxis should not be given simultaneously with live attenuated vaccine.

d) Preferred vaccines for immunodefectives and pregnant women are inactivated vaccines.

e) Subvirion vaccines may be live-attenuated or inactivated vaccine.

ANSWERS TO REVIEW QUESTIONS

1. *e*

2. *a*

3. *d*

4. *e*

5. *d*

6. *c*

7. *e*

8. *d*

9. *e*

VIRUS MUTATION AND INTERACTION

Like bacteria, viruses also undergo variations during replication. Variations of viruses may be grouped according to the following three categories: mutation, genetic interaction, and nongenetic interaction. Nongenetic interaction is unique to viruses; it does not occur with prokaryotic or eukaryotic cells.

MUTATION

Mutations refer to changes within the genome of a single virus due to errors in its replication. The changes may be base substitutions, deletions, or rearrangements. Unlike the replication of DNA genomes, there is no proofreading mechanism during the replication of RNA genome. Without this proofreading mechanism to reduce the frequency of errors in replication, the frequency of **mutations of RNA viruses can be very high.** A frequency of 10^{-2} per replication has been described for certain markers of RNA viruses.

A mutation is said to be conditional if the mutation is phenotypically expressed under one set but not under another set of experimental conditions. For example, if a mutation in the viral polymerase gene renders the polymerase defective at elevated temperature ($ 38°C), the mutant would not replicate at elevated body temperature but would replicate at normal body temperature. Such a mutant is a **temperature-sensitive mutant,** a type of **conditional mutation.** In general, temperature-sensitive mutants are less virulent for the human host. The selection of a temperature-sensitive mutant is one way of attenuating viruses for use in the preparation of live attenuated virus vaccine.

Mutations may affect the viral gene that codes for surface proteins important in the attachment of the virion to the cell receptor. Such a mutation would render the preexisting neutralizing antibodies ineffective or less effective in intercepting the viral replication cycle at the stage of attachment. Mutation of the genes that code for the peplomers of the influenzavirus is responsible for its **antigenic drift.**

Drug resistant mutants are readily isolated under experimental conditions and occasionally demonstrated in clinical materials. Unlike drug resistant bacteria, **drug resistant viruses** (amantadine-resistant influenza A virus, acyclovir-resistant herpes simplex virus, or zidovudine-resistant HIV) rarely cause diseases in a new host who is immunocompetent.

Deletion mutants are a common type of mutation that affect a large number of RNA and DNA viruses. A deletion mutant has lost a portion of its genome that codes for certain essential functions such as the polymerase and capsid protein. By itself, the deletion mutant cannot replicate, but if the same cell is also infected by the wild virus, the wild virus would provide the missing component and, thereby, permits the deletion mutant to replicate. Because both the deletion mutant and the wild virus are competing for a finite amount of the essential component, the amount of wild type of virus formed is reduced. For this reason, deletion mutants are also known as **defective interfering particles** (see Fig. 35.1). In cell cultures, defective interfering particles affect the time course and severity of infections and contribute to the establishment of persistent infection. There is no convincing evidence that defective interfering particles play a significant role in virus infections of humans.

There is increasing interest in minor differences in base sequences of virus strains within a species. Some of these minor differences are brought about by silent mutations that affect the sites of action of restriction endonucleases. Digestion of DNA genomes of different virus strains by restriction endonucleases may generate DNA fragments of different length; each strain may have a characteristic pattern of fragments. The digestion of DNA into fragments is known as **fragment length polymorphism** and has been used extensively in epidemiology (see Fig. 35.2).

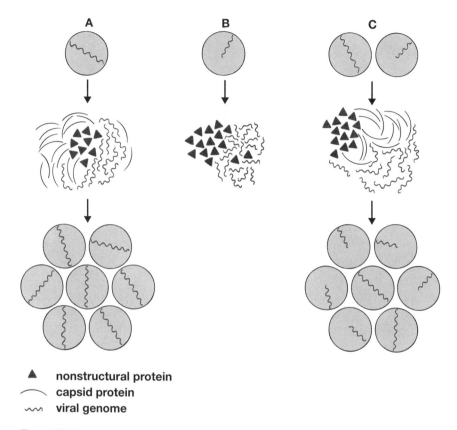

▲   nonstructural protein
⌒   capsid protein
∿   viral genome

Figure 35.1.

Example of interference on virus growth by deletion mutants (defective interfering particles). Parts A and B depict key steps (denoted by solid line arrows) in the growth cycles of a wild strain of virus (A) and its deletion mutant (B). Note 3 key products (nonstructural proteins, capsid proteins, and viral genomes) in the synthetic phase of A and the absence of capsid proteins in B. Part C depicts key events in a cell infected by both the wild strain and its deletion mutant. Due to this competition of capsid proteins, the number of progeny virions of the wild strain is reduced.

GENETIC INTERACTION

Genetic interaction requires the simultaneous replication of two identifiable strains of the same species of virus within the same cell. Genomes of the two strains may recombine to form a new strain that has the characteristics of both parental strains. This phenomenon is known as **genetic recombination.** Like bacteria and eukaryotes, genetic recombination between viruses occurs through the breakage and reunion of a homologous pair of genes or through **gene reassort-**

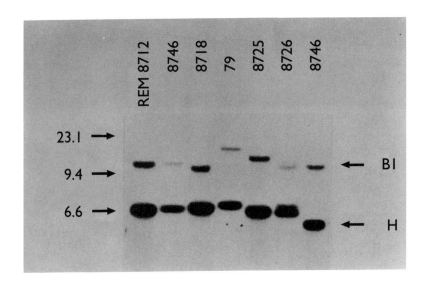

Figure 35.2.

Southern blots of DNAs from seven isolates of Epstein-Barr viruses. Molecular weight markers in thousands are shown at the left. Note different sizes of the B1 and H fragments of the seven isolates. [Reprinted with permission from Lung ML, Chang RS, and Jones JH (1988): Genetic polymorphism of natural Epstein-Barr virus isolates from infectious mononucleosis patients and healthy carriers. J Virol 62:3865.]

ment (see Fig. 35.3 A and B). Only viruses that have **segmented genomes** (e.g., influenzavirus) can undergo genetic recombination through the reassortment of their genes. In general, the frequency of genetic recombinants from breakage and reunion is low while that from reassortment is extremely high. To facilitate description, genetic recombination through gene reassortment is simply referred to as gene reassortment.

Two variations of gene reassortment are **marker rescue** and **multiplicity reactivation** (see Fig. 35.4). In marker rescue, one parental strain A cannot replicate by itself because one of its essential genes X is defective. When the same cell is infected by a homologous but nondefective strain B some of the progeny virus will be reassortants that have the genome of strain A except for the replacement of its defective X gene by the nondefective X gene from strain B. The reassortant is now capable of multiplying by itself and have most of the characteristics of strain A; therefore, many of the genes (markers) of strain A have been ''rescued.'' Multiplicity reactivation is similar to marker rescue except that both parental strains have defective genes at different loci (e.g., strain A is defective at the X locus and strain B, the Y locus). When a cell is infected simultaneously by both defective viruses, some of the progeny virus will be the reassortant that have the X of strain B and Y of strain A. The reassortant is ''reactivated'' and can multiply by itself. Marker rescue and multiplicity reactivation are interesting laboratory phenomena and are probably unimportant in clinical medicine.

The principle of gene reassortment between two identifiable strains of influenza virus has major medical relevance. The construction of reassortant influenza

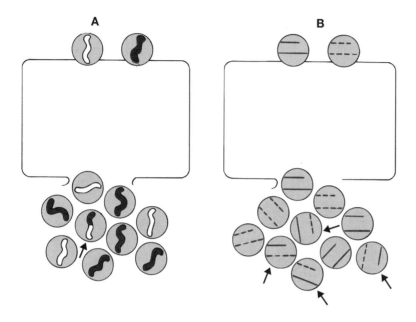

Figure 35.3.
(A) Genetic recombination. (B) Gene reassortment. Arrows identify the recombinant in A and reassortant in B.

virus with specified characteristic for vaccine production is achieved through gene reassortment. Gene reassortment in nature may be responsible for **antigenic shift** of the influenzavirus. Antigenic shift is the sudden emergence of a new antigenic variant that usually precedes an influenza pandemic.

NONGENETIC INTERACTION

When a single cell is infected by two viruses, the viruses may interact in ways other than genetic recombination. In nongenetic interaction, **genomes of the progeny virus** are the same as the parental viruses. Also, the two **interacting viruses need not be viruses of the same species.** Nongenetic interaction is unique to viruses. It requires the intermixing of gene products of the interacting viruses during replication. The more important nongenetic interactions are complementation, interference, and phenotypic mixing.

Complementation

One virus is **defective** and incapable of completing its cycle of replication. The defectiveness is generally due to the deletion of, or a defect in, a gene that codes for an essential protein. This essential protein may be provided by a second

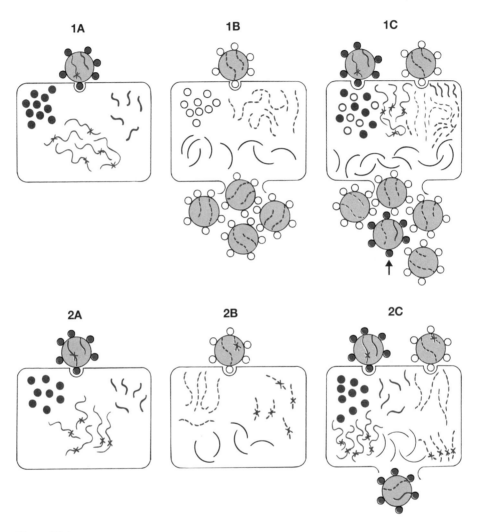

Figure 35.4.

Principle involved in marker rescue and multiplicity reactivation. Replication cycle (1A) of a virus with segmented genome and a defect in its long segment; note absence of capsid protein due to the defect and of progeny virions. Replication (1B) of a homologous virus without defect. A cell infected simultaneously by the defective and nondefective pair of virus (1C); note one of the progeny virion (identified by the arrow) contains the functional short segment of the defective virion. This virion will breed true in subsequent replication. In multiplicity reactivation (2A, B, and C) the same principle is involved except that both viruses are defective and the defects involve different gene segments.

virus during its replication in the same cell. Thus, the defect of one virus is complemented by a second virus. For example, the δ hepatitis virus is defective because it lacks the gene for the surface protein. When the same cell is infected by the hepatitis B virus, the surface protein (coded for by the hepatitis B virus) is formed in abundance and is used by both viruses for virion formation (see Fig. 35.5). In this example, hepatitis B virus complements the defect of the δ hepatitis virus by providing it with the surface protein. Hepatitis B is also known as the **helper virus.** Another important example involves those retroviruses that carry an oncogene. Retroviruses that carry an oncogene are defective because the oncogene has replaced one of its own genes. The defect can usually be complemented by a nondefective retrovirus (Chapter 42). The formation of defective interfering particles also depends on complementation.

Interference

Two species of viruses may compete for the **same binding sites** on the surface of a susceptible cell. One virus may occupy all the binding sites and prevents the other virus from establishing an infection. For example, immunizing

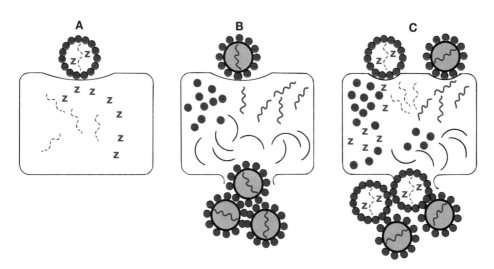

Figure 35.5.

Principle of complementation. Delta hepatitis virus by itself does not form progeny virions due to lack of surface proteins (A). Replication of hepatitis B virus (B). A cell infected by both viruses (C). Note, in C, that the cell releases both the hepatitis B and δ hepatitis viruses, that progeny and parental viruses are genetically the same and that the progeny δ hepatitis virus has acquired the surface protein of hepatitis B virus.

an infant with live attenuated oral polio vaccine while the infant is having an enterovirus infection may be ineffective. A possible explanation is that the enterovirus and poliovirus compete for the same binding site on intestinal epithelium; that the enterovirus has already occupied all the binding sites on the cell surface by the time the poliovirus reaches the intestine; and that the vaccine poliovirus cannot establish an infection.

Interference by deletion mutants, also known as **autointerference,** has already been described (see Deletion mutants, p. 634). Interference of virus replication by interferons (Chapter 34) is not a nongenetic interaction between two viruses, since this phenomenon does not involve the simultaneous infection of a single cell by two viruses.

Phenotypic Mixing

Mixed infection of a single cell by two viruses with distinguishable but related surface proteins, such as peplomers and capsid proteins, may result in production of progeny that have the genome of one virus and part or all of the surface protein supplied by the other virus. **Phenotypic mixing** can drastically alter the host range and/or antigenicity of a virus for a single replication cycle (see Fig. 35.6).

SUMMARY

1. Viruses, like prokaryotic and eukaryotic cells, undergo variations during replication.

2. One type of variation is mutation characterized by a change in the structure of the viral genome during one replication cycle of a single virion. Mutations are commonly due to base substitution or deletion. Because of the lack of a proofreading mechanism, RNA viruses generally have a much higher frequency of mutation than DNA viruses.

3. When a single cell is infected by two strains of viruses of the same species, genetic recombination may occur. Both strains of virus contribute a part of their genomes to the recombinant. In a virus with a nonsegmented genome, genetic recombination occurs by the "breakage and reunion" type of reaction. The frequency of such a reaction is usually very low. In a virus with a segmented genome, recombination also occurs through the reassort-

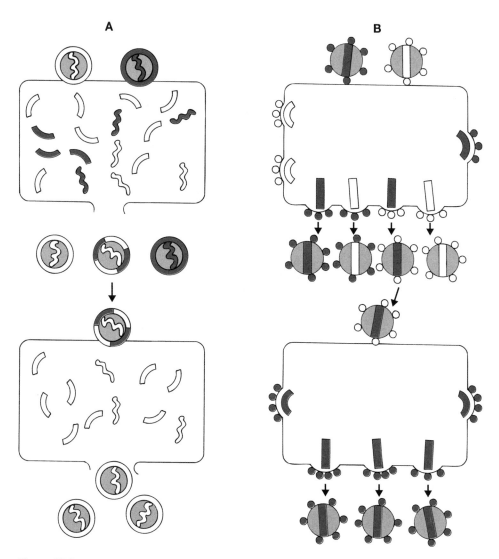

Figure 35.6.

The principle of phenotypic mixing. A cell infected by types 1 and 2 polioviruses (A). Progeny virions will consist of type 1 and type 2 virions plus a few particles whose capsids contain capsid proteins from both types. These rare particles are phenotypically mixed (identified by the short arrow). A cell infected by two different enveloped viruses, red and blue (B). On rare occasions, the blue genome may be wrapped in a red envelope (or red genome in a blue envelope). These are phenotypically mixed; their host range may drastically change for the next replication cycle.

ment of genomic segments. The frequency of recombinants through gene reassortment is extremely high.

4. When a single cell is infected by two strains of viruses that need not be the same species, nongenetic interaction may occur. In nongenetic interaction, the genomes of progeny virions are derived entirely from the parental virions without changes (except for possible mutations). Nongenetic interactions of medical importance include complementation, interference, and phenotypic mixing.

5. In complementation, the defect in one virus is complemented by the other virus.

6. In interference, both viruses compete for a limiting amount of viral or cell protein essential for virus replication. Consequently, the formation of progeny virions from one or both parental viruses is partially or completely inhibited.

7. In phenotypic mixing, the genome of a virus may be wrapped in proteins supplied partly or completely by the other virus. In some situations, cellular tropism of the phenotypically mixed virion may be expanded.

REFERENCES

Carman W, Thomas H, Domingo E (1993): Viral genetic variation: hepatitis B virus as a clinical example. Lancet 341:349.

Gateley A et al. (1990): Herpes simplex virus type 2 meningoencephalitis resistant to acyclovir in a patient with AIDS. J Inf Dis 161:711.

Hayden FG et al. (1989): Emergence and apparent transmission of rimantadine-resistant influenza A virus in families. N Engl J Med 321:1696.

Joklik WK (1992): The Genetics of Animal Viruses. In Joklik WK, Willet HP, Amos DB, Wilfert CM (eds): Zinsser Microbiology, Chap 57. 20th ed. Norwalk, CT: Appleton & Lange, pp 843–853.

Larder BA, Kemp SD (1989): Multiple mutation in HIV-1 reverse transcriptase confer high level resistance to zidovudine (AZT). Science 246:1155.

Lusso P et al. (1990): Expanded HIV-1 cellular tropism by phenotypic mixing with murine endogenous retroviruses. Science 247:848.

Morse SS, Schluederberg A (1990): Emerging viruses: the evolution of viruses and viral diseases. J Inf Dis 162:1.

Tudor-Williams G et al. (1992): HIV-1 sensitivity to zidovudine and clinical outcome in children. Lancet 339:15.

REVIEW QUESTIONS

For questions 1 to 4, choose the ONE
BEST answer or completion.

1. Which of the following viruses is expected
   to have the highest mutation rate during replication?
   a) Herpes simplex virus
   b) Poliovirus
   c) Adenovirus
   d) Papillomavirus

2. A cell is infected simultaneously by two virions of the same species. The two virions
   are distinguishable by genetic markers.
   Which of the following viruses is expected
   to have the highest frequency of genetic recombinants (including reassortants) among
   the progeny virions?
   a) Herpes simplex virus
   b) Adenovirus
   c) Poliovirus
   d) Influenzavirus
   e) Rubellavirus

3. A human CD4 positive lymphocyte is put
   into culture medium that contains zidovudine in therapeutic concentration. The cell is
   then infected by two human immunodeficiency virions. One virion is sensitive to zi-

dovudine and the other is resistant. Among
the progeny virions released, one finds both
zidovudine-sensitive and zidovudine-resistant virions. The most likely theoretical explanation for the presence of zidovudine-sensitive progeny virions is
a) genetic recombination
b) mutation
c) complementation
d) phenotypic mixing
e) multiplicity reactivation

4. A strain of mouse leukemia virus is infectious for human CD4 positive lymphocytes
   and human fibroblasts; and, a strain of HIV
   virus is infectious for the CD4 positive lymphocyte but not the fibroblast. You infect a
   CD4 lymphocyte with both strains of viruses
   and study the characteristics of individual
   progeny virions. You encounter one virion
   that has the genome of the HIV and is infectious for the fibroblast. Progeny virions released by this infected fibroblast are no
   longer infectious for fibroblasts but fully infectious for CD4 lymphocytes. This observation is known as
   a) autointerference
   b) marker rescue
   c) phenotypic mixing
   d) genetic reassortment
   e) conditionally lethal mutation

ANSWERS TO REVIEW QUESTIONS

1. **b** The fidelity of DNA replication is enhanced by a proofreading mechanism. RNA replication does not have this proofreading mechanism. Therefore, one expects more errors in mutations during RNA replication than during DNA replication. Of the four viruses listed, only polio (**b**) is an RNA virus.

2. **d** Genetic reassortment occurs at very much higher frequency than genetic recombination. However, only viruses with segmented genomes (multiple molecules of nucleic acid) can undergo gene reassortment. Of the five listed viruses, only the influenzavirus (**d**) has a segmented genome.

3. **c** Zidovudine targets the reverse transcriptase of HIV. A zidovudine-sensitive HIV virion obviously cannot replicate in a cell exposed to zidovudine. But, when the same cell is also infected by a zidovudine-resistant HIV virion, the reverse transcrip-

tase of the resistant virion will synthesize the genome of the resistant as well as the sensitive variant. The sensitive virion is ''defective'' in a zidovudine-positive environment and this ''defect'' is corrected by the reverse transcriptase from the resistant variant.

4. **c** A few progeny HIV virions released from the lymphocyte infected by both the HIV and mouse leukemia virus (MLV) will have acquired peplomers of the MLV. Through the MLV peplomer, these few HIV virions can attach to fibroblasts and initiate a cycle of replication. Since there is no genetic information for MLV peplomers introduced into the fibroblasts, progeny HIV virions from the infected fibroblasts will have HIV but not MLV peplomers. Hence, they are no longer infectious for the fibroblast. This phenomenon does not involve genetic change; it is phenotypic mixing.

VIRUS PATHOGENESIS

Virus pathogenesis deals with the induction of diseases by virus infections. The basic question is how do viruses injure the human host. Since there are literally hundreds of species of viruses pathogenic for humans and since viruses are a heterogenous group of infectious agents, one expects that there may be a large variety of pathogenic mechanisms for disease induction by viruses. Nevertheless, there are general concepts that adequately describe the host's responses to virus multiplication both at the cell and the organism levels. This chapter describes the general concepts. Specific details are found in subsequent chapters on specific virus families. The complex process of virus pathogenesis can be described under the following headings: effects of virus replication on the human cell, responses of the human host to virus infections, target organs, virus persistence, and virus oncogenesis. It is useful to review immunologic injury in your immunology text at this time.

EFFECTS OF VIRUS REPLICATION ON A HUMAN CELL

Virus replication in a human cell may be **cytocidal** or **noncytocidal.** In a cytocidal infection, the cell dies while the replication cycle is being completed. Hundreds of progeny virions are released into extracellular space and are ready to infect other susceptible cells. In cell culture studies, the replication cycle of some viruses, such as the poliovirus, is completed in about 4 h. The exact mechanism for cell death is not known; it may be due to **inhibition of the synthesis of cell components by virus proteins.** Most pathogenic human viruses are cytocidal to human cells in cell culture studies.

In noncytocidal infection, the cell is not killed but is usually altered. Two best known alterations are the **appearance of virus proteins on the cell surface and changes in growth characteristics.** One should recall that enveloped viruses mature in and exit from the cell through the ''budding'' out process (Chapter 33). At the site of budding, cell membrane proteins are replaced by viral proteins (the peplomer). Such a cell is recognized by the host as foreign and can be killed by the host's specific immune response. Changes in growth characteristics are usually due to the binding of virus proteins to certain specific sites of the host cell chromosome. This binding presumably alters certain control mechanisms resulting in rapid and persistent cell multiplication (at least in vitro). For example, the human B lymphocyte undergoes no more than a few cycles of multiplication in the cell culture system. After infection by the Epstein-Barr virus, however, the B lymphocyte will multiply rapidly (cell generation time of 1 day) and indefinitely (for years). This process is known as **transformation** or **immortalization.**

RESPONSES OF THE HUMAN HOST TO VIRUS INFECTION

Interferon Release at the Site of Infection

This response occurs within a few hours of virus implantation. It is the first and an important response of the host to suppress the infection.

Specific Immune Responses

Specific immune responses to the virus are usually demonstrable at about the time virus multiplication has reached its height. The most important antibody in overcoming the infection is the neutralizing antibody. This antibody binds onto the surface protein of virions in extracellular space and, thereby, inactivates the virion. It may also facilitate the phagocytosis of extracellular virions and the killing of those virus-infected cells that have peplomers on the cell membrane. Antibodies also form immune complexes that incites acute inflammatory response. Excessive or persistent formation of intravascular complexes can be quite damaging to the host. Enhancing antibodies are those that facilitate infections of the host cell (usually macrophage). Specific cytotoxic T lymphocytes play a key role in the killing of virus-infected cells. This killing releases virions into the extracellular space where they are neutralized by antibodies.

Inflammation

One important host response is acute inflammation at sites of virus multiplication and tissue damage. The response is to quench the infection and repair tissue damage. Inflammatory cells are predominantly lymphocytes and macrophages.

Immune Suppression

This response usually occurs during acute generalized infections, such as measles, infectious mononucleosis, and so on. The suppression usually involves the cell-mediated component and is transient. A mechanism for, and the clinical significance of, this transient immune suppression are unclear. This type of immune suppression is different from that due to infection by HIV (see Chapter 43).

TARGET ORGANS

Primary Target Organs

Primary targets are sites where the virus first multiplies. These targets are usually the site of implantation of the virus and/or the lymphoid tissue draining such a site. Viruses land on mucosa or traumatized skin, multiply at the site of deposition, and spread contiguously. Examples are the multiplication of influenzavirus on mucosa of the respiratory tract and papillomavirus on traumatized skin. The primary target organs for influenzaviruses and papillomaviruses are respiratory tract mucosa and skin, respectively.

Secondary Target Organs

Some viruses first multiply at the primary sites and then spread to distant organs by way of the blood, lymph, or peripheral nerve. Distant organs so involved are **secondary targets.** For example, ingested hepatitis A virus multiplies first on intestinal mucosa (primary target) and then spreads to the liver (secondary target) causing hepatitis. With some viruses, multiplication at primary sites may be minimal or difficult to detect. The distinction between primary and secondary target organs may be difficult.

Organ Tropism

Many viruses have an affinity for specific cell types. This affinity is determined by specific virus receptors on the cell surface. For example, the receptor for HIV is the CD4 molecule of T lymphocytes; the virus is, therefore, T lymphotropic. Receptors for parvovirus B19 are erythrocyte P antigens; people who lack this antigen are resistant to infection by parvovirus B19.

Pathology

The pathology and clinical manifestations of infection by a specific species of virus depend on the target organ involved. Severity of the infection depends on the extent of damage to the target organ. The extent of damage is determined by the virulence of the virus, its dosage, and host factors. These determinants are difficult to quantify in clinical setting. In general, virus infections are more severe among infants and adults than among children. If virus components are spilled into the blood during infection, intravascular immune complexes may be formed. These complexes will be deposited in small blood vessels and incite acute inflammation at the site of deposition.

VIRUS PERSISTENCE

Infections by most viruses are acute. The virus multiplies in the target organ; the host mounts an immune response; the immune response eliminates completely the virus from the host's tissue. The host becomes partially or completely immune to subsequent infection by the same species of virus. There are two important exceptions to this generalization. First, the virus or its genome may persist in a host cell in a nonreplicative state. No virus protein is found on the cell surface; hence, the host immune system cannot recognize the cell as one that harbors a virus. This phenomenon is known as **latency.** During latency, there is no virus replication, no tissue damage, and no associated clinical manifestations. Latency can be reactivated into active infection during which there is virus multiplication, tissue destruction, and associated clinical manifestations. Factors that determine latency and reactivation have not been clearly defined. Viruses of the herpesvirus family have a propensity toward latency. Second, the host may not form neutralizing antibody and/or expand the T cytotoxic cell population capable of recognizing the virion surface. Such a deficiency permits the persistent replication of the virus and is known as **persistent or chronic infection.** In a persistent infection, there is continuous virus replication and tissue damage. The best known example is chronic active hepatitis following acute hepatitis B infection.

VIRUS ONCOGENESIS

Virus oncogenesis is a type of virus persistence that leads to cell proliferation rather than cell death. Virus-induced cell proliferation may be due to any of the following mechanisms:

Binding of virus early gene products to chromosome or regulatory proteins of the host cell. The genome of DNA viruses is transcribed in blocks sequentially by a host cell transcriptional mechanism. **Early gene products** are generally regulatory proteins while late gene products are structural proteins. For certain DNA viruses within certain cells, only the early genes are transcribed. Some of the early gene products have been shown to **bind onto certain regulatory proteins or onto specific chromosomal sites** of the host cell. These bindings are believed to interfere with regulatory mechanisms of the host cell leading to cell proliferation.

Insertion of an oncogene. During the replication of a retrovirus, a portion of viral genome may be replaced by a host gene. If the host gene codes for a protein with a regulatory function, the host gene ''captured'' in the virus genome is known as an **oncogene.** A retrovirus positive for an oncogene may infect a cell and its genome is reverse transcribed into proviral DNA. Some of the proviral DNA are inserted into the host cell DNA. The site of proviral DNA may not be optimal for the regulation of oncogene expression. This results in excessive amount of oncogene product within the cell. Since products of many oncogenes are cell growth factors, it is conceivable that excessive concentration of oncogene products lead to abnormal cell proliferation.

Release of ''growth factor.'' A virus-infected cell may release virus-coded proteins that stimulate neighboring cells to proliferate. Kaposi sarcoma in patients with AIDS is believed to be due to the stimulation of endothelial cells by the transactivating protein of HIV.

Insertion mutation. Virtually all oncogenic viruses can insert their genomes into host cell genomes. The insertion produces gene mutation at the insertion site. The affected gene may be inactivated. The expression of the host genes downstream from the insertion site may be altered. One important outcome of **insertion mutation** is disturbance in the cell regulatory mechanism. This disturbance may in turn lead to abnormal cell proliferation.

It is difficult to obtain conclusive proof of virus oncogenesis in humans. Epidemiologic studies, however, have revealed strong association between the following pairs of virus and cancer: hepatitis B virus and hepatoma, human T lymphotropic virus and adult T cell leukemia, Epstein-Barr virus and African Burkitt's lymphoma, Epstein-Barr virus and nasopharyngeal carcinoma, and human papillomavirus and cervical carcinoma. Characteristics common to these four viruses are viral DNA or proviral DNA commonly integrate (insert) into host DNA; and, virus gene expression depends on the host cell's transcriptional machinery.

SUMMARY

1. Virus replication leads to death of the infected cell (cytocidal infection). Cell death may occur as early as 4 h after infection. Hundreds of progeny virions are released from each infected cell. The exact mechanism of cell death is not known; presumably it is due to interference of some essential cell functions by virus proteins.

2. A few species of viruses, such as the Epstein-Barr and hepatitis B viruses, cause noncytocidal infection. Infected cells are usually modified. Important modifications include the appearance of virus proteins on cell membrane and stimulation of cell growth.

3. The human host responds to virus invasion by first releasing interferon at the site of virus multiplication, then mounting specific immune responses, and finally reacting with acute inflammation at the site of tissue injury.

4. A primary target organ is the organ through which the virus enters the body and at which the virus multiplies initially. Virus in the primary target may spread to distant organs through the blood, lymph, or peripheral nerve. Distant organs so infected are secondary target organs.

5. A virus may have affinity for a specific cell type. This affinity is determined by specific virus receptors on the cell surface. The virus receptor for the Epstein-Barr virus is the CR2 molecule on B lymphocytes. Therefore, the Epstein-Barr virus is B lymphotropic.

6. Pathology of a specific virus infection depends on the target organs. Severity of pathological changes is determined by the size of virus inoculum, virulence of the virus, the virus species, and host factors.

7. Viruses within the host are completely inactivated after the host has mounted its immune responses against the virus. The infection is quenched and the host is immune to reinfection by the same species of virus. But, a few species of viruses have the propensity to persist in the host.

8. Latency is one type of persistence in which the virus or its genome remains in a cell in the nonreplicative state. The affected cell is not modified by the virus and is not recognized by the host's immune system as foreign. Latency may be reactivated.

9. Chronic or persistent infection is a second type of virus persistence in which the host is incapable of mounting an adequate immune response (especially forming neutralizing antibody) against the virus and the virus continues to replicate.

10. There is no conclusive evidence that viruses induce cancers in humans. But there are epidemiologic data that show strong association between hepatitis B virus and hepatoma, human T lymphotropic virus and adult T-cell leukemia, Epstein-Barr virus and nasopharyngeal carcinoma, Epstein-Barr virus and African Burkitt's lymphoma, and human papillomavirus and cervical carcinoma.

11. A virus may stimulate cell growth by any of the following mechanisms: (1) the binding of early gene products onto regulatory proteins or chromosome of the host cell, (2) introducing oncogenes into the host cell, (3) producing insertion mutation, and (4) the release by a virus-infected cell of virus-coded proteins that stimulate the growth of neighboring uninfected cells. All viruses capable of stimulating cell growth are DNA viruses or those RNA viruses whose genomes are reversed transcribed into proviral DNA.

REFERENCES

Berns KI, Whitley RW (1991): Latency by herpes simplex viruses. Intervirology 32:69.
Brown KE et al. (1994): Resistance to parvovirus B19 infection due to lack of virus receptor. N Engl J Med 330:1192.
Editorials (1992): Transposons: friends or foes? Lancet 339:215.
Klinken SP (1989): Oncogenes: past present and future. Clin Exp Pharmacol Physiol 16:505.
Marx JL (1989): How DNA viruses may cause cancer. Science 243:1012.
Mims CA (1987): The pathogenesis of infectious diseases. 3rd ed. London: Academic Press.
Spector S, Bendinelli M, Friedman H (1992): Neuropathogenic viruses and immunity. New York: Plenum Press.
Stevens JG (1989): Human herpesviruses: a consideration of the latent state. Microbiol Rev 53:318.

REVIEW QUESTIONS

For questions 1 to 7, choose the ONE
BEST answer or completion.

1. All but one of the following statements about
   cell responses to virus multiplication are correct:
   a) Some viruses kill the cell within several
      hours after infection and produce hun-
      dreds of progeny virions.
   b) Some viruses modify the host cell by in-
      serting virus surface proteins on the cell
      membrane.
   c) A few species of viruses immortalize the
      host cell in vitro.
   d) A few species induce the host cell to re-
      lease exotoxins capable of damaging a
      distant organ.

2. Host responses important in the quenching
   of a virus infection include all but one of the
   following:
   a) release of interferons at the site of virus
      implantation
   b) the formation of neutralizing antibodies
   c) the generation of virus-specific cytotoxic
      T lymphocytes
   d) the formation of antibodies against virus
      polymerase

3. All but one of the following statements about

the host immune response to a virus infection
are correct:
   a) Virus-specific antibodies may damage the
      host through the formation of intravas-
      cular immune complexes.
   b) Certain types of antibodies (e.g., enhanc-
      ing antibody) may facilitate virus dissem-
      ination.
   c) Virus-specific cytotoxic T lymphocytes
      damage the target organ as they attempt
      to kill the virus-infected cells.
   d) Transient immunosuppression during
      systemic infections by viruses other than
      HIV results in frequent opportunistic in-
      fections.

4. Pathology (clinical manifestations) of a virus
   infection depends on all but one of the following factors:
   a) tissue tropism of the virus
   b) certain host factors
   c) virulence of the virus
   d) dosage of the virus
   e) size of the viral genome

5. Some viruses may persist in host tissue for
   many months or years after the acute infection. This persistence of virus may be due to
   all but one of the following:
   a) virus latency (the presence of virus in a
      nonreplicative state within a host cell)

b) unexplained failure of the host to mount effective immune responses against virus surface proteins
c) acquired or congenital immunodeficiency
d) infection by unconventional viruses (prions)
e) mutation to interferon resistance

6. Possible mechanism(s) for the stimulation of cell growth by viruses include all but one of the following:
   a) the binding of virus proteins to the host's regulatory proteins or DNA
   b) insertion mutation
   c) inserting an exogenous oncogene
   d) release of unusual or of excessive amount

of cell growth factors into extracellular spaces
e) replacement of cell DNA polymerase by viral DNA polymerase

7. Association between viruses and human cancers has been indisputably established for all but one of the following:
   a) hepatitis B virus and hepatoma
   b) Epstein-Barr virus and African Burkitt's lymphoma and nasopharyngeal carcinoma and salivary gland carcinoma
   c) human T lymphotropic virus type 1 and adult T-cell leukemia
   d) papillomavirus type 16 and carcinoma of the uterine cervix and vulva
   e) cytomegalovirus and Kaposi sarcoma

ANSWERS TO REVIEW QUESTIONS

1. *d* Viruses may induce cells to release biological modifiers that act on cells at the site of infection. However, there is no evidence that a virus-infected cell releases toxins that damage tissue at distant sites.

2. *d* To interfere with virus replication, the antibody against viral polymerase must react against the polymerase within the virion or in the infected cell. Since the antibody cannot penetrate viral envelope virus capsid or cell membrane, it cannot interfere with virus replication.

3. *d* Immune response is a two-edged sword. It is essential for the quenching of virus infection, but at the same time, it damages the host. The significance of transient immune suppression is not known. There is no evidence that opportunistic infections occur more frequently.

4. *e* The size of the viral genome has nothing to do with pathology.

5. *e* Interferon-resistant mutant of clinical significance has not been demonstrated to

date. [Infection by the unconventional virus *invariably* results in a chronic persistent infection. The unconventional virus is a unique group of virus-like agents (see Chapter 48). It does not form virions and the host does not mount the customary immune response.]

6. *e*

7. *e*

DIAGNOSIS OF VIRUS DISEASES

Virus diseases are exceedingly common in humans. In the United States, disability (person-day lost from work) due to virus infections of the respiratory tract is more than that due to heart diseases, cancers, and strokes combined. Because the vast majority of virus diseases are acute and self-limiting and because effective antiviral therapies are available for only a few species of viruses, it is generally sufficient in clinical setting to determine if an acute infectious condition is due to a virus infection. Proving infection by a specific virus is generally expensive, time consuming, and difficult to achieve in most clinical settings. Therefore, laboratory tests to prove infections by specific viruses are reserved for those situations where the results will contribute significantly to management of the infections. Situations where specific virologic diagnosis is important are described in chapters on individual virus families.

GENERAL CHARACTERISTICS OF VIRUS DISEASES

Presenting symptoms of virus infections can be quite variable; these symptoms depend on the target organ involved. There are, however, some features that are characteristic of virus diseases in general. With a few exceptions, virus diseases tend to be acute in onset and brief in duration (<2 weeks). Inflammatory exudate, if any, is nonpurulent. White blood count generally shows no abnormality, absolute or relative lymphocytosis and not neutrophilia. Knowing the probability that a clinical syndrome in question is due to a virus infection is also useful. For example: (1) virus infections are responsible for virtually all cases of aseptic meningitis, acute encephalitis, acute hepatitis, mononucleosis, and acute nonpurulent conjunctivitis; (2) over 80% of acute respiratory infections and about one-half of all acute watery diarrhea have viral etiologies; and (3) many of the acute exanthemata are virus induced. Sometimes the diagnosis of a virus disease is established by exclusion. Especially important is the exclusion of those diseases for which specific laboratory diagnostic procedures are readily available and against which specific treatments are indicated. For example, the exclusion of bacterial infection is of utmost importance in the differential diagnosis of acute meningitis. Histories of past infections and/or immunization are also important especially in the exclusion of a specific virus disease. For example, a past history of infectious mononucleosis is strong evidence against the diagnosis of infectious mononucleosis for the present illness. A record of adequate polio vaccination would virtually eliminate poliomyelitis in the differential diagnosis of a paralytic disease.

LABORATORY DIAGNOSIS OF SPECIFIC VIRUS DISEASES

There are a wide variety of laboratory tests for the diagnosis of diseases caused by a specific virus. These tests may be grouped into four categories: morphology, serology, virus isolation, and nucleic acid technology. Choice of the optimal test for a specific clinical situation can be quite complex. It is generally useful to consult with a clinical virologist regarding the collection of appropriate clinical material for testing and the selection of tests to be used.

Morphology

In a morphologic test, one directly examines the clinical specimen for evidence of virus. A morphologic test can usually be completed within a few hours but requires a high concentration of virions or virus components in the clinical specimen. Morphologic tests, useful in clinical practice, include: electron microscopic examination of vesicular fluid for poxviruses and herpesviruses, electron microscopic examination of feces for rotaviruses, immunofluorescent test of respiratory secretion for the respiratory syncytial virus, and examination of brain material for the rabiesvirus by immunofluorescence. In general, a positive morphologic test establishes the diagnosis while a negative test does not exclude the diagnosis.

Serology

In a serologic test, one examines the serum directly for viral antigen or antibody with procedures that are based on the principle of antigen-antibody reaction. Commonly used serologic tests include the testing of acute and convalescent phase sera for a significant rise in antibody titers against a specific virus antigen, the testing of acute phase serum for specific IgM, and the testing of serum for viral antigen, such as in the diagnosis of hepatitis B. Students are advised to review immunology lectures on serologic diagnosis of infectious diseases.

Virus Isolation

In this procedure, one inoculates appropriate clinical material into cell cultures or laboratory animals and then observes for evidence of virus replication. This technique is most sensitive procedure in detecting viruses in clinical materials providing that cell cultures or laboratory animals susceptible to infection by the virus under study are available. In general, virus isolation is a slow and expensive process and is not commonly used in clinical practice except in the diagnosis of herpes simplex.

Nucleic Acid Technology

Virus genomes in tissues or secretions can be detected by the **hybridization** technique. This technique is not a sensitive procedure; it generally requires 10^5 genome equivalents to give a positive test. The sensitivity of this test can be vastly enhanced by amplifying the virus genome prior to hybridization. This amplification is achieved by the **polymerase chain reaction (PCR).** In theory, PCR can amplify a single copy of virus genome into millions. The place of PCR in the diagnosis of virus diseases in clinical practice is being intensely investigated. One major area of concern is a false positive reaction.

FRAGMENT LENGTH POLYMORPHISM AND EPIDEMIOLOGY

Restriction endonucleases hydrolyze viral DNA into fragments known as **restriction fragments.** Each restriction nuclease cuts DNA molecules at specific nucleotide sequences. Therefore, the number of restriction fragments and the length of each fragment for two strains of viruses should be the same if the viral DNA are hydrolyzed with the same restriction nuclease and if both viral strains are genomically identical. Interestingly, many species of viruses show marked genomic diversity as determined by restriction fragment length analysis. For viruses, such as the Epstein-Barr (EB) and HIV, epidemiologically unrelated strains are genomically different (Figs. 37.1 and 37.2 for illustration). This information is useful in epidemiologic study, such as in tracing the source of a virus isolate. For example, if the HIV isolated from the blood of a laboratory technician and that used in the laboratory are genomically distinct, it is very unlikely that the technician acquired the infection from the laboratory.

DISEASE CAUSATION IN MICROBIOLOGY

To establish an etiologic relationship between an infectious agent and a disease, one generally depends on **Koch's postulates.** The postulates state: ''The microorganisms must be regularly isolated from cases of illness, it must be grown

Figure 37.1.

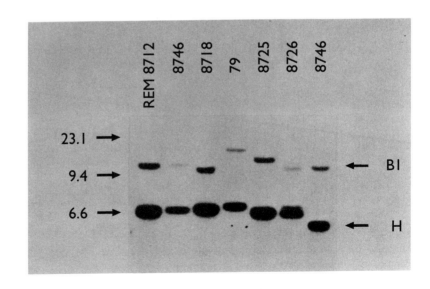

Fragment length polymorphism of seven isolates of EB virus from students at the University of California at Davis. Note that molecular weights (lengths) of their B1 and H fragments are different. (Molecular weight markers in 10^3 are shown at the left margin.) [Reproduced with permission from Lung ML, Chang RS, and Jones JH (1988): Genetic polymorphism of natural Epstein-Barr virus isolates from infectious mononucleosis patients and healthy carriers. J Virol 62:3862.]

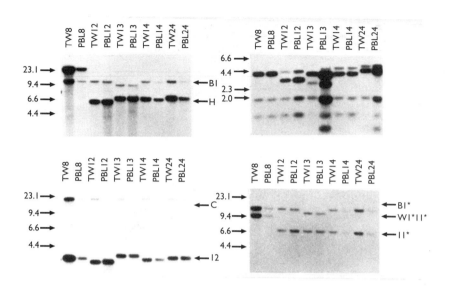

Figure 37.2.
Fragment length polymorphism of EB virus isolated from the throat wash (TW) and peripheral blood lymphocyte (PBL) of five infectious mononucleosis patients at the University of California at Davis. Probes for viral DNA fragments are indicated on the right and molecular weights in 10^3 on the left. Note that viruses from each patient are different but viruses from the same patient are the same. [Reproduced with permission from Lung ML, Chang RS, and Jones JH (1988): Genetic polymorphism of natural Epstein–Barr virus isolates from infectious mononucleosis patients and healthy carriers. J Virol 62:3862.]

in pure culture in vitro, inoculation of the pure culture into susceptible animals must result in typical disease, and the microorganism must be re-isolated from experimentally induced disease.'' These postulates can be very difficult to fulfill when the infectious agent is a virus because: (1) humans may be the only susceptible hosts for the virus under study (e.g., AIDS), and/or (2) the virus under study may not replicate outside the human host (e.g., hepatitis B virus).

To overcome the aforementioned difficulties, **modifications of Koch's postulates** have been proposed. One modified version states: ''If a virus is etiologically associated with a disease, the virus must be found regularly in the target organ of the diseased but not of the healthy subjects; this association must be present at different times and places.'' Difficulties with this version are (1) how regularly will the virus be found in the target organ of the diseases depends on sensitivity of the available technique, and (2) the virus may also be found in the target organ of the healthy because the virus may cause subclinical infections, may have a very long incubation, or may persist.

Another modified version is that specific antibody must be absence prior to the disease and must appear during illness. An extension of this version is that the disease should be preventable with a specific vaccine.

In some situations, it is virtually impossible to fulfill Koch's postulates, original or modified. In such situations, one simply states that there is an association between a virus and a disease (without specifying the nature of the association). For example, the human papillomavirus is found in most of the cervical carcinoma and some of the normal cervical tissues. One simply states that the human papillomavirus is associated with cervical carcinoma in humans.

SUMMARY

1. With some important exceptions, the diagnosis of virus diseases are generally based on clinical impression. Proving infections by a specific virus using laboratory procedures is generally unnecessary. The exceptions include any situations where the diagnosis of infection by a specific virus is important in management of the infection.

2. Virus diseases tend to be acute in onset and brief in induration (<2 weeks), produce nonpurulent exudate, and induce absolute or relative lymphocytosis not neutrophilia.

3. Virus infections cause virtually all cases of acute hepatitis, mononucleosis, acute nonpurulent conjunctivitis, aseptic meningitis, and acute encephalitis; most cases of acute infections of the respiratory tract; and, many cases of acute watery diarrhea and of acute exanthemata.

4. Diagnosis of infection by a specific virus generally depends on the demonstration of virions or viral components in the target organ or secretion-excretion of the target organ.

5. Diagnosis of a specific virus infection can also be established by demonstrating antibody rise during the convalescent phase of illness or specific IgM during the acute phase of illness.

6. Polymerase chain reaction (PCR) is a procedure that amplifies specific DNA sequences. Theoretically, it can detect a single copy of the DNA viral genome. Because of this exquisite sensitivity, its specificity needs thorough evaluation.

7. Viral DNA can be hydrolyzed by restriction nucleases at specific nucleotide sites into restriction fragments. The length of restriction fragments of epidemiologically unrelated isolates of certain species of viruses have been found to be different. This difference is known as fragment length polymorphism, which is a useful tool in epidemiologic study.

8. In proving etiologic relation between a virus and a disease, Koch's postulates are difficult to fulfill. Modified versions of Koch's postulates are used. One modified version states that the virus must be present regularly in the target organ of the diseased but not of the healthy subject at different times and places. Another version states that specific antibody must be absent prior to the disease and must appear during illness.

9. When a virus is found more frequently in the target organ of diseased than that of healthy subjects, the virus is said to be associated with the disease. The nature of this association need not be etiological.

REFERENCES

Lennette EH, Halonen P, Murphy FA (eds.) (1988): Laboratory Diagnosis of Infectious Diseases. New York: Springer-Verlag.

Tomkins LS (1992): Current concepts: the use of molecular methods in infectious diseases. N Engl J Med 327:1290.

REVIEW QUESTIONS

For questions 1 to 6, choose the ONE BEST answer or completion.

1. Proving infection by a specific virus in clinical practice is NOT generally done for all but one of the following reasons:
   a) The required procedure is generally expensive and slow.
   b) The required procedure is frequently not available in an average clinical laboratory.
   c) The result usually contribute little to management of the infection.
   d) Even if one establishes the etiologic diagnosis, there is little that a physician can do to arrest the disease regardless of the species of virus that causes the disease.

2. All but one of the following findings are consistent with an acute virus disease:
   a) Purulent exudate from the target organ.
   b) Lymphocytosis, absolute or relative.
   c) A generalized maculopapular eruption lasting no more than 7 days.
   d) A brief course lasting less than 2 weeks
   e) Palpable posterior occipital lymphnodes bilaterally without evidence of infection of the scalp.

3. Diagnosis of an acute infection by a specific virus can be achieved by any one of the following procedures, *except*
   a) demonstration of viral antigens by immunofluorescence
   b) demonstration of infectious virus by virus cultivation
   c) demonstration of viral genome by nucleic acid hybridization
   d) demonstrating specific antibody rise during the course of illness
   e) demonstration of specific IgG

4. About polymerase chain reaction in detecting viral genome in tissues, all but one of the following statements are correct:
   a) Its principle is based on amplification of specific gene sequences.
   b) Oligonucleotide primer needed in the reaction is specific for each species of virus.
   c) It is an exquisitely sensitive procedure; false positive reaction (due to carrying over) is a major concern.
   d) A biopsy that is positive for the genome of herpes simplex virus by the polymerase chain reaction is also positive for live infectious herpes simplex virus.

5. About fragment length polymorphism, all but one of the following statements are correct:
   a) The restriction fragment pattern of a virus depends on the restriction endonuclease used in hydrolyzing the viral genome.
   b) The restriction fragment pattern of certain species of virus (e.g., Epstein-Barr) can be so diverse that virtually no two epidemiologically unrelated strains have identical patterns.
   c) A difference in fragment pattern indicates a difference in genomic structure.
   d) If the restriction fragment patterns of two isolates of HIV are identical, it is reasonable to assume that the two isolates come from the same source.
   e) Fragment length polymorphism is a useful marker for virulence.

6. Identify the correct statement on postulation of causation.
   a) All patients with nasopharyngeal carcinoma are positive for Epstein-Barr virus antibody; therefore, the EB virus is the etiological agent of nasopharyngeal carcinoma.
   b) Persons infected with the hepatitis B virus are at least 100 times more likely to develop hepatoma. Therefore, hepatitis B virus is the etiological agent of hepatoma.
   c) Kaposi's sarcoma is common among young persons ($<$45 years) infected by HIV virus but exceedingly rare among those not infected by HIV. Therefore, HIV is the etiologic agent of Kaposi's sarcoma.
   d) All pre-illness and postillness sera from infectious mononucleosis patients are, respectively, negative and positive for Epstein-Barr virus antibody; therefore, the EB virus is the etiologic agent of infectious mononucleosis.

ANSWERS TO REVIEW QUESTIONS

1. *d* While most of the virus infections are non-responsive to antiviral therapy, there are a few important exceptions. For examples, acyclovir is effective in treating diseases caused by the herpes simplex and varicella viruses; zidovudine in AIDS; ribavirin, in acute bronchiolitis caused by the respiratory syncytial virus, and so on.

2. *a* Purulent exudate is characteristic of infections by pyogenic bacteria not viruses.

3. *e* Specific IgG indicates infection by the virus, now or in the past.

4. *d* Polymerase chain reaction amplifies viral gene sequences regardless of the infectiousness of the virus.

5. *e*

6. *d* Only *d* has fulfilled a modification of Koch's postulates. *a, b,* and *c* are incorrect because the data have established an association that may or may not be an etiologic one. It is exceedingly difficult to prove etiologic association between a virus and a disease that has long incubation period (in years), such as cancer.

THE HERPESVIRUS FAMILY: HERPES SIMPLEX AND VARICELLA-ZOSTER VIRUSES

The herpesvirus family is one of the most important family of viruses in medical practice. These viruses are ubiquitous, infect virtually every person, induce a wide variety of diseases, respond to antiviral therapy, and enter into latency after recovery from primary infections. There are six species of human pathogens in this family of viruses: herpes simplex 1, herpes simplex 2, varicella-zoster, Epstein-Barr, cytomegalo, and human herpes 6.

FAMILY CHARACTERISTICS

Genomic Chemistry

The genome of the herpesvirus consists of a single molecule of linear double-stranded DNA ($\sim$ 120–220 kbp in size). The ends are flanked by terminal repeats that enable the molecule to circularize. There is little DNA homology among these six human herpesviruses except for the 50% homology between herpes simplex 1 and 2.

Morphology

The virion has four structural components. The core consists of internal proteins on which the viral DNA is wrapped. The capsid is icosahedral and 100 nm in diameter. The envelope has surface projection (peplomers). In between the capsid and envelope are the matrix protein (see Figs. 32.1A, 32.2, and 32.4).

Replication

It follows the general scheme of an enveloped DNA virus. Briefly, glycoproteins (peplomers) on the envelope attach to specific virus receptors on the surface of susceptible cells. The nucleocapsid enters through fusion of the virus envelope and the cell membrane. After uncoating by an unidentified host enzyme, the viral DNA is transcribed by host DNA dependent RNA polymerase. The viral genome is transcribed in three blocks sequentially, immediate early, delayed early, and late genes. Immediate early genes coded mostly for regulatory proteins; delayed early genes, enzymes, such as DNA polymerase and thymidine kinase; and late genes, structural proteins. Once the structural proteins are formed in sufficient quantity, the synthesis of host proteins is shut off and the cell eventually died. Structural proteins condense on viral DNA and form nucleocapsids. The nucleocapsid is then budded out thereby acquiring an envelope, which is a portion of the cell membrane whose proteins are almost entirely replaced by viral glycoproteins. One important variation of this scheme for the herpesviruses is that certain host cells are capable of preventing the transcription of delayed early and late genes. In such a cell, the viral genome persists, the virus does not replicate, and the cell does not die. This is an example of **viral latency.** Note also that the herpesvirus is one of the few DNA virus families that code for their own DNA polymerases. These **viral DNA polymerases are targets for antiviral drugs.**

Biologic Characteristics

These include propensity to latent infections, formation of intranuclear inclusion in permissive cells, and ubiquity.

Antigenic Relation

There is no, or only minimal (no clinical significance), antigenic similarity among the six species except for herpes simplex 1 and 2 viruses (see next paragraph).

HERPES SIMPLEX VIRUSES

Herpes simplex viruses types 1 and 2 (HSV 1 and HSV 2) show about 50% DNA homology and have common and type-specific antigens. Infection by one type provides partial immunity to the other type. Infections in or around the oral cavity are more likely to be due to type 1 than type 2. The reverse is true for infections in the genital area. Herpes simplex virus types 1 and 2 can be easily distinguished in the laboratory by serology using type-specific monoclonal antibodies.

Pathogenesis

Infections occur through contacts with herpetic lesions directly or indirectly. The virus multiplies at the site of implantation and spreads contiguously, by way of sensory nerve, by way of lymphatics, and rarely by way of blood circulation. The primary target is epithelial cells at the site of the virus implantation. Important secondary targets are neurons of the dorsal root sensory ganglion, brain, and meninges. Recovery from the first infection results in **latency,** near complete immunity from reinfection by homologous type, and partial immunity against the heterologous type. **Reactivation** of latent infection is common.

A typical skin lesion consists of a small (1–2 mm) **erythematous vesiculopapules.** Clustering and coalescing of lesions are common. The vesicular fluid is rich in virions. Vesicles dry in several days, form scabs, and drop off without a scar. Lesions are usually not painful unless irritated. On moist areas, herpetic lesions usually ulcerate forming shallow ulcers. Common sites for herpetic lesions are the skin around the oral and genital orifices, the oral cavity, the cornea, the vagina and cervix, the anal canal, and the urethra. All superficial herpetic lesions should heal in less than 3 weeks without treatment unless the host is immunologically defective.

Herpetic whitlows is a special type of herpetic infection of the skin. It involves the finger, may be quite painful, and is common among health care personnel.

Important secondary targets are the brain and meninges. **Herpes simplex virus encephalitis** is the most common encephalitis in the United States. It is a very severe disease with high mortality and permanent residual damages. Prompt diagnosis and treatment with acyclovir are critical. The temporal lobes are the main sites of infection. Herpes simplex virus meningitis comprises about 1% of severe aseptic meningitis; it is severe but self-limiting and without sequela.

Neonatal HSV infection is a primary infection in an immunologically immature host. This infection can be very serious and is preventable. Its incidence is about 14 cases per 10^5 live births in the United States (70% develop disseminated infections). Mortality is very high (>50%) and sequelae (CNS) common. Prompt treatment reduces mortality. It is usually acquired through contact with HSV in the birth canal. Postnatal contact is less common and intrauterine infection is rare. Key risk factor for neonatal herpes appears to be a lack of passive immunity (maternal antibody). Abdominal delivery to avoid the HSV contaminated birth canal is recommended.

Diagnosis

The diagnosis is usually based on clinical manifestations except for the following three situations: (1) encephalitis [early treatment with acyclovir important], (2) suspected active genital herpes in a near-term pregnant woman (neonatal herpes preventable by Cesarean section), and (3) keratitis (responds to treatment with a variety of antiherpes drugs). In these situations, confirmation of clinical impression by laboratory procedures is crucial in management of the infection. The laboratory procedure of choice is **virus isolation.**

Treatment

The drug of choice is **acyclovir.** Acyclovir is an acyclic purine nucleoside analog (see Fig. 34.1A). It is a potent inhibitor against HSV 1 and HSV 2 and is virtually nontoxic to humans. It is not available for cell metabolism until phosphorylated by herpesvirus-specified thymidine kinase. Acyclovir monophosphate is converted by a host enzyme into acyclovir triphosphate, which then acts as a competitive inhibitor against deoxyguanosine triphosphate in DNA synthesis. When acyclovir phosphate is incorporated into an elongating DNA, chain elongation is interrupted (acyclovir does not have an -OH group in the 3′ position). Acyclovir triphosphate also has a higher affinity for the virus than the host DNA polymerase. Acyclovir resistant HSV has been isolated from patients on prolonged

ACV therapy. Resistant forms are due to mutation in genes coding for thymidine kinase or DNA polymerase. Acyclovir resistant HSV infections are uncommon in clinical practice except in patients with AIDS.

Vidarabine, idoxuridine, and trifluridine have all been approved for treatment of HSV associated diseases. All are nucleoside analogs and are phosphorylated by host enzymes. Therefore, they are quite toxic to the host. Idoxuridine and trifluridine are approved for topical use only. For internal use, acyclovir is the drug of choice. The only toxicity of acyclovir is the crystallization of acyclovir in the kidney when large doses are given intravenously in patients whose fluid balance is inadequately attended to.

Epidemiology and Prevention

Sources of HSV are the **active herpetic lesions.** The vesicle fluid has HSV in high concentration. Prevalence of HSV seropositive adults vary from 50 to 100% depending on the socioeconomic status of the population. Infections by the HSV can be prevented by avoiding direct or indirect contacts with herpetic lesions. There is no FDA approved HSV vaccine.

VARICELLA-ZOSTER VIRUS

Varicella-zoster virus (VZV) infects virtually every human subject and the infection is almost always recognizable as chickenpox. Hence, the average annual incidence of chickenpox should be about the same as the average annual incidence of live births (several million cases a year in the United States!). While chickenpox is mostly a childhood disease and is generally mild in immunocompetent children, VZV infections can be severe and even fatal in **high risk groups.** Such high risk groups include neonates, immunocompromised persons, and susceptible adults. Much can be done to protect these high risk subjects. Recovery from primary infections leads to latency. **Reactivations** are common and result in **herpes zoster** (shingles). Shingles can be a painful and debilitating disease.

Pathogenesis

The HSV primarily induces a localized infection; but VZV invariably causes widely disseminated diseases. The portal of entry of VZV is the respiratory tract. It is believed that significant viral replication occurs in regional lymphnodes. This replication results in **viremia** during which the virus is widely disseminated. The clinically significant organ systems affected are the **skin, mucosa of the respiratory tract,** and the nervous system.

Incubation is 10–20 days. The first evidence of disease is the appearance of vesiculopapules on the skin. The skin lesions become generalized within 24 h. New lesions appear on the next 2 or 3 days. Individual skin lesions appear similar to those induced by the HSV. Vesicles soon dry and form a scab. Scabs generally drop off by the seventh day after onset leaving no scar.

In adults, the vesicular eruption is usually much more severe and dyspnea (due to **varicella pneumonitis**) may occur on the third or fourth day after onset. In immunocompromised subjects and in neonates, the disease tends to be more severe.

Recovery from the first infection results in latency that may be reactivated as herpes zoster (shingles). Clinically, herpes zoster is similar to chickenpox except that the vesiculopapules are localized with **dermatomal distribution,** are larger, last longer, and are preceded by dysesthesia. There may be **protracted pain.** Herpes zoster is a **neuronitis.** A second attack of shingles is rare among immunocompetent subjects.

Diagnosis

The characteristic clinical and epidemiologic features are usually sufficient for establishing the diagnosis of chickenpox and herpes zoster. The vesicle fluid is rich in VZV and should be used in laboratory diagnosis if necessary.

Treatment

Acyclovir is inhibitory to the VZV through the same inhibitory mechanisms for HSV and has been approved by the FDA for treatment of chickenpox. It should be used for treatment of infections in high risk subjects.

Epidemiology and Prevention

Chickenpox is a **highly contagious disease.** About 95% of susceptible household contacts acquire the disease. It is acquired through inhalation of respiratory secretions containing VZV or through direct contact with varicella or zoster lesions. The first infection usually occurs during childhood; but up to 5%

of adults in the United States may still be susceptible. In immunocompetent subjects, one infection confers **solid lifelong immunity** to a second attack of chickenpox. Immunity is generally determined by a test for antibodies against envelope glycoproteins known as fluorescein **antibody to membrane antigen (FAMA).**

Herpes zoster tends to occur among older subjects. Unlike HSV reactivation, only 10–20% of all persons develop herpes zoster during their lifetime and second attacks of herpes zoster are rare.

Varicella-zoster immune globulin (VZIg) is effective in reducing the severity of chickenpox if given soon after exposure. It should be given to high risk subjects. A reasonably **effective live attenuated vaccine** is available. It is recommended for immunocompromised subjects who are susceptible to the VZV. There is no agreement whether susceptible children should receive VZV vaccine.

SUMMARY

1. **The herpesvirus is a large DNA virus, has icosahedral nucleocapsid, and an envelope.**

2. **Its replication strategy is similar to all enveloped DNA virus. It codes for its own DNA polymerase.**

3. **The herpesvirus family includes six species pathogenic for humans. The species are herpes simplex type 1, herpes simplex type 2, varicella-zoster, Epstein-Barr, cytomegalo, and human herpes type 6. There is no DNA homology among these six viruses except for the 50% homology between herpes simplex virus types 1 and 2. There is also no common antigen of clinical significance shared by the six viruses except for shared common antigens between herpes simplex virus types 1 and 2.**

4. **Herpesviruses are ubiquitous, infecting virtually every person, induce a wide spectrum of clinical syndromes, respond to antiviral therapy and enter into latency after recovery form primary infections, and induce intranuclear inclusion in permissive cells.**

5. **Herpes simplex viruses 1 and 2 are closely related viruses. They show a 50% DNA homology, share common antigens, and induce similar pathology. Infection by one type provides partial immunity to infection by the other type.**

6. **Primary targets of HSV are the skin and mucosa. The virus multiplies at the implantation site, damages the tissue, and forms a vesiculopapule. Most**

of the HSV infections around the oral and genital orifices are due to HSV 1 and HSV 2, respectively. Dissemination of the virus to secondary targets is uncommon (except for the dorsal root ganglion). One important secondary target is the brain.

7. Herpes simplex virus encephalitis is a serious disease with high mortality. Prompt diagnosis and treatment with acyclovir are crucial.

8. Neonatal herpes is usually a disseminated infection with high mortality. It is usually acquired by the neonate during passage through a birth canal contaminated by the HSV. Neonatal herpes can be prevented by avoiding the HSV contaminated birth canal during delivery (i.e., Cesarean section). Prompt diagnosis of genital herpes in a near term pregnant woman is exceedingly important.

9. Herpes simplex virus infections are acquired through direct or indirect contacts with herpetic lesions. The vesicle fluid contains HSV in high concentration.

10. Herpes simplex virus travels to the dorsal root ganglion by way of the sensory nerve and remains latent in the neuron. Reactivations are common. Factors responsible for reactivation are not well defined.

11. Varicella-zoster virus infections are highly contagious. Infection results in chickenpox, which is characterized by a generalized vesiculopapular eruption. The primary target is believed to be the regional lymphnode where the VZV multiplies. The virus then enters the blood stream and is localized in distant secondary targets. Key secondary targets are the skin and respiratory tract.

12. Chickenpox is a mild self-limiting disease among children. It can be severe and even fatal in adults, neonates, and the immunodeficient. Severity of chickenpox among these high risk subjects can be reduced by administration of VZV antibody (VZIg) during incubation and acyclovir.

13. Varicella-zoster virus may also remain latent in the dorsal root ganglion. Reactivation results in shingles (herpes zoster). A second attack of shingles is rare.

14. A live attenuated varicella vaccine has been approved by the FDA for immunizing immunodeficient children.

15. The best test for immunity to VZV is known as fluorescein antibody to membrane antigen (FAMA).

16. Acyclovir is an acyclic analog of guanosine. It is a potent inhibitor against the HSV and VZV and is virtually nontoxic to the host. It has high affinity for viral DNA polymerase. It is not effective until it has been converted into the triphosphate derivative. The first step in this conversion requires a virus-coded thymidine kinase.

REFERENCES

Allen WP, Hitchcock PJ (1991): Herpes simplex vaccine workshop. Rev Inf Dis 13:S891.

Asano Y et al. (1990): Severity of viremia and clinical findings in children with varicella. J Inf Dis 161:1095.

Brown ZA et al. (1991): Neonatal HSV infection in relation to asymptomatic maternal infection at the time of labor. N Engl J Med 324:1247.

Corey L, Spear PG (1986): Infections with herpes simplex viruses. N Engl J Med 314:686 and 314:749.

Gershon A (1992): The first international conference on VZV. J Inf Dis 166 (suppl 1):S1.

Gibbs RS, Mead PB (1992): Preventing neonatal herpes—current strategies. N Engl J Med 326:946.

Gilden DH (1994): Herpes zoster with post-herpetic neuralgia. N Engl J Med 330:932.

Hardy I, Gershon AA, Steinberg SP, LaRussa P (1991): The incidence of zoster after immunization with live attenuated varicella vaccine. N Engl J Med 325:1545.

Kost RG et al. (1993): Recurrent acyclovir-resistant genital herpes in an immunocompetent patient. N Engl J Med 329:1777.

Stevens JG (1989): Human herpesviruses: a consideration of the latent state. Microbiol Rev 53:318.

Straus SE et al. (1988): Varicella-zoster virus infections. Biology, natural history, treatment and prevention. Ann Intern Med 108:221.

Whitley R, Arvin A, Prober C (1991): A controlled trial comparing vidarabine with acyclovir in neonatal herpes simplex virus infection. N Engl J Med 324:444.

Whitley JR, Gnann JW (1993): Drug therapy: Acyclovir: A decade later. N Engl J Med 327:782.

REVIEW QUESTIONS

For questions 1 to 12, choose the ONE
BEST answer or completion.

1. All but one of the following statements about
   herpesviruses are correct:
   a) Infections by the herpesviruses are very
      common.
   b) These viruses induce a wide variety of
      diseases.
   c) Some herpesvirus-induced diseases are
      responsive to antiviral therapy.
   d) These viruses may persist indefinitely in
      the host after recovery from acute infec-
      tion.
   e) FDA-approved vaccines are available
      against most of the herpesviruses.

2. One of the following is not characteristic of
   the herpesvirus family:
   a) being large DNA viruses
   b) coding for own DNA polymerases
   c) having an envelope
   d) no sharing of antigens of clinical signifi-
      cance among the following species: her-
      pes simplex virus (HSV), varicella-zoster
      virus (VZV), Epstein-Barr virus (EBV),
      cytomegalovirus (CMV), and human her-
      pesvirus type 6 (HHV 6)
   e) over 50% DNA homology among the fol-
      lowing species: EBV, CMV, and HHV 6

3. One of the following statements about herpes
   simplex viruses 1 and 2 is incorrect:
   a) They share antigens of clinical signifi-
      cance.
   b) Recovery from primary infection by type
      1 virus results in partial immunity to in-
      fection by type 2 virus.
   c) Type 1 virus is more likely to be isolated
      from herpetic lesions around the mouth
      than type 2 virus; and type 2 virus, from
      herpetic lesions on the external genitalia
      than type 1 virus.
   d) Type 2 virus is more virulent than type 1
      virus.
   e) HSV encephalitis may be caused by type
      1 or 2 viruses.

4. Identify the incorrect statements on the pathogenesis of herpes simplex virus infections.
   a) Herpes simplex virus usually multiplies
      and induces pathology at the site of im-
      plantation without spreading to other dis-
      tant organs (except the dorsal root gan-
      glion).
   b) Herpes simplex virus lesion is typically a
      vesiculopapule.
   c) Herpes simplex virus infection may oc-
      casionally spread to the brain and cause
      acute encephalitis.
   d) Herpes simplex virus associated diseases
      are more likely to undergo remission (la-
      tency) and clinical reactivation than dis-
      eases associated with other herpesviruses.

e) Herpes simplex virus reactivation is due to a decrease in specific neutralizing antibody.

5. Identify the incorrect statement about herpes simplex virus transmission.
   a) The main source of HSV is the vesicle fluid of a herpetic lesion.
   b) Infections are generally acquired by direct or indirect contacts with a herpetic lesion.
   c) About 50% of middle class young adults in the United States have not yet been infected by the HSV.
   d) Solid immunity to HSV infection can be induced by a live attenuated FDA-approved HSV vaccine.
   e) Neonatal herpes is more likely to be due to type 2 than type 1 HSV.

6. Identify the incorrect statement about neonatal herpes.
   a) It is usually an infection with high mortality.
   b) It is usually acquired during passage through a birth canal contaminated with the HSV.
   c) It can usually be prevented by Cesarean delivery.
   d) Of the disseminated variety, it is more likely to occur when the parturient woman has primary genital herpes than reactivated genital herpes.
   e) Of the disseminated variety, treatment with acyclovir reduces the mortality to less than 10%.

7. Identify the incorrect statement about acyclovir.

a) It is a acyclic analog of deoxyguanosine.
b) It is not active until it is phosphorylated to triphosphate derivative.
c) It cannot be converted to acyclovir monophosphate by the host enzyme (kinase).
d) Its triphosphate has higher affinity for viral (HSV) than for host DNA polymerase.
e) It is toxic to dorsal root ganglion cells that harbor latent HSV genomes.

8. Identify the incorrect statement about acyclovir.
   a) It is recommended for the treatment of selected herpes simplex virus and varicella-zoster virus infections but not Epstein-Barr or cytomegalovirus infections.
   b) Resistant HSV has been isolated from patients on prolonged acyclovir therapy.
   c) Resistant HSV is uncommon except in patients with AIDS.
   d) Resistant HSV are usually the results of point mutations affecting the gene that codes for thymidine kinase or DNA polymerase.
   e) Suppression of the bone marrow is an important complication during prolonged acyclovir therapy.

9. Identify the incorrect statement about varicella-zoster virus.
   a) Its primary target organ is believed to be the regional lymphnode.
   b) Viral multiplication in its primary target is clinically inapparent.
   c) Its secondary targets include the skin and respiratory mucosa.
   d) It reaches the secondary targets through hematogenous spread.
   e) Latent VZV are found in the skin of most VZV seropositive persons.

10. Identify the incorrect statement about chickenpox.
    a) It is a mild self-limiting disease in children.
    b) Its individual skin lesion is similar to a herpetic lesion.
    c) High risk groups for severe disease include VZV seronegative adults, neonates, and immunodeficient persons.
    d) Its reactivation results in herpes zoster.
    e) Pneumonitis is a rare (<0.1%) but fatal complication of chickenpox in adults.

11. Varicella-zoster immune globulin
    a) given parenterally during incubation should block partially or completely the spread of VZV from primary to secondary targets
    b) should be given to all susceptible persons after known exposure to VZV
    c) is prepared from the outdated blood from blood banks
    d) given during the prodroma of herpes zoster has been shown to abort or reduce the severity of shingles

12. Immunity to varicella-zoster virus
    a) is best determined by testing for antibodies against its peplomers
    b) is best induced by administration of live attenuated VZV vaccine to all susceptible persons
    c) are present in about 70% of young adults in the United States
    d) its level is predictive of the development of herpes zoster

ANSWERS TO REVIEW QUESTIONS

1. *e*

2. *e*

3. *d* There is no evidence that virulence is related to types.

4. *e* The cause of HSV reactivation is not known.

5. *d* There is no approved HSV vaccine.

6. *e* A recent study showed the mortality for neonates suffering from disseminated herpes and treated with acyclovir was about 50%.

7. *e* Latent HSV genome does not express the thymidine kinase gene. Hence, ACV cannot be phosphorylated.

8. *e* Acyclovir, in therapeutic dose, is nontoxic.

9. *e* The important point is that, unlike HSV, VZV infection regularly results in viremia and involvement of secondary target organs. The administration of specific antibodies prior to or during viremia should be considered in any virus diseases with viremia. Latent VZV are in the dorsal root ganglion, not skin.

10. *e* One study showed that greater than 10% of adult patients developed pneumonitis. Clinical manifestations of varicella pneumonitis may be alarming (high fever and dyspnea) but rarely fatal.

11. *a* Only those at high risk of developing severe diseases should be given VZIg. In nonhigh risk groups, chickenpox is a mild self-limiting disease. The antibody VZIg is expensive and the supply is limited (it is prepared from the blood of persons known to have VZV antibodies in high titers). It is not clear what causes the reactivation of latent VZV infection into shingles. There is no evidence that it is due to a loss of VZ antibody. Also reactivation into shingles does not involve a viremic phase; therefore, administration of antibodies would not be useful.

12. *a* The most reliable test for immunity to VZV is the detection of antibody against VZV membrane antigens (FAMA). Membrane antigens are viral glycoproteins on the envelope, which is the same as peplomers. An effective VZV vaccine is available; but, it should be used to protect persons at high risk for severe disease. For persons not at high risk it is better to acquire immunity through natural infection, since the natural infection is mild and presumably induces more solid immunity. Several surveys showed that greater than or equal to 95% of young adults in the United States had VZV antibodies.

THE HERPESVIRUS FAMILY: EPSTEIN-BARR, CYTOMEGALO VIRUSES, AND HUMAN HERPESVIRUS TYPE 6

EPSTEIN-BARR VIRUS

Like other herpesviruses, the Epstein-Barr virus (EBV) is ubiquitous and worldwide in distribution. Virtually all humans are infected by the EBV. In addition to being the etiologic agent of infectious mononucleosis (IM), the EBV has been strongly associated with other diseases. Chief among these EBV-associated diseases are hairy leukoplakia, nasopharyngeal carcinoma, African Burkitt's lymphoma, salivary gland carcinoma, Hodgkin's disease, and chronic fatigue syndrome. Because of its ability to immortalize human B lymphocytes in vitro, the EBV is extensively used as a reagent in biomedical research.

In Vitro Characteristics

The main difference between EBV and HSV is in their replication strategy. **B lymphocytes** are the only proven cells susceptible to infection by the EBV in vitro. The B lymphocytes have **CR2 receptors** that can bind both EBV and C3d fragments. After EBV infection of B lymphocytes in vitro, only the early genes are transcribed. The infection is a **nonproductive** one. Instead of releasing progeny virions and disintegrating, the infected B cell multiplies rapidly and persistently (**immortalization** or transformation). Because EB virions have been recovered from secretions of salivary glands and the pharynx, it is believed that the epithelium of these organs are susceptible to productive infection by the EBV. Knowing the properties of EBV transformed cells is the key to understanding the pathogenesis of IM.

Each EBV-immortalized B lymphocyte has up to several hundred EBV genomes and the early gene products. Key early products are the **EBV-associated nuclear antigens (EBNAs)** and **latent infection membrane protein (LMP).** The EBNA have affinity for host DNA. Presumably, the binding of EBNA to specific sites of host chromosome is responsible for the immortalization. Latent infection membrane protein is found on the surface of immortalized cells. Through LMP, the immortalized cell is recognized as foreign by the host's immune mechanism.

Functionally, **EBV-immortalized B lymphocytes** multiply rapidly and persistently in vitro (and presumably in vivo) and are powerful activators of T lymphocytes. These two attributes probably account for lymphoproliferation in IM. Immortalized B lymphocytes also release immunoglobulins and are probably responsible for the transient immunoglobulinopathy in IM.

Pathogenesis

The primary target of the EBV is the **oropharynx** (salivary glands?) where susceptible cells are permissively infected. Infection of the primary target is subclinical. The B lymphocytes circulating through the primary target become infected. Infected B lymphocytes spread by way of lymphatics and blood to **distant lymphoid** and **parenchymal organs** where **foci of lymphoproliferation** are formed. The foci consist of proliferating EBV infected B and activated (also proliferating) T lymphocytes. The T lymphocytes activated by EBV infected B lymphocytes will in turn destroy the activator cells. This process results in inflammation followed by resolution. Quenching of infection is incomplete since occasional EBV-infected lymphocytes can be regularly found in the blood of EBV infected persons.

Infectious mononucleosis is a **self-limiting lymphoproliferative disease;** its basic pathology is lymphoproliferation. The main pathology is found in the lymphoid organs although other parenchymal organs can also be damaged. Hepatocellular damages are common in IM. **Transient immunoglobulinopathy** is also common (due to polyclonal activation of B lymphocytes by EBV).

Reactivation of latent EBV infection is theoretically possible; but, clinical manifestations of reactivation are not well defined. The nature of association between the EBV and other EBV associated diseases is not clear.

Oncogenic Potential

This EBV is said to have **oncogenic potential** based on the following observations. It immortalizes B lymphocytes in vitro; it induces lymphoma in marmosets; it induces a self-limiting lymphoproliferative disease in humans; and it is associated with African Burkitt's lymphoma, nasopharyngeal carcinoma, and salivary gland carcinoma. There is no conclusive evidence that the EBV is oncogenic in humans, but such evidence are difficult to obtain.

Diagnosis

The diagnosis of IM is based on **clinical evidence of lymphoproliferation, absolute lymphocytosis** ($>4000/mm^3$), and positive reaction in the **heterophile antibody test** (Monospot test). Heterophile antibodies are agglutinins of sheep or horse erythrocytes. These antibodies are removed by absorption with ox erythrocytes but not with guinea pig kidney powder.

Heterophile antibody test is an empirical test. These antibodies do not react with EBV antigens and disappear soon after recovery from IM. It is a highly specific test for IM but has low sensitivity. About 15% of IM cases among young adults are heterophile antibody negative (the percentage of negatives is higher among children). In heterophile antibody-negative cases, **testing for EBV antibodies** is useful in confirming the diagnosis. Three tests are required: IgG antiVCA (viral capsid antigen), IgM antiVCA, and antiEBNA. Interpretations are described in Table 39.1.

Treatment

No specific antiviral therapy is effective. Acyclovir inhibits virus excretion but has no effect on the clinical course.

TABLE 39.1. Interpretation of EBV Serologic Test[a]

AntiVCA			
IgG	IgM	AntiEBNA	Interpretation
0	0	0	Not yet infected (susceptible)
+	0	+	Past infection (immune)
+	+	0	Current infection
0	+	0	Current infection
+	+	+	Current or recent infection
+	0	0	Current or recent infection

[a] Sera collected during the first 3 weeks after onset of illness.

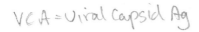

VCA = Viral Capsid Ag

Epidemiology and Prevention

There are numerous genomic variants (based on restriction fragment length, p. 658) but presumably **only one serotype.** A second attack of IM is rare. The EBV is ubiquitous; at least 10% of the healthy adults in the United States are EBV excreters.

Primary EBV infections in children are generally subclinical or too mild to be recognized as IM. Depending on the socioeconomic status and geographic locations, 50–100% of the children in a community have already been infected by the EBV. Primary EBV infections in teenagers and adults are more severe; about 50% are diagnosed as IM.

Effective vaccine is not available. Prevention is unnecessary for immunocompetent persons.

CYTOMEGALOVIRUS

Virtually all cytomegalovirus (CMV) infections in immunocompetent persons are **subclinical.** In immunologically immature subjects or immunodeficient subjects, CMV infections can have major health consequences. The CMV infections are the most important cause of **congenital infections** in the United States and a major **opportunistic infection** in organ transplant recipients and in patients with AIDS.

Pathogenesis

The infection is a **systemic infection.** The virus is **widely disseminated** throughout the body during a primary infection. This dissemination is presumably hematogenous since CMV has been demonstrated in blood cells (mostly in monocytes). The CMV is epitheliotropic. Infected cells are frequently swollen and have large intranuclear inclusions. During the infection, CMV has been demonstrated in **many body secretions,** such as urine, saliva, milk, semen, and cervical secretion. The development of CMV immunity results in latency. Latency can be **reactivated by immunosuppressive agents** and during pregnancy.

Primary CMV infections are generally subclinical. Rarely, it may manifest as **CMV mononucleosis** (a condition similar to IM except that the heterophile antibody is invariably negative).

In immunocompromised subjects, CMV frequently causes severe diseases, such as retinitis, pneumonitis, and gastroenteritis.

Cytomegalovirus is one of the most common causes of intrauterine infections. Severity varies from fetal death to inapparent infection. Determinants for severity of fetal infection have not been identified except for immunity status of the pregnant woman. Severe fetal infections **(cytomegalo inclusion diseases)** occur chiefly in pregnant women suffering from primary CMV infections. Fetal infections may also occur during CMV reactivation in pregnancy, but the infections are usually mild or subclinical. In severe fetal infections, there are multiorgan involvement (including the brain).

Diagnosis

The procedure of choice is to demonstrate the CMV in body secretions. Antibody study is useful in differentiating EBV from CMV mononucleosis.

Treatment

Ganciclovir has been approved for the treatment of **CMV retinitis.** It is an analog of deoxyguanosine. The concentration of its triphosphate derivative is 10 times higher in CMV-infected cells than in uninfected cells. The mode of action of ganciclovir triphosphate is similar to that of acyclovir triphosphate. **Foscarnet** (phosphonoformate) has also been approved by the FDA for treatment of CMV retinitis.

Epidemiology and Prevention

Cytomegalovirus infection is acquired primarily through the **contact** of the mucosal surface with body secretion that contain the CMV. Other important modes of transmission are **transplacental, perinatal** (during parturition and breast feeding) blood **transfusion,** and organ **transplantation.** In general, the CMV infection is acquired earlier in life among populations with lower socioeconomic status (e.g., 90% of the population in developing countries are seropositive by the age of 6 years as compared to <30% in the United States and western Europe). In the United States, the high income population is less likely to be CMV seropositive than low income population. In one study of pregnant women, 65% of the high and 23% of the low income groups remained CMV seronegative. About **0.5% of all infants** in the United States have congenital CMV infections.

A person with primary CMV infection may be excreting CMV for months in the saliva and urine. **Day care centers** are a notorious source of CMV in the United States. Surveys have shown that over 25% of the children in day care centers are viruric.

Prevention is unnecessary except for the fetus and organ transplant recipients. Attempts should be made by CMV seronegative pregnant women to avoid mucosal contact with the CMV. Careful attention to **personal hygiene** should significantly reduce interpersonal transmission of CMV (e.g., CMV seronegative nurses are no more likely to acquire CMV than seronegative young women in the community). For CMV seronegative organ transplant recipients, organs from CMV seronegative donors should be used if possible. There is suggestive evidence that chemoprophylaxis with ganciclovir may reduce CMV morbidity in homograft recipients.

HUMAN HERPESVIRUS TYPE 6

Human herpesvirus type 6 (HHV6) is infectious for a wide variety of human cells, including the CD4-positive T lymphocyte. HHV6 is the etiologic agent of erythema subitum (a mild acute infectious exanthematous disease among children) and may be responsible for occasional cases of mononucleosis and hepatitis. In immunocompromised hosts, HHV6 may cause pneumonitis encephalitis and other disseminated infections. HHV6 infections are generally subclinical; over 90% of the adults in the United States have HHV6 antibodies.

SUMMARY

1. The Epstein-Barr virus (EBV) is the etiologic agent of infectious mononucleosis (IM). It is also associated with nasopharyngeal carcinoma, African Burkitt's lymphoma, hairy leukoplakia, chronic fatigue syndrome.

2. Receptor for EBV is the complement receptor 2 (CR2), which is also the receptor for C3d. The CR2 is found on human B lymphocyte and may also be present on oropharyngeal epithelium.

3. In the B lymphocyte, only the early genes of the EBV are expressed. Early gene products are the EBV associated nuclear antigen (EBNA) and latent infection membrane proteins (LMP). The EBNA has affinity for host DNA and LMP present itself on the cell surface.

4. The EBV infected lymphocytes multiply rapidly and persistently (immortalized or transformed) are positive for EBNA and LMP and release immunoglobulins.

5. The primary pathology of IM is lymphoproliferation. Parenchymal organs, such as liver, brain, and other parenchymal organs, may be secondarily involved.

6. Diagnosis of IM is based on clinical evidence of lymphoproliferation, absolute lymphocytosis, and appearance of heterophile antibody.

7. A heterophile antibody is an agglutinin against the sheep or horse erythrocytes; it is removed by absorption with ox erythrocytes, but not by guinea pig kidney powder; it does not react with the EBV; it is highly specific but rather insensitive in the diagnosis of IM.

8. About 15% of IM cases in adults are negative for the heterophile antibody. In such cases, EBV serology is helpful.

9. The EBV serology includes the following three tests: IgM antiVCA (viral capsid antigen), IgG antiVCA, and antiEBNA. Most IM cases are positive in IgM antiVCA and IgG antiVCA, but negative for antiEBNA.

10. Acyclovir inhibits EBV replication in vitro, suppresses EBV excretion by IM patients, but has no effect on the clinical course.

11. There are numerous genomic variants but presumably only one serotype of EBV. Over 90% of adults over 30 years old are already infected by the EBV. A second attack of IM is rare.

12. Cytomegalovirus (CMV) infections are also common. The infection is usually subclinical except among the immunodefectives and the fetuses. Among the immunocompetent CMV rarely results in heterophile-negative mononucleosis.

13. Among the immunodefectives (AIDS patients, homograft recipients, lymphoma patients, etc.), the CMV infection is usually generalized. Pneumonitis, gastroenteritis, and retinitis are common.

14. Intrauterine CMV infections among fetuses are common (1 in 200 live birth) and vary in severity from subclinical to severe or fatal generalized infection, known as cytomegalic inclusion disease.

15. Diagnosis of CMV infection is usually based on the demonstration of CMV in body secretion (saliva, cervical, or milk) or excretion (urine).

16. Ganciclovir and foscarnet have been approved for treatment of CMV retinitis by the FDA.

17. The HHV-6 may be responsible for exanthema subitum (a mild acute exanthema), an occasional case of acute hepatitis, and a few cases of heterophile-negative mononucleosis. Over 90% of adults in the United States have HHV 6 antibody.

REFERENCES

Agut H (1993): Puzzles concerning the pathogenesis of HHV6. N Engl J Med 329:203.

Hirsh MS (1992): The treatment of cytomegalovirus in AIDS—more than meets the eye. N Engl J Med 326:264.

Ho M (1991): Cytomegalovirus New York: Plenum Press.

Jarrett RF, Clark DA, Josephs SF, Onions DE (1990): Detection of HHV6 DNA in peripheral blood and saliva. J Med Virol 32:73.

Kendell RE (1991): Chronic fatigue, viruses and depression. Lancet i:160.

Knox KK, Carrigan DR (1994): Disseminated active HHV6 infections in patients with AIDS. Lancet 343:577.

Murph JR, Baron JC, Brown CK, Ebelhack CL, Bak JF (1991): The occupational risk of cytomegalovirus infection among day care providers. JAMA 265:603.

Niedobitek G, Young L (1994): EBV persistence and virus-associated tumors. Lancet 343:333.

Schlossberg D (1989): Infectious mononucleosis. 2nd ed. New York: Springer-Verlag.

Schmidt GM et al. (1991): A randomized controlled trial of prophylactic ganciclovir for CMV pulmonary infection in recipients of allogeneic bone marrow transplants. N Engl J Med 324:1005.

Sobue R et al. (1991): Fulminant hepatitis in primary human HHV6 infection. N Engl J Med 324:1290.

Stevens JG (1989): Human herpesviruses: a consideration of the latent state. Microbiol Rev 53:318.

Stewart JA (1990): HHV6: basic biology and clinical associations. Med Virol 9:163.

Yow MD (1989): Congenital cytomegalovirus disease: A NOW problem. J Inf Dis 159:163.

REVIEW QUESTIONS

For questions 1 to 10, choose the ONE BEST answer or completion.

1. The Epstein-Barr virus is the etiological agent for
   a) nasopharyngeal carcinoma
   b) African Burkitt's lymphoma
   c) chronic fatigue syndrome
   d) infectious mononucleosis
   e) hairy leukoplakia

2. One of the following statements about Epstein-Barr virus replication is incorrect:
   a) The virus receptor is a complement receptor known as CR2.
   b) The EBV receptor is found on B lymphocytes and may also be present on epithelium of oropharynx.
   c) The EBV infection of the B lymphocyte is usually nonproductive.
   d) The EBV infection of epithelium of oropharynx is believed to be productive.
   e) The EBV infected epithelial cells are immortalized.

3. One of the following statements about Epstein-Barr virus infected B lymphocytes is incorrect:
   a) They multiply rapidly and persistently in vitro.

b) They contain early viral gene products: the EBV associated nuclear antigens and latent infection membrane protein.
   c) They release immunoglobulins.
   d) They activate T lymphocytes in an autologous host.
   e) They are completely eliminated from the host within 1 year after recovery from infectious mononucleosis.

4. One of the following statements about heterophile-positive mononucleosis is incorrect:
   a) Its basic pathology is lymphoproliferation.
   b) There may be foci of lymphoproliferation in parenchymal organs, such as liver, brain, and so on; these foci may damage the involved organs.
   c) Immunoglobulinopathy is common.
   d) The etiologic agent may be Epstein-Barr virus, cytomegalovirus, or human herpesvirus type 6.

5. The diagnosis of infectious mononucleosis
   a) is based generally on clinical evidence of lymphoproliferation, absolute lymphocytosis, and positive Monospot test (heterophile antibody)
   b) is excluded by repeatedly negative Monospot tests
   c) can be confirmed by IgG versus EBV capsid

d) can be excluded by clinical evidence of acute myocarditis

6. Heterophile antibody diagnostic of infectious mononucleosis
    a) agglutinates sheep or horse erythrocytes and is removed by absorption with ox erythrocyte powder
    b) binds specifically to the surface antigens of Epstein-Barr virions
    c) is positive in all infectious mononucleosis cases among adults
    d) may also be positive in cytomegalovirus mononucleosis

7. About the epidemiology of Epstein-Barr virus infections:
    a) there is presumably one serotype of EBV
    b) there is presumably one genomic type of EBV
    c) less than 50% of adults (>30 years old) in the United States have EBV antibodies)
    d) the main source of EB virions is the EBV-infected B lymphocyte

8. Cytomegalovirus infections
    a) are invariable subclinical in immunocompetent persons
    b) can be severe among patients with AIDS and among homograft recipients
    c) among fetuses usually result in cytomegalic inclusion diseases
    d) occur in about 0.05% of live births in the United States

9. One of the following descriptions of ganciclovir is not correct:
    a) It is approved by the FDA for the treatment of cytomegalovirus retinitis.
    b) It is an analogous of deoxyguanosine.
    c) It acts by a mechanism similar to acyclovir.
    d) It, like acyclovir, is virtually nontoxic to the host cell.

10. Human herpesvirus type 6
    a) antibodies are present in over 80% of the adults in the United States
    b) shares common antigens with the EBV
    c) has been associated with lymphoma
    d) is a nonenveloped DNA virus

ANSWERS TO REVIEW QUESTIONS

1. *d* The EBV is associated with nasopharyngeal carcinoma, African Burkitt's lymphoma, hairy leukoplakia, and chronic fatigue syndrome; but, the association has not met with modified Koch's postulates for etiologic association.

2. *e* In vitro multiplication of EBV in epithe-

lial cells has not been demonstrated; therefore, it is not possible to demonstrate immortalization.

3. *e* There are always a few EBV infected lymphocytes in the blood of EBV seropositive persons.

4. *d* Both CMV and HHV 6 have been shown to cause heterophile-negative mononucleosis and the correct names are CMV mononucleosis and HHV 6 mononucleosis.

5. *a* About 15% of IM are repeatedly negative for heterophile antibody; a positive Monospot test proves but negative tests do not exclude IM. In IM, virtually any parenchymal organ (including myocardium) can be involved by foci of proliferating lymphocytes. The IgG vs. EBV capsid is a marker of EBV infection (past or current).

6. *a* Heterophile antibody is probably due to immunologically nonspecific polyclonal activation of B lymphocytes by the EBV; it does not react with any EBV antigen. The heterophile antibody or Monospot test is never positive in mononucleosis induced by viruses other than EBV.

7. *a* There are numerous genomic variants (as determined by restriction fragment length study) of EBV. The EBV infection of B lymphocytes are nonproductive; therefore, there is no release of progeny virions. Oropharynx secretion (saliva) are the main source of EB virions. Over 95% of persons 30 years old or older in the United States have EBV antibodies.

8. *b* Primary CMV infections occasionally result in CMV mononucleosis. Most CMV infections of fetuses are subclinical. About 0.5% live births in the United States have CMV in urine.

9. *d* Ganciclovir is quite a toxic drug. Its triphosphate derivative is found in higher concentrations in CMV infected than in uninfected cells. Nevertheless, unlikely acyclovir triphosphate, ganciclovir triphosphate is found in uninfected cells (hence, its toxicity).

10. *b* The HHV-6 does not share an antigen with other species of herpesviruses. It is a herpesvirus and, therefore, has an envelope. It induces erythema subitum and heterophile-negative mononucleosis but has no relation to lymphoma.

THE ORTHOMYXOVIRUS FAMILY

Orthomyxoviruses are the etiologic agent of influenza. Influenza is one of the last few major epidemic diseases that inflict humans. In the 1918 pandemic, it killed over 0.5 million persons in the United States. In some of the more recent severe epidemics in the United States, influenza attacked over 25% of the population and killed over 40,000 persons. There is much a physician can do to reduce the morbidity and mortality of influenza. Unfortunately, preventive measures against influenza are not widely practiced, possibly due to the mistaken belief that influenza is a relative mild and self-limiting disease and that influenza immunization is not particularly effective. Influenza is a very serious disease among high risk subjects. Influenza immunization is at least 80% effective.

FAMILY CHARACTERISTICS

Genomic Chemistry

The genome of the orthomyxovirus is RNA, **segmented** (eight segments), single stranded, and negative sense. Each segment codes for a polypeptide.

Morphology

The orthomyxovirus is an enveloped virion with helical nucleocapsid. It is pleomorphic and about 100 nm in diameter. The peplomers on the envelope are the **hemagglutinin** and **neuraminidase** molecules (see Figs. 32.1B and 32.5).

Replication Strategy

The envelope of the orthomyxovirus contains two species of glycoproteins: the hemagglutinin and neuraminidase. Infection is initiated by the attachment of virion hemagglutinin to a specific receptor on the cell surface. After uncoating, the virus-specified RNA dependent RNA polymerases, which remain attached to the uncoated viral genes, transcribe the viral genes into positive sense RNA. This positive sense RNA serves as viral mRNA, which is then translated by the host into structural proteins and polymerases. The positive sense RNA also serve as templates for progeny viral genes. Maturation and release presumably proceed as with other enveloped viruses.

Species

Three species (influenzaviruses A, B, and C) are human pathogens. Domestic animals, such as swine, horses, and ducks, also carry many species of influenzaviruses. These animal viruses can infect humans but spread poorly from one person to another. In wild ducks influenzaviruses replicate preferentially in cells lining the intestinal tract, cause asymptomatic infections, and are excreted in high concentrations (up to 10^9 infectious doses per gram of feces). **Wild ducks** may be the main reservoir of influenzaviruses.

Antigenic Composition

Knowing the antigenic composition of the influenzavirus is important in understanding its epidemic behavior (Figure 40.1). Each virion has three important antigens:

1. **Internal proteins** consist mostly of capsid protein, some matrix protein, and a few molecules of polymerase. **Type specificity** depends on these proteins

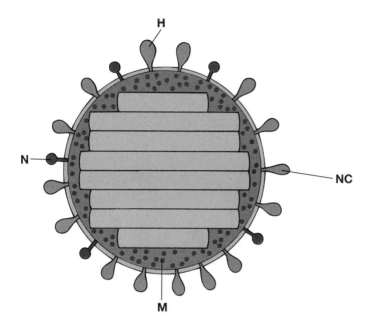

Figure 40.1.

Diagram of an influenzavirus. Hemagglutinin is (H), neuraminidase is (N), matrix proteins is (M), and nucleocapsid is (NC).

and they are unimportant in immunity (because they are internal). These proteins cause toxic symptoms.

2. **Hemagglutinin** (H) is an envelope antigen that can attach to erythrocytes and cause agglutination. It is the attachment ''organ'' of the virion. Blocking hemagglutinin with an antibody will prevent its attachment to a susceptible cell **(a very important factor in immunity).** A hemagglutination-inhibition titer of greater than or equal to 1/40 is believed to be protective.

3. **Neuraminidase** (N) is an envelope protein with an enzyme activity (liquify mucus). It **facilitates the local spread of virions.** Specific antibodies do not prevent infection but do reduce their severity (slow down the spreading of virions).

ANTIGENIC VARIATIONS

Influenzaviruses have a propensity of undergoing **antigenic variations.** Immunity acquired through infection by one virus is frequently insufficient to prevent infection by a variant. This antigenic variation is the main reason why it is difficult to prevent influenza through immunization and why recurrences of influenza in the same person are common. Key points to understand about antigenic variation are:

1. *The hemagglutinin (H) and neuraminidase (N) genes of the type A but not type B and type C virus are* **polymorphic.** The H gene of type A virus has 14 alleles each coding for a serologically noncross reacting hemagglutinin (designated as H1 to H14). The N gene has 9 alleles each also coding for a serologically noncross reacting neuraminidase (N1 to N9). So far, only H1, H2 and H3, and N1 and N2 have been found in type A human influenzavirus. In describing a type A virus, it is crucial to name the H and N components. For example, the 1993-1994 influenza vaccine contain the A (H1N1), A (H3N2), and B viruses.

2. *A type A virus can change its H and/or N gene through* **gene reassortment.** When such an event occurs under natural conditions [A (H1N1) to A (H2N1)], the virus has undergone an **antigenic shift.** Immunity against one type of H is not protective against another type. Antigenic shift usually precedes a major epidemic or pandemic.

3. *The H and N gene of types A and B viruses have the propensity of undergoing* **point mutation.** The mutation changes the configuration of the epitope against which neutralizing antibodies reacts. The extent of change is measured by the reciprocal inhibition test. The key point is that antibodies against the parental H or N is now less effective in inhibiting the mutated (progeny) H or N. When a significant mutation occurs under natural conditions, the prevailing virus has undergone **antigen "drift."** If the drift is big, one expects an influenza epidemic to appear. Rarely, a mutation may affect a glycosylating site of the H or N antigens. A new glycosylated site near an epitope may mask the epitope. This results in antigenic camouflage.

DESCRIPTION OF A STRAIN OF INFLUENZAVIRUS

Because of the high degree of **antigenic diversity** of the influenzavirus, it is useful to include the antigenic contents in the designation of an isolate. The conventional designation is to include the type, place, and time of isolation and the H and N content, if it is a type A virus. For example, A/Bangkok/3/79 (H3N2) denotes, respectively, type A, isolated in Bangkok, local laboratory designate of no. 3, first isolated in 1979, and envelope antigens of H3N2. A major drawback of this method of description is the lack of information on the extent of antigenic difference between two strains with the same H or N. Such differences may be considerable due to antigenic drift.

INFLUENZAVIRUS TYPE A

Pathogenesis

Target cells are the **epithelium of the respiratory tract.** The virus is deposited on the respiratory tract through inhalation of droplets that contain the virus or through indirect contact with respiratory secretion positive for the virus. Virus multiplies rapidly at the site of implantation and spreads contiguously and through the respiratory tract. Infected cells are damaged by virus multiplication. Virus-induced pathology includes **desquamation of epithelium** and **submucosal inflammation.** Incubation is only 1–3 days. Viremia is rare but has occurred.

Due to impairment of mucociliary clearance and of phagocyte function, **secondary bacterial pneumonias** are the most important and serious complication. Bacterial pneumonia usually occur 5–50 days after onset of influenza and are due mostly to *Streptococcus pneumoniae* or *Staphylococcus aureus.*

Diagnosis

Diagnosis is usually based on the sudden onset of fever, myalgia, nonproductive cough, and retrosternal discomfort or pain (especially during coughing). Specific virologic procedures are seldom necessary in clinical practice, but are important in epidemiologic settings (e.g., to determine if an epidemic of acute respiratory infections is due to the influenzavirus). The virus can be readily isolated from respiratory secretion collected 1 or 2 days before and after onset of illness.

Treatment

In most cases, treatments are chiefly **supportive** and **symptomatic.** Also important is the prompt recognition and treatment of **secondary bacterial pneumonias. Amantadine,** if given within 1 or 2 days after onset, is effective in shortening the course and reducing the severity. It should be given to high risk subjects.

Amantadine is a synthetic amine that specifically inhibits influenza A replication by blocking virus penetration or uncoating. Rimantadine is a derivative of amantadine; it is as effective as amantadine but may be less toxic. Resistant virus has been isolated from persons on prolonged therapy but has not yet caused a serious epidemic.

Epidemiology and Prevention

An **epidemic** occurs every winter in the United States. The severity of epidemics varies greatly from year to year. Introduction of a "contagious" strain into a population with little or no immunity against the strain will result in a major epidemic. It is not clear why epidemics in the United States (all temperate zones?) always occur in the winter. In the tropics, influenza is a year-round disease.

Source of virus is the **respiratory secretion** from infected persons (including subclinical infection and during incubation). Chronic carriers and latency have not been demonstrated. Infections by influenzavirus from domestic animals occur occasionally but interpersonal transmission of animal influenzavirus is inefficient.

Annual immunization with current vaccine is an effective preventive measure. Current vaccine contains inactivated purified virions of strains specified by the CDC in the Spring of each year. For example, the vaccine for the 1994–1995 influenza season contains A/Texas/36/91 (H1N1), A/Shangdong/9/93 (H3N2), and B/Panama/45/90 viruses. The vaccine is at least 80% effective. The vaccine is recommended for high and moderate risk subjects, health care personnel with patient care activity and, if available, to anyone who wishes to be vaccinated. **High risk subjects** include persons with chronic conditions, such as cardiovascular diseases, pulmonary diseases, metabolic disease, renal dysfunction, anemia, asthma, and immunosuppression. Healthy subjects over 65 years old are moderate risk subjects. Amantadine is an effective **chemoprophylactic agent** against influenza. It may be used during an epidemic to protect high risk persons who have not yet received their annual immunization. **Subvirion vaccine** contains only the peplomers and is less toxic.

INFLUENZAVIRUS TYPE B

Pathogenesis, diagnosis, treatment, epidemiology, and prevention of type B virus infections are similar to type A virus infections except: (1) amantadine is ineffective against type B virus and (2) genes that code for the hemagglutinin and neuraminidase of the type B virus are monomorphic. Therefore, type B virus does not undergo antigenic shift and does not cause pandemic.

INFLUENZAVIRUS TYPE C

Type C virus infections are uncommon and have little medical importance.

SUMMARY

1. The genome of orthomyxovirus is single-stranded negative-sense and segmented RNA.

2. The virion of orthomyxoviruses is enveloped, has helical nucleocapsid, and contains RNA dependent RNA polymerase.

3. Three species of orthomyxoviruses pathogenic for humans are influenzavirus types A, B, and C. The three species do not share common antigen. Infections by the type C virus are uncommon.

4. Each virion has three important antigens: internal proteins, hemagglutinins (H), and neuraminidase (N). The internal proteins account for type specificity, cause toxic symptoms, but are unimportant in immunity. The H, a peplomer, is the attachment site of the virion and is the most important antigen in inducing immunity. The N, also a peplomer, facilitates local spread of infection; it induces immunity that reduces the severity of infection.

5. The H and N genes of type A, but not types B or C, are polymorphic.

6. Antigenic variations are common with influenzaviruses. The antigenic variations are responsible for the recurrent epidemics.

7. Antigenic shift is due to the replacement of one H (or N) gene by another. The shift is due to gene reassortment. After the shift, H of the virion is totally different immunologically from those before the shift. A pandemic of influenza may appear after antigenic shift. Antigenic shift occurs with type A virus only.

8. Antigenic drift is due to mutation of the H (or N) gene. Immunity acquired through infection with the parental virus is less effective against the mutant virus.

9. An influenzavirus isolate is designated according to its type, place and time of isolation, and the H and N content, if it is a type A virus. Examples: A/Beijing/89 (H3N2), B/Taiwan/86. The extent of antigenic differences due to antigenic drift is not specified by this designation.

10. The primary target of the influenzavirus is the respiratory tract. Secondary targets are exceedingly rare. Bacterial pneumonia is the most important complication.

11. Diagnosis is usually based on clinical manifestations.

12. Early diagnosis and prompt treatment of secondary bacterial pneumonia are important in the management of influenza. Amantadine given soon after onset must be considered in high risk subjects.

13. Annual administration of influenza vaccine (inactivated) provides about 80% protection. Persons at high risk of severe disease should receive annual immunization. High risk persons include anyone with chronic respiratory or cardiovascular diseases, immunologically defective, other chronic diseases, and healthy subjects over 65 years old.

14. Chemoprophylaxis with amantadine provides transient protection.

REFERENCES

Belshe RB, Burk B, Newman F, Cerruti RL, Sim IS (1989): Resistance of influenza A virus to amantadine and rimantadine: Results of one decade of surveillance. J Inf Dis 159:430.

Chapman LE et al. (1992): Influenza—United States, 1989-90 and 1990-91 seasons. MMWR SS3:35.

Centers for Disease Control (1994): Update: Influenza activity—U.S. and worldwide and the composition of the 1994–1995 influenza vaccine. MMWR 43:179.

Douglas Jr RG (1990): Prophylaxis and treatment of influenza. N Engl J Med 322:443.

Immunization Practices Advisory Committee (1994): Prevention and control of influenza. MMWR 43(RR9):1.

Webster RG, Bean WJ, Gorman OT, Chambers TM, Kawaoka Y (1992): Evolution and ecology of influenza A viruses. Microbiol Rev 56:152.

Wells DL et al. (1991): Swine influenza virus infections. JAMA 265:478.

REVIEW QUESTIONS

For questions 1 to 8, choose the ONE BEST answer or completion.

1. One of the following is not characteristic of orthomyxoviruses:
   a) The genome is negative sense and segmented RNA.
   b) The virion has an envelope.
   c) The virion contains a polymerase.
   d) Swine influenzaviruses are not pathogenic for humans.

2. One of the following statements about the functions of antigens (components) of orthomyxoviruses is incorrect:
   a) The internal proteins specify type specificity and cause toxic symptoms.
   b) The hemagglutinin initiates the cycle of replication by binding onto cell receptor.
   c) The neuraminidase facilitates the local spread of infection.
   d) The polymerase is essential in the initiation of synthetic phase.
   e) The capsid protein is the key component in the subvirion vaccine.

3. One of the following statements about antigenic variations of influenzavirus is incorrect:

   a) A(H1N1) to A(H2N1) or A(H3N1) to A(H3N2) are descriptive of antigenic shifts.
   b) Immunity acquired through a prior infection with A (H3N1) virus is ineffective in preventing infection by A(H2N1) virus.
   c) A/Taiwan/79 (H1N1) and A/Japan/89 (H1N1) may have antigenic differences due to antigenic drift.
   d) The bigger the antigenic drift, the less effective the previously acquired immunity.
   e) Antigenic shift is due to point mutation of the hemagglutinin gene.

4. One of the following statements about influenza is incorrect;
   a) The principal target organ of the virus is respiratory epithelium.
   b) Involvement of myocardium following viremia may occur, but this is exceedingly rare.
   c) Damage to respiratory epithelium is an important predisposing factor for secondary bacterial infection.
   d) Most deaths during an influenza epidemic are due to secondary bacterial pneumonia.
   e) Type A virus is invariably more virulent than type B virus.

5. Amantadine
   a) is approved by the FDA for the prevention and treatment of infections by all influenzaviruses
   b) is a nucleoside analog
   c) interrupts virus replication by inactivating virus specified RNA dependent RNA polymerase
   d) is a relatively nontoxic drug and can be used in chemoprophylaxis

6. During an influenza epidemic, the diagnosis of influenza
   a) is usually based on clinical manifestations
   b) must be confirmed by the demonstration of influenzavirus in respiratory secretion
   c) must be verified by the demonstration of IgM anti-influenza
   d) must be confirmed by a therapeutic response to amantadine
   e) must be supported by other cases of acute respiratory diseases in the same household

7. During an influenza epidemic, a 70-year-old man, who has not yet received his annual immunization against influenza, seeks your advice regarding protection from influenza, the best advice should be
   a) getting the annual immunization right away
   b) getting the annual immunization right away but using twice the usual dose of vaccine
   c) taking amantadine daily until the epidemic has subsided
   d) getting the annual immunization right away and at the same time taking amantadine for 2 weeks
   e) avoiding contact with persons suffering from influenza

8. FDA-approved influenza vaccine
   a) contains live attenuated influenzavirus
   b) contains one type A and one type B virus
   c) confers lifelong immunity similar to live polio vaccine
   d) is recommended for persons with AIDS

ANSWERS TO REVIEW QUESTIONS

---

1. *d* Statements *a, b,* and *c* describe the most important characteristics of the orthomyxoviruses. *d* is incorrect. Swine influenzaviruses frequently infect humans although the transmission of swineviruses from one person to another is inefficient.

2. *e* Statements *a, b, c,* and *d* describe the functions of four important proteins of the influenzavirus. Influenza subvirion vaccine contains the peplomers, not capsid proteins.

3. *e* Antigenic shift is achieved through gene reassortment between two viruses.

4. *e* There is no relation between type and virulence.

5. *d* Although amantadine inhibits the growth of all species of influenzaviruses in vitro, it is effective (in clinical trials) in the prevention and treatment of infections by type A virus only. Amantadine is not a nucleoside analog; it interferes with penetration or uncoating.

6. *a* There is no rapid and dependable laboratory procedure for the diagnosis of influenza. During an epidemic of influenza, it is highly probable that an acute upper respiratory tract infection is due to influenza.

7. *d* A 70-year-old person who has not yet received the annual flu immunization is at high risk of getting severe infection. The person must be protected right away. Flu immunization requires about 1-2 weeks to become effective. During the 1-2 weeks, while the host immune system is responding to the immunization, the person must be protected with amantadine. Amantadine will not interfere with the immunization because flu vaccine contains inactivated virions or virion components (peplomers).

8. *d* The FDA-approved flu vaccines are inactivated or subvirion vaccine. The vaccine composition may vary from year to year; the 1993 vaccine contained two type A and 1 type B viruses. Immunity following flu vaccination is transient; annual revaccination is recommended. Being an inactivated or subvirion vaccine, flu vaccination of persons with AIDS carries no risk of progressive disease. How much immunity the vaccination induces depends on the immune status of the person with AIDS.

HEPATITIS A, B (HEPADNAVIRUS FAMILY), C, D, AND E VIRUSES

Acute hepatitis is a common disease; most are due to virus infections. Viruses that are primarily hepatotropic are frequently referred to as hepatitis viruses. There are at least five hepatitis viruses pathogenic for humans; they are hepatitis A, B, C, D, and E viruses. There may be other unidentified hepatitis viruses. Hepatitis A virus is a picornavirus and will be described in Chapter 44. Hepatitis B virus is an hepadnavirus. Hepatitis C, D, and E viruses have not yet been sufficiently characterized to be designated to virus families. This chapter deals with the hepatitis B, C, D, and E viruses. Hepatitis B virus (HBV) is an exceedingly important virus in medical practice. HBV infections are common and worldwide in distribution. Infections by the HBV may result in acute hepatitis, chronic hepatitis, cirrhosis, and hepatoma. Chronic carrier state is also common; there are more than 200 million HBV carriers in the world. Effective immunoprophylactic procedures, both active and passive, are available. Some cases of chronic hepatitis respond to treatment with interferons. Hepatitis C virus (HCV) infections have become a very important subject because our knowledge of HCV infections is expanding constantly over the last few years. This expanding knowledge is made possible through the cloning of HCV genome. The availability of HCV genome leads to a proliferation of specific assays for studying HCV infection.

HEPADNAVIRUS FAMILY CHARACTERISTICS

Morphology

The hepadnavirus is spherical and measures about 42 nm in diameter. It consists of an outer shell that surrounds a hexagonal inner core 27 nm (nucleocapsid) in diameter (Fig. 41.1). Analysis shows that the outer shell consists of virus-specified glycosylated proteins and lipid. Removal of the outer shell by detergents results in the loss of infectivity. It appears that this outer shell has the chemical composition and function of the envelope. Thus, the hepadnavirus is technically an enveloped virus with icosahedral capsid symmetry. In clinical practice, virus proteins on the outer shell are known as **surface antigens (HB$_s$Ag);** the capsid proteins, as **core antigen (HB$_c$Ag);** and the name **"e antigen" (HB$_e$Ag)** is given to a derivative of the core antigen.

Genomic Chemistry

The genome is made up of two strands of DNA of unequal length. The long strand is constant in length (1.6 kb) while the short strand may vary in length. The long (minus) strand carries all the protein-coding capacity of the virus. **Four open reading frames** have been identified on this long strand. Presumably these

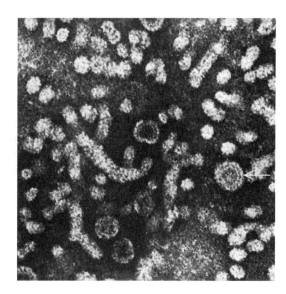

Figure 41.1.

Electron micrograph of HBV from the blood of a patient with HB. Note the three types of particles: smaller spheres 20 nm in diameter, filamentous object 20 nm wide, and larger spheres 42 nm in diameter. The larger sphere (arrow) is the HBV; others are aggregates of HB$_s$ Ag. [Reproduced with permission from Melnick JL, Dreesman GR, Hollinger FB (1977): Viral Hepatitis. Sci Am 237(no. 1):45.]

open reading frames correspond to genes that code for the surface antigen, core antigen, polymerase, and an ''x'' protein of unknown function.

Replication Strategy

Attachment is believed to occur through the binding of viral envelope glycoprotein (surface antigens) to receptors on the surface of hepatocytes. Penetration and uncoating presumably proceed as with other enveloped viruses. After uncoding, the virion-associated DNA polymerase repairs the short strand, thereby converting the partial double strand into a double-stranded DNA. The host's DNA dependent RNA polymerase then transcribes the negative sense (the long strand before repair) strand into multiple copies of mRNA. These mRNAs are translated into HB_sAg, HB_cAg, DNA polymerase, and ''x'' proteins. While the translation is in progress, the mRNA and gene products are packaged into core structures in the cytoplasm. The packaged mRNA is now called pregenomic RNA and is **reverse transcribed by the viral DNA polymerase** into the long strand of viral DNA. The same enzyme then replaces the pregenomic RNA with the short-stranded DNA. (Apparently, the viral DNA polymerase can function not only as a DNA polymerase but also as a reverse transcriptase and RNAse). This core structure then acquires its outer shell (envelope) of surface antigens (possibly by a process other than ''budding off'' from the cell membrane).

Species

Only one species of hepadnavirus, the HBV, is a human pathogen.

HEPATITIS B VIRUS

Pathogenesis

The clinically significant target cell of the hepatitis B virus (HBV) is the hepatocyte and the basic pathology is **hepatocellular damage.** It is generally assumed that HBV is not cytocidal to the hepatocyte. It is the host **immune response** that kills HBV-infected cells. Biopsies of liver infected by the HBV reveal HB_sAg and HB_cAg in abundance on the cell surface and in the cytoplasm. These excess antigens are released into the circulation and may reach a high concentration of 10^{13} particles (aggregates of HB_sAg) per milliliter of blood. These circulating antigens combine with antibodies to form **intravascular complexes** that are then deposited in small blood vessels (such as glomeruli) and, thereby, incites a local inflammation. Virtually all clinical manifestations of acute hepatitis B can be explained by virus-induced hepatocellular damages and deposition of the intravascular immune complex. In some cases, the intravascular immune complexes are cryoglobulins and not complexes of HB_sAg and antiHB$_s$Ag. HBV replication in many extrahepatic tissues have also been described.

One important characteristic of HBV infection is that many infected persons are unable to quench the infection; such persons become **chronic carriers.** About 10% of healthy adults and at least 85% of young infants infected by HBV become HBV carriers. A carrier is defined as one who is HB_sAg positive for 6 months or more. About 10–30% of the chronic carriers develop **chronic active hepatitis** (progressive destruction of hepatocytes) that eventually end in hepatic failure. The rest remain apparently healthy carriers. The HBV carriers are 20–200 times more likely to develop **hepatoma** later on in life.

Chronic HBV infections and hepatoma are strongly associated. Evidence for this association include (1) a striking correspondence between areas where hepatoma is common and where HBV is hyperendemic, (2) a prospective study showing that HBV carriers are about 100 times more likely to develop hepatoma than matched controls, and (3) animal experimental data showing that woodchucks inoculated with a woodchuck hepadnavirus at birth often become chronic carriers of the hepadnavirus and that all carriers eventually develop hepatoma. It is not clear how HBV induces hepatoma. Viral DNA, RNA, and proteins have been found in tumor tissues. Integration of viral DNA into the genome of tumor cells (as well as nontumor cells) has been demonstrated. Sites of integration appear to be random.

Diagnosis

Acute hepatitis is usually diagnosed by clinical manifestations and biochemical evidence of hepatocellular injuries. Clinical diagnosis does not distinguish hepatitis due to the different hepatitis viruses. Such a distinction is important in many clinical situations because the prognosis and the management of contacts depend on the hepatitis virus that causes the infection. For the etiologic diagnosis of hepatitis B, a variety of **serologic markers** are available (Table 41.1). In a typical HBV infection, the following serologic markers appear sequentially: HB_sAg, HB_eAg or HB_cAg, antiHB$_c$Ag, and then antiHB$_s$Ag. There are temporal overlapping of these markers.

TABLE 41.1. Serologic Markers of HBV Infection

Marker	Interpretation
HB_s	Active infection
HB_e or HB_c	Blood is infectious
antiHB$_s$	Immunity
IgM antiHB$_c$	Current or recent infection
IgG antiHB$_c$	Current or past infection

Treatment

There is no antiviral substance that has been approved by the FDA for the treatment of acute hepatitis B. **Interferon-α** has been found effective in the treatment of some cases of chronic HBV hepatitis.

Epidemiology and Prevention

There is only **one serotype** of HBV; therefore, recovery from one HBV infection results in solid immunity to reinfection. However, detailed analysis of the HB$_s$Ag has revealed at least four subtypes. The HB$_s$Ag has three major antigenic determinants (a, d, or y and w or r), which permit four combinations of antigens (adw, adr, ayw, and ayr). Further refinements have shown that the w determinant can be subdivided into w_1, w_2, w_3, and w_4. Subtyping is very useful in epidemiologic study.

The source of HBV is the **blood** of HBV infected persons. The concentration of HBV in some blood can be very high (still infectious after 1–10^6 dilution!). Saliva and semen may also contain HBV, but in lower concentrations. Transmission occurs through **percutaneous and permucosal routes.** It is similar to HIV except that HBV transmission is more efficient; hence, persons at high risk for HIV infections are also at high risk for HBV infections (e.g., IV drug users and homosexual males). Because of mandatory screening and discarding of HBV contaminated blood transfusion associated HBV infections have now been reduced to one case per 300 units. Genomic analysis of HBV has provided evidence for **intrafamilial nonsexual transmission** of HBV.

The percentages of the adults who are immune to HBV infections or are carriers of HBV vary from country to country (Table 41.2). In countries of **low HBV endemicity,** such as in the United States, HBV infections are not infections of the general population but infections of high risk groups. For example, the prevalence rates of serologic HBV markers among IV drug users, homosexually active males, inmates of institutions for the mentally retarded, and sex partners of HBV carriers are very much higher than the general population. Health care workers with frequent blood contact, household contacts of HBV carriers, patients on hemodialysis, and staff of institutions for the mentally retarded are also more likely to be positive for HBV markers than the general population. In **highly endemic regions** (e.g., Polynesia, western Pacific and sub-Sahara Africa), over 80% of the adults are infected and 10–15% of the infected are chronic carriers. Immigrants from highly endemic regions are expected to have high percentages of positive antiHB$_s$Ag and positive HB$_s$Ag. The immigrants presumably acquired HBV infections in countries of origin.

For prevention, effective **HBV vaccines** and **HB immunoglobulins (HBIg)** are available. The HBV vaccine, which contains HB$_s$Ag harvested from chronic carriers or prepared by recombinant DNA technology, are recommended for preexposure immunization of the high risk groups listed in the preceding paragraph. Travelers to countries of high endemicity of HBV may be suitable candidates for preexposure vaccination. Since HBV vaccination of HBV carriers or HBV immune subjects produce no adverse effects, prevaccination screening for susceptibility is an issue of cost. If prevaccination screening is indicated, antiHB$_c$Ag is the marker of choice. Postexposure immunoprophylaxis for hepatitis B (simultaneous administration of HBV vaccine and HBIg) is recommended in the following situations: (1) perinatal exposure of an infant born to a HB$_s$Ag-positive mother, (2) accidental percutaneous or permucosal exposure to HB$_s$Ag positive blood, and (3) sexual exposure to a HB$_s$Ag positive person. **Universal childhood HBV immunization** has been recommended recently.

TABLE 41.2. Seroprevalence of HBV Markers Among Healthy Adults Residing in Regions of High and Low Endemicity

Marker	Endemicity	
	High[a] (%)	Low[b] (%)
antiHB$_s$	>80	5–10
HB$_s$	10–15	0.1–0.5

[a] China, Taiwan, Southeast Asia, Pacific islands, and subSahara Africa.
[b] United States and western Europe.

HEPATITIS C VIRUS

Hepatitis C virus (HCV) is the predominant agent of posttransfusion hepatitis. Little is known about its characteristics except that: (1) it is serially transmissible in chimpanzees and induces hepatitis in chimpanzees; (2) it is 30–60 nm in diameter (based on filtration study); (3) its genome is a positive-sense single-stranded RNA; and (4) its infectivity is destroyed by treatment with organic solvent (suggesting that it is enveloped). Based on these findings, one may speculate that HCV is a togovirus or a flavivirus. There may be more than one immunotypes.

Pathogenesis

Relatively little is known. It may be **similar to hepatitis B.** Chronicity followed by cirrhosis is common in HCV infections but **association with hepatoma has not been established.** Some cases of cryoglobulinemia are associated with HCV infections. Apparently, HCV persists for many years in the host after clinical recovery.

Diagnosis

Diagnosis is usually established by exclusion of hepatitis A and B. The HCV antigens produced recently by recombinant DNA technology appear to be specific and sensitive in detecting antiHCV. But about 10% of infected persons do not develop antiHCV. The sensitivity and specificity of HCV antigen and RNA detection are being evaluated; preliminary results appear promising.

Treatment

Prolonged administration of **interferon-α** to chronic HCV patients has been found beneficial in about 50% of the patients. Its use has been approved by the FDA.

Epidemiology and Prevention

The source and the mode of transmission is presumed to be the same as HBV, except that **HCV is less efficiently transmitted than HBV.** The concentration of HCV in the blood of HC patients is much lower than that of HBV in

HB patients. In the United States HCV amounts for about 30% of all acute hepatitis and is the most common transfusion-associated hepatitis. The risk of acquiring HCV infection after blood transfusion is less than 0.5% in the United States. Sexual and perinatal transmission are uncommon. Prevention must be directed at the interception of transmission.

HEPATITIS D VIRUS

Hepatitis D virus (HDV) is **defective.** It requires helper functions from HBV for replication. Therefore, a single cell must be simultaneously infected by both viruses in order for HDV to multiply. The HDV particles are a little smaller than HBV; its outer layer (envelope?) consists entirely of **HB$_s$Ag.** Within this envelope is a molecule of single-stranded RNA slightly larger than 1.5 kb. The RNA is complexed with a HDV-specific protein without forming any specific morphology, such as nucleocapsid of virus (see Fig. 35.5). There are similarities between the genome of HDV and **viroids:** they are small in size (the genome of the smallest RNA virus is 7 kb); they have many regions of internal complementarity that permit the formation of stable rodlike structures and circularization; and, they have a similarity in base sequences to group I introns (see Table 48.2).

Since HDV requires helper functions from HBV, HDV infections are intimately linked to HBV infections. This linkage can be a **coinfection** (simultaneous acute infections by both viruses) or a **superinfection** (acute HDV infection in a chronic HBV carrier). In general, this dual infection increases the severity and worsens the prognosis of the resultant hepatitis. For example: the mortality rates of acute hepatitis D and B were, respectively, 2–20% and less than 1%; and the probability of developing cirrhosis and portal hypertension was 70% for chronic hepatitis D and 20% for chronic hepatitis B. Coinfection generally has a better prognosis than superinfection.

The diagnosis of hepatitis D generally rests on the finding of **antiHDV** and **HB$_s$Ag** in the serum. Coinfection can be distinguished from superinfection by IgM antiHB$_c$Ag. An antibody study will distinguish an acute from a chronic infection: IgM antiHD signifies acute infection and antiHD in high titer plus negative or low titer IgM antiHD indicates chronic infection. There are about 70,000 cases of chronic HDV infections in the United States.

Interferon-α is effective against chronic HDV infections; presumably, FDA approval is forthcoming. The source of HDV is the blood of persons with active HDV infection. The mode of transmission is believed to be similar to HBV (including sexual transmission). The HDV infections are prevalent among HB$_s$Ag positive persons in the Mediterranean area and Middle East but are uncommon in

Southeast Asia and China where HB$_s$Ag-carrier rates are high. In the United States, HDV infections are seen predominantly among **IV drug users** and their sex partners.

Prevention of HDV infection is best achieved by immunizing HBV-susceptible persons with HBV vaccine. For persons who are already HB$_s$Ag carriers, there is no effective preventive measures other than intercepting transmission.

HEPATITIS E VIRUS

There is still another type of nonA nonB hepatitis that occurs primarily in less developed countries and in epidemics. This type of infection is **enterically transmitted** and is caused by a nonenveloped RNA virus about 30 nm in diameter. It does not cross react serologically with hepatitis A, B, C, or D viruses. It has been tentatively named hepatitis E virus (HEV) and may be a **calicivirus.** Endogenous hepatitis E has not yet been encountered in the United States.

Pathogenesis may be similar to hepatitis A (see Chapter 44). Diagnosis is based on epidemiology and exclusion of other hepatitis. In research laboratories, immunoelectron microscopic examination of feces is useful.

Hepatitis E has a high mortality (30%) among **pregnant women** in some epidemics. Specific antiviral treatment is not available. Prevention depends on strategy for minimizing fecal-oral transmission of infectious agents.

SUMMARY

1. Viruses that are primarily hepatotropic are known as hepatitis viruses. There are at least five species of hepatitisviruses: A, B, C, D, and E. Hepatitis A virus is a picornavirus; hepatitis B virus, a hepadnavirus; and hepatitis C, D, and E viruses (HCV), (HDV), and (HEV) are unclassified.

2. Hepadnaviruses are small enveloped DNA viruses. The only species pathogenic for humans is the HBV. There is only one serotype of HBV, but there are many subtypes.

3. The replication of hepadnaviruses is unique in that viral genomes (DNA) are synthesized by reversed transcription of viral mRNA. This reversed transcription is performed by the virus-coded DNA polymerase.

4. Basic pathology of HBV is hepatocellular damage and the formation of intravascular immune complexes.

5. The HBV is not cytocidal. Infected hepatocytes synthesize viral components in great excess and spill viral components into the blood. Consequently, infected hepatocytes have viral components on the cell surface and the host immune system recognizes such cells as foreign. Excess viral components form intravascular immune complexes with antiHBV.

6. Chronicity of HBV infections occur in about 10% of infected adults and at least 85% of infected infants.

7. Hepatoma and HBV are strongly associated. The HBV carriers are about 100 times more likely to develop hepatoma than noncarriers.

8. Diagnosis of HBV infections is based on HBV serologic markers. The HB_sAg signifies virus multiplication; HB_eAg or HB_cAg signify the presence of HB virions; $antiHB_sAg$ signifies immunity; IgM $antiHB_cAg$ signifies current or recent infection; and IgG $antiHB_cAg$ is evidence of HBV infection.

9. In hyperendemic areas (China, Southeast Asia, etc.), over 80% of the adults have been infected by the HBV and 10–15% are chronic carriers. Among adults in the United States 5–10% are $antiHB_sAg$ positive and 0.1–0.5% HB_sAg positive.

10. The blood of HBV-infected persons contains HBV in high concentration; saliva and semen contain HBV in low concentrations. Modes of transmission are similar to HIV (percutaneous and permucosal) except that HBV transmission is more efficient and there is evidence for transmission resulting from close but nonsexual contacts.

11. An effective subvirion HBV vaccine (containing HB_sAg) is available. Passive immunization with HBIg is effective in certain situations. Interferon-α is beneficial in some cases of chronic HB.

12. Hepatitis C virus is the predominant cause of posttransfusion nonA nonB hepatitis. It has the characteristics of a togavirus but remains unclassified.

13. Pathogenesis and epidemiology of HCV are believed to be similar to HBV except that HCV is less efficiently transmitted than HBV and association with hepatoma has not been established.

14. Diagnosis of HCV is usually established by exclusion of hepatitis A and B, and by testing for antiHCV or HCV RNA (if the test is available). Vaccine or Ig effective against hepatitis C are not available. Interferon-α has been approved by the FDA for the treatment of chronic HCV.

15. Hepatitis D virus is a defective virus; its envelope is composed of HB$_s$Ag. No progeny HDV is released from an infected cell unless the same cell is also infected by HBV.

16. Coinfection by HDV and HBV or superinfection of HDV in an HBV carrier results in severe hepatitis with high mortality.

17. Diagnosis of HDV depends on the presence in serum of HB$_s$ and antiHD.

18. Prevention of HDV is best achieved by preventing HBV.

19. Hepatitis E virus is the etiologic agent of enterically transmitted nonA nonB hepatitis. The virus is unclassified, but it has some characteristics of a calicivirus.

20. Hepatitis E usually occurs in epidemics in less developed countries, and has high mortality among pregnant women. Infections are seen occasionally in the United States among travelers returning from countries endemic for HEV. Diagnosis is based on epidemiology, exclusion of hepatitis A, and antibody study.

21. Interferon therapy is effective in chronic virus hepatitis.

REFERENCES

Alter MJ et al. (1990): The changing epidemiology of hepatitis B in the United States. JAMA 263:1218.

Alter MJ et al. (1992): The natural history of community acquired hepatitis C in the U.S. N Engl J Med 327:1899.

Bloch KJ (1992): Cryoglobulinemia and HCV. N Engl J Med 327:1521.

Centers for Disease Control (1993): Hepatitis E among U.S. travellers. MMWR 42:1.

Centers for Disease Control (1991): Hepatitis B virus: a comprehensive strategy for eliminating transmission in the U.S. through universal childhood vaccination. MMWR 40(RR13):1.

DiBisceglie AM (1994): Interferon therapy for chronic viral hepatitis. N Engl J Med 330:137.

Dodd RY (1992): The risk of transfusion-transmitted infection. N Engl J Med 327:419.

Hoofnagle JH (1990): Chronic hepatitis B. N Engl J Med 323:337.

Hoofnagle JH (1989): Type D (delta) hepatitis. JAMA 261:1321.

Koretz RL et al. (1993): NonA nonB post transfusion hepatitis. Looking back in the second decade. Ann Int Med 119:110.

Lai ME et al. (1994): HCV in multiple episodes of acute hepatitis in polytransfused thalassemic children. Lancet 343:388.

NIH Conference (1988): Hepatocellular carcinoma. Ann Intern Med 108:390.

Perrillo RP, Mason Al (1993): Hepatitis B and liver transplantation. N Engl J Med 329:1885.

Shapiro CN (1994): Transmission of hepatitis viruses. Ann Int Med 120:82.

Stevens CE et al. (1990): Epidemiology of hepatitis C virus. JAMA 263:49.

VanderPoel CL et al. (1991): Confirmation of HCV infection by new four-antigen recombinant immunoblot assay. Lancet 337:317.

REVIEW QUESTIONS

> For questions 1 to 11, choose the ONE BEST answer or completion.

1. Hepatitis
   a) viruses include all viruses that are capable of damaging the hepatocyte
   b) induced by hepatitis A, B, C, and E viruses have similar prognoses
   c) A and E viruses are both picornaviruses
   d) diagnosis should include the determination of the specific type of hepatitisvirus responsible for the infection

2. About hepadnaviruses:
   a) its genome is double-stranded DNA
   b) the synthesis of its genome depends on the host's DNA dependent DNA polymerase
   c) the polymerase coded for by its genome functions both as a DNA dependent DNA polymerase and as a RNA dependent DNA polymerase
   d) its genome integrates into host DNA at a single specific site

3. Identify the incorrect statement about the structure of hepatitis B virus.
   a) Virus proteins on the HBV envelope are known as surface antigens (HB$_s$Ag).
   b) Hepatitis B virus nucleocapsid contains the core antigen (HB$_c$Ag).

   c) Hepatitis B virus e antigen is a derivative of the core antigen.
   d) A serum positive for HB$_c$Ag is almost always positive for DNA polymerase.
   e) The 20-nm particles present in blood in great abundance are the HB virion.

4. Identify the incorrect statement about the pathogenesis of hepatitis B virus infection.
   a) Its basic pathology is hepatocellular damage and formation of intravascular immune complexes.
   b) Hepatitis B virus kills hepatocytes by interfering with the synthesis of proteins and mRNA.
   c) Chronicity is probably due to inadequate immune response mounted by the host.
   d) Integration of virus DNA into host DNA has been demonstrated in cancerous and noncancerous hepatocytes.

5. Identify the incorrect statement about serologic markers of hepatitis B virus infections.
   a) HB$_s$Ag signifies active infection.
   b) AntiHB$_s$Ag signifies resistance to reinfection.
   c) A serum positive for both HB$_s$Ag and antiHB$_c$Ag is rare.
   d) A serum positive for HB$_e$Ag is considered as positive for HB virion.
   e) AntiHB$_c$Ag indicates present or past infection.

6. Hepatitis B virus vaccine
   a) is a subvirion vaccine
   b) contains HB_cAg as its chief component
   c) is recommended for universal usage
   d) containing subtype adw induces stronger immunity against subtype adw than subtype ayr

7. Identify the incorrect statements about the epidemiology of hepatitis B virus.
   a) The mode of transmission of HBV is similar to HIV except that it is transmitted more efficiently and household nonsexual contacts are also at risk of acquiring HBV infection.
   b) The carrier rate is 10–15% in hyperendemic regions (Taiwan and Vietnam) and less than 0.5% in low endemic regions, such as the United States.
   c) The blood of an HBV-infected person may contain HBV in very high concentration (infectious at 1 to 10^6 dilution).
   d) Population groups at high risk of acquiring HBV infections in the United States include health care workers with frequent exposure to blood, persons having multiple sex partners, and Vietnamese children who are $antiHB_cAg$ negative.
   e) The risk of infection for infants of HB_sAg-pos and HB_eAg-neg women is about the same as that of the general population.

8. Identify the incorrect statements about hepatitis B virus and hepatoma.
   a) Hepatoma occurs more frequently in Taiwan than in the United States.
   b) Persons positive for $antiHB_sAg$ are more likely to develop hepatoma later on in life than persons negative for $antiHB_sAg$.

   c) Persons having chronic HBV infections are about 100 times more likely to develop hepatoma than matched controls.
   d) Hepatoma may occur in persons without HBV serologic marker.

9. Identify the incorrect statements.
   a) Hepatitis C virus is responsible for most but not all cases of posttransfusion hepatitis in the United States.
   b) Hepatitis C virus is an unclassified virus but has some of the characteristics of togavirus (envelope, positive-sense single-stranded RNA genome, <80 nm in diameter).
   c) Hepatitis C virus infection is diagnosed by exclusion of HAV and HBV infections and also by testing for antiHCV or HCV RNA.
   d) Hepatitis C virus infections in the United States are reduced chiefly by the identification and avoidance of blood donated by HCV-infected donors.
   e) There is no effective antiviral against HCV infections.

10. Identify the incorrect statement about hepatitis D virus.
    a) Infection of a human hepatocyte by HDV does not result in the release of progeny virion.
    b) Dependence of HDV on HBV is an example of nongenetic interaction known as complementation.
    c) A serum positive for antiHDV and negative for HB_sAg probably indicates recovery from HDV infection.
    d) One method of preventing HDV infections is to immunize $antiHB_cAg$ negative subjects with HBV vaccine.

e) Incidence of HDV infections in the United States is the highest among immigrants from Vietnam.

11. Identify the incorrect statement about hepatitis E and C viruses.
   a) Both are unclassified and induce nonA nonB hepatitis.

b) The mode of transmission of HEV is similar to HAV (fecal-oral route) and that for HCV is similar to HBV.
c) Endogenous HEV infection has not yet occurred in the United States; HCV infection is common in the United States.
d) Chronicity is common in infection by both viruses.

ANSWERS TO REVIEW QUESTIONS

---

1. **d** Hepatitisviruses include only those viruses that are primarily hepatotropic. There are many other viruses (e.g., herpes simplex, Epstein-Barr, and yellow fever) that are capable of damaging the hepatocyte; hepatocytes are not their primary targets; therefore, these viruses are not called hepatitis viruses. Prognosis for HA and HE is excellent; mortality is virtually nil and recovery is complete. Prognosis for HB is not as good; about 10% of those infected develop chronic infections, which may lead to cirrhosis and hepatoma (HB). Hepatitis E is unclassified; it may be a calicivirus not a picornavirus.

2. **c** The HBV genome is a partial double-stranded DNA. The synthesis of the HBV genome is unique in that the genome is transcribed first into viral mRNA and viral genomes are synthesized from viral mRNA by reverse transcription. Therefore, synthesis of HBV genomes depends on the host's DNA dependent RNA polymerase and the virus' DNA polymerase, which has reverse transcriptase function. The integration appears to be random and there are many integration sites.

3. **e** The 20-nm particles are aggregates of HB_sAg.

4. **b** Virus growth modifies the cell surface by inserting virus proteins on the cell membrane; modified cells are recognized as foreign and are destroyed by the host's immune system.

5. **c** Serum HB_sAg originates from HB_sAg synthesized in HBV-infected hepatocytes; therefore, HB_sAg indicates HBV replication in acute or chronic infection. $AntiHB_cAg$ signifies past or present in-

fection by HBV and not immunity to HBV. Therefore, the presence in sera of HB_s and antiHB$_c$Ag is common during acute or chronic infections.

6. *a* A subvirion vaccine is one that contains only viral components. The HBV vaccine is a subvirion vaccine; it contains HB_sAg.

7. *e* These infants have a 50% chance of infection during the first 5 years of life.

8. *b* AntiHB$_s$Ag positive persons have completely quenched the HBV infection and are immune to reinfection by HBV.

These persons are no more likely to develop hepatoma than matched controls since hepatoma is associated with chronic HBV infection. Hepatoma has occurred in low endemic areas in persons not infected by HBV; presumably hepatoma in these antiHB$_c$ negative subjects are due to exposure to hepatotoxins.

9. *e* Interferon-α is approved by the FDA for the treatment of chronic HC.

10. *e* Hepatitis D virus infections in the United States are found mostly in IV drug users.

11. *d* Chronicity is common for HCV but not for HEV infections.

THE RETROVIRUS FAMILY: HUMAN T LYMPHOTROPIC VIRUSES TYPES 1 AND 2

Retroviruses are a unique family of viruses. These viruses utilize DNA as a replicative intermediate. Genetic information flows from its RNA genome to DNA and then back to RNA again. This reverse flow of genetic information depends on a virion-associated virus-specified polymerase, the reverse transcriptase. Host species specific retroviruses are found in many species of vertebrates. Many are oncogenic, causing leukemia sarcoma and mammary carcinoma. Before the onset of the AIDS epidemic and the discovery of HIV as the etiology of AIDS, retroviruses were of major interest to experimental oncologists but were of minor importance in medical practice. The AIDS epidemic has brought the retroviruses to the forefront of medical virology.

FAMILY CHARACTERISTICS

Morphology

The retrovirus is an enveloped virus with a **nucleocapsid of unknown symmetry.** It measures about 100 nm in diameter. Thin sections of a mature virion reveal a nucleoid surrounded by a membrane. The location (centrally or eccentrically located) and shape (round or cylindrical) of the nucleoid have diagnostic value (Fig. 42.1).

Genomic Chemistry

The genome is a nonsegmented single-stranded positive-sense RNA. Each virion contains **two identical molecules of the RNA.** Each RNA has three structural and several regulatory genes that are flanked by the lateral terminal repeats.

Replication Strategy

The retrovirus follows the same general scheme for enveloped viruses except for the early steps of the synthetic phase. After the internalized nucleocapsid is uncoated, the virion-associated **reverse transcriptase** transcribes the viral genome into viral DNA. Some of the viral DNA are then integrated into the host's DNA and are called **provirus.** The provirus is transcribed by the host's DNA dependent RNA polymerase into viral genome (full-length transcript) and viral mRNA (transcripts of one or more genes with or without splicing).

Infection by the retrovirus may disturb cellular DNA metabolism in at least four ways. (1) A retrovirus may pick up a host regulatory gene (**oncogene**) and transduce the oncogene into a host cell in its next cycle of replication. This transduced oncogene may no longer be under the host cell's usual regulatory control and may have excessive expression. (2) There are **many integration sites** on the host DNA for the provirus. The provirus may integrate near a regulatory gene of the host, and through its powerful enhancer and promoter elements, the provirus may increase the expression of the regulatory genes in the immediate vicinity of viral integration site. (3) Virus integration may inactivate a host gene through **insertion mutation.** If the inactivated gene has a suppressor function, excessive expression of other genes may occur. (4) The virus specified **transactivating protein** may transactivate certain cellular gene and thereby stimulate the growth

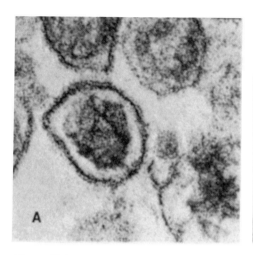 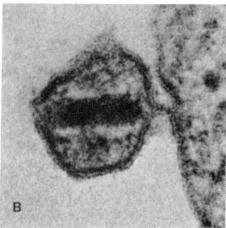

Figure 42.1.

Electron micrograph of the oncornavirus HTLV 1 (A) and the lentivirus HIV 1 (B). Note centrally located round nucleoid or type C morphology in (A) and cylindrical nucleoid or type D morphology in (B). [Reproduced with permission from Schupbach J (1984): Serological analysis of a subgroup of human T lymphotropic retroviruses associated with AIDS. Science 224:504.]

of uninfected cells (see Chapter 43). The final outcome of these four mechanisms of altering the host cell's DNA metabolism may be abnormal cell growth.

Because of its proven ability to transduce genes from one to another mammalian cell, the retrovirus is a useful **vector** in introducing a foreign gene into a human cell.

Species

There are many species of retroviruses that are grouped into three subfamilies. Only two subfamilies (*Oncornavirinae* and *Lentivirinae*) are medically important. Human T lymphotropic virus types 1 and 2 (HTLV 1 and HTLV 2) are **oncornaviruses** while HIV types 1 and 2 (HIV 1 and HIV 2) are **lentiviruses.** Oncornaviruses have a **centrally located nucleoid** (type C morphology) and are oncogenic. Lentiviruses have a **cylindrical nucleoid** (type D morphology), are not oncogenic, but cause chronic diseases that often involve the CNS (Fig. 42.1). A species of the third subfanily, *Spumaviridae,* has been claimed to be associated with chronic fatigue syndrome; but, this claim has not been substantiated by recent data.

Antigenic Relatedness

Species within each subfamily may share antigens. It is usually the internal protein, **p24** (a protein of 24 kDa), that shows antigenic cross-reactivity.

THE ONCORNAVIRUSES (HTLV 1 AND 2)

The term "oncornavirus" is derived from the phrase "oncogenic RNA virus." There are numerous species, most of which are pathogens of nonhuman vertebrates. Some of these animal oncornaviruses have been studied extensively. These viruses cause leukemia and sarcoma in the natural host; some variants cause a chronic degenerative disease of the CNS; and some are transmitted to a new host through the germ cell (a virus so transmitted is known as an **endogenous virus** and such a mode of transmission is known as **vertical transmission**).

There are only two species of human oncornaviruses, **HTLV 1** and **HTLV 2.** The HTLV 1 is etiologically associated with **adult T-cell leukemia (ATL)** and is also associated with a chronic degenerative neurologic disease known as **tropical spastic paralysis (TSP)** in the Caribbean and **HTLV 1 associated myelopathy (HAM)** in Japan (TSP and HAM are probably the same disease). Both ATL and TSP/HAM are rare in the United States. The importance of HTLV 1 in the United States is primarily theoretical. Some believe that HTLV 1 is the only human virus that has fulfilled modified Koch's postulate for etiologic association with a human cancer. It may be the etiologic agent of a chronic degenerative neurological disease. Also, there is an alarming increase of HTLV 1 and 2 infections among IV drug users in the United States.

The HTLV 2 is closely related to HTLV 1. There is extensive serologic cross-reactivity between HTLV 1 and HTLV 2. It has about 65% genomic homology with HTLV 1. Little is known about the pathogenesis and epidemiology of HTLV 2. The remainder of this chapter will be devoted to HTLV 1.

Pathogenesis

The genome of HTLV 1 consists of four genes: the *gag, env, pol,* and *pX,* which are flanked by terminal repeats. The *pX* **gene** codes for a **transactivator protein,** known as p40 *tax;* it enhances the transcription of the provirus and certain specific host genes. The *pX* is the early gene while *gag, env,* and *pol* are late genes. The *pX* product is believed to be essential in leukemogenesis.

The HTLV 1 is a **cell-associated virus;** the infected cell seldom releases progeny virions into extracellular space. Consequently, transmission of the virus from one cell to another is achieved chiefly by cell-to-cell contact. The HTLV 1 is infectious for a wide variety of human and mammalian cells by **cocultivation.** (Cocultivation is the mixing of HTLV 1 positive and negative cells in culture.) But, only infected T lymphocytes become **immortalized.** Some, but not all, of these immortalized T lymphocytes express viral antigens. In the human host, the HTLV 1 immortalized T lymphocytes proliferate and stimulate HTLV 1 specific immunity. The host immune system will kill HTLV 1 infected T lymphocytes that express viral antigens. Infected T lymphocytes that do not express viral antigens are spared. These cells proliferate and cause leukemia in the host. Indeed, the most characteristic pathologic finding in ATL is **rapid proliferation of abnormal T lymphocytes.** The HTLV 1 also persists indefinitely in an infected person.

The pathogenetic mechanism of ATL must be more complex than that described in the preceding paragraph. The described mechanism cannot explain the monoclonicity and exceedingly long incubation of ATL. (Most people acquire HTLV 1 infection during birth; yet, the average age of ATL patients is 55 years.)

Etiologic association of HTLV 1 and ATL is based on the following observations: HTLV 1 proviral DNA are found regularly in ATL neoplastic cells; all ATL patients are positive for HTLV 1 antibodies; and areas of high incidence of ATL correspond closely with those of high prevalence of HTLV 1 infections.

Little is known about the pathogenesis of TSP/HAM. Since HTLV 1 is infective for a wide variety of human cells, it is possible the TSP/HAM is the result of infection of the nervous system by HTLV 1. Indeed, HTLV 1 has been demonstrated in the blood and cerebrospinal fluid of a few patients with TSP/HAM. So far, the association between HTLV 1 and TSP/HAM has not met with the modified Koch's postulate for *etiologic* association. Recent data suggest that HTLV 1 infections may be associated with other conditions such as uveitis, monoclonal gammopathy, etc.

Diagnosis

The HTLV 1 infections can be readily detected by **antibody testing** with standard serologic procedures, such as immunofluorescence and immunoenzyme assay. The HTLV 1 can be demonstrated in the peripheral blood mononuclear cells by cocultivation or gene amplification.

Treatment

No specific antiviral therapy against the HTLV 1 is available.

Epidemiology and Prevention

The source of HTLV 1 is the **T lymphocyte** of infected persons. Blood, semen, milk, and cervical secretion contain T lymphocytes; therefore, one expects these body fluid from HTLV 1 infected persons to be positive for HTLV 1. Since the virus is cell associated, the **efficiency of interpersonal transmission is low.**

These HTLV 1 infections are common in **endemic regions,** such as southern Japan, the Caribbean islands, and some areas of Africa. Population surveys in endemic areas have shown that up to 20% are positive for the HTLV 1 antibody. In the United States, HTLV 1 antibodies are detected with increasing frequency among the **IV drug users;** the seroprevalence rates range from 5 to 50%. Homosexual males and hemophiliacs are no more likely to be positive for HTLV 1 antibody than the general population.

Transmission by **blood transfusion** is well documented; about two-thirds of recipients of contaminated blood acquire the infection. Injection of plasma or plasma fraction has not resulted in infection. Transmission among IV drug users must be due to the sharing of needles and syringes contaminated with infectious blood. Mother-infant transmission occurs primarily but not exclusively through **breast feeding;** about 25% of breast-fed infants of seropositive mothers are infected. **Sexual transmission** appears to be inefficient but does occur (especially from male to female). In a recent study, 7 out of 97 acquired infections from their spouses in 5 years.

Adult T-cell leukemia is rare in the United States (10 cases per year). In endemic areas of Japan, about 2% of infected persons develop ATL. Because most HTLV infections are acquired early in life, the incubation period for ATL must be years or decades. If the HTLV 1 infection in the United States is confined to the IV drug users, it may remain as an insignificant medical problem.

Prevention is achieved by the identification and destruction of infected blood and by stopping the practice of breast feeding by HTLV 1 seropositive mothers.

SUMMARY

1. Retroviruses are enveloped. The genome is a dimeric single-stranded positive-sensed RNA. The virion contains a polymerase, the reverse transcriptase.

2. The synthetic phase of retrovirus replication is unique in that its RNA genome is reverse transcribed by the virion-associated polymerase into viral DNA and the viral DNA is integrated into host DNA as a provirus. The pro-

viral DNA is transcribed by host's DNA dependent RNA polymerase into viral mRNA and viral genomes.

3. Retroviruses may have important effects on the host cell DNA metabolism. These retroviruses may transduce an oncogene; they may enhance the expression of regulatory genes in the vicinity of the insertion site of the provirus; they may inactivate a suppressor gene through insertion mutation; and, their transactivating protein may stimulate abnormal cell growth. The outcome is a disturbance in the regulation of DNA metabolism.

4. Retroviruses are divided into three subfamilies, two of which (oncornaviruses and lentiviruses) are medically important. Oncornaviruses have type C morphology (centrally located nucleoid) and are oncogenic; lentiviruses have type D morphology (cylindrical nucleoid), are not oncogenic but cause chronic diseases that often involve the CNS.

5. The medically important oncornavirus is human T lymphotropic virus type-1 (HTLV 1). The HTLV 1 is etiologically associated with adult T-cell leukemia and is statistically associated with tropical spastic paralysis (a chronic degenerative disease).

6. The HTLV 1 infects a wide variety of human cells in vitro but it immortalizes only the T lymphocyte. It is this immortalization that leads to adult T-cell leukemia. The incubation is very long (decades). Presumably, HTLV 1 persists for life in an infected person.

7. The HTLV 1 may be found in the blood, semen, milk, or cervical secretion of an infected person. The virus is found in the lymphocyte in these body secretion. Interpersonal transmission is inefficient except among recipients of contaminated blood.

8. The HTLV 1 infections are endemic in southern Japan, the Caribbean islands, and some parts of Africa. It is rare in the United States except among IV drug users. Only about 2% of HTLV 1 infected persons in Japan develop adult T-cell leukemia.

9. The HTLV 2 is probably an antigenic variant of HTLV 1.

REFERENCES

Centers for Disease Control (1990): HTLV1 screening in volunteer blood donors. MMWR 39:915.
Centers for Disease Control (1993): Inability of retroviral test to identify persons with chronic fatigue syndrome. MMWR 42:183.

Druker BJ, Mamon HJ, Roberts TM (1989): Oncogenes, growth factors and signal transduction. N Engl J Med 321:1383.

Hayes CG, Burans JP, Oberst RB (1991): Antibodies to HTLV1 in a population from the Philippines: evidence for cross-reactivity with *Plasmodium falciparum*. J Inf Dis 163:257.

Hinuma Y (1990): HTLV-1 infections. Med Virol 9:147.

Khabbaz RF, et al. (1992): Seroprevalence of HTLV-1 and HTLV-2 among intravenous drug users and persons in clinics for sexually transmitted diseases. N Engl J Med 326:375.

Levy JA (1992): The Retroviridae. New York: Plenum Press.

Stuver SO et al. (1993): Heterosexual transmission of HTLV 1 among married couples in Southwestern Japan. J Inf Dis 167:57.

Yamaguchi K (1994): HTLV 1 in Japan. Lancet 343:213.

REVIEW QUESTIONS

For questions 1 to 5, choose the ONE BEST answer or completion.

1. Retrovirus
   a) is a nonenveloped virus
   b) genome consists of a molecule of single-stranded, positive-sense RNA
   c) virion contains a polymerase, the reverse transcriptase
   d) is transmitted vertically through the germ cell

2. About the synthetic phase of retrovirus multiplication:
   a) the uncoated virus genome must be reverse transcribed to proviral DNA for replication to proceed
   b) drugs that block reverse transcription also interfere with the synthesis and release of progeny virions from cells positive for provirus

   c) successful transfection of proviral DNA has not been demonstrated
   d) like all single-stranded positive-sense RNA viruses, retrovirus genomes (stripped of all virus proteins) have been successfully transfected in mammalian cells

3. Identify the incorrect statement about transduction and oncogene.
   a) Retroviruses are commonly used as vectors in transducing a foreign gene into a human cell.
   b) An oncogene is, for practical purposes, a cell regulatory gene that has been integrated into the genome of a retrovirus.
   c) An oncogene-positive retrovirus virion is presumably defective and requires for its replication helper function from a nondefective virion of the same species.
   d) A retrovirus without an oncogene may also stimulate the host cell to multiple rapidly.

e) Transduction bypasses the first step (attachment) of the virus replication cycle.

4. Identify the incorrect statement about human T lymphotropic virus type 1 infections.
   a) It is extremely rare in the United States except among the IV drug users.
   b) The probability of developing adult T-cell leukemia in the lifetime of a HTLV 1 infected person is about 2%.
   c) The interval between HTLV 1 infection and onset of adult T-cell leukemia has been shown to be as long as several decades.
   d) Persons most likely to get infected are recipients of blood contaminated with HTLV 1 and infants breast-fed by HTLV 1-seropositive women.
   e) Zidovudine prolongs the life of patients with adult T-cell leukemia.

5. Patients with tropical spastic paralysis
   a) are invariably positive for human T lymphotropic virus type 1 antibody
   b) are more likely to be positive for HTLV 1 antibody than matched controls
   c) also develop severe immunodeficiency similar to patients with AIDS
   d) are positive for HTLV 1 in nerve tissues

ANSWERS TO REVIEW QUESTIONS

---

1. *c*

2. *a*

3. *e* Transduction is the introduction of a host gene carried in a virion; it cannot bypass the attachment step.

4. *e*

5. *b* About two-thirds of patients with TSP and 5% of matched controls have HTLV 1 antibodies. The HTLV 1 has been demonstrated in the nerve tissue of a few cases of TSP; therefore, *d* is too general a statement.

THE RETROVIRUS FAMILY: HUMAN IMMUNODEFICIENCY VIRUSES TYPES 1 AND 2

THE LENTIVIRUSES (HIV 1 AND 2)

Acquired immunodeficiency syndrome (AIDS) was first reported in the United States in 1981. By 1989, about 100,000 AIDS cases and 50,000 AIDS deaths had been recorded. Over 10^5 cases were reported to the Centers for Disease Control in 1993. The number of persons infected by the AIDS viruses (HIV 1 and HIV 2) is not known. Rough estimates are that in 1989 there were 1–2 million HIV-infected persons in the United States. Globally, over 12 million persons were HIV-infected in 1992. Of these, 8 million were in Africa. Today, it is in Thailand, Burma, and India that the AIDS pandemic is most volatile. In just a few years, the Thai epidemic has involved over 400,000 persons.

The human immunodeficiency virus belongs to the lentivirus subfamily (see Chapter 42). Two species, **HIV 1** and **HIV 2,** are medically important. Both HIV 1 and HIV 2 show a **50% nucleic acid homology.** Their **p24 cross-react** in serologic tests. Both cause AIDS in humans but infections by HIV 2 tend to be less severe and spread less efficiently. The HIV 2 infections are found mostly in

West Africa while HIV 1 are now worldwide in distribution. Simian immunodeficiency virsuses **(SIV)** are lentiviruses indigenous to monkeys in Africa but capable of inducing immunodeficiency in Asiatic monkeys. SIVs are genomically and antigenically related to HIV 2. Seroconversion against the SIV among laboratory workers has been reported.

HIV Genome and Gene Products

The HIV genome contains three structural genes (*gag, pol,* and *env*), four **regulatory genes** (*tat, rev, nef,*, and *vif*), and two or more genes of unknown functions (Fig. 43.1). These genes are flanked by regulatory sequences **(lateral terminal repeats or LTR).** A virus-specified protease cleaves the product of *gag* gene into three core proteins (one of which is **p24**); the product of the *pol* gene, into three enzymes **(reverse transcriptase, protease,** and **integrase);** and the product of *env* gene **(gp160),** into two envelope antigens **(gp120** and **gp41).** The **tat** protein transactivates HIV expression, rev protein upregulates virus expression, nef protein down regulates virus expression while vif protein is necessary for the production of infectious virions. The replication of HIV is intricately controlled. After integration, the **proviral DNA** can exist in a latent or productive state depending on how these regulatory proteins interact.

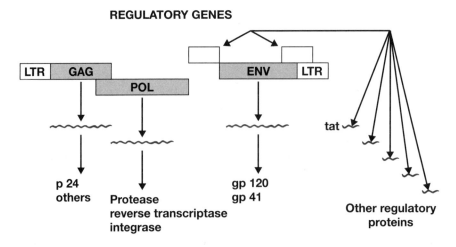

Figure 43.1.

Diagram of the genome of HIV showing the key genes and gene products. Note the proteolytic cleavage of *gag* gene product into p24 and other proteins; *pol* gene product into protease, RT, and integrase; and *env* gene product into gp120 and gp41.

After integration of the proviral DNA into the host DNA, the synthetic phase of virus replication proceeds much like DNA viruses. Some of the regulatory genes, such as *tat* (transactivator) and *nef* (negative factor) are presumably the early genes. The LTR region is extremely complex. This region contains **enhancer and suppressor sequences.** Following binding of the tat protein to one of these regulatory sequences, transcription of the viral genome is enhanced by several thousand-folds. It is believed that, in resting T lymphocytes, *tat* gene is for practical purpose not expressed; that, without tat protein, viral genome is expressed at a very low level (if at all); and that the HIV is latent in resting T lymphocytes. Upon the activation of a latently infected T lymphocyte, the *tat* gene is activated. Expression of the *tat* gene initiates a sequence of events that result in the release of many progeny virions, the infection of many new cells, and death of the original cell. Most likely, the regulation of virus growth is much more complex than what has just been described. Host proteins are also involved in this regulation.

HIV Virion and Key Components

At least seven species of proteins have been found in the virion (Fig. 43.2). Important ones are the **gp120, gp41, p24,** and **RT.** The peplomer of the virion is made of the gp120 and gp41. The gp120 protein is the attachment site for the virion, and it is antibodies against gp120 that neutralize the virus. The gp41 protein

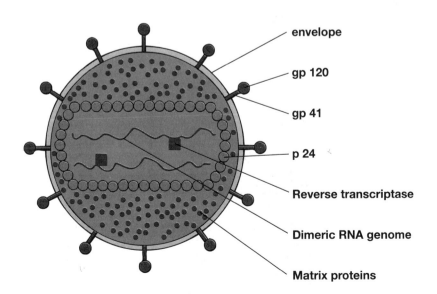

envelope

gp 120

gp 41

p 24

Reverse transcriptase

Dimeric RNA genome

Matrix proteins

Figure 43.2.

Diagram of a human immunodeficiency virion showing the key components.

causes the viral envelope to fuse with the cell membrane; it is also a key antigen in the diagnosis of HIV infection. The p24 protein is the main capsid protein; it is also a key antigen in the diagnosis of HIV infection. The p24 of HIV 1 and HIV 2 cross-react in serologic test. Reverse transcriptase (RT) is the virion-associated polymerase that is essential in initiating the synthetic phase of the HIV replication cycle.

Biologic Serologic and Genomic Heterogeneity

Restriction fragment length analysis of epidemiologically unrelated HIV isolates have shown that each isolate is genomically distinct. The coexistence at one time point of a large number of related but **genomically distinct HIV isolates** in the same person has also been reported. It is well known that HIV **mutates at very high frequency** during its replication. Presumably, the mutations occur during the reverse transcription of the viral genome to proviral DNA.

Mutations affecting the DNA sequence that codes for the attachment site of gp120 occur frequently. As a consequence, HIV isolates vary in **susceptibility to neutralizing antibody.** Mutations affecting the *pol* gene are also common. Some of these mutants become **resistant to zidovudine.**

Virus isolates may differ in **cell tropism.** For examples, some isolates grow chiefly in CD4 lymphocytes, others grow chiefly in macrophages, and still others grow in both CD4 lymphocytes and macrophages. Virus isolates may also vary in their ability to **productively infect cells.** Some isolates replicate rapidly and release a large number of progeny virions while other replicate slowly and release a small number of progeny virions.

Pathogenesis

The principal cell receptor for HIV attachment is the **CD4 molecule.** As expected, cells rich in CD4 molecules, such as **CD4 lymphocytes** and a subpopulation of **macrophages,** are the principal target cells of HIV. In **nonactivated T cells,** the HIV presumably exists in the **latent state.** Once the infected resting T cell is activated, viral latency is converted into productive infection, many progeny virions are released, and the cell is killed. The progeny virions, unless neutralized by antibody, will infect other cells. Cell death is accelerated through **cell fusion** and formation of multinucleated cells. Cells fuse through the binding of gp120 on the surface of a productively infected CD4 cell to CD4 molecules on uninfected CD4 cells. In the macrophage, HIV may replicate without killing the cell. In situ hybridization studies indicate that the **glial cell** in the brain and **enterochromaffin cells** of the intestinal epithelium are also susceptible to HIV infection.

The most important outcome of HIV infection is the depletion of T4 helper cells and **immunodeficiency,** particularly the cell mediated aspect of immunity. It is generally agreed that the direct destruction of T4 cells by HIV replication alone cannot explain the immunodeficiency; there are too few HIV infected T4 cells in an infected person.

Involvement of the brain is common among persons infected by the HIV. Many believe that **brain damage** is due to the migration of HIV-infected macrophage into the brain and to the release by these macrophages of cytokines toxic to brain cells and the myelin.

Diagnosis

The diagnosis of HIV infection is generally achieved through **antibody detection** with a variety of serologic tests. Persons infected by the HIV develop a detectable antibody within 6–12 weeks; but, there are rare exceptions. **Indeterminate tests** refer to those sera that react only with the p24. Such a test is not indicative of HIV infection. In situations where antibody detection is not meaningful (e.g., young infants), the demonstration of HIV by **virus culture** or of **HIV gene sequences** (with or without prior gene amplification) is generally used. Knowledge of HIV infection status is useful because it allows infected persons to seek antiretroviral treatment and to avoid infecting others.

The diagnosis of AIDS is established by the following two criteria: (1) laboratory evidence of HIV infection, and (2) a disease indicative of a defect in cell-mediated immunity in a person with no known cause for diminished resistance to disease. Indicator diseases include *Pneumocystis carinii* pneumonia, Kaposi's sarcoma, HIV encephalopathy, extrapulmonary tuberculosis, disseminated histoplasmosis, and serious opportunistic infections. In 1992, the CDC proposed that the diagnosis of AIDS be based on the following criteria: **laboratory evidence of HIV infection plus a CD4 cell count of less than 200/mm³.**

Three laboratory tests are now being used to measure the severity of HIV infection—**CD4 lymphocyte count, p24 antigenemia,** and serum level of β_2 **microglobulin.** Uninfected persons and many healthy HIV-infected subjects have a CD4 lymphocyte count of greater than or equal to 500/mm³ while most patients with AIDS have less than 200/mm³. Presence of measurable p24 in the blood is an indication of increasing virus production as the host defense wanes. The β_2 microglobulin is a component of the major histocompatibility complex found on all cells. Its serum level rises with advanced disease (possibly due to increase in lymphocyte destruction).

In considering the diagnosis of HIV infections and AIDS, it is useful to know the natural history of the HIV infection (Fig. 43.3). A small number of persons with CD4 T lymphocyte depletion, but without evidence of HIV infection, have been reported. The basis for this CD4 lymphocyte depletion is not known at this time. This **idiopathic CD4⁺ T lymphocytopenia** is believed to be a rare syndrome, noninfectious, and distinct from AIDS epidemiologically.

Treatment

Zidovudine and **interferon-α** have been approved by the FDA for the treatment of AIDS. Zidovudine reduces the mortality, partially restores immunity, and improves performance in patients with AIDS. It does not cure the infection and is myelotoxic. Interferon-α has been shown to induce complete or major regression of Kaposi's sarcoma in about 40% of treated patients. Other 2′,3′-deoxynucleosides, such as **didanosine** and **zalcitadine,** have also been approved by the FDA

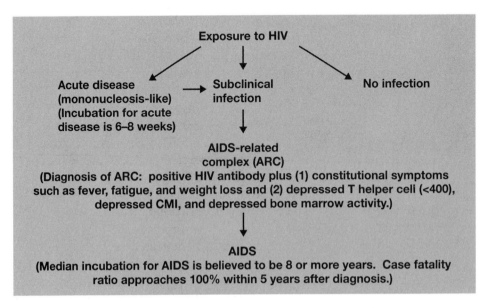

Figure 43.3.

Natural history of HIV infection.

for the treatment of AIDS. Curing HIV infection is a very difficult task because of the **provirus in latency.** To rid the host of all latent provirus, one must be able to identify and selectively kill all cells that carry latent provirus. There is to date no known way of accomplishing this task.

Zidovudine, didanosine, and zalcitadine are nucleoside analogs. After conversion to the triphosphate derivative, they inhibit the reverse transcriptase. They are also incorporated into elongating DNA and, thereby, prevent further chain elongation.

Epidemiology and Prevention

The principal sources of HIV are the **blood** and **genital secretions** of HIV infected persons. Other body secretions or fluids may contain HIV in low concentrations and are probably unimportant in transmission. Three main modes of transmission have been recognized: (1) **sexual contact** with an infected person, (2) **inoculation of blood or blood products** contaminated by HIV (mainly through needle sharing among IV drug users), and (3) **perinatal transmission** from an infected woman to her fetus or infant. No other mode of transmission has been firmly established. While intact skin definitely protects against HIV infection, it is not clear whether intact mucosa provides similar protection. A recent report documented HIV transmission from one child to another; it is unclear how this transmission occurs.

Over 80,000 cases of AIDS in the United States had been reported to the CDC as of December 31, 1988. A projected number of cases by December 1992 is about 365,000. In the United States, the distribution of AIDS cases varies according to **age, sex, geographic location,** and **race.** As of December 31, 1988, 98% were in adults; 91% of the adult cases were in men; most were in urban areas; and Blacks and Hispanics are three times more likely than Whites to acquire AIDS. Heterosexually acquired AIDS is increasing in frequency in the United States in recent years. For example, there were 9288 cases attributed to heterosexual transmission in 1993, compared to 4045 in 1992.

The CDC has estimated that about 0.5% of the United States population is infected by the HIV. Note that the percentages of positives vary greatly among population groups and in geographic locations (Table 43.1).

Immunoprophylaxis and chemoprophylaxis against HIV are ineffective; therefore, prevention depends on the **interception of transmission.** Fortunately, the sources of HIV and its modes of transmission are well established. In principle, it is easy to prevent HIV infections by avoiding the type of behavior that permits HIV transmission, such as sharing a needle with another person, having sex with

TABLE 43.1. Human Immunodeficiency Virus Antibody Prevalence Among Population Groups in the United States[a]

Population characteristics	HIV antibody-positive (%)
A. General Population	
Blood donors (1988)	0.01
Civilian applicants for military service (1985–1988)	0.14
Parturient women: California	0.1
New York	0.7
College students	0.2
Sentinel hospital patients	0.1–0.8[b]
B. High-Risk Populations	
Male prostitutes: New York City	50
Female prostitutes: South Florida	41
San Francisco	5
Las Vegas	0
Memphis	0
Homosexual/bisexual: San Francisco	50
Albuquerque	12
IV drug users: New York	50
San Antonio	1
Heterosexual partners of HIV-infected: California, females	24
California, males	0
New York City, females	45
New York City, males	50
Wives of HIV-infected hemophiliacs	14

[a] Data from St. Louis ME et al. MMWR 1987; 36:S-6 and 1989; 38:S-4.
[b] A recent publication [(St. Louis ME, et al. (1990): Seroprevalence rates of human immunodeficiency virus infection at Sentinel Hospitals in the United States. N Engl J Med 1990;323:213)] reported seroprevalence rates as high as 7–8% (average 1–3%).

a person known to be at risk for HIV infection, avoiding sex with casual partners and with multiple partners, avoiding anal intercourse, and using condoms. Blood prescreened for HIV antibodies appears to be quite safe; the risk of transmission is less than 1/40,000 units. The antihemophiliac factor, prepared by approved procedures, is now free from the HIV.

SUMMARY

1. **Human lentiviruses include human immunodeficiency viruses 1 and 2 (HIV 1 and HIV 2). These two viruses show a 50% nucleic acid homology. Their p24 antigens cross-react in serologic tests. Both cause AIDS in humans**

but HIV 2 infections tend to be less severe. The HIV 2 infections are found chiefly in West Africa, while HIV 1 infections are now worldwide in distribution. SIVs are monkey lentiviruses genetically and antigenically related to HIV 2. Accidental innoculation of SIV may result in seroconversion in humans.

2. The HIV genome consists of three structural genes (*gag*, *pol*, and *env*) and several regulatory genes (*tat*, *nef*, etc.) flanked by regulatory sequences known as lateral terminal repeats (LTR).

3. *Gag* gene product is cleaved by a virus specified protease into three core proteins, one of which is the p24 antigen; *pol* gene product, into three enzymes (reverse transcriptase, protease, and endonuclease); and *env* gene product, into two envelope antigens (gp 120 and gp41).

4. Key virion proteins are gp 120 (virion attachment), gp 41 (fusion factor), p24 (core component), and reverse transcriptase (initiation of synthetic phase). Antibodies against gp41 and p24 are important in the diagnosis of HIV infection. The p24 of HIV 1 and HIV 2 cross-react serologically.

5. After uncoating, the viral genome is reverse transcribed to proviral DNA. Proviral DNA is integrated into host DNA as provirus. The expression of provirus is highly regulated. The tat protein (early gene product) binds on to a regulatory sequence on LTR and, thereby, enhances the expression of provirus by more than 1000-folds. In resting CD4 lymphocytes carrying the provirus, *tat* gene is for practical purpose not expressed and the provirus is also not expressed (latency). When the CD4 lymphocyte is activated, the *tat* gene is also expressed. The tat protein will then enhance expression of the provirus; this results in the formation of numerous progeny virions and the infection of a new crop of cells.

6. The HIV mutates at very high frequency during reverse transcription; therefore, HIV isolates are very heterogenous genomically, serologically, and biologically. The coexistence of genomically distinct (by restriction fragment length study) HIV in the same patient has been documented. Mutation may affect the *env* gene (coding for gp120) and produces mutants that are poorly neutralized by existing neutralizing antibody. Variants differing in cell tropism and rapidity of replication are known. Zidovudine-resistant mutants have become troublesome clinically.

7. The CD4 molecules bind firmly to gp120. Therefore, cells rich in CD4 molecules (T helper lymphocytes and a subpopulation of macrophages) are

the principal but may not be the exclusive target cells of HIV. In activated CD4 lymphocytes, HIV replicates rapidly releasing many progeny virions and killing the infected cell. In macrophages, HIV multiplies slowly without killing the cell. End results are the slow depletion of CD4 lymphocytes, immunodeficiency, and encephalopathy. Encephalopathy is probably due to migration of HIV infected macrophages to the brain and the release by these macrophages of cytokines toxic to the brain.

8. The median interval between HIV infection and clinical evidence of immunodeficiency is about 8–10 years. Clinical evidence of immunodeficiency includes opportunistic infections and Kaposi's sarcoma.

9. Diagnosis of HIV infection is usually based on a serologic test for the HIV antibody. Diagnosis of AIDS is established by positive tests for HIV or HIV antibody and a disease indicative of impairment in cell-mediated immunity in a previously healthy person. (Recently, proposed criteria for the diagnosis of AIDS consist of laboratory evidence of HIV infection and a CD4 cell count of less than 200.)

10. The CD4 lymphocyte is an important marker of immunodeficiency. Uninfected persons and many healthy HIV-infected subjects have a CD4 lymphocyte count of greater than or equal to $500/mm^3$; most AIDS patients have less than $200/mm^3$.

11. Zidovudine, didanosine, and zalcitadine temporarily arrests the progression of HIV infections. Interferon-α is useful in treating Kaposi's sarcoma. Because no drug (approved or experimental) can destroy the provirus, the curing the HIV infection appears unlikely in the foreseeable future.

12. The main sources of HIV are the blood and genital secretion of HIV infected persons. Modes of transmission are sexual intercourse with infected persons, inoculation of blood or blood products contaminated by HIV, and perinatal transmission from an infected woman to her fetus or neonate.

13. Immuno- and chemoprophylaxis are ineffective; therefore, prevention depends on interception of HIV transmission.

14. Idiopathic $CD4^+$ T lymphocytopenia is a rare syndrome with the following characteristics: (1)CD4 lymphocyte depletion; (2) no serologic evidence of HIV infection; and, (3) no known explanation for the depletion of CD4 lymphocyte. This condition is known as idiophatic CD4 lymphocytopenia.

REFERENCES

Bartlett JG (1993): Zidovudine now or later? N Engl J Med 329:351.

Borkowsky W et al. (1992): Early diagnosis of HIV infection in children <6 months of age: comparison of polymerase chain reaction, culture, and plasma antigen capture techniques. J Inf Dis 166:616.

Centers for Disease Control (1992): Projections of the number of persons diagnosed with AIDS and the number of immunosuppressed persons, United States 1992–1994. MMWR 41 (RR18):1.

Centers for Disease Control (1992): 1993 revised classification system for HIV infection and expanded surveillance case definition for AIDS among adolescents and adults. MMWR 41(RR17):1

Centers for Disease Control (1993): Update: Investigations of patients who had been treated by HIV-infected health care workers. MMWR 42:329.

Centers for Disease Control (1993): Impact of the expanded AIDS surveillance and case definition on AIDS case reporting. MMWR 42:308.

Centers for Disease Control (1993): Use of vaccines and immune globulins in persons with altered immunocompetence. MMWR 42 (RR4):1.

Centers for Disease Control (1994): Heterosexually acquired AIDS—United States, 1993. MMWR 43:155.

Centers for Disease Control (1994): HIV transmission in household settings. MMWR 43:347.

Daar ES et al. (1991): Transient high levels of viremia in patients with primary HIV-1 infection. N Engl J Med 324:961.

Essex M (1994): SIV in people. N Engl J Med 330:329.

European Collaborative Study (1991): Children born to women with HIV-1 infection: natural history and risk of transmission. Lancet 337:253.

Fauci AS (1993): CD4+ T-lymphocytopenia without HIV infection—no lights, no camera, just facts. N Engl J Med 328:429.

Farzadegan H et al. (1993): Detection of HIV 1 infection by polymerase chain reaction in a cohort of seronegative IV drug users. J Inf Dis 168:327.

Greene WC (1991): The molecular biology of HIV-1 infection. N Engl J Med 314:308.

Heagarty MC, Abrams EJ (1992): Caring for HIV infected women and children. N Engl J Med 326:887.

Hirsch MS, D'Aquila RT (1993): Therapy for HIV infections. N Engl J Med 328:1686.

Hughes MD et al (1994): Within-subject variation in CD4 lymphocyte count in asymptomatic HIV infection: implications for patient monitoring. J Inf Dis 168:28.

Jackson JB et al. (1990): Absence of HIV infection in blood donors with indeterminate western blot tests for antibody to HIV-1. N Engl J Med 322:217.

Letvin NL (1993): Vaccines against HIV—progress and prospects. N Engl J Med 329:1400.

Mann JM (1993): AIDS in the 1900s: A global analysis. The Pharos 56 (3):2.

Simonds RJ, Roger MF (1993): HIV prevention—bring the message home. N Engl J Med 329:1883.

REVIEW QUESTIONS

For questions 1 to 9, choose the ONE BEST answer or completion.

1. Human immunodeficiency virus type 2
   a) and HIV 1 are both lentiviruses
   b) is an antigenic variant of HIV 1
   c) and HIV 1 infections are prevalent worldwide

2. About the HIV proviral genome:
   a) it contains three structural genes, several regulatory genes, two or more genes of unknown function, and the lateral terminal repeats
   b) a mutation of that portion of *pol* gene that codes for the reverse transcriptase (assuming that the mutation results in defective reverse transcriptase) should suppress expression of the proviral DNA and the release of progeny virion
   c) tat protein enhances expression of virion RNA
   d) lateral terminal repeats protein is essential for maintaining the proviral DNA in the integrated state

3. Identify the incorrect statements about HIV proteins in the virion.
   a) A virion with defective reverse transcriptase can initiate but cannot complete the virus replication cycle.
   b) The HIV protease is responsible for post-translation modification of polypeptides.
   c) Attachment and penetration steps require the gp120 and gp41 of the virion.
   d) A positive serologic reaction to p24 is diagnostic of human immunodeficiency virus type 1 infection.

4. Identify the incorrect statements about heterogeneity of HIV isolates.
   a) The high frequency of errors in the reverse transcription of the viral genome by reverse transcriptase is believed to be responsible for the heterogeneity.
   b) Like many other viruses, epidemiologically unrelated virus isolates are genomically distinct (based on restriction fragment length analysis) but isolates from the same person over time remain genomically identical.
   c) Despite the presence of neutralizing antibody in high titer in an AIDS patient, it is possible (occasionally) to obtain from the blood of the same patient an HIV isolate that is not neutralizable by the patient's serum.
   d) The HIV isolates may have different degrees of tropism for T helper lymphocytes and macrophages.

5. Identify the incorrect statement about the pathogenesis of HIV infection.

a) Principal target cells are the CD4 + macrophages and lymphocytes.
b) Immunodeficiency is due primarily, but not exclusively, to the slow destruction of T helper lymphocytes.
c) The prolonged persistence of HIV is due to its ability to remain latent in nonactivated CD4 + lymphocytes, or its ability to replicate in but without killing the macrophages or both.
d) Encephalopathy in AIDS is believed to be due to the migration of HIV-infected macrophages to the brain and the release of cytokines by these macrophages.
e) The most reliable predictor of the severity of immunodeficiency is the serum level of p24.

6. About the diagnosis of HIV infection:
   a) it is usually based on antibody study
   b) the absence of HIV antibody invariably excludes HIV infection
   c) human immunodeficiency viruses types 1 and 2 infection cannot be distinguished by antibody testing
   d) the presence of HIV antibody invariably proving HIV infection

7. The diagnosis of AIDS is established by
   a) a positive HIV antibody test
   b) a serious opportunistic infection
   c) a positive blood culture for HIV
   d) both a laboratory evidence of HIV infection and a disease indicative of impaired cell mediated immunity

8. Identify the incorrect statement on zidovudine.
   a) zidovudine triphosphate interferes with reverse transcription of HIV genome.
   b) zidovudine temporarily arrests or slow down the progression of AIDS.
   c) zidovudine is not expected to destroy the provirus.
   d) Resistant HIV mutants are common in AIDS patients on prolonged therapy.
   e) zidovudine invariably prevents HIV infections when used in postexposure chemoprophylaxis.

9. Identify the least accurate statement about HIV transmission.
   a) The main sources of HIV are the blood and sexual secretion of HIV-infected persons.
   b) The principal modes of transmission include sexual intercourse with HIV-seropositive persons, inoculation of HIV-contaminated blood or blood products, and mother to fetus during perinatal period.
   c) Intercepting transmission is the most effective way of preventing HIV infection.
   d) Transmission from health care providers to patients have been documented despite stringent adherence to precautionary measures.

ANSWERS TO REVIEW QUESTIONS

1. *a* Both HIV 1 and HIV 2 are distinct species; they show only 50% homology. Only the p24 antigens cross-react. The HIV 2 is confined largely to West Africa. Therefore, *b* and *c* are incorrect.

2. *a* Once the proviral DNA is formed, RT is no longer necessary for the completion of the viral replication cycle. The tat protein does not act on virion RNA; it acts on the provirus. The LTR is the regulatory sequence in which are found enhancer, suppressor, and promoter regions; it does not code for protein. Therefore, *b, c,* and *d* are wrong.

3. *d* The p24 antigens of HIV 1 and HIV 2 cross-react; therefore, antibody to p24 may be due to HIV 1 or HIV 2 infection. Occasionally, a person who is not at risk for HIV infection may have a positive reaction to p24 only; such a reaction is called "indeterminate."

4. *b* The second half of *b* is incorrect; the coexistence of a large number of related but genomically distinct HIV in the same person has been reported.

5. *e* The CD4 lymphocyte count is the most reliable predictor.

6. *a* It usually takes 6–12 weeks for an infected person to develop HIV antibody (*b* is wrong). Both HIV 1 and HIV 2 infections can be distinguished by testing for antibodies against the gp41 (*c* is wrong). Maternal antibody in young infants complicates the interpretation of HIV testing in young infants; only about one-third of HIV seropositive young infants are infected by the HIV (*d* is wrong).

7. *d* Both *a* and *c* indicate HIV infection not AIDS. *b* Indicates impairment of cell mediated immunity that may be due to diseases other than AIDS. (In 1992, the CDC proposed that the diagnosis of AIDS be based on laboratory evidence of HIV infection in a person with a CD4 cell count of less than 200.)

8. *e* There were three reports (N Engl J Med 1991;324:1062) of accidental or intentional inoculation of HIV-positive blood and prompt treatment with zidovudine (0.75–6 h after inoculation). All three subjects developed symptoms and signs of acute HIV infection and HIV antibodies 6–12 weeks after blood inoculation.

9. *d* There was a report (see reference) of HIV transmission from a dental surgeon to three of his patients; but the investigators could not be absolutely certain about stringent adherence to precautionary measures. Of the four statements, *d* is the least accurate.

THE PICORNAVIRUS FAMILY

The picornavirus (pico rna viruses) family includes over 150 "species" that are pathogenic for humans. Infections by these viruses are common throughout the world. While most infections are inapparent or minor, severe infections are not uncommon. Among the severe infections are encephalitis, poliomyelitis, aseptic meningitis, acute myocarditis, and hepatitis. Effective active and passive immunoprophylaxis are available for the prevention and modification of some of these infections.

FAMILY CHARACTERISTICS

Morphology

The picornaviruses are small (~27 nm in diameter). These viruses have icosahedral capsid symmetry and are not enveloped.

Genomic Chemistry

The genome is a nonsegmented single-stranded positive-sense RNA of about 8 kb.

Replication Strategy

The **genomic RNA** and **viral mRNA** are identical. Hence, after uncoating, the genomic RNA is translated into a **polyprotein.** This polyprotein is cleaved presumably by a **virus-specified protease** into a RNA replicase and capsid proteins. The RNA replicase then synthesizes a negative-sense RNA that complexes with the original positive-sense RNA to form a **replicative intermediate.** Using this replicative intermediate as a template, many positive-sense RNAs are synthesized. The positive-sense RNAs are translated into capsid and other proteins. When capsid proteins have reached a critical concentration, they will condense on the positive-sense RNA to form nucleocapsids. In this type of replicative strategy, the naked gene is infectious and virion-associated polymerase is unnecessary.

"Species"

There are over 150 medically important species. These species are grouped into two genera: **enteroviruses** and **rhinoviruses.** Enteroviruses primarily inhabit the human intestines and are stable at low pH, such as in gastric juice. This genus includes polioviruses 1, 2, and 3, coxsackieviruses A (many types), coxsackieviruses B (many types), echoviruses (many types), hepatitis A virus or (HAV) (1 type), and enteroviruses (many types). Rhinoviruses inhabit the human upper respiratory tract and are unstable in acidic pH; there are over 100 types of rhinoviruses. The picornaviruses are typed by **reciprocal cross-neutralization.** Generally, there is no cross-reactivity between types as determined by this test. Viruses so typed are frequently referred to as **serotypes** or **immunotypes.** There is virtually complete immunity to homologous immunotype and little or no immunity to heterologous immunotypes. There is no agreement whether each type is equivalent to a species. However, it is useful to remember whether a virus has one, few, or many serotypes. Specific virologic diagnosis and the feasibility of vaccine production are more difficult for viruses that have many serotypes. Also, the frequency of infections by a specific virus in a lifetime depends on the number of serotypes.

Interference

Interference of the growth of one enterovirus by another enterovirus has been observed in the human host.

Example 1: Active multiplication of a vaccine poliovirus prevents the growth of a superinfecting wild poliovirus (an important point to remember in epidemic control).

Example 2: After receiving the first dose of trivalent polio vaccine, not all three types of polioviruses will successfully establish infection, hence immunity, in the vaccinated person (an explanation why primary polio immunization requires a series of three doses).

Example 3: A vaccine poliovirus fed to a child with an active enterovirus infection may not successfully establish an infection.

This interference among enteroviruses is believed to be due to the blocking of virus receptors by the first virus.

ENTEROVIRUSES

Pathogenesis

Infections occur primarily through ingestion of **contaminated food** or drinking **contaminated water.** The primary target is the **intestinal mucosa** including the **lymphoid tissue.** (For HAV or enterovirus 72, the primary target may be some lymphoid tissues of the GI tract rather than intestinal mucosa.) Multiplication in the primary target may be followed by a transient **viremia** and dissemination of virus to **secondary targets.** Important secondary targets are:

1. Brain and spinal cord (polioviruses 1, 2 and 3, and enterovirus 71).
2. Meninges (all enteroviruses).
3. Hepatocyte (enterovirus 72 also known as HAV).
4. Muscles (coxsackieviruses).
5. Myo- and pericardium (coxsackievirus).
6. Skin resulting in acute exanthema (coxsackieviruses and echoviruses).
7. Pancreas (coxsackievirus).

All infections are **acute** in nature in immunocompetent persons; chronic or latent infections do not occur. But **fecal excretion** of viruses may persist for up to 2 months after recovery. In immunologically immature subjects (young infants), coxsackievirus infections tend to be severe and generalized (involving the CNS, heart, and liver).

Diagnosis

It is difficult to establish specific virologic diagnosis of enterovirus infections because of the large number of serotypes. However, in **paralytic disease** (polio or polio-like), **acute hepatitis,** and **acute encephalitis,** etiologic diagnosis is essential. In paralytic disease, one must know if paralysis is due to wild poliovirus, vaccine poliovirus, enterovirus 71, or other enteroviruses. Etiologic diagnosis can be achieved by culturing the virus in feces and typing the virus. In acute hepatitis, it is important to determine which of the hepatitis viruses causes the hepatitis. If it is due to HAV, IgM antiHAV is almost always positive. The following four tests are usually required in the etiologic diagnosis of acute hepatitis: IgM antiHAV, IgM antiHB$_c$, HB$_s$, and IgM antiHD (see also Chapter 41). For acute encephalitis, see Chapter 45 on togavirus.

Treatment

Specific antiviral agents are not available.

Epidemiology and Prevention

Infections usually occur through the eating of contaminated food or drinking of contaminated water. The main source of enteroviruses is **fecal materials** from infected persons. It is useful to remember that an infected person may excrete virus for many weeks after infection, that the enterovirus is stable in the environment, and that gastric juice cannot inactivate the virus. Enteroviruses are widely distributed throughout the world. In communities with **poor hygienic practices,** infections by most ''species'' occur early in life. In the United States, surveys for antibody against a specific enterovirus have shown that about one-third of healthy adults are immune to that virus. An important source of enteroviruses in the United States is the **child day care center.**

As with all infectious agents transmitted by the fecal-oral route, the chance of acquiring infections by the enterovirus can be minimized by attendance to personal hygiene and avoidance of food or water that have a high chance of fecal contamination. Enteroviruses can be reliably destroyed by boiling.

Active immunoprophylaxis against polioviruses and passive immunoprophylaxis against the HAV are available (see sections on polio immunization and human Ig in HAV infection). There is an effective experimental HAV vaccine (inactivated) that is awaiting approval by the FDA.

RHINOVIRUSES

Pathogenesis

The primary target is the **epithelium of the upper respiratory tract,** especially that of the nasal cavity. The nasal secretion of an infected person is the main source of rhinovirus. The virus reaches its target usually through indirect contact or aerosolized nasal secretion. There is **no secondary target;** but, on rare occasion, the virus may spread to the lower respiratory tract. Rhinoviruses cause common cold, a minor illness except in patients with severe asthma.

Diagnosis

Specific virologic diagnosis is difficult and unnecessary.

Treatment

There is no specific antiviral treatment.

Epidemiology and Prevention

There are more than 100 immunotypes of rhinoviruses. Presumably, every person can expect infections by most of the rhinoviruses. Because young subjects have fewer experiences with the rhinovirus than older persons, common colds are more common among young children than older adults. Avoiding contact with nasal secretions of infected persons reduces the chance of infections. Experimental application of interferon locally also reduces the chance of rhinovirus infection. Because of the large number of immunotypes, the preparation of a vaccine against rhinovirus infection is impractical.

POLIOVIRUS VACCINES

The introduction of polio vaccines is one of the major advances of modern medicine. The average annual incidence of poliomyelitis in the United States has dramatically declined from over 15,000 to about 10 cases since the introduction of polio vaccines. Most of the poliomyelitis cases seen nowadays in the United

States are vaccine associated. Prevention of poliomyelitis in the United States requires the maintenance of adequate levels of community immunity against the poliovirus through immunization.

Two types of polio vaccines are currently licensed in the United States: **oral polio vaccine (OPV)** and **inactivated polio vaccine (IPV).** The OPV contains live attenuated poliovirus types 1, 2, and 3 and is given orally, while IPV contains inactivated viruses (also types 1, 2, and 3), but must be given subcutaneously. Both are effective in preventing poliomyelitis, but OPV is the preferred vaccine for primary immunization of children in the United States. The OPV is preferred because it is simpler to administer, is well accepted by patients, induces intestinal immunity that provides resistance to reinfection by wild poliovirus, results in immunization of some contacts of the vaccinated person, and interferes with simultaneous infection by wild poliovirus. But OPV has been associated with paralytic disease in the vaccinated person or their close contacts. The incidence of vaccine-associated poliomyelitis in the United States is 1 per 1 to 3 million doses of vaccine distributed or 8/year. Adults appear to be more susceptible to vaccine-associated poliomyelitis. Relative advantages and disadvantages of OPV and IPV are summarized in Table 44.1.

Primary immunization with OPV should be started as soon as possible after 6 weeks of age. It consists of three doses at intervals of 8 weeks. A supplementary dose just prior to school entry is recommended. The schedule for primary immunization with IPV is the same as OPV except that a fourth dose is given 12 months after the third dose. Additional supplementary doses once every 5 years are recommended when IPV is used in primary immunization.

Routine primary polio immunization of adults ($\geq$ 18 years old) residing in the United States is unnecessary because most are already immune and have only a small risk of exposure to wild poliovirus in the United States. For adults who

TABLE 44.1. Advantages and Disadvantages of OPV and IPV

Characteristic	OPV	IPV or EIPV
Route of administration	Oral	Subcutaneous
Acceptability to the vaccinated person	Well accepted	Not acceptable
Supplementary dose after the primary course	One	Every 5 years
Intestinal immunity	Yes	Less so than OPV
Interference with simultaneous infection by wild poliovirus	Yes	No
Vaccine-associated poliomyelitis among:		
vaccinated persons	Yes	No
household contacts of the vaccinated person	Yes	No

had not been immunized and are at increased risk of exposure to wild poliovirus, primary immunization with IPV is recommended. Persons who are at increased risk of exposure to wild poliovirus include: members of a community with disease caused by wild poliovirus, travelers to areas where poliomyelitis is epidemic or endemic, persons who handle materials may contain wild poliovirus, and that workers in close contact with patients who may be excreting wild poliovirus.

Inactivated polio vaccine is recommended for the immunization of immunodeficient patients and their household contacts. In principle, one avoids immunizing pregnant women; but, if immediate protection against poliomyelitis is needed, OPV is recommended. There is no convincing evidence for adverse effect of OPV on developing fetuses.

Enhanced potency inactivated polio vaccine (EIPV) is a refinement of IPV. EIPV produces higher seroconversion rates and higher serum antibody levels than IPV and OPV. EIPV is the preferred vaccine in all situations where IPV is indicated.

PASSIVE IMMUNIZATION IN HEPATITIS A VIRUS

The natural history of HAV infection consists of the following four sequential stages: **virus multiplication at the primary target** without clinical manifestation, a brief **viremic phase,** virus multiplication in and injury to **secondary targets,** and **quenching** of the infection. Severity of the disease depends on the **extent of injury to the secondary target,** which is the hepatocyte. In this type of infection, it is often possible to reduce the severity or even abort the development of the disease by placing a **barrier between the primary and secondary targets** before the viremic phase. Indeed, by inoculating persons exposed to HAV with human immunoglobulins (i.e., passive immunization) early in the incubation, the severity of acute hepatitis is significantly reduced. For persons at higher risk of HAV infections (e.g., new workers in a setting where the level of hygienic practice among the indigenous populations is low) administration of HAV antibody (i.e., human immunoglobulins) is recommended.

POSTPOLIO SYNDROME

This syndrome refers to symptoms of new weakness, fatigue, and pain after recovery from acute poliomyelitis. Typically 25–35 years after the original attack, some begin to develop insidiously new fatigability, weakness, loss of muscle bulk, and at times, unusual pain. These symptoms usually affect the previously involved muscles but may also occur in muscle groups believed to be unaffected in the original attack of poliomyelitis. There is evidence of active denervation and muscle atrophy. What causes the abnormality is not known.

SUMMARY

1. Picornaviruses are small and nonenveloped and have nonsegmented single-stranded positive-sense RNA.

2. Its genome and mRNA are the same. The first step in its synthetic phase is the translation of uncoated viral gene into viral proteins. One viral protein is a RNA replicase (RNA dependent RNA polymerase). This enzyme synthesizes a negative-sense RNA that complexes with the original genome to form a double-stranded RNA (known as replicative intermediate). From this replicative intermediate, many copies of viral mRNA (viral genomes) are formed.

3. Naked picornavirus RNA are infectious (can be transfected). Virion-associated polymerase is unnecessary.

4. There are more than 150 species (or types) of pathogenic picornaviruses. Species are distinguished by cross-neutralization. There is little or no cross-reactivity between species.

5. Picornaviruses are divided into two genera: enteroviruses and rhinoviruses. Enteroviruses are stable in acidic environment and multiply primarily in intestinal epithelium. Rhinoviruses are unstable in acidic environment and multiply primarily in epithelium of the upper respiratory tract. Medically important species of enteroviruses are polioviruses (3 serotypes) coxsackieviruses (many serotypes), echoviruses (many serotypes), and enteroviruses (many serotypes). Enterovirus 72 is the hepatitis A virus (HAV).

6. Enterovirus infections may have a viremic phase during which the virus reaches secondary target organs. Important secondary targets include the CNS, the meninges, the liver, the muscle (including myocardium), and the skin.

7. Etiologic diagnosis is usually unnecessary except in the following three conditions: poliomyelitis (to determine if the disease is due to wild or vaccine poliovirus or to other enteroviruses), acute hepatitis (to determine if it is due to hepatitis A, B, C, D, or E viruses) or acute encephalitis (see Chapter 46).

8. Enteroviruses are transmitted primarily by the fecal-oral route.

9. Live attenuated or inactivated poliovaccine induces solid immunity against infection by poliovirus types 1, 2, and 3.

10. Postpolio syndrome refers to symptoms of new weakness, fatigue, and pain years after recovery from acute poliomyelitis. What causes this reappearance of symptoms is not known.

11. Administration of human Ig during incubation reduces the severity of hepatitis due to HAV.

12. Interference among enteroviruses is responsible for the occasional failure of the attenuated poliovirus to establish infection in the vaccinated person.

13. The small number of poliomyelitis cases seen annually in the United States are mostly due to infections by vaccine poliovirus.

14. Rhinoviruses cause acute upper respiratory infections (usually acute rhinitis or common cold). There are over 100 serotypes of human rhinoviruses.

REFERENCES

Abraham R et al. (1993): Shedding of virulent poliovirus revertants during immunization with OPV and with EIPV. J Inf Dis 168:1105.

Alexander JP et al. (1994): Enterovirus 71 infections and neurologic disease—U.S.A., 1977 to 1991. J Inf Dis 169:905.

Al-Nakib W, Tyrrell DAJ (1988): *Picornaviridae*: rhinoviruses—common cold viruses. In Lennette EH, Halonen P, Murphy FA (eds): Laboratory Diagnosis of Infectious Diseases Principles and Practice, Vol. 2. New York: Springer-Verlag, pp 723–742.

Bancroft WH (1992): Hepatitis A vaccine. N Engl J Med 327:488.

Berlin LE et al. (1993): Aseptic meningitis in infants <2 years of age: diagnosis and etiology. J Inf Dis 168:888.

Center for Disease Control (1990): Update: progress toward eradicating poliomyelitis from the Americas. MMWR 39:557.

Immunization Practices Advisory Committee (1982): Poliomyelitis prevention. MMWR 31:22.

Lemon SM (1985): Type A viral hepatitis. N Engl J Med 313:1059.

Kapsenberg JG (1988): *Picornaviridae*: the enteroviruses (polioviruses, coxsackieviruses, echoviruses). In Lennette EH, Halonen P, Murphy FA (eds): Laboratory Diagnosis of Infectious Diseases Principles and Practice, Vol. 2. New York: Springer-Verlag, pp 692–722.

Munsat TL (1991): Poliomyelitis—New problems with an old disease. N Engl J Med 324:1206.

Nkowane BM, Wassilak SGF, Orenstein WA, Bart KJ, Schonberger LB, Hinman AR, Kew OM (1987): Vaccine-associated paralytic poliomyelitis. JAMA 257:1335.

Robertson BH, Khanna B., Nainan OV, Margolis HS (1991): Epidemiologic patterns of wild-type HAV determined by genetic variation. J Inf Dis 163:286.

Tyrrell DAJ (1988): Hot news on the common cold. Annu Rev Microbiol 42:35.

REVIEW QUESTIONS

> For questions 1 to 9, choose the ONE
> BEST answer or completion.

1. Picornavirus
   a) is an enveloped virus
   b) genome is single-stranded negative-sense RNA
   c) RNA is infectious (can be transfected)
   d) virion contains a RNA replicase

2. One of the following statements on enteroviruses is incorrect. Enteroviruses include
   a) poliovirus types 1, 2, and 3
   b) many types of coxsackieviruses
   c) many types of echoviruses
   d) the hepatitis A virus
   e) the hepatitis E virus

3. Identify the incorrect statement about enterovirus infections.
   a) Enteroviruses may localize primarily in the intestinal epithelium and/or adjacent lymphoid tissues.
   b) Enteroviruses may have a viremic phase.
   c) Enteroviruses may involve secondary target organs distant from the primary site of virus replication.
   d) Enteroviruses are frequently subclinical.
   e) Human Ig has been found effective in treating coxsackievirus-related myocarditis.

4. Strong association has not been established between
   a) enterovirus 71 and poliomyelitis-like disease
   b) coxsackievirus and acute myocarditis
   c) many species of enteroviruses and aseptic (viral) meningitis
   d) many species of enteroviruses and acute exanthema
   e) enteroviruses and heterophile-negative mononucleosis

5. In medical practice in the United States etiologic diagnosis (identifying the virus responsible for the infection) must be established in
   a) all cases of aseptic (viral) meningitis
   b) all cases of acute myocarditis
   c) all cases of acute exanthema
   d) all cases of poliomyelitis or polio-like diseases

6. About the epidemiology and prevention of enterovirus infections:
   a) virus is no longer present in the feces of a person who has just recovered from an acute infection
   b) a person who has no immunity against the HAV and who plans to work a day care center for preschool children should receive a preemployment dose of human immunoglobulin.

c) a medical student who has received all immunizations required for employment in a teaching hospital in the United States need not receive further immunoprophylaxis (active or passive) prior to departure to rural Mexico for 3 months of medical training.

7. One of the following statements on trivalent oral poliovaccine is incorrect. Trivalent oral poliovaccine

a) is recommended for all U.S. residents who are less than 21 years old, have not received polio vaccination, and have no past history of poliomyelitis

b) have caused poliomyelitis in a small number ($<1/0.5$ million) of vaccinated persons.

c) given in one single dose, is sufficient to induce immunity against the three types of poliovirus

d) is the recommended vaccine for inducing immunity against poliomyelitis in persons <21 years old in the United States

8. The cause of postpolio syndrome is

a) reactivation of poliovirus in latency

b) mutation of poliovirus that persists in the spinal cord

c) immune-mediated damage

d) metabolic exhaustion

e) unknown

9. Rhinovirus infection

a) always results in acute rhinitis

b) is equally likely to occur among senior citizens or preschool children

c) may aggravate the symptoms of asthma

d) vaccine is not available because of the difficulty of growing common cold virus in cell culture

ANSWERS TO REVIEW QUESTIONS

1. *c*

2. *e* There are similarities between HAV and HEV. But HEV has not been sufficiently characterized to be assigned to a family or genus.

3. *e* Passive immunization with Ig are effective in the prevention or modification of certain

virus infections, but not in treatment of virus diseases.

4. *e*

5. *d* Virologic diagnosis must be performed in all cases of poliomyelitis or polio-like disease. The purpose is to determine if the disease is caused by wild or vaccine po-

liovirus or by a nonpolio enterovirus. Isolation of wild poliovirus from the feces of such a patient indicates that wild poliovirus is circulating in the community and that the level of immunity among the community members against the poliovirus may be inadequate.

Aseptic meningitis and acute exanthema may be caused by any one of a large number of virus species and by a few nonviral agents. It is time consuming to establish etiologic diagnosis by virologic procedure. Since the diseases (if they are due to viruses) are usually self-limiting and do not respond to antiviral agents, it is generally sufficient to exclude nonviral infectious agents as the etiologic agent.

There is increasing evidence that some species of coxsackievirus are the etiologic agent of a sizable percentage of acute myocarditis and pericarditis. Since there is no effective antiviral therapy against the coxsackievirus and it is difficult to obtain appropriate clinical material for virologic testing, virological diagnosis of acute myocarditis is interesting academically but has no practical value.

6. *b* A day care center for preschool children is a notorious source of common infectious agents. Reasons: preschool children have no immunity to most of the common agents; when infected, the infection tends to be subclinical; and, having poor hygienic practice, they tend to spread the infections to one another and to contaminate the environment. The situation is similar to those of a developing country with high population density and poor hygienic practice. New workers in a day care center for preschool children should be considered to be at high risk of acquiring HAV infection and should be protected with passive immunization. Therefore, *b* is correct. *a* is correct for HAV infection but incorrect for virtually all other enterovirus infections (virus may be found in feces for up to 2 months after recovery from the acute illness). *c* is incorrect because pre-employment immunization for a teaching hospital in the United States does not include passive immunization against HAV infection.

7. *c* Due to interference, one single dose is not sufficient to induce immunity against all three types.

8. *e* The cause of postpolio syndrome is unknown at this time. Choices *a, b, c,* and *d* are ''candidate'' theories.

9. *c* Rhinovirus infections may be subclinical and may also involve the lower respiratory tract (*a* is wrong). Senior citizens have already been infected by, and are immune to, many serotypes of rhinoviruses; therefore, they are less likely to catch a common cold (*b* is wrong). Common cold vaccine is unavailable because it is impractical to prepare a vaccine that contains 100 or more serotypes of viruses (*d* is wrong).

THE PARAMYXOVIRUS, TOGAVIRUS, AND FLAVIVIRUS FAMILIES

THE PARAMYXOVIRUS FAMILY

This family of viruses includes the following human pathogens: measles, mumps, respiratory syncytial, and parainfluenzaviruses. Measles and mumps are now uncommon diseases in the United States due to the widespread use of effective vaccines. The physician's responsibility is to achieve and maintain a high level of immunity against these two diseases. Respiratory syncytial and parainfluenzaviruses continue to be important respiratory pathogens especially among young infants. Ribavirin, administered by aerosolization, is effective in the treatment of severe lower respiratory tract infection by the respiratory syncytial virus among young infants.

FAMILY CHARACTERISTICS

Morphology

These viruses are **enveloped,** have helical nucleocapsid, and vary from 100 to 300 nm in diameter.

Genomic Chemistry

The genomes of the paramyxovirus family are single-stranded, negative-sense, and nonsegmented RNA.

Replication Strategy

In general, it is similar to other enveloped RNA virus whose genome is single stranded and negative sense. A **virion-associated polymerase** is essential in initiating the synthetic phase. A **fusion protein** on the envelope that mediates the fusion of the viral envelope and the cell membrane has been well characterized. The matrix (M) protein is essential for the maturation of virions.

Species

There are four medically important species: the **measlesvirus (1 serotype),** the **mumpsvirus (1 serotype),** the **respiratory syncytial virus (2 serotypes ?),** and the **parainfluenzavirus (4 serotypes).** These viruses are antigenically distinct except for the cross-reactivity between the mumps- and parainfluenzaviruses.

THE MEASLESVIRUS

Pathogenesis

The portal of entry is the **upper respiratory tract.** Presumably, the virus multiplies locally at sites of implantation without signs or symptoms of infection. Local multiplication is followed by a **viremic phase** during which the virus is widely disseminated. The virus lodges and multiplies in the mucosa of the respiratory alimentary and urinary tracts, the endothelial cell of small blood vessels, and the lymphatics. The CNS may also be invaded. The **characteristic skin rash** is believed to be due to damage inflicted by **immune T lymphocytes** on virus-infected endothelial cells.

One rare but conceptually important complication is **subacute sclerosing panencephalitis (SSPE).** In SSPE, the virus has invaded the brain. But the brain cell cannot support the formation of progeny virions because of the **deficiency in the synthesis of M proteins.** Without the release of progeny virions, the infection can only spread slowly by cell-to-cell contact through the action of the fusion protein. Consequently, SSPE is characteristically a **"slow virus infection"** with long incubation and a slow but relentless progression terminating in death. The deficiency in M protein synthesis may be due to host cell restriction of viral gene expression or the emergence of a viral mutant.

Diagnosis

No specific virologic diagnosis is required. Clinical manifestations are sufficient for the diagnosis of measles. The presence of measles antibody in cerebrospinal fluid is diagnostic of SSPE.

Treatment

There is no specific antiviral agent against the measlesvirus.

Epidemiology and Prevention

Sources of the measlesvirus are the **respiratory secretions** of persons infected by the virus. Chronic or intermittent excreters have not been described. Transmission occurs through the respiratory route or indirect contact with respiratory secretions positive for the virus.

Measles is a common and **highly contagious disease.** It is worldwide in distribution and is primarily a childhood disease. One attack confers lifelong immunity. Subclinical infections are rare. In countries where universal immunization against measles is rigorously enforced (e.g., the United States), measles is an uncommon disease. In 1991 less than 10^4 cases are reported in the United States; and 20% were among persons older than 19 years. Preventive measures include **preexposure immunization, postexposure immunization,** and the administration of **immunoglobulins** after exposure.

Measles vaccine contains live **attenuated measlesvirus.** It is generally administered together with live attenuated mumps- and rubellaviruses as the measles, mumps, and rubella (MMR) vaccine. **Two doses of MMR** vaccine given at least 1 month apart are recommended for all persons who are **15 months old** or more and have no immunity against measles. Immunity to measles is proven by (1) evidence of the measles antibody, (2) a past history of measles diagnosed by a physician, (3) birth date before 1957 (the older persons should have acquired natural measles infection), or (4) documentation in medical record of having received two doses of measles or MMR vaccine at least 1 month apart. Measles immunization is at least 95% effective. If the first dose is given before 15 months of age, its efficacy may be reduced (presumably because of interference by residual maternal antibody of the growth of vaccine measlesvirus). In persons who are not immune and have recent exposure to measles, measles vaccine given within 3-days postexposure or immunoglobulins given within 6 days postexposure will prevent or reduce the severity of infection.

THE MUMPSVIRUS

Pathogenesis

The primary target is the **upper respiratory tract** and regional lymphnodes where the infection is asymptomatic. Two weeks after the successful establishment of infection, there is a **viremic phase** during which the virus is **widely disseminated.** Clinically important secondary targets are the **salivary glands; the testes,** meninges, and brain may also be involved.

Diagnosis

Clinical manifestation of mumps **(acute parotitis)** is quite characteristic. In a situation where specific virologic diagnosis is indicated (as in acute meningoencephalitis), serology is the method of choice. Serology includes the demonstration of specific IgM or antibody rise.

Treatment

Specific treatment is not available.

Epidemiology and Prevention

The source of the virus is the **oropharyngeal secretion** from subjects with current infections. Chronic or intermittent excreters are not known. The route of transmission is through direct or indirect contact with secretions positive for the virus. Mumps is a common childhood disease, which is worldwide in distribution. In countries where universal immunization is rigorously enforced, mumps is no longer a common disease. For example, the number of reported cases of mumps in the United States was about 5000 in 1988.

The mumps vaccine contains **live attenuated mumpsvirus** that is usually administered together with measles and rubella vaccine viruses as the MMR vaccine. It is at least 95% effective and is recommended for all persons who are born after 1957, have no immunity against mumps, and are 15 months old or more. Vaccine-associated meningitis has been reported in about $1/10^5$ of the vaccinated persons; the meningitis is usually mild and self-limiting.

THE RESPIRATORY SYNCYTIAL VIRUS

Pathogenesis

The primary target of the respiratory syncytial virus (RSV) is the epithelium of the respiratory tract. Virus replication injures cells and evokes local inflammatory response. Spread of infection from the upper to the lower respiratory tract is common. Infection of the **lower respiratory tract** tends to be severe, especially among young infants. A mortality rate of 35% has been reported for **young infants with congenital heart disease** and who are infected by the RSV. Distant secondary targets have not been demonstrated. Reinfection is not uncommon, but it tends to involve only the upper respiratory tract.

Diagnosis

Because infections of the lower respiratory tract (acute bronchiolitis) in young infants by the RSV can be severe and because specific antiviral treatment is available, **etiologic diagnosis** of acute bronchiolitis is important. The diagnosis is achieved by detecting RSV antigens in nasopharyngeal aspirate using monoclonal antibody known to be reactive against all strains of RSV.

Treatment

Aerosolized ribavirin is effective in the treatment of RSV infection of the lower respiratory tract.

Epidemiology and Prevention

Sources of the viruses are the **respiratory tract secretion** of subjects with current infections. Chronic or intermittent virus excreters are not unknown. Transmission occurs through the respiratory route or indirect contact with virus-positive respiratory secretion. Infections are common especially among infants and young children and are worldwide in distribution. **Nosocomial infections** by the RSV is common. There is no effective vaccine. Attempts to prevent nosocomial transmission should be encouraged. **RSV-specific immune globulins** appear to be effective in protecting infants from severe disease.

PARAINFLUENZAVIRUSES

Pathogenesis

The parainfluenzaviruses are similar to RSV. These viruses are important pathogens associated with acute lower respiratory tract illness and infants and children.

Diagnosis

Etiologic diagnosis is not necessary in clinical practice because effective antiviral therapy and prevention are not yet available.

Treatment

Specific antiviral treatment is not available.

Epidemiology and Prevention

These viruses are similar to RSV in general.

THE TOGAVIRUS FAMILY

This family of viruses includes two genera that are of medical importance in the United States: the rubivirus and the alphavirus genera. Diseases caused by these viruses are now rare, but they are medically important because effective preventive measures against these diseases are available.

FAMILY CHARACTERISTICS

Morphology

The virus is spherical and about 60 nm in diameter. It has an icosahedral capsid symmetry and an envelope.

Genomic Chemistry

The genome of the togavirus is a single-stranded positive-sense RNA.

Replication Strategy

Attachment, penetration, maturation, and release are in general similar to other envelopes viruses. The synthetic phase is similar to the picornavirus.

Medically Important Species

Togaviruses are divided into four genera, but only two (the rubivirus and alphavirus genera) are important medically. The sole species of the rubivirus genus is the **rubellavirus.** The alphavirus genus includes seven species, only two of which are important in the United States **(Western and Eastern equine encephalitis viruses).** All alphaviruses share common antigens and are transmitted by insect bites.

RUBELLAVIRUS

Pathogenesis

The primary target is the **nasopharyngeal mucosa** and regional lymphnodes. Viral multiplication at the primary site (asymptomatic) is followed by a **viremic**

phase during which the virus is widely disseminated. The virus has been isolated from urine, feces, joint fluid, uterine cervical secretion, and fetal tissue (besides nasopharyngeal and pharyngeal swabs) during rubella. The **generalized maculopapular rash** seen in most cases of rubella is believed to be due to injury of virus-infected endothelial cells inflicted by the **host's immune system.** Rubella is a mild **self-limiting disease except for the fetus.** Virtually all fetuses are born with **congenital defects** (heart malformation, deafness, cataract, and mental retardation) if infection occurred during the **first trimester** of pregnancy. Congenital defects are less likely for infection during the second trimester, and are seldom seen for infection during the third trimester. The rubellavirus is teratogenic.

Diagnosis

Virus isolation is useful for confirming congenitally acquired rubella. An infant showing congenital malformation and excreting virus is referred to as having **congenital rubella syndrome (CRS).** Pregnant women who have no documented immunity to rubella and are exposed to rubella or have illness suggestive of rubella during the first trimester should have the diagnosis of rubella excluded or confirmed by serology.

Treatment

No specific treatment for rubella is available.

Epidemiology and Prevention

Sources of rubellavirus are the **respiratory secretion** of subjects having current infections. Chronic or intermittent virus excreters are not known except for infants with CRS. The body secretions and excretions from these infants may contain the virus for many months. Transmission occurs through the respiratory route and indirect contact with virus-positive secretions or excretions. Due to the rigorous enforcement of universal immunization against rubella in the United States and many other countries, rubella is now an uncommon disease. In 1987, there were about 300 reported cases of rubella and 3 confirmed cases of CRS in the United States.

Rubella vaccine contains **live attenuated rubellavirus** that is usually administered with measles and mumps vaccine viruses as the MMR vaccine. It is highly effective in preventing viremia of wild rubellavirus and is recommended for all nonimmune women of child bearing age unless contraindicated. The presence of rubella antibody or documentation of prior rubella vaccination are accepted as immunity. Contraindications are immunodeficiency or **pregnancy.** In the United States and many other countries, the vaccine is given to all children at the age of 15 months. Side effects of rubella immunization in adult females are common: (1) 15% developed arthralgia lasting 1–10 days (<2%, arthritis and a few develop chronic or recurrent arthralgia); (2) report on six postpartal vaccinated persons having chronic arthralgia 2–7 years, frequent episodes of paresthesia, blurred vision or painful limbs, chronic viremia (virus in mononuclear cells) for up to 6 years, and, virus in milk for 1 year. Between 1979 and 1988, 272 susceptible pregnant women were inadvertently inoculated with the rubella vaccine; none of the 212 live-born infants had defects indicative of CRS.

WESTERN AND EASTERN EQUINE ENCEPHALITIS VIRUSES

Pathogenesis

The viruses of western equine encephalitis (**WEE**) and eastern equine encephalitis (**EEE**) are inoculated into the body through the **bite of an infected mosquito.** Where the virus multiplies initially is not clear, but a viremic phase usually follows. During **viremia,** the virus may lodge in the **brain** resulting in **acute encephalitis.**

Diagnosis

Etiologic diagnosis must be attempted in **all cases of acute encephalitis,** which are almost always caused by viruses. Many species of viruses are capable of causing acute encephalitis. Some, such as HSV-1 and HSV-2, respond to acyclovir; others, such as mumps and Epstein-Barr, generally induce self-limiting encephalitis with complete recovery; still others, such as the arboviruses, are epidemic in nature and require prompt community action to deal with the epidemic. Etiologic diagnosis of acute encephalitis due to WEE and EEE viruses is usually established by serology.

Treatment

There is no specific antiviral therapy against encephalitis due to the alphaviruses.

Epidemiology and Prevention

The EEE and WEE viruses are maintained perennially in a cycle between birds and mosquitoes. Occasionally, a human may be bitten by an infected mosquito. In situations where the mosquito population is large and the number of infected mosquitoes is also large, an epidemic may emerge. For example, there were over 3000 WEE cases in humans and over 3×10^5 cases among horses in 1941. In 1987, less than 100 cases were reported. For each case of WEE, there are many subclinical infections. Control of EEE and WEE virus infections is achieved by **mosquito abatement program.**

THE FLAVIVIRUS FAMILY

The flaviviruses differ from the togaviruses in the sizes of the virion (40 instead of 60 nm in diameter) and the RNA genome (10 instead of 12 kb). There are over 70 ''species,'' many of which are human pathogens. The species seen in the United States is the **St. Louis encephalitis (SLE)** virus. Other species now not present in the continental United States are the **denguevirus** and **yellow fever virus. Japanese B encephalitis virus** is endemic primarily in Japan, Korea, China, and Southeast Asia; an inactivated vaccine is available from travelers to these endemic areas. Denguevirus is endemic in the Caribbean, Mexico, Central and South America, the Pacific basin, Southeast Asia, and central Africa. Imported cases are seen in southern United States and Hawaii. Yellow fever virus is endemic in tropical Africa and tropical South America; an effective live-virus vaccine is available.

The pathogenesis, diagnosis, treatment, epidemiology, and prevention of St. Louis encephalitis virus are similar to those of WEE virus.

SUMMARY

1. Paramyxoviruses are enveloped and have single-stranded negative-sense nonsegmented RNA genome. Medically important species include measles (1 serotype), mumps (1 serotype), respiratory syncytial (2 serotypes?), and parainfluenzaviruses (4 serotypes).

2. Measlesvirus multiplies at sites of implantation (upper respiratory). This multiplication is followed by a viremic phase during which the virus is

widely disseminated throughout the body. It causes damage to these secondary targets resulting in measles.

3. Subacute sclerosing panencephalitis is a rare but conceptually important complication of measles. In this disease, the virus has invaded the brain but spreads slowly by cell-to-cell contact. This slow spread is due to a deficiency in the production of matrix proteins, which is essential for the maturation and release of enveloped viruses. This slow spread of virus results in a slow virus infection characterized by a long incubation and a slow but relentless progression toward death.

4. The widespread use of measles vaccine in the United States has changed measles from a common and highly contagious childhood disease into an uncommon disease. The maintenance of a high level of measles immunity in the community is of utmost importance.

5. Measles vaccine contains the live attenuated measlesvirus. The virus is usually administered with live attenuated mumps- and rubellaviruses as the measles, mumps, and rubella (MMR) vaccine. Two doses of MMR vaccine, given at least 1 month apart, are recommended for all persons who are 15 months old or older and have no immunity against measles.

6. In susceptible persons, active immunization within 3 days of postexposure or passive immunization with human Ig within 6 days of exposure will prevent or reduce severity of measles.

7. Mumpsvirus multiplies at implantation site (upper respiratory tract and regional lymphnodes). This asymptomatic virus multiplication is followed by a viremic phase during which the virus is widely disseminated. Clinically important secondary targets include salivary glands, testes, meninges, and the brain.

8. Like measles, the incidence of mumps in the United States has been drastically reduced through the widespread use of the mumps vaccine and the maintenance of community immunity against mumps is important. Usage of mumps vaccine is similar to that of measles vaccine.

9. Respiratory syncytial and parainfluenzaviruses produce superficial infections of the respiratory tract and are important pathogens associated with acute lower respiratory tract illnesses in infants and children.

10. Acute bronchiolitis induced by the respiratory syncytial virus in infants is a serious disease that responds to aerosolized ribavirin. Therefore,

etiologic diagnosis of acute bronchiolitis in infants is important. The procedure of choice is to demonstrate respiratory syncytial virus antigens in nasopharyngeal aspirate. RSV-specific Ig may be effective in preventing serious infections among infants.

11. Togaviruses are enveloped and have a single-stranded positive-sense nonsegmented RNA genome. Medically important species include the rubella, western equine encephalitis (WEE), and eastern equine encephalitis (EEE) viruses.

12. The pathogenesis of rubella is similar to measles except that it is a mild disease. However, fetal infections especially during the first trimester result in severe congenital defects. Therefore, the strategy in dealing with rubellavirus infection is to protect fetuses from infection by wild rubellavirus.

13. Rubella vaccine contains live attenuated rubellavirus. This vaccine virus is a component of the MMR vaccine. It is highly effective in preventing viremia during rubellavirus infection. Through its wide spread use, the incidence of rubella and congenital rubella syndrome in the United States have been reduced, respectively, to less than 1000 and less than 5 cases per year. The maintenance of a high level of community immunity against rubella is crucial to the prevention of congenital rubella syndrome. Immunization programs for the prevention of measles and mumps by the use of MMR vaccine should be adequate for the prevention of rubella.

14. The MMR or monovalent rubella vaccine should not be given to pregnant women or women planning to conceive within 2 months because of the theoretical risk of fetal infection by the vaccine virus.

15. Western and eastern equine encephalitis viruses may cause acute encephalitis; they are arboviruses (see Chapter 46). Mosquito abatement program is useful in preventing or terminating an epidemic.

16. The flavivirus of importance in the United States is the St. Louis encephalitis (SLE) virus. It is also an arbovirus. The mosquito abatement program is useful in preventing or terminating an epidemic.

17. Two other flaviviruses, yellow fever and Japanese B encephalitis, are endemic, respectively, in certain parts of South America and Africa and in the western Pacific. Effective vaccines are available against these two viruses. Travelers to the endemic regions needs to consider immunization prior to departure.

18. Denguevirus, another flavivirus, is endemic in the Caribbean, Mexico, Central and South America, the Pacific basin and Southeast Asia. Imported cases are occasionally seen in the United States.

REFERENCES

Anderson LJ (1990): Strains of respiratory syncytial virus: implication for vaccine development. Med Virol 9:187.

Centers for Disease Control (1989): Measles prevention. MMWR 38 (5–9):1.

Centers for Disease Control (1989): Rubella vaccination during pregnancy. MMWR 38:289.

Centers for Disease Control (1989): Measles—U.S. and 1st 20 weeks 1990. MMWR 39:353.

Centers for Disease Control (1990): Rubella prevention. MMWR 39(RR-15):1.

Centers for Disease Control (1991): St. Louis encephalitis outbreak—Arkansas 1991. MMWR 40:605.

Denning DW, Kaneko K (1987): Should travellers to Asia be vaccinated against Japanese encephalitis? Lancet i:853.

Editorial (1989): Mumps meningitis and MMR vaccination. Lancet ii:1015.

Greenberg BL et al. (1991): Measles-associated diarrhea in hospitalized children in Lima, Peru: pathogenic agent and impact on growth. J Inf Dis 163:495.

Heilman CA (1990): Respiratory syncytial and parainfluenza viruses. J Inf Dis 161:402.

Immunization Practices Advisory Committee (1984): Yellow fever vaccine. Ann Intern Med 100:540.

Kingsbury DW (1991): The Paramyxoviruses. New York: Plenum Press.

McIntosh K (1993): RSV-successful immunoprophylaxis at last. N Engl Med 329:1572.

Whitley RJ (1990): Viral encephalitis. N Engl J Med 323:242.

REVIEW QUESTIONS

> For questions 1 to 12, choose the ONE BEST answer or completion.

1. Paramyxoviruses
   a) are not enveloped
   b) have a virion-associated polymerase
   c) have a positive-sense RNA genome
   d) include measles-, mumps-, and rubella-viruses
   e) have matrix protein of unknown function

2. All but one of the following statements about the pathogenesis of measles are correct. Identify the incorrect statement.
   a) Multiplication of virus at the primary target site is asymptomatic.
   b) A viremic phase occurs in virtually all infections.
   c) Clinical manifestations of measles are the consequence of virus multiplication in secondary targets.
   d) Acute encephalitis occurs in about 10% of all measles cases.
   e) Subacute sclerosing panencephalitis is a very rare complication of measles ($<1/10^5$ cases of measles).

3. During an outbreak of measles in your community, human immunoglobulins should be given to

   a) patients who have had symptoms of measles for less than 48 h
   b) all persons who are over 65 years old and have cardiorespiratory insufficiency
   c) young children between the age of 6 and 14 months
   d) intravenous drug users who have AIDS
   e) women in first trimester of pregnancy

4. Identify the incorrect statement about the pathogenesis of mumps.
   a) Multiplication of the virus at the primary target site is asymptomatic.
   b) A viremic phase occurs in virtually all infections.
   c) Clinical manifestations of mumps are due to virus multiplication in secondary target organs.
   d) Acute meningoencephalitis is an important complication in mumps.
   e) Acute orchitis and parotitis occur in about equal frequency during infection by the mumpsvirus.

5. Mumps and measles vaccine are similar, *except*
   a) mumps vaccine contains inactivated virus while measles vaccine contains live attenuated virus
   b) mumps vaccine is 99% effective while measles vaccine is 85% effective
   c) mumps but not measles vaccine may in-

duce meningitis in a small number of vaccinated persons (1/10⁵)

d) universal immunization against measles but not mumps is recommended in the United States

e) it is more important for a traveler to a foreign country to have measles antibody than mumps antibody

6. Identify the incorrect statement about the measles vaccine. The measles vaccine
   a) contains live attenuated measlesvirus
   b) should be given to all persons who are born after 1957, who are 15 months old or more, and have no immunity against measles
   c) should be given to asymptomatic HIV-infected persons if there are indications for measles vaccination
   d) virus is known to cause fetal infections if given to pregnant women who have no immunity against measles

7. Accepted as proof of immunity against measles are
   a) the presence of serum antibody against the measlesvirus
   b) a past history of measles (based on mother's recollection)
   c) a birth date before 1970
   d) having received one dose of measles, mumps, and rubella at the age of 16 months as documented in medical record

8. About lower respiratory tract infections in young infants by the respiratory syncytial and parainfluenzaviruses
   a) the infections can be differentiated by clinical manifestations

b) the infections are usually distinguished by the demonstration of specific virus antigen in respiratory secretion

c) infections by parainfluenza but not by respiratory syncytial viruses are effectively prevented by preexposure immunization

d) infections by respiratory syncytial and by parainfluenzaviruses respond to aerosolized ribavirin treatment

9. Rubella
   a) and Western equine encephalitis viruses are both togaviruses.
   b) and Western equine encephalitis viruses are both arbovirus.
   c) virus infections are innocuous
   d) infections of fetuses almost always result in spontaneous abortion

10. Rubella
    a) vaccine is recommended for all nonimmune women of child bearing age unless contraindicated
    b) immunity is established by past history of physician-diagnosed rubella
    c) vaccination does not cause unpleasant side effects
    d) vaccination during pregnancy results in congenital malformation of about 10% of the fetuses

11. Identify the incorrect statement about Western equine encephalitis and St. Louis encephalitis viruses. These viruses
    a) are transmitted by bites of infected mosquitos
    b) are some of the viruses capable of causing acute encephalitis

c) cause diseases that may occur in epidemics

d) cause diseases that are preventable by preexposure immunization

12. Identify the incorrect statement about acute encephalitis.

a) Most are caused by virus infections.

b) Specific etiologic diagnosis is important.

c) Cases caused by the herpes simplex virus usually respond to acyclovir therapy.

d) Cases caused by the mumpsvirus usually recovered completely without sequelae.

e) Over 50% of HIV-infected persons eventually develop acute encephalitis.

ANSWERS TO REVIEW QUESTIONS

---

1. **b**

2. **d** Acute encephalitis is a rare ($<1/10^5$) but serious complication of measles.

3. **c** Children of this age may no longer be protected by maternal antibody and none has received the MMR vaccine. Also, the disease among nonimmune young children (6–14 months) tend to be severe. Passive immunization within 1 week of exposure is important.

4. **e** Acute orchitis occurs only in postpubertal males; and, in postpubertal males with mumps, less than 20% develop acute orchitis.

5. **c**

6. **d** d is incorrect—measles vaccination is not recommended for pregnant woman because of *theoretical* consideration of fetal infection. There is no proof that fetal infection has occurred.

7. **a** Past history of measles must be measles diagnosed by a physician; recollection of the person's mother is insufficient; therefore, **b** is wrong. Persons born in 1957 or earlier are considered immune to measles because of natural measles infections (measles vaccine was first approved for universal usage in early 1970s); therefore, **c** is wrong. Since 1989, the official recommendation is that each child must receive two doses of measles vaccine (preferably MMR vaccine), one at 15 months of age and another just prior to school entry; therefore, **d** is wrong.

8. **b** Infections of the respiratory tract can be

due to any one of a large number of viruses. While the anatomical locations of infection can be easily differentiated by clinical manifestations (e.g., acute bronchiolitis vs. acute laryngitis), infections of the same anatomical location by different viruses can only be distinguished by virological diagnostic procedures.

9. *a* Rubellavirus is not an arbovirus; therefore, *b* is wrong. (This is one situation where the virus classification seems to have failed; the two viruses belong to the same family, yet they have totally different epidemiology.) Rubella is a mild infection except among fetuses 16 weeks old or less; therefore, *c* is wrong. Fetal infections during the first trimester may result in fetal death and spontaneous abortion (frequency unknown) but infections during the second or third trimester seldom result in spontaneous abortion; therefore, *d* is wrong.

10. *a* Clinical diagnosis of rubella, even by a physician, is not sufficiently dependable to be accepted as evidence of rubella immunity. Side effects (arthralgia and arthritis) are common among adult female rubella vaccinated persons. Rubella vaccination during pregnancy should be avoided. This avoidance is based on theoretical consideration of possible damage to the fetus and not on actual evidence of fetal damage. Indeed, over 250 pregnant women were inadvertently inoculated with rubella vaccine; none of the live-born infants had defects indicative of congenital rubella syndrome.

11. *d* There is no FDA-approved vaccine against WEE and SLE viruses.

12. *e* Persons with HIV infection seldom develop acute encephalitis. Many of them do have slowly progressing degeneration of the brain (encephalopathy).

THE RHABDOVIRUS, REOVIRUS, AND OTHER RNA VIRUS FAMILIES

THE RHABDOVIRUS FAMILY

The only medically important species of rhabdovirus in the United States is the rabiesvirus. Rabies is rare among humans in the United States; there are less than 2 confirmed cases per year since 1980. But, animal rabies is still quite prevalent; about 5000 cases were reported in 1987 in the United States. Since rabies is transmitted by animal bites and is uniformly fatal, and since postexposure immunoprophylaxis is quite effective, the possibility of exposure to the rabiesvirus must be considered by the attending physician in every instance of animal bite. Because human rabies is extremely rare in the United States, the diagnosis is difficult especially in the absence of an exposure history. It is important to consider rabies in the differential diagnosis of acute encephalitis.

FAMILY CHARACTERISTICS

Morphology

Rhabdoviruses are enveloped and have helical capsid symmetry. These viruses have a **bullet-shaped morphology** that is unique for this family (Fig. 46.1).

Genomic Chemistry

The genome is a single-stranded negative-sense RNA.

Replication Strategy

This virus is presumed to be similar to all other enveloped virions with negative-sense RNA genome. The synthetic phase is initiated by a virion-associated polymerase that transcribes the negative-sense into positive-sense RNA (mRNA).

Species

There are numerous isolates of rhabdoviruses, many of which have not been sufficiently characterized for classification. Only one species, the **rabiesvirus,** is important medically in the United States. There is only **one immunotype** of rabiesvirus (i.e., vaccine prepared from a standard strain induces immunity against all others). By antigenic analysis with monoclonal antibodies, several antigenic variants have been identified. Knowledge of these antigenic variants are useful in epidemiology. The rabiesvirus is also known as lyssavirus serotype 1.

RABIESVIRUS

Pathogenesis

The rabiesvirus enters the human body through the **bite of rabid animals.** The virus multiplies in muscle cells at the **site of inoculation** and then enters the nervous system by way of the **myoneural junction.** It moves passively to the CNS through the motor nerve. In the CNS, the virus multiplies extensively and

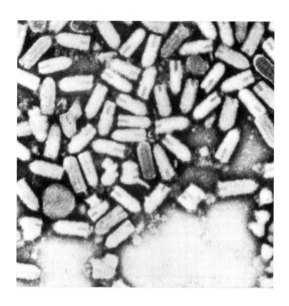

Figure 46.1.
Electromicrograph of a rhabdovirus. Note its bullet shape. (Courtesy of Dr. Y.C. Zee.)

then descends to the peripheral organs through peripheral nerves. The **acetylcholine receptor** may serve as a receptor for the virus. The host's immune response is intimately associated with symptomatology of rabies. The main pathology is **acute encephalitis.** The incubation period is usually 20–60 days but may be less than 10 days to over 1 year. It is not clear why the **incubation period varies** so widely.

Diagnosis

In the management of animal bites, it is crucial to know if the biting animal is rabid. The method of choice is to detect **rabies antigens in the brain** smear of the suspected animal by immunofluorescence. As mentioned in Chapter 45, etiologic diagnosis of all cases of acute encephalitis must be attempted. The **demonstration of rabies antibody** is the method of choice in patients not previously given rabies immunoprophylaxis.

Treatment

Specific antiviral treatment for rabies is not available.

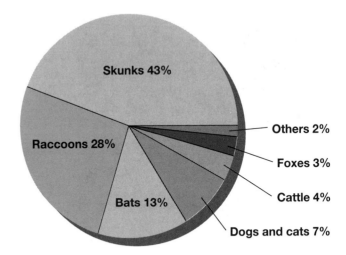

Figure 46.2.
Animal rabies in the United States in 1987. [Data taken from Fishbein DB, Dobbins JG, Bryson JH, Pinsky PF, Smith JS (1988): Rabies surveillance, United States, 1987. MMWR 37(SS4):12.]

Epidemiology and Prevention

An epidemiologically important source of rabiesvirus is the **saliva** of infected animals. Distribution of 4729 reported cases of rabies among animal species in the United States in 1987 is shown in Figure 46.2. Key points to note are (1) **skunks, raccoons, foxes,** and **bats** accounted for 87%; (2) dogs and cats, only 7%; and (3) none among small agile mammals, such as mice, chipmunks, squirrels, and rabbits. In many developing countries, most of the animal rabies are among dogs. For example, in 1987, there were about 15,000 reported cases of dog rabies in Mexico, a number about 30 times higher than in the United States.

Prevention of rabies in humans is achieved by (1) mandatory immunization of dogs and cats, (2) preexposure immunization of persons at high risk of animal bites (e.g., veterinarians, park rangers, animal handlers, etc.), and (3) postexposure immunoprophylaxis of persons exposed to rabies. Postexposure immunoprophylaxis consists of the local infiltration and parenteral administration of human rabies immunoglobulins and a course of rabies vaccine. **Rabies vaccine** for human use contains **inactivated rabiesvirus.** The alum-adsorbed type induces acceptable level of rabies neutralizing antibody in over 99% of the vaccinated persons.

THE REOVIRUS FAMILY

Viruses of this family are unique in that their genomes consist of double-stranded RNA. There are many species in this family, but only the rotaviruses produce significant human diseases in the United States. The rotavirus is a major cause of diarrhea among infants and young children. A specific prevention or treatment for rotavirus diarrhea is not available.

FAMILY CHARACTERISTICS

Morphology

The virion is not enveloped, it has **double layers of capsids** that are icosahedral in symmetry. The arrangement of capsomeres gives the virion a **"wheel-like" appearance** that is especially striking for the genus *Rotavirus* (Fig. 46.3).

Genomic Chemistry

The genome consists of segmented **double-stranded RNA.**

Replication Strategy

The virion contains a polymerase that initiates the synthetic phase by transcribing the viral genome into viral mRNA.

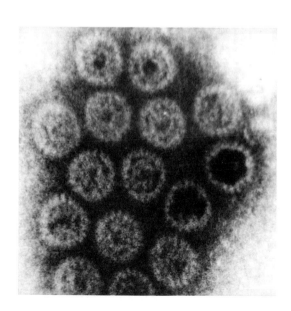

Figure 46.3.

Electronmicrograph of a rotavirus. Note its resemblance to a wheel. (Courtesy of Dr. Andrew Dean.)

Species

Reoviruses are divided into several genera. Three are pathogenic to humans found in the United States. The three genera are *Reovirus, Rotavirus,* and *Orbivirus.* Species of the genus *Reovirus* induce minor illnesses or subclinical infections. Colorado tick fever virus (an orbivirus) infections of humans are uncommon. Only species of the genus ***Rotavirus*** are important in medical practice in the United States.

ROTAVIRUS

Pathogenesis

The primary target is **intestinal epithelial cells.** Virus multiplication damages the epithelial lining resulting in **watery diarrhea,** which can lead to dehydration in infants.

Diagnosis

Rotavirus is present in high concentration in feces. **Virions or viral antigens in feces** can be readily detected by electron microscopy or serology. Etiologic diagnosis is seldom necessary in medical practice.

Treatment

There is no specific antiviral treatment.

Epidemiology and Prevention

The source of the virus is the **feces** of infected persons. Transmission is through the **fecal-oral route.** Rotavirus infections are common. In the United States, over 90% of preschool children have rotavirus antibody and rotavirus diarrhea usually occurs among **infants** in the **winter.** There are four major serotypes of human rotaviruses. Recovery from infection by one type provides partial immunity against reinfection by the same type. **Nosocomial infections** among infants are not uncommon. Such infections should be minimized by attending to procedures that prevent fecal-oral transmission.

OTHER RNA VIRUS FAMILIES

This subchapter deals with the remaining five families of RNA viruses. These viruses are relatively unimportant because they cause self-limiting diseases against which there is no effective preventive measure or specific treatment; or, because infections are rare in the United States.

THE BUNYAVIRUS FAMILY

The bunyavirus family includes over 200 species most of which are arboviruses. Only two species, the **LaCrosse encephalitis** virus and **hantavirus,** are of medical importance in the United States. Like other arboviruses, LaCrosse virus is transmitted from its nonhuman vertebrate hosts (small mammals, and birds) to human by the **bites of mosquitoes.** LaCrosse encephalitis is an uncommon disease in the United States; it occurs chiefly in the states bordering the Great Lakes.

The hantavirus infects primarily rodents and is found in the **excreta of infected rodents.** Humans in **close contact** with infected rodents acquire infections through the **respiratory tract.** Severe infections, known as **hantavirus pulmonary syndrome,** have occurred in western United States and Florida and have a mortality of over 50%. Serologic surveys reveal a seroprevalence of 1% in some parts of the United States. In some other countries, severe infections may manifest as **hemorrhagic fever with renal syndrome.**

THE CORONAVIRUS FAMILY

Coronaviruses are one of the several groups of viruses capable of causing **acute respiratory infections** in humans. Specific virologic diagnosis is unnecessary. Effective vaccine and antiviral against the coronavirus are not available.

THE CALICIVIRUS FAMILY

Caliciviruses are one of the several groups of viruses capable of causing **acute gastroenteritis** in humans. Specific virologic diagnosis is unnecessary. There are no effective vaccines or antiviral agents against this family of viruses.

THE ARENAVIRUS FAMILY

Lymphocytic choriomeningitis virus (LCMV) is the only arenavirus of medical importance in the United States. This virus is one of the many viruses capable of causing **aseptic meningitis** or **meningoencephalitis** in humans. The LCMV induced meningitis or meningoencephalitis are usually self-limiting and are rare in the United States. There are no effective vaccines or antiviral agents against LCMV. Infection by LCMV occurs through contact with **urine of infected rodents.**

Lassa fever virus infections are endemic in tropical **West Africa; imported cases** have been reported from the United States and other countries. Lassa fever is a **severe systemic infection** with high mortality and is responsive to **ribavirin** therapy.

THE FILOVIRUS FAMILY

This family of viruses includes two species that are highly pathogenic for humans, the **Marburg** and the **Ebola hemorrhage fever viruses.** These two viruses are indigenous to Africa and the Philippines and were **imported** to Europe and the United States through **infected monkeys.** In one importation to Europe, 25 workers who handled blood and tissues from infected monkeys acquired the infection; 7 died. There were also 6 secondary cases, but none of the animal caretakers became infected. In the importation of infected monkeys from the Philippines to the United States, many of the imported monkeys died during quarantine. The Ebolavirus was detected in many of the dying animals. No human was infected in this importation. It appears that these filoviruses are of importance to workers in facilities that handle imported monkeys.

The filoviruses are negative-sense single-stranded RNA viruses. These viruses are enveloped and have a unique bacilliform morphology (Fig. 46.4).

ARBOVIRUSES

Arboviruses is a term frequently used in medical literature. This term is derived from *arthropod-bo*rne viruses. Arboviruses include all viruses that are **transmitted between vertebrate hosts by the bite of arthropod vectors.** To be a "successful" arbovirus, the virus must have a **viremic phase of high intensity** in the vertebrate host and the capability of **multiplying in the arthropod vector.** This grouping of viruses by the mode of transmission is an **epidemiologic clas-**

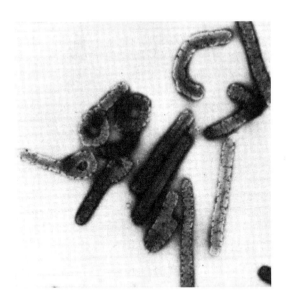

Figure 46.4.
Electronmicrograph of a filovirus. Note its resemblance to a bacillus. [Reproduced with permission from MP Kiley (1988): Laboratory Diagnosis of Infectious Diseases: Principles and Practice, Vol. 2. Viral Rickettsial and Chlamydial Diseases. New York: Springer-Verlag.]

sification. Arboviruses include **species in five families of RNA viruses** (togavirus, flavivirus, rhabdovirus, reovirus, and bunyavirus). The more important arboviruses in the United States cause acute encephalitis in humans. These viruses are St. Louis, La Crosse, Western and Eastern equine encephalitis viruses; belong to the togavirus, flavivirus, and bunyavirus families; and are controlled by mosquito abatement program.

SUMMARY

1. **Rhabdoviruses have a unique morphology (bullet shaped).**

2. **The rabiesvirus is the only medically important species of rhabdoviruses in the United States.**

3. **The rabiesvirus is transmitted to humans through the bite of rabid animals. The virus multiplies at the site of inoculation, enters the CNS through the myoneural junction and the motor nerve, and induces a rapidly progressing acute encephalitis. The incubation period curiously varies from less than 10 days to over 1 year.**

4. **Virological diagnosis of rabies is important to determine if the biting animal is rabid and in the differential diagnosis of rapidly progressing acute**

encephalitis. To determine if the biting animal is rabid the method of choice is to demonstrate rabies antigens in the brain. In the differential diagnosis of acute encephalitis in humans, the method of choice is the demonstration of rabies antibody in the patient's serum (providing that the patient had not received rabies immunoprophylaxis).

5. Rabies in the United States is primarily a disease of the wildlife mammals. Skunks, raccoons, foxes, and bats accounted for 87% of reported rabies in animals in 1987; dogs and cats only 7%.

6. Prevention of rabies in humans in achieved by mandatory rabies immunization of dogs and cats, preexposure immunization of persons at high risk of animal bites, and postexposure immunoprophylaxis of persons exposed to rabies.

7. Rabies vaccine for human use contains inactivated rabiesvirus. Postexposure immunoprophylaxis consists of the administration of human rabies Ig and a course of rabies vaccine.

8. The morphology of reoviruses is unique in that the arrangement of capsomeres gives the appearance of a wheel, especially striking for the genus *Rotavirus*.

9. The genome of reoviruses is also unique in that it is double-stranded RNA (also segmented).

10. The more medically important reoviruses in the United States are the rotaviruses that cause winter infantile diarrhea.

11. The target of rotaviruses is the intestine epithelium.

12. The feces of infected persons contains rotavirus in high concentration. The virus is transmitted by the fecal-oral route. Over 90% of preschool children in the United States have rotavirus antibodies. Little is known about immunity to reinfection by the homologous and heterologous types.

13. Rotaviruses are the major but not the sole cause of viral gastroenteritis in the United States.

14. Bunyaviruses of medical importance in the United States are the LaCrosse encephalitis and the hantaviruses. The former is an arbovirus occuring primarily in the Great Lakes region. The latter causes a severe infection (hantavirus pulmonary syndrome); the infection is acquired through close contact with infected rodents.

15. Coronaviruses are respiratory pathogens of minor medical importance.

16. Some caliciviruses (Norwalk virus) are capable of causing acute gastroenteritis.

17. The arenavirus of medical importance in the United States is the lymphocytic choriomeningitis virus. It is capable of causing aseptic meningitis and encephalitis. Humans acquire infections through contact with the urine of infected rodents.

18. The Marburg and the Ebola hemorrhagic fever viruses (filoviruses) cause severe infections and high mortality in humans. They are indigenous to Africa and the Philippines, and have been imported to Europe and the United States via infected monkeys. Handlers of blood and tissues from infected momkeys are at high risk of acquiring the infection. To date, human infection has not been documented in the United States.

19. Arboviruses (*ar*thropod-*bo*rne viruses) include all viruses that are transmitted between vertebrates by bites of arthropod vectors. These viruses have a viremic phase in the vertebrate host and also multiply in the arthropod vector. The more important arboviruses in the United States cause acute encephalitis in humans (St. Louis, Western and Eastern equine, and LaCrosse encephalitis viruses); belong to the togavirus, flavivirus, and bunyavirus families; and are controlled by mosquito abatement program.

REFERENCES

Blacklow NR, Greenberg HB (1991): Viral gastroenteritis. N Engl J Med 252.

Cavanagh D, Brown TDK (1990): Coronaviruses and their diseases. In Advances in Experimental Medicine and Biology, Vol. 276. New York: Plenum Press.

Centers for Disease Control (1993): Compendium of animal rabies control 1993. MMWR 42(RR7):1.

Centers for Disease Control (1990): Update: filovirus infection associated with contact with non-human primates or their tissues. MMWR 39:404.

Centers for Disease Control (1994): Hantavirus pulmonary syndrome—U.S., 1993. MMWR 43:45.

Centers for Disease Control (1992): Arboviral disease—U.S. 1991. MMWR 41:545.

Duchin JS et al. (1994): Hantavirus pulmonary syndrome: a clinical description of 17 patients with a newly recognized disease. N Engl J Med 330:949.

Estes MK, Cohen J. Rotavirus gene structure and function. Microbiol Rev 1989;53:410–449.

Fishbein DB, Robinson LE (1993): Rabies. N Engl J Med 329:1632.

Holmes GP et al. (1990): Lassa fever in the U.S. N Engl J Med 323:1120.

Kiley MP (1988): Filoviridae in Laboratory Diagnosis of Infectious Diseases, Vol. II, In Lennett EH, Halonen P, Murphy FA (eds): Viral Rickettsial and Chlamydial Diseases. New York: Springer-Verlag pp 595–601.

Ing D, Glass RI, LeBaron CW, Lew JF (1992): Laboratory based surveillance for rotavirus, U.S. Jan 89–May 91. MMWR 41(SS3):47.

Salvato MS (1992): The arenaviridae. New York: Plenum Press.

Smith JS, Fishbein DB, Rupprecht CE, Clark K (1991): Unexplained rabies in 3 immigrants in the U.S. N Engl J Med 324:205.

Ward RL, Bernstein DI, and the U.S. Rotavirus Vaccine Efficacy Group (1994): Protection against rotavirus disease after natural rotavirus infection. J Inf Dis 169:900.

REVIEW QUESTIONS

> For questions 1 to 9, choose the ONE BEST answer or completion.

1. Rhabdovirus
   a) infections among U.S. residents are common (>1% of the adult population)
   b) is an arbovirus
   c) of major medical importance in the United States is the LaCrosse encephalitis virus
   d) has the morphologic appearance of a bullet
   e) all of the above

2. Rabiesvirus
   a) infections in the United States are more common in dogs than in skunks
   b) infections in the United States are more common in humans than in cats
   c) is a rhabdovirus
   d) infections in humans have an incubation period of about 3 weeks

e) infections may become latent in the human host

3. About the pathogenesis of rabies:
   a) its principal pathology is acute encephalitis
   b) a viremic phase precedes the encephalitis
   c) parenteral administration of rabies Ig during incubation reduces the severity of rabies
   d) the highest concentration of rabiesvirus in an infected mammal is in the salivary gland
   e) all of the above

4. Rabies
   a) vaccine for human use contains inactivated rabiesviruses
   b) virus isolates in the United States belong to one serotype as determined by neutralization test
   c) in the United States occurs chiefly among wildlife mammals

d) transmission from a patient with rabies to health care workers has not been documented
e) all of the above

5. Effective rabies prevention measures include
   a) mandatory rabies vaccination of dogs and cats
   b) preexposure immunization of persons at high risk of animal bits
   c) avoid playing with stray dogs or with wild mammals that appear to be unafraid of humans
   d) postexposure immunoprophylaxis of persons exposed to rabies.
   e) all of the above

6. Virologic confirmation of clinical impression (diagnosis) of rabies
   a) in animals is generally established by the demonstration of rabies antigens in the brain of the animal
   b) in a practicing veterinarian is usually established by the demonstration of serum antibody against the rabiesvirus
   c) in a medical student is generally established by the demonstration of rabies antigen in a biopsy of the brain
   d) needs not be performed in a patient with acute encephalitis and without a history of animal bite
   e) all of the above

7. Rotavirus
   a) belongs to the reovirus family
   b) have capsomeres that are so arranged that the virion appears like a wheel
   c) is the etiologic agent of infantile winter diarrhea in the United States
   d) has a double-stranded RNA genome
   e) all of the above

8. Rotavirus
   a) is found in high concentration in the feces of an infected person
   b) antibody is present in over 90% of preschool children in urban areas of the United States
   c) is transmitted between persons by the fecal-oral route
   d) is the major but not the sole cause of viral gastroenteritis
   e) all of the above

9. Identify the incorrect statement about arboviruses.
   a) Viruses that are transmitted between vertebrate hosts by the bite of arthropod vectors and are capable of multiplying in the arthropod vector are known as arboviruses.
   b) The HIV is not an arbovirus because it cannot multiply in the arthropod.
   c) Most of the medically important arboviruses in the United States are encephalitis viruses.
   d) The most effective method of preventing any arbovirus infectior is a mosquito abatement program.

10. Hantavirus
    a) was introduced into the United States by Korean war veterans
    b) infection invariably leads to adult respiratory distress syndrome
    c) is introduced into the human body through bites of infected mice
    d) infections are confined to the boundary area of New Mexico, Utah, Colorado, and Arizona
    e) respiratory syndrome is characterized by flu-like syndrome followed by rapidly progressing respiratory failure

ANSWERS TO REVIEW QUESTIONS

1. *d*

2. *c*

3. *a*

4. *e* (all are correct).

5. *e* (all are correct).

6. *a* All practicing veterinarians have rabies antibodies because of preexposure immunoprophylaxis. If the medical student had not received rabies immunoprophylaxis prior to onset, the method of choice is demonstration of rabies antibody. If the student had prior immunoprophylaxis, then antigen detection is the method of choice. For antigen detection; skin biopsies, corneal impression smears, and cell sediment from saliva are generally used. It is important to remember that patients with rabies do not always give histories of animal bites.

7. *e* (all are correct).

8. *e* (all are correct).

9. *d* (1, 2, and 3 are correct). Mosquito abatement is effective when the vector is a mosquito living in an urban environment, such as the vector of St. Louis encephalitis virus. If the vector is a tick (e.g., Colorado tick fever) or a mosquito that lives in the forest (e.g., jungle yellow fever), mosquito abatement program is ineffective or impractical.

10. *e*

THE ADENOVIRUS, PAPOVIRUS, AND PARVOVIRUS FAMILIES

THE ADENOVIRUS FAMILY

This family of viruses includes over 40 ''species'' or ''serotypes'' capable of infecting humans. Most of them produce superficial infections of the respiratory and/or intestinal tracts. A few occasionally infect the urinary tract and the meninges. Specific antiviral therapy against, and practical measure for the prevention of, adenovirus infections are not available.

FAMILY CHARACTERISTICS

Morphology

Adenovirus virions are nonenveloped, have icosahedral capsid symmetry, and measure about 80 nm in diameter. Except for the 12 vertex capsomeres, the capsid is formed by the capsomeres known as **hexons.** The vertex capsomer is known as the **penton.** From each penton is a fiber projection known as the **fiber antigen** (Fig. 47.1).

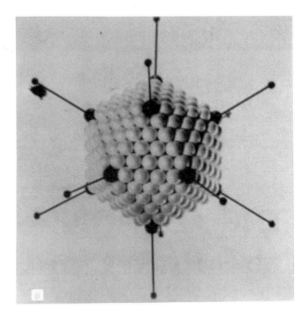

Figure 47.1.

Diagram of an adenovirus showing the hexon, penton, and fiber antigens. [Reproduced with permission from Horne RW (1974): Virus Structure. New York: Academic Press.]

Genomic Chemistry

The genome consists of a single molecule of double-stranded DNA.

Replication Strategy

The **fiber antigen** attaches to a specific **cell receptor** and, thereby, initiates the replication cycle. Six **early** and one **late transcription region** have been identified within the genome. The early regions yield products that are essential for the replication of viral DNA and the transcription of the late transcription region, which codes for structural proteins. Like all true DNA viruses, transcription of viral genes depend on the **host's polymerases.** The virus codes for its own DNA dependent DNA polymerase.

Species

There are numerous species that are pathogenic for humans, nonhuman mammals, and avian species. They are grouped into genera, subgenera, and types (species). Based on the neutralization test, there are **over 40 types of human adenoviruses.**

Antigens

The hexon of all mammalian adenoviruses contains cross-reacting epitope. The tip of the **fiber antigen is serotype specific.** The penton is toxic to cultured human cells.

HUMAN ADENOVIRUSES

Pathogenesis

Primary targets are the **epithelium of the respiratory and/or the intestinal tracts.** Virus multiplication damages the cells and incites inflammation locally. Rarely, the virus may reach the urinary tract and meninges presumably during a transient viremic phase. Diseases associated with adenovirus infections include **acute respiratory infection, conjunctivitis** and **keratoconjunctivitis, enteritis,** acute hemorrhagic cystitis, and aseptic meningitis. Except for the involvement of the lower respiratory tract, all adenovirus infections are benign and self-limiting. Chronic symptomatic infection or latent infection have not been described.

Diagnosis

Specific virologic diagnosis is seldom indicated in medical practice.

Treatment

Specific antiadenovirus treatment is not available.

Epidemiology and Prevention

Sources of adenoviruses are the **respiratory secretions** and **feces** of infected persons. Portals of entry are the respiratory and alimentary tracts. Modes of transmission include the respiratory and fecal-oral routes. Some infected persons may excrete the virus in feces for many months. **Nosocomial infections** of the conjunctiva are not uncommon. There are more than 40 serotypes of human adenoviruses. Presumably, infection by one serotype induces solid immunity to reinfection by the homologous type only; therefore, adenovirus infections are common.

Vaccines against two serotypes are available, but they are not in general use. Practical procedures for intercepting transmission are not available except in nosocomial infections. **Epidemics of acute keratoconjunctivitis** are sometimes associated with visits to eye clinics. Such epidemics are due to indirect transfer of virus with contaminated fingers and instruments. The routine use of disposable gloves and the washing of hands and instruments with soap and water should prevent the occurrence of such epidemics.

THE PAPOVAVIRUS FAMILY

Several members of the papovavirus family are common infectious agents of humans. Except for the papillomavirus, they rarely induce significant diseases in immunocompetent persons. The main interest in this family of viruses is their **oncogenic potential.** The papillomavirus was the first DNA virus proven to be carcinogenic in the laboratory; a mouse polyomavirus when inoculated into newborn mice was shown to induce more than 20 types of cancer; and a monkey polyomavirus (simian virus 40) was capable of transforming human epithelium and fibroblasts in vitro. Certain types of human papillomaviruses have been associated with carcinoma of the cervix.

FAMILY CHARACTERISTICS

Morphology

They are nonenveloped spherical viruses with icosahedral nucleocapsid symmetry. Virions measure 45–70 nm in diameter.

Genomic Chemistry

The genome consists of a single molecule of double-stranded and circularized DNA.

Replication Strategy

The genome consists of an **early region** that codes for **two T proteins,** a **late region** that codes for the **capsid protein,** and a **noncoding region** that contains the T protein binding site, origin of DNA replication, and transcription control sequences. The virus does not code for any polymcrase. The DNA synthesis and transcription **depend on the host's polymerases.** After uncoating, the early region is transcribed and translated into two proteins known as T and t. The **T protein then binds onto the noncoding region** and, thereby enables the host's polymerases to transcribe the late genes and synthesize DNA. The **T protein also interacts with cellular components,** which results in the enhancement of host DNA replication.

Medically Important Species

The papovaviruses are divided into two genera: the **papillomaviruses** and the **polyomaviruses.** The papillomavirus is larger than the polyomavirus (70 vs. 45 nm). The genome of the papillomavirus is also longer (8 vs. 5 kbp). Papillomaviruses are classified according to host range (e.g., human, bovine, etc.) and nucleic acid relatedness. By definition, isolates showing **less than 50% DNA homology are considered as independent types.** There are **at least 60 types of human papillomaviruses.** Due to our inability to grow the virus in the laboratory, little information is available on antigenic relatedness of the papillomavirus. Little is known about immunity to reinfection by homologous or heterologous types. However, it is known that papillomaviruses and polyomaviruses do not cross-react serologically. There are two species of human polyomavirus: the **JC** and **BK viruses.**

HUMAN PAPILLOMAVIRUSES

Pathogenesis

The target is the **cutaneous and mucosal squamous epithelium.** Cell infection results not in cell death but in **cell proliferation.** Cell proliferation leads to **circumscribed tumor** (wart), which almost always regress spontaneously. **Long persistence of viral gene** sequences in and around the regressed tumor is common. The carcinogenic potential of human papillomavirus is under active investigation. There are reports of association between **anogenital carcinoma and human papillomaviruses** (especially types 16 and 18).

Diagnosis

Virological confirmation of clinical diagnosis of warts is unnecessary.

Treatment

The general principle is to destroy as much wart and as little normal tissue as possible. **Interferon-α** has been approved by the FDA for treatment of severe anogenital wart (condyloma acuminata) by local infiltration.

Epidemiology and Prevention

The source of the virus is the **wart tissue.** Transmission occurs through **direct contact** with the virus. **Sexual transmission** is common. Two-thirds of sexual contacts of infected persons eventually become infected. In one recent survey of healthy college women undergoing annual gynecological examination, 46% were positive for viral gene sequences by a PCR-based method. The only effective preventive measure is the avoidance of contact with wart tissue.

HUMAN POLYOMAVIRUSES

Pathogenesis

Presumably, the portal of entry is the respiratory tract. After some replication, there is a brief viremic phase during which the virus lodges in the kidney. The virus multiplies in the urinary tract and may produce viruria. In immunocompetent persons, the infection is asymptomatic. Despite their oncogenicity in laboratory animals, there is no evidence for proliferative response in humans. Despite extensive searches, the **JC or BK viruses have not been associated with cancers in human. Latency is common.**

Rarely, and only in immunodefective subjects, the JC virus may cause **progressive multifocal leukoencephalopathy.** This illness is a chronic progressive degenerative disease of the CNS with multiple foci of demyelinization.

Diagnosis

Etiologic diagnosis is not required.

Treatment

Specific antiviral therapy is not available.

Epidemiology and Prevention

The exact source and mode of transmission are not known, although viruses are frequently demonstrated in the **urine of infected subjects.** A limited number of serologic surveys suggested that many acquire infections during childhood. About 70% of healthy adults are seropositive. Effective preventive procedures are not available and probably not necessary.

THE PARVOVIRUS FAMILY

This family includes two genera that are of some interest: the **parvovirus** and the **dependovirus.** The parvovirus B19 is the etiologic agent of a common childhood disease (erythema infestiosum), but may cause more serious complications, such as transient aplastic crisis, chronic anemia, and fetal death. Dependoviruses are defective and require helper function of the adeno- or herpesviruses. Dependoviruses do not cause disease in humans.

FAMILY CHARACTERISTICS

Morphology

Parvovirus virions are nonenveloped, have icosahedral capsid symmetry, and measure about 20 nm in diameter. These viruses are the **smallest virions** known to be infectious for humans.

Genomic Chemistry

The genome consists of one molecule of **single-stranded DNA** only about 5 kb in size. Some virions encapsidate the positive strand and others, encapsidate the negative. Parvovirus is the only family of human viruses that has single-stranded DNA as genome.

Replication Strategy

Not much is known about the synthetic phase. Other phases of the replication cycle are presumably the same as other nonenveloped virions.

Medically Important Species

This family includes two genera infectious for humans, the parvo- and dependoviruses. A major difference between them is that dependoviruses are defective in humans and parvoviruses are not. Only the parvoviruses cause diseases in humans.

PARVOVIRUS B19

Pathogenesis

This parvovirus is the etiologic agent of a self-limiting common exanthema (**erythema infectiosum**) that occur predominantly among children. The infection has been studied in human volunteers. Several days after intranasal inoculation of the B19 virus, there is an **intensive viremia** (virus titer in the blood may reach 10^{11} virus particles per milliliter!). At the same time, the virus is found in the throat. At the time the skin rash appears, infectious virus can no longer be detected in the blood or throat. The skin rash, arthralgia, and arthritis are presumably due to the formation of **intravascular immune complexes.** Target cells that release this large number of virions have not yet been identified.

The B19 virus does replicate in and presumably destroy dividing **erythroid precursor cells.** Bone marrow aspirates obtained during incubation show a marked reduction of erythroid cells of all development stages. In previously normal subjects, this destruction results in a transient and clinically **insignificant anemia.** In subjects with chronic hemolytic anemia in whom the life-span of the erythrocyte is markedly reduced, the destruction of erythroid cells may result in **severe anemia.** In immunodefective persons, B19 infection may persist with chronic anemia as the consequence. There is suggestive evidence for B19-associated fetal death. Congenital anomalies associated with B19 intrauterine infections have not been proven.

Diagnosis

In day-to-day clinical practice, virologic confirmation of clinical diagnosis is unnecessary. In situations when virologic diagnosis is desired, the test of choice is the assay for **IgM antibody against the B19.**

Treatment

Specific antiviral therapy against the B19 virus is unavailable.

Epidemiology and Prevention

The source of the virus is the **respiratory secretion** of infected persons during the incubation period. Although the blood may contain the virus in high concentration, it is not an important source, presumably because the viremic phase is transient. The chief mode of transmission is presumably close personal contact. The B19 infections occur worldwide. Surveys have revealed the B19 antibody in over 30% of healthy adults. Erythema infectiosum is a mild self-limiting disease and does not require prevention except among the following three groups of high risk subjects: persons with chronic hemolytic anemia, immunodefective subjects, and pregnant women. Active or passive immunoprophylaxis are not available; therefore, prevention depends on avoiding contact with infected persons.

SUMMARY

1. Adenoviruses are nonenveloped DNA viruses. At least 40 serotypes are infectious for humans. The capsid consists of three antigens: the hexon, penton, and fiber antigen. The hexon of all mammalian adenoviruses cross-reacts in serological tests, while the fiber antigen is type specific. It is through the fiber antigen that the virion attaches to the cell receptor.

2. Primary targets are the epithelium of the respiratory and/or intestinal tract. Diseases caused by adenoviruses include acute respiratory infection, conjunctivitis, keratoconjunctivitis, and gastroenteritis. Rarely, the virus may reach distant secondary targets through the blood circulation.

3. Virologic diagnosis is unnecessary in clinical practice and specific antiviral treatment is not available.

4. Papovaviruses are also nonenveloped DNA viruses. The medically important viruses belong to the genus *Papillomavirus*. There are many species or types of papillomaviruses; at least 60 types are infectious for humans. Typing is based on DNA homology; virus isolates showing less than 50% homology are considered as independent types.

5. The primary target of human papillomavirus is the squamous epithelium of the skin and mucosa. Virus multiplication results in cell proliferation, and cell proliferation results in circumscribed tumor (wart). Warts almost always regress spontaneously. Viral gene sequences persist for many years at the site of regressed tumor. The relationship between anogenital carcinoma and type 16 virus and between anogenital carcinoma and type 18 virus is under active investigation.

6. Interferon-α, infiltrated locally, is effective in the treatment of condyloma acuminata (severe anogenital wart).

7. Human papillomavirus is transmitted by contact, especially sexual contact. In a survey of university students attending gynecological clinic, 46% were positive for the virus (by a PCR-based method).

8. Parvoviruses are also nonenveloped DNA viruses. These viruses are the smallest known human viruses (20 nm). The genome is unique in that it consists of single-strand DNA. The DNA is only 5 kb in size.

9. Only one species, the parvovirus B19, is of medical importance. The B19 virus is the etiologic agent of erythema infectiosum, a common self-limiting acute exanthemata diseases occurring predominantly among children.

10. The B19 virus first multiplies in the upper respiratory tract. This step is followed by a very intensive viremia, which may reach 10^{11} virions per milliliter of blood. Finally, generalized exanthematous eruption, arthralgia, and arthritis appear. These manifestations are presumably due to the formation of intravascular immune complexes.

11. The B19 virus also multiplies in and destroys the multiplying erythroid precursor cells. This results in a transient, but clinically insignificant, anemia. In subjects having chronic hemolytic anemia, this transient destruction of erythroid cells may lead to severe anemia. In immunocompromised persons, parvovirus B19 may persist as a chronic infection with anemia as a consequence and B19-associated fetal deaths have been reported.

12. Parvovirus B19 infections are common. Over 30% of the healthy adult population have B19 antibody. Virologic diagnosis is unnecessary. Specific treatment and immunoprophylaxis are not available.

REFERENCES

Anderson LJ (1990): Human parvoviruses. J Inf Dis 161:603.

Bauer HM et al. (1991): Genital human papilloma virus infection in female university students as determined by a PCR-based method. JAMA 265:472.

Editorial Human papillomaviruses and the PCR (1990): Lancet i:1051.

Jernigan JA et al. (1993): Adenovirus type 8 epidemic keratoconjunctivitis in an eye clinic: risk factors and control. J Inf Dis 167:1307.

Jha PK et al. (1993): Antibodies to human papillomavirus and to other gential infectious agents and invasive cervical cancer risk. Lancet 341:1116.

Markowitz RB et al. (1993): Incidence of BK virus and JC virus viruria in HIV infected and uninfected subjects. J Inf Dis 167:13.

Munoz N, Bosch X, Kaldor JM (1988): Does human papilloma-virus cause cervical cancer? The state of epidemiological evidence. Br J Cancer 57:1.

Pillay D, et al. (1992): Parvovirus B19 outbreak in a children's ward. Lancet 339:107.

Reichman RC, Strike DG (1989): Pathogenesis and treatment of human genital papillomavirus infections: a review. Antiviral Res 11:109.

Serjeant GR et al. (1993): Human parvovirus infection in homozygous sickle cell disease. Lancet 341:1237.

Singer A, Jenkins D (1991): Viruses and cervical cancer. Br Med J 302:251.

Villareal LP (1989): Common Mechanisms of Transformation by Small DNA Tumor Viruses. American Society of Microbiology. Washington, DC.

Wadell G (1988): Adenoviridae in Laboratory Diagnosis of Infectious Diseases Principles and Practice, Vol. II. In Lennette EH, Halonen P, Murphy FA (eds): (1991): Viral Rickettsial and Chlamydial Diseases. New York: Springer-Verlag pp 284–300.

REVIEW QUESTIONS

For questions 1 to 8, choose the ONE BEST answer or completion.

1. About human adenoviruses:
   a) there are at least 40 serotypes
   b) typing is based on the neutralization test
   c) neutralizing antibody reacts with epitope(s) on the fiber antigen of the virion
   d) antibody reactive against the hexon capsomeres of type 2 virus in human serum is also reactive against the hexons of types 1, 5, 9, and 13 viruses
   e) all of the above

2. Human adenovirus
   a) generally causes superficial infection of the respiratory and/or the intestinal tract
   b) may cause conjunctivitis, keratoconjunctivitis, pharyngitis, and/or acute diarrhea
   c) associated conjunctivitis and/or keratoconjunctivitis may be due to nosocomial infections at eye clinics
   d) type-specific vaccines are effective but are available only against a few types
   e) all of the above

3. Papovaviridae
   a) are of medical importance primarily because of their oncogenic potential
   b) are DNA viruses
   c) are divided into two genera: the papillomaviruses and polyomaviruses
   d) infections in humans are common (>10% of the adult females in the United States have evidence of infection past or present)
   e) all of the above

4. About human papillomaviruses:
   a) there are at least 50 types of viruses
   b) they are typed by DNA homology
   c) their primary target is the squamous epithelium of the skin and mucosa
   d) multiplication in target cells results in cell proliferation rather than cell death
   e) all of the above

5. About human papillomaviruses:
   a) they are transmitted from person to person exclusively through sexual contacts
   b) persistence of virus genomes in tissue after clinical recovery is uncommon
   c) recovery from infection by type 1 virus induces solid immunity to infection by all other types
   d) type 16 virus is more likely to be found in cervical carcinoma than in normal cervix

6. The parvoviruses
   a) are the smallest virion known to be infectious for humans

b) are about the size of a ribosome (20 nm in diameter)
c) have single-stranded DNA genome
d) have a genome of only 5 kb in size
e) all of the above

7. The human parvovirus B19
   a) is the etiologic agent of erythema infectiosum
   b) induces a transient but very intense viremia in the infected person
   c) associated clinical manifestations (exanthema and arthralgia) are presumably due to the formation of intravascular immune complexes
   d) antibody is present in at least 30% of the healthy adult population in the United States

e) all of the above

8. About the parvovirus B19 infection in humans:
   a) it multiplies in and destroys multiplying erythroid cells
   b) there may be depletion of erythroid cells in bone marrow during incubation of erythema infectiosum
   c) transient but clinically insignificant anemia is present in most cases of erythema infectiosum
   d) population groups at high risk of developing severe infections include persons with chronic hemolytic anemia, immunodefective subjects and the fetuses (pregnant women)
   e) all of the above

ANSWERS TO REVIEW QUESTIONS

---

1. *e*

2. *e*

3. *e*

4. *e*

5. *d* Warts may occur in areas other than the anogenital region; infections may occur through activity other than sexual intercourse. For example, laryngeal papilloma in young children is due to passage through a birth canal contaminated with the papillomavirus during birth. The persistence of viral gene sequences is very common. Very little is known about the immunologic relationship between the different types of papillomaviruses. Therefore, only *d* is correct.

6. *e*

7. *e*

8. *e*

POXVIRIDAE, VIROIDS, AND PRIONS

This chapter briefly describes three groups of "virus-like" infectious agents. Whether these virus-like agents are true viruses depends on definition and usage.

POXVIRIDAE

The poxviruses are recognized as true viruses by the International Committee on Nomenclature of viruses despite the fact that many of their basic characteristics are uniquely different from those of the true viruses. The important differences are summarized in Table 48.1. Some virologists have questioned the validity of classifying the poxviruses as viruses.

Three species are of medical interest: **smallpox, vaccinia,** and **molluscum contagiosum** viruses. Smallpox has been **eradicated** through a worldwide coordinated effort of vaccination, case identification, and quarantine. The World Health Organization (WHO) declared in 1980 that the world is free of smallpox. **Vacciniavirus is the smallpox vaccine virus.** Smallpox vaccination is **not an innocuous procedure** and is no longer recommended for universal usage. The vacciniavirus is now used extensively as **vectors for selected genes** (e.g., HB$_s$Ag, HIV

TABLE 48.1. Major Differences in the Basic Characteristics of the Poxviruses and All Other Medically Important Families of Viruses

Characteristic	Other virus families	*Poxviridae*
Size	Submicroscopic (<200 nm in diameter)	Visible with a light microscope
Shape	Mostly spherical (excepting rhabdo-and filoviruses)	Brick shaped
Basic architecture	Nucleic acids wrapped in a protective layer of capsid protein that may be surrounded by an outermost envelope	Very much more complex (Fig. 32.6)
Uncoating	By host enzymes	Require virus-specified uncoating enzymes
Synthetic phase	Transcription of viral DNA by host's polymerase; transcription in the nucleus	Transcription of poxviral DNA by virus-specified transcriptase; whole replication cycle in the cytoplasm
Maturation and release	Envelope virions mature and release through "budding out" of cell membrane	Acquires its outermost envelope in the cytoplasm; viruses released through cell death.
Envelope essential?	The envelope of all enveloped viruses is essential in initiating the replication cycle	Poxviruses without the envelope can initiate the replication cycle

gp 120, etc.) in experimental **recombinant vaccine.** Molluscum contagiosum virus cause molluscum contagiosum, which is a benign self-limiting skin condition characterized by **umbilicated pearl-like nodules.** The disease is acquired by direct contact with the virus.

VIROIDS

Viroids are small molecules of single-stranded RNA less than 0.5 kb in size and are capable of replicating in susceptible cells. The RNA have regions of internal complementarity allows for self-anneal by internal base pairing, thereby yielding stable rodlike structures (Fig. 48.1). Complementarity at both ends of the RNA molecule permits circularization. It is not clear if viroids code for viroid specific proteins. Since the host does not have RNA replicase and the viroid genome is too small to code for such an enzyme, how viroids multiply remains unresolved. There is some similarity in base sequences between viroids and group I intron, which codes for ribosomal RNA and mitochondrial mRNA. Viroids are conceptually but not medically important since all viroids identified thus far are

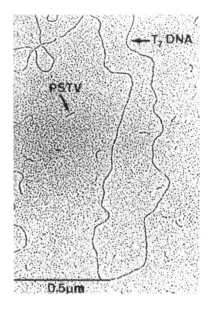

Figure 48.1.

Electronmicrograph of a plant viroid (PSTV) and the DNA of a T7 coliphage. [Reproduced with permission from Diener TO (1979): Viroids and viroid diseases. New York: Wiley.]

plant pathogens. Virusoids are similar to viroids except that the virusoid is encapsidated in an RNA virus and that the virusoid needs helper function from the RNA virus for replication.

There is suggestive evidence that the **hepatitis D virus (HDV) may be a viroid.** Similarities and differences between viroids and HDV and between HDV and the smallest RNA virus are outlined in Table 48.2 (see also Chapter 41 regarding HDV).

PRIONS

Prion is an acronym derived from **"*pr*oteinaceous *in*fectious particles."** Infectivity of prions is destroyed by most procedures that modify proteins but not by most that modify nucleic acids. The term ''prion'' has not yet been universally accepted; some refer to this group of infectious agents as **unconventional virus** or **agents of spongioform encephalopathies.** The more important prions are the infectious agent of **scrapie** (laboratory animal model) and **Creutzfeldt-Jakob disease** (humans). Prion-associated diseases are chronic degenerative diseases of the brain, known as **spongioform encephalopathies.**

Prions from scrapie-infected hamster brains have been extensively studied. Its infectivity is associated with or inseparable from a purified protein known as prion protein (PrP), which has a molecular weight of 27–30 kDa. The PrP is

TABLE 48.2. Similarities and Differences Among Viroids, δ Hepatitis Agent (Hepatitis D Virus), and the Smallest RNA Virus (Picornaviruses)

Characteristics	Viroid	HDV	Picornavirus
Genome			
Size (in kilobarns)	0.5	1.7	7
Internal complementarity	Yes	Yes	No
circularization	Yes	Yes	No
rodlike morphology	Yes	Yes	No
Homology with group I intron	Yes	Some	No
Virus-specified			
RNA replicase	No	No	Yes
antigens	No	Yes	Yes
Nucleocapsid	No	No	Yes
Needing helper function from a helper virus for replication	No	?[a]	No

[a] There is speculation that the helper function provided to the HDV by the HBV is for transmission and not for replication.

derived from the host glycoprotein. In contrast to glycoprotein from uninfected host, PrP is resistant to hydrolysis by proteinase K. The PrP may aggregate into "prion rods" or "scrapie-associated fibrils" about 10–20 nm in diameter and 100–200 nm long. Prion protein is weakly antigenic; specific antibody has been produced. Similar PrP have also been isolated from the brain of patients with prion-associated diseases, such as Creutzfeldt-Jakob disease (Fig. 48.2).

There are two types of PrP, **PrP^C** and **PrP^{SC}**. PrP^C are **products of the *PrP* gene** of host cells, found on **cell surface, precursor molecules** of PrP^{SC}, and degraded by proteinase K. PrP^{SC} initiate the **conversion of PrP^C to PrP^{SC},** are found **within the cell,** is resistant to **proteinase K,** and is responsible for the **spongeoform appearance** of affected cells.

Creutzfeldt-Jakob disease is rare; its prevalence rate (United States and worldwide) is 1 per million. Modes of transmission are not known, but cornea transplantation, brain surgery, and parenteral administration of growth hormone extracted from human pituitary glands, and dura matter transplantation have been implicated. The brain of a Creutzfeldt-Jakob patient may contain up to 10^{10} LD$_{50}$ prions per gram. Diagnosis is based on the clinical picture and may be confirmed after death by the characteristic spongiform degeneration in the brain. There is no specific treatment. Prevention is limited to those transmitted iatrogenically. It is useful to remember that complete inactivation of prions requires autoclaving at 132°C in a steam autoclave for 1 h or soaking in 1 N sodium hydroxide at room temp for 1 h. Soaking in 2.5% sodium hypochlorite for 1 h at room temperature **almost but not quite completely** inactivate prions.

Fatal familial insomnia has been claimed to be a prion-associated disease.

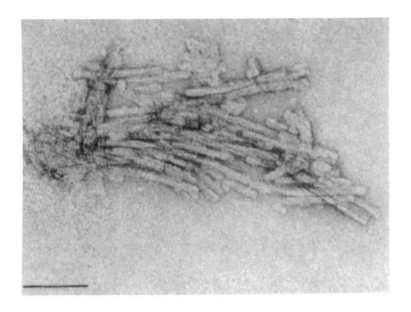

Figure 48.2.
Electronmicrograph of prion rods from Creutzfeldt-Jakob disease. Bar = 100 nm. [Reproduced with permission from Buckman JM, Kingsbury DT (1985): Creutzfeldt-Jakob disease prion proteins in human brains. N Engl J Med 312:76, fig. 3C.]

SUMMARY

1. Many of the basic characteristics of the poxviruses are uniquely different from those of other viruses (see Table 48.1 for these differences). Some virologists have questioned the validity of classifying the poxviruses as viruses.

2. Smallpox has been eradicated through a worldwide effort of vaccination case finding and quarantine.

3. Smallpox vaccination with the vacciniavirus is not an innocuous procedure and should not be used any more in medical practice.

4. Vaccinavirus is now used as a vector for selected genes in experimental recombinant vaccine.

5. Molluscum contagiosum virus causes a benign self-limiting skin lesion characterized by umbilicated pearllike nodules.

6. Viroids are small RNA molecules capable of replicating in susceptible cells.

7. The RNA has regions of internal complementarity, which allows for self-annealing to form stable rod and to circularize.

8. There is base homology between viroids and group 1 intron.

9. All viroids identified thus far are plant pathogens.

10. The δ hepatitis agent (hepatitis D virus) has some similarities to viroids (see Table 48.2).

11. Prions are proteinaceous infectious agents whose infectivity is destroyed by many procedures that destroy proteins and not by procedures that destroy nucleic acids.

12. The basic pathology of prion-associated diseases is spongiform encephalopathy.

13. Infectivity of prions is inseparable from a prion protein. This protein has a molecular weight of 27–30 kDa, derives from the host's glycoprotein, but is not hydrolyzed by proteinase K.

14. The most important prions in medicine are the scrapie (animal model) and Creutzfeldt-Jakob disease prions.

15. Creutzfeldt-Jakob disease is rare (prevalence of 1 per million). The brain of a patient dying from this disease may contain 10^{10} LD_{50} per gram of tissue. Transmission has been associated with cornea or transplantation, brain surgery, administration of growth hormone (extract from human pituitary glands), and transplantation of dura matter.

16. Destruction of prions requires autoclaving at 132°C for 1 h or soaking in 1 N sodium hydroxide also for 1 h.

REFERENCES

Centers for Disease Control (1991): Vaccinia (Smallpox) vaccine. MMWR 40:1.

Cooney EL et al. (1991): Safety and immunological response to a recombinant vaccinia virus vaccine expressing HIV envelope glycoprotein. Lancet 337:567.

Brown P, Liberski PP, Wolff A, Gajdusek DC (1990): Resistance of scrapie infectivity to steam autoclaving, after formaldehyde fixation, and limited survival after ashing at 360°C: practical and theoretical implications. J Inf Dis 161:467.

Fradkin JE et al. (1991): Creutzfeldt-Jakob disease in pituitary growth hormone recipients in the U.S. JAMA 265:880.

Hsiao K et al. (1991): Mutation of the prion protein in Libyan Jews with Creutzfeldt-Jakob disease. N Engl J Med 324(16):1091.

Medori R et al. (1992): Fatal familial insomnia, a prion disease with a mutation at codon 178 of the prion protein gene. N Engl J Med 326:444.

Safar J, Ceroni M, Gajdusek DC, Gribbs CJ (1991): Differences in membrane interaction of scrapie amyloid precursor proteins in normal and scrapie- or Creutzfeldt-Jakob disease-infected brains. J Inf Dis 163:488.

Prusiner SB (1989): Scrapie prions. Annu Rev Microbiol 43:345.

REVIEW QUESTIONS

For questions 1 to 9, choose the ONE
BEST answer or completion.

1. Poxviruses
   a) are brick shaped
   b) are visible with a light microscope
   c) have an envelope
   d) have neither a helical nor an icosahedral
      nucleocapsid
   e) all of the above

2. About the replication cycle of poxviruses:
   a) attachment depends on a virus glycopro-
      tein on the viral envelope
   b) uncoating depends entirely on host en-
      zyme
   c) early genes are transcribed by the host
      RNA polymerase II (DNA-dependent
      RNA polymerase)
   d) maturation and release through "bud-
      ding" from infected cell membrane have
      not been documented

3. About medically important poxviruses:
   a) smallpox has been eradicated from the
      planet Earth through vaccination case
      finding and quarantine
   b) the vacciniavirus was used in inducing
      immunity against smallpox
   c) the vacciniavirus is now used as a vector

   for HB_s gene in experimental recombinant vaccine
   d) molluscum contagiosum over the genital
      area is seen with increasing frequency
      among adults having multiple sex part-
      ners
   e) all of the above

4. Viroids
   a) are small molecules of single-stranded
      RNA capable of forming circles
   b) are capable of replicating in susceptible
      cells
   c) show some degree of homology with
      group I intron
   d) are plant pathogens
   e) all of the above

5. Key similarity between viroids and δ hepatitis agent (hepatitis D virus) include
   a) genomes consisting of small single-
      stranded 0.5-kb RNA
   b) coding for only one antigen
   c) some homology with group I intron
   d) requirement for helper function from an-
      other virus in order to replicate

6. Prion
   a) is a proteinaceous infectious agent
   b) is also known as unconventional virus
   c) associated diseases consist pathologically
      of spongiform encephalopathy

    d) of Creutzfeldt-Jakob disease is infectious for humans

    e) all of the above

7. Prion protein

    a) has a molecular weight of no more than 30 kDa

    b) and prion infectivity are inseparable

    c) is a derivative of the host glycoprotein but is resistant to digestion by proteinase K

    d) is found in the brain of animal infected by the scrapie prion or of human dying of Creutzfeldt-Jakob disease

    e) all of the above

8. Creutzfeldt-Jakob

    a) disease has a prevalence of about $1/10^6$ in the United States

    b) disease prions may be found in the brain of a patient dying of the disease in concentration as high as 10^{10} LD_{50} (50% lethal doses for hamster) per gram of tissue

    c) disease has been transmitted between persons through transplantation of cornea or dura matter, during brain surgery, and inoculation of growth hormone extracted from human pituitary glands

    d) disease transmission between spouses has not been documented

    e) all of the above

9. Creutzfeldt-Jakob disease prion

    a) in the brain is still infectious after storing the brain in 10% formalin for 3 years

    b) contaminated surgical instruments still have infectious prions after autoclaving at 110°C for 10 min (this is the usual procedure for sterilizing solution)

    c) on a surgical instrument is not completely destroyed by soaking the instrument in 2.5% bleach (sodium hypochlorite) for 1 h at room temperature

    d) contaminated surgical instruments must be autoclaved at 132°C for 1 h or immersed in 1 *N* sodium hydroxide for 1 h to be absolutely certain that the prion has been destroyed

    e) all of the above

ANSWERS TO REVIEW QUESTIONS

1. *e*

2. *d* *a, b,* and *c* are correct for all enveloped DNA viruses; but the poxvirus is an exception.

3. *e*

4. *e*

5. *c* The genome of δ hepatitis agent is much larger than 0.5 kb. There is no evidence that viroids code for any antigen; and there is evidence that δ hepatitis agent codes for two antigens. Viroids do not require helper function from another virus for replication.

6. *e*

7. *e*

8. *e*

9. *e* The resistance of prions to destruction by the usual disinfectants have been a difficult problem for Hospital Infection Control Committee. Conditions known to completely inactivate prions are also detrimental to delicate instruments.

PARASITOLOGY

PARASITOLOGY

Although the term **"parasite"** may be applied broadly to all infectious agents, including bacteria, viruses, and fungi, it is traditionally reserved for parasitic protozoa, helminths (worms), and arthropods. The classification of parasites used in this chapter is simplified and uses common terminology.

CLASSIFICATION

Protozoa

Protozoa are single-cell animals. A list of the various groups of protozoa follows:

Amebae (Sarcodina) move by the use of cytoplasmic protrusions called pseudopods. Reproduction is asexual. An example of this group is *Entamoeba histolytica,* the cause of amebic dysentery.

Flagellates (Mastigophora) use specialized whiplike structures called flagella for motility. Reproduction is asexual. Examples are the intestinal flagellate, *Giardia lamblia,* and the blood flagellates, *Trypanosoma* species.

Apicomplexa (also called Sporozoa) are intracellular parasites that contain several organelles organized into an "apical complex." This structure functions in the penetration of host cells. Reproduction involves both sexual and asexual cycles. The malaria parasites and the intestinal parasite, *Cryptosporidium,* are examples of this group.

Ciliates (Ciliophora) are represented by only a single species that is parasitic in humans, *Balantidium coli.* Ciliates move by the use of cilia that cover the organism's surface. Cilia resemble short flagella in their structure and function. Reproduction may be asexual and also may occur through the exchange of nuclear material between organisms during conjugation.

Microsporidia (also called Microsporida) are very small, intracellular organisms that produce spores containing a characteristic coiled polar tube. Almost all human infections occur in immunocompromised individuals.

Helminths

Helminths are multicelled worms, which are classified as flatworms and roundworms.

Flatworms (Platyhelminthes) that parasitize humans are classified into two major groups: flukes and tapeworms. **Flukes (Trematodes)** are leaf-shaped, dorsoventrally flattened, and possess oral and ventral suckers for attachment. All species excepting the schistosomes are hermaphroditic. **Tapeworms (Cestodes)** are ribbon-shaped with an anterior attachment organ, the scolex, and a segmented body. Each segment contains both male and female sex organs.

Roundworms (Nematodes) are cylindrical and possess a well-developed intestinal tract. The sexes are separate.

Arthropods

The arthropods have chitinous exoskeletons with jointed appendages. Arthropods of major medical importance are classified as insects or arachnids.

Insects have a body that is divided into the head, thorax, and abdomen. Three pairs of legs originate from the thorax. An example of an insect parasite is the body louse. Many species of insects are not, by strict definition, parasites, but they serve as vectors for a wide variety of diseases. For example, mosquitoes transmit malaria, filariasis, and many arboviruses. **Arachnids** have four pairs of legs in the adult stage. The body is divided into the cephalothorax and abdomen. This group contains mites, ticks, spiders, and scorpions. Mites and ticks appear unsegmented because the the cephalothorax is fused with the abdomen.

DEFINITIONS

Below are definitions of terms that are used in describing parasite life cycles and host-parasite interrelationships:

Host: An organism that harbors or nourishes another organism.

Definitive Host: A host that harbors the adult or sexual form of the parasite.

Intermediate Host: A host that harbors larval or asexual stages of the parasite.

Reservoir Host: A nonhuman host that can maintain the infection in nature in the absence of human hosts.

Adult: The sexually mature stage of helminths and arthropods.

Larva: Immature stages of helminths and arthropods.

Vector: An arthropod that is responsible for the transmission of an infection. Mechanical vectors transmit disease by transferring organisms from contaminated body parts to the host or by having the organisms pass through the intestinal tract of the vector and be excreted in its feces. An example would be houseflies contaminating food with typhoid bacilli. Biologic vectors are essential in the multiplication or development of the organisms to infectious levels or stages. Examples are the multiplication of plague bacilli in the rat flea and the development of infectious stages of malaria parasites in mosquitoes.

Symbiosis: Organisms that are "living together." This arrangement may offer benefits to one or both organisms or may be detrimental to one organism. Symbiosis may be divided into categories. The categories pertinent to human parasitology are:

Commensalism: "Eating at the same table." There is benefit to one organism but no significant effect on the other. This term is most frequently used when referring to intestinal protozoa that have no pathologic effects on the host. These organisms are called **"commensals."**

Parasitism: One organism (the parasite) benefits at the expense of the other (the host).

Endoparasite: A parasite that lives inside the host, such as intestinal parasites. Endoparasites cause **infections.**

Ectoparasite: A parasite that lives on the surface of the host, such as the head louse. Ectoparasites cause **infestations.**

In Chapters 49–61, the major parasitic organisms are discussed in detail. Less common parasites may be mentioned briefly or displayed in tabular form. In general, the discussion of each parasite will focus on the following areas:

Organism: The scientific name of the organism and common name when one exists. The name of the disease caused by the organism.

Transmission: A discussion of how the infection is acquired by humans.

Geographic Distribution and Epidemiology: This information provides a listing of countries or general areas where the parasitic infection is found in humans with a brief discussion of the factors that influence the distribution and prevalence.

Habitat: A description of where the parasites are found in the human body.

Properties of the Organism: Provides a description of the parasite and its stages of development.

Clinical Manifestations: A brief listing of the major signs and symptoms associated with the infection.

Laboratory Diagnosis: A discussion of the appropriate laboratory tests used to arrive at a definitive diagnosis.

Treatment: A very brief mention of the approach to treatment of the infection. No attempt is made to provide drug regimens and dosages.

These chapters provide illustrations of the most important parasites. However, the student is encouraged to supplement the reading with other sources of visual material (see the reference section).

DIAGNOSTIC TECHNIQUES FOR PARASITIC INFECTIONS

Although there may be specific diagnostic techniques that are mentioned in the discussion of individual parasites, there are some general techniques that will be discussed here.

Fecal Examination

Fecal examination for ova and parasites is used for most intestinal parasites. In clinical jargon, this is often referred to as "stool for O and P" when an order is written to collect fecal specimens for parasitologic examination. The most practical method for collection of stool specimens is to use preservatives. A collection kit consisting of two vials is often recommended. One vial contains polyvinyl alcohol (PVA) with fixative, and the other contains buffered formalin solution. The PVA vial is used to make permanent stained preparations and the formalin vial is used to make concentrates.

Wet mounts can be made from fresh fecal specimens. These preparations allow the detection of movement of protozoan trophozoites. Studies have shown that, in comparison to data derived from permanent stained slides and concentrates, the wet mount contributes little information.

Permanent stained slides can be made from fresh fecal specimens or from specimens preserved in PVA. Gomori trichrome stain is commonly used. The stained preparation allows the visualization of diagnostic morphologic features of intestinal protozoa. It is an essential component of the fecal examination.

Fecal concentration techniques attempt to concentrate ova of helminths and cysts of protozoa from relatively large amounts of stool. The method used by most laboratories is called the formalin-ethyl acetate sedimentation method. Ethyl acetate removes fatty substances and some debris from the stool specimen. Repeated decanting and resuspending the sediment following centrifugation provides a small amount of sediment that is rich in ova and cysts. Another technique, the zinc sulfate flotation method, is similar except that the final step suspends the sediment in a zinc sulfate solution of precise specific gravity. After centrifugation, the surface film of the solution, which contains the ova and cysts, is removed with a loop and examined.

Antigen detection systems are new and promising supplements to the microscopic examination of stool. These systems rely on the use of antibodies to specific antigens excreted in the stool of infected individuals. Antigen in the stool binds to antibody. Enzyme techniques that produce a visible colored product are used to detect the bound antibody.

Blood Films

Blood films may be stained to demonstrate parasites. Giemsa stain is preferred for most parasitic infections.

Thin films are made by drawing out a drop of blood on a microscope slide so that the red cells form an even layer that is one cell thick. The film is then fixed and stained. This preparation allows optimal determination of the morphology of the parasites, especially malaria organisms.

Thick films are made by stirring several drops of blood on a microscope slide into a single circular area. The blood is allowed to dry. The slide is placed in water that removes hemoglobin from the RBCs. The slide is then stained. This technique allows the concentration of organisms in a small area for easier detection.

Serologic Tests

Serologic tests, which detect antibody to the parasite, are becoming increasingly valuable as specific antigens are identified and used in sensitive tests, such as ELISA and in immunoblotting methods. Tests have also been developed that distinguish between the classes of antibody, usually IgM and IgG. This test is useful, in some parasitic diseases, for separating acute infection from prior exposure or chronic infection. Identification of specific antigens also allows the development of labeled **monoclonal antibodies,** which can be used in diagnostic tests even with fecal specimens. This technique is currently practical for a limited number of parasitic infections. Some newly developed serologic tests are available through the Centers for Disease Control and Prevention in Atlanta, Georgia.

Molecular Techniques

Molecular techniques may eventually replace microscopic examinations in the detection of parasitic infections. Probes that recognize specific sequences of nucleotides have been developed for some parasitic organisms. Probes can be used to detect DNA or RNA that is specific for a given organism. The use of the PCR promises to make these probes exquisitely sensitive. These techniques may become practical for the clinical laboratory in the near future.

SUMMARY

1. Parasites of humans are classified into three major groups: protozoa (single-cell animals), helminths (worms), and arthropods (jointed appendages, chitinous exoskeleton).

2. Parasitic protozoa are classified as amebae, flagellates, apicomplexa, ciliates, and microsporidia.

3. The major parasitic helminths are found in the two groups called flatworms (flukes and tapeworms) and roundworms.

4. Arthropods of major medical importance are classified as insects (lice, flies, mosquitoes, etc.) or arachnids (mites, ticks, spiders, scorpions). Some arthropods serve as vectors that transmit infectious diseases.

5. A parasite requires a host for nourishment or protection. Definitive hosts harbor the adult or sexual stages of the parasite; intermediate hosts

harbor the larval or asexual stages of the parasite. Reservoir hosts maintain the life cycle of a parasite in the absence of humans.

6. Symbiosis refers to organisms living together. Commensalism is a form of symbiosis with one organism benefitting without causing harm to the other. Parasitism is a symbiotic relationship where one organism (the parasite) benefits at the expense of the other (the host).

7. Parasites that live within the host are called endoparasites; those that live on the surface of the host are called ectoparasites.

8. Fecal examination for ova and parasites may be performed on fresh material or preserved specimens. The examination must include permanent stained slides and a concentration technique. Wet preparations may be used, but are not essential.

9. Other general diagnostic techniques for parasitic infection include antigen detection systems, thick and thin blood films, and serologic tests. Molecular techniques, including the polymerase chain reaction are under development for the detection and identification of parasitic infections.

REFERENCES

Ash LR, Orihel TC (1990): Atlas of Human Parasitology. 3rd ed. New York: Raven Press.

Binford CH, Connor DH (eds) (1976): Pathology of Tropical and Extraordinary Diseases. Vols 1 and 2. Washington DC: Armed Forces Institute of Pathology.

Peters W, Gilles HM (1989): Colour Atlas of Tropical Medicine and Parasitology. 3rd ed. Boca Raton, FL: CRC Press.

Price DL (1994): Procedure Manual for the Diagnosis of Intestinal Parasites. Boca Raton, FL: CRC Press.

Salfelder K (ed) (1988): Protozoan Infections in Man: Colour Atlas. New York: Alan R. Liss.

Zaman V (1979): Atlas of Medical Parasitology. Philadelphia: Lea & Febiger.

REVIEW QUESTIONS

For questions 1 to 2, choose the ONE BEST answer or completion.

1. Which of the following examinations is essential for an accurate fecal examination for ova and parasites?
   a) Antigen detection by the use of specific antibody.
   b) Direct wet mount for motility of the organisms.
   c) Permanent stained slide.
   d) Use of DNA probes for specific sequences of nucleotides.
   e) Polymerase chain reaction to amplify the DNA prior to the use of specific probes.

2. Which of the following use pseudopods for locomotion?
   a) Amebae
   b) Flagellates
   c) Ciliates
   d) Microsporidia
   e) Arachnids

For questions 3 to 8, a list of lettered options is followed by several numbered items. For each numbered item, select the ONE lettered option that is most closely associated with it. Each lettered option may be selected once, more than once, or not at all.

A) Commensals
B) Vectors
C) Microsporidia
D) Flagellates
E) Amebas
F) Roundworms
G) Flukes
H) Tapeworms
I) Arachnids
J) Ectoparasites
K) Endoparasites
L) Intermediate host
M) Definitive host
N) Reservoir host
O) Helminth

For each definition below, select the appropriate term.

3. Organisms that cause infestations of the surface of the host.

4. Organisms that dwell within the intestine of the host but produce no deleterious effect.

5. A general term that includes all worm parasites.

6. A host that harbors the larval or asexual stages of a parasite.

7. The term applied to arthropods that transmit infections.

8. Ribbonlike helminth parasites.

ANSWERS TO REVIEW QUESTIONS

---

1. *c* The permanent stained slide is essential for the adequate detection and identification of intestinal protozoa. Direct wet mounts allow observation of motility but are not optimal for detection or morphologic identification. Polymerase chain reaction and DNA probes have not yet developed to the practical application stage for fecal examinations. Antigen detection is now being used for some intestinal protozoa but has not replaced morphologic identification by permanent stained preparations.

2. *a* Amebae move by means of pseudopods.

3. *J* Ectoparasites cause infestations of the surface of the host.

4. *A* Commensals have no pathologic effect on the host.

5. *O* Helminth is a general term for all worms.

6. *L* The intermediate host harbors the larval or asexual stage of a parasite; the definitive host harbors adult parasites or sexual stages; a reservoir host serves as an alternate host for stages found in humans.

7. *B* An arthropod that transmits an infection is called a vector.

8. *H* Tapeworms are ribbonlike. Flukes are usually dorsoventrally flattened and leaf shaped. Roundworms are cylindrical.

AMEBIASIS AND INFECTIONS WITH FREE-LIVING AMEBAE

AMEBIASIS

Organism

Amebiasis is caused by infection with the intestinal ameba, *Entamoeba histolytica.*

Transmission

Infection is acquired through the fecal-oral route. The major source of infection is the asymptomatic person who is passing cysts in his or her feces. The infectious cysts are ingested in contaminated food, beverages, or from fomites. Flies and cockroaches can be mechanical vectors. Transmission also occurs through sexual practices that foster ingestion of fecal organisms.

Geographic Distribution and Epidemiology

The infection occurs worldwide with increased prevalence in areas of poor hygiene and sanitation. It is estimated that 480 million infections exist with about 10% of that number representing invasive disease. Prevalence rates in the United States are 2–3%, with higher rates in southeastern states and in male homosexuals. Invasive disease is more common in tropical areas but may also be found in temperate and arctic zones.

Habitat

E. histolytica is found in the colon. It may invade the colon wall and may be found in liver abscesses and other sites.

Properties of the Organism

Morphologic terms that apply to amebae and to other protozoa are briefly defined below:

Trophozoite: The motile, actively feeding form that reproduces by binary fission.

Cyst: The infectious stage that has a protective cyst wall and is resistant to adverse environmental conditions.

Cytoplasm: Cell contents exclusive of the nucleus. It is divided into endoplasm, the granular portion that often contains vacuoles, and ectoplasm the portion that is clear.

Pseudopod: A protrusion of cytoplasm, the ''false foot.'' Usually clear ectoplasm is extended in a blunt or fingerlike projection followed by the flowing of endoplasm into the pseudopod. This process is the method of locomotion in amebae.

Nucleus: The spheroid body in the cell having morphologic features that are characteristic for the species. The nucleus is bounded by a nuclear membrane.

Chromatin: The stainable material within the nucleus.

Karyosome or **endosome:** Condensed chromatin within the nucleus.

Peripheral chromatin: Chromatin deposited on the inside of the nuclear membrane.

Vacuoles: Spaces or cavities within the cytoplasm.

The trophozoite of *E. histolytica* contains a single nucleus that has a small central karyosome and peripheral chromatin, which is evenly distributed on the nuclear membrane in small granules (Fig. 50.1). The cytoplasm is usually finely granular, and, in invasive disease, it often contains vacuoles with ingested RBCs. Trophozoites vary in size from 12 to 60 μ in diameter. The cyst is the resistant stage that is excreted in the stool. The mature cyst has a refractile cyst wall and contains four nuclei that resemble the nuclei of the trophozoites. Young cysts often contain deeply staining bundles of crystalline RNA that are called **chromatoidal bodies.** Cysts range in size from 10 to 20 μ in diameter. *E. histolytica* contains microfilaments and microtubules, but has no mitochondria or Golgi complex. Scanning electron microscopic (SEM) studies of *E. histolytica* trophozoites have shown cuplike indentations of the surface, which appear to function as sites of phagocytosis.

When cysts are ingested, the cyst walls break down in the small intestine. Trophozoites, newly formed from the cytoplasm and nuclei of the cyst, colonize the colonic lumen and begin reproducing. When conditions are suitable, some trophozoites will transform into cysts by becoming spherical, forming a cyst wall, and showing division of the nuclei. The cysts are excreted in the stool. Trophozoites are found in the tissues in invasive disease. Cysts do not form in tissues.

Studies of isoenzymes of *E. histolytica* and the use of DNA probes indicate that there are identifiable strains of the ameba that are associated with invasive disease and other strains that are nonpathogenic. Although the pathogenic and nonpathogenic strains are morphologically indistinguishable, other differences are of such magnitude that some authorities are designating the nonpathogenic strain as a separate species, *Entamoeba dispar.*

Trophozoites in the colon may feed and reproduce without causing disease. However, in some circumstances that are poorly understood, they may penetrate

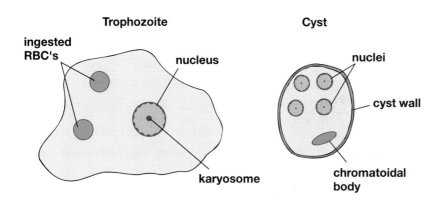

Figure 50.1.
Trophozoite and cyst of *E. histolytica.*

the mucosa of the colon. Pathogenic strains have a surface lectin or adhesin that is inhibited by galactose, *N*-acetyl-D-galactosamine, and colonic mucin. This adhesin appears key in the sequence of adherence and subsequent killing and phagocytosis of mammalian cells in vitro. Experiments show an early intense infiltrate with neutrophils. The death of the neutrophils caused by the amebae may release toxic substances that damage surrounding cells. Trophozoites also contain a variety of enzymes that may participate in the lysis of host cells. Erosion of colonic mucosa begins in the base of the crypts and progresses to ulceration. The ulcers may extend into the submucosa and undermine the normal mucosa to produce flask-shaped lesions. The mucosa between the ulcers may appear normal. The deeper portions of adjacent ulcers may merge and cause the sloughing of large areas of overlying mucosa. In rare instances, necrosis, granulation tissue, and fibrosis may produce a localized mass lesion or colonic wall thickening, which is called an **ameboma.** Amebomas usually occur in the cecum or rectosigmoid.

Invasive trophozoites can enter venules of the colon wall and can be carried to the liver by the portal vein. This process may lead to the development of an **amebic liver abscess.** Complications of an amebic liver abscess are rupture or extension into the pleural space, pericardium or lung through the diaphragm, to the exterior through the chest wall, or into the peritoneal cavity. Amebic liver abscesses occur more frequently in the right lobe of the liver. The abscess is often solitary, but multiple abscesses are not uncommon. The abscess contains brownish material that represents cellular debris. Few intact neutrophils are present in amebic ''pus.'' Pulmonary involvement is usually caused by the extension of a liver abscess through the diaphragm to produce either an intrapulmonary abscess, a bronchohepatic fistula, or a pleural effusion. Liver abscesses may extend to any adjacent organ and may rupture into the peritoneal cavity or through the chest wall. Rarely, amebic brain abscesses develop from organisms carried by the blood to the brain, usually from a liver abscess.

Clinical Manifestations

Colonic amebiasis may be divided into the following four categories:

The **asymptomatic carrier** or ''cyst passer'' produces formed stools that contain infective cysts. There is no evidence of tissue invasion and the individual is free of symptoms.

Nondysenteric colitis is associated with nonspecific symptoms, such as intermittent diarrhea and constipation, or abdominal pain. Cysts are found in formed stools and trophozoites are seen during times of diarrhea.

Dysentery (acute amebic colitis) is associated with diarrhea containing blood, mucus, and amebic trophozoites. There may be 6–10 or more gelatinous stools per day. Tenesmus is present if the rectum is involved. Fever is low grade or absent. Leukocytosis is usually mild. The disease may progress to colonic perforation with peritonitis, or diffuse, severe involvement of the colon may produce dilatation and paralysis of the colon resembling the "toxic megacolon" of ulcerative colitis.

An **ameboma** may have insidious onset with gradual narrowing of the colonic lumen. Progressive constipation and the presence of a mass or constriction of the bowel lumen mimics carcinoma.

Amebic liver abscess may have either an insidious onset or begin abruptly with chills and fever. Fever is nearly always present. Pain in the right upper quadrant of the abdomen or in the right lower chest is common. Cough and right shoulder pain usually indicate involvement of the diaphragm. The liver is usually enlarged and tender. Leukocytosis may be high. Jaundice and liver function impairment is uncommon.

Liver abscess may occur as a complication of amebic colitis, but frequently develops in the absence of colonic symptons. Less than 50% of patients with liver abscess have a history of significant diarrhea.

Cutaneous amebiasis may develop as an extention of rectal disease to the perianal skin. It also may occur at colostomy sites or around draining hepatic abscesses.

Laboratory Diagnosis

Tests used to detect infection with *E. histolytica* are as follows:

The primary method of testing involves demonstration of the parasite. *E. histolytica* must be differentiated morphologically from other intestinal protozoa. There are other species of *Entamoeba* that resemble *E. histolytica,* such as the common commensal organisms, *Entamoeba hartmanni* and *Entamoeba coli.* Other related amebae are *Entamoeba gingivalis,* which is found in the human mouth, usually in association with gum disease, and *Entamoeba polecki,* a parasite of pigs, which occasionally infects the intestinal tract of humans. Other commensal intestinal amebae are *Iodamoeba bütschlii* and *Endolimax nana.*

1. Fecal examination is the primary diagnostic test in colonic amebiasis. In

order to increase the likelihood of finding organisms, it is usual to order three stool specimens, which should be collected on separate days. Less than 50% of patients with amebic liver abscesses will have amebae demonstrable in their stools.

2. Proctosigmoidoscopy allows direct visualization of the colonic mucosa. Rectal biopsy can be done and should be stained with PAS stain to highlight amebic trophozoites. Scrapings of the mucosa can be made and stained with trichrome stain.

3. Aspirate of material from liver abscesses may be examined microscopically for motile trophozoites.

Serologic tests are commercially available including indirect hemagglutination, immunofluorescence, countercurrent immunoelectrophoresis, ELISA, and gel diffusion. These tests, which are sensitive and highly specific, are especially valuable in differentiation of amebic from bacterial liver abscesses. Serologic tests are less helpful in colonic disease and may give false positive results in individuals who have been infected in the past.

Tests under development that are able to detect specific amebic antigens or DNA sequences in stool specimens may eventually replace microscopic examinations. These tests will also be able to differentiate pathogenic and nonpathogenic strains.

Imaging techniques, such as ultrasound and computed tomographic (CT) scanning, are effective in localizing liver abscesses, but cannot distinguish between an amebic abscess and a bacterial abscess.

Treatment

The treatment of amebiasis has two major components: the elimination of tissue invading organisms and the elimination of organisms from the lumen of the intestine. The drugs that are most commonly used for tissue invasion are metronidazole, emetine, or dehydroemetine and chloroquine. Metronidazole (a nitroimidazole compound) is considered the drug of choice in symptomatic colonic amebiasis and in amebic liver abscess. None of the drugs used for symptomatic, invasive disease are very effective in eliminating amebae from the colonic lumen. Drugs that are used to treat the luminal organisms are iodoquinol and diloxanide furoate. The latter drug is only available in the United States for investigational use. Treatment regimens are complex and usually require the use of two drugs to eliminate both the lumen dwelling organisms as well as those in the tissues.

FREE-LIVING AMEBAE THAT CAUSE DISEASE IN HUMANS

There are several species of amebae that live in soil or water and only rarely cause disease in humans. *Naegleria fowleri* has morphologic features of both amebae and flagellates and is called an ameboflagellate. It causes primary amebic meningoencephalitis (PAM). Infection is probably acquired when contaminated water gets into the nose during swimming or diving in ponds, lakes, and so on. The organism is found worldwide in collections of warm, stagnant water. The ameboid form of *N. fowleri* has a single nucleus with a prominent karysome. Only the trophozoite is found in pathologic lesions. A flagellated form occurs in water, and cysts are found in nature but not in tissues. Amebae gain access to the CNS by the nasal mucosa and olfactory nerves through the cribiform plate to the olfactory bulbs, and produce meningitis and hemorrhagic necrosis of brain tissue. Early symptoms of fever, headache, and sometimes disturbance of smell or taste, rapidly progress to frank meningitis with confusion followed by coma. Death usually occurs within 3–6 days from the onset of symptoms. Examination of fresh cerebrospinal fluid reveals motile organisms. The organisms can be cultured and identified by the formation of flagella in water. Very few patients have survived. Treatment with intrathecal amphotericin B appears essential. Other drugs that may be synergistic with amphotericin B should also be used.

Acanthamoeba species cause granulomatous amebic encephalitis (GAE), keratitis, and skin ulcerations. The infection is acquired by inhalation or by direct contact with soil, water, or solutions containing the organism. Cysts may be carried by air currents and may easily contaminate the entire environment. Granulomatous amebic encephalitis is usually found in individuals that have some compromise of their immunity. Keratitis (corneal ulceration) is usually seen in contact lens wearers who have not used sterile saline solutions. Chronic granulomatous skin lesions are probably the result of accidental inoculation or contamination of a traumatic wound. The organism is found worldwide and has been isolated from freshwater, brackish water, soil, dust, hot tubs, and sewage.

Acanthamoeba species are frequent contaminants in tissue cultures. These organisms may be found in normal respiratory tracts and occur in a trophozoite and a cyst form. Trophozoites in tissue resemble *Naegleria*, but flagellated forms do not develop in water. Cysts of *Acanthamoeba* are commonly found in infected tissues.

Granulomatous amebic encephalitis has an insidious onset and resembles a bacterial brain abscess in its signs and symptoms. The course is much longer than for PAM caused by *Naegleria.* Corneal and skin ulcerations may be chronic and progressive.

The diagnosis is made by finding amebae in biopsies, scrapings, or in fresh cerebrospinal fluid. Characteristic cysts of *Acanthamoeba* may be found in infected tissues. Cultured organisms are differentiated from *Naegleria* by their failure to form flagella in water. Sulfa drugs have been effective in experimental infections, but do not seem to work well in clinical situations. In GAE, amphotericin B should be tried with other drugs as in PAM. Keratitis may respond to topical drugs followed by corneal transplantation.

SUMMARY

1. Amebiasis is caused by *Entamoeba histolytica* and is acquired by the ingestion of cysts excreted in the feces of infected humans.

2. Amebiasis is found worldwide but it is more common in areas of poor sanitation and hygiene.

3. The parasites are located in the colon where the trophozoites may invade the tissues of the colon causing ulcers and bloody diarrhea (amebic dysentery). Infections may also be asymptomatic when the trophozoites live as noninvasive commensal organisms.

4. Isoenzyme patterns and DNA probes have separated strains of *E. histolytica* into pathogenic and nonpathogenic categories. Some authorities feel that the nonpathogenic strain should be considered as a separate species.

5. Amebic liver abscess may complicate colonic amebiasis but frequently develops in the absence of colonic symptoms.

6. The diagnosis of colonic amebiasis relies on identification of the organism in stool or colonic mucosal scrapings.

7. Amebic liver abscess is usually associated with pain, tender hepatomegaly, and leukocytosis. Serologic tests are used to differentiate amebic from bacterial liver abscesses. Fecal examinations are often negative for organisms in patients with amebic liver abscesses.

8. Treatment of amebiasis often requires two drugs. One to kill amebae in the tissues, and a second to eliminate the amebae in the colonic lumen.

9. *Naegleria fowleri*, a free-living ameba found in stagnant water, causes a rapidly fatal infection of the brain called primary amebic meningoencephalitis.

10. *Acanthamoeba* species are free-living amebae that may cause corneal ulcers or skin lesions. Immunocompromised individuals may develop a lesion in the brain, called granulomatous amebic encephalitis, which resembles a brain abscess.

11. In *Naegleria fowleri* and *Acanthamoeba* infections of the CNS, the diagnosis is made by examination of the cerebrospinal fluid for motile trophozoites. *Acanthamoeba* trophozoites and cysts may be found in scrapings or biopsies of skin or corneal lesions.

REFERENCES

Adams EB, MacLeod IN (1977): Invasive amebiasis. I. Amebic dysentery and its complications. Medicine 56:315.

Adams EB, MacLeod IN (1977): Invasive amebiasis. II. Amebic liver abscess and its complications. Medicine 56:325.

Aucott JN, Ravdin JI (1993): Amebiasis and ''nonpathogenic'' intestinal protozoa. Infect Dis Clin North Am 7:467.

Kretschmer RR (1990): Amebiasis: Infection and Disease by *Entamoeba histolytica.* Boca Raton, FL: CRC Press.

Ma P, Visvesvara GS, Martinez AJ, Theodore FH, Daggett PM, Sawyer TK (1990): Naegleria and Acanthamoeba infections: review. Rev Infect Dis 12:490.

Martinez AJ (1985): Free-Living Amebas: Natural History, Prevention, Diagnosis, Pathology, and Treatment of Disease. Boca Raton, FL: CRC Press.

Martinez-Palomo A (1987): The pathogenesis of amoebiasis. Parasitol Today 3:111.

Ravdin JI (ed) (1988): Amebiasis. Human Infection with Entamoeba histolytica. New York: Wiley.

REVIEW QUESTIONS

For questions 1 to 3, choose the ONE BEST answer or completion.

1. The best technique used to differentiate an amebic liver abscess from a bacterial liver abscess is
   a) computed tomography of the liver
   b) the magnitude of leukocytosis and fever
   c) ultrasound examination of the liver
   d) a serologic test for antibody to *Entamoeba histolytica*
   e) the presence or absence of *E. histolytica* in the stool of the patient

2. An ameboma causes
   a) a mass lesion in, or constriction of the lumen of the colon
   b) tenesmus
   c) a mass within the liver
   d) an ulcer of the perianal skin
   e) a brain abscess

3. Pathogenic strains of *E. histolytica* have been differentiated from nonpathogenic strains by
   a) the arrangement of chromatin on the nuclear membrane
   b) isoenzyme analysis
   c) the glycogen content of cysts
   d) the presence of bacteria in the cytoplasm of trophozoites
   e) The size of the trophozoites

For questions 4 to 10, a list of lettered options is followed by several numbered items. For each numbered item, select the ONE lettered option that is most closely associated with it. Each lettered option may be selected once, more than once, or not at all.

A) *Naegleria fowleri*
B) *Acanthamoeba*
C) *Entamoeba histolytica*
D) *Entamoeba coli*

For each condition or characteristic, select the appropriate organism.

4. Amebic dysentery

5. Primary amebic meningoencephalitis

6. Granulomatous amebic encephalitis

7. Nonpathogenic organism

A) Trophozoite
B) Cyst
C) Chromatin
D) Vacuole
E) Karyosome

F) Chromatoidal body
G) Pseudopod
H) Peripheral chromatin

8. Bundles of crystalline ribonucleic acid

9. Resistant infectious stages of amebae

For each definition, select the correct term.

10. Motile, reproducing stage of amebae

ANSWERS TO REVIEW QUESTIONS

1. *d* The serologic test is specific for infection with *Entamoeba histolytica*. Patients with liver abscesses usually have very high titres of antibody. Ultrasound and computed tomography detect abscesses but cannot differentiate amebic and bacteriologic causes. Leukocytosis and fever are common to both conditions. Patients with amebic liver abscesses often have no *E. histolytica* demonstrable in their stools.

2. *a* Amebomas result from a localized tissue reaction in the colon which produces an intralumenal mass or a constriction of the lumen. Tenesmus is caused by inflammation and ulceration of the rectum.

3. *b* Isoenzyme analysis has been used to differentiate pathogenic and nonpathogenic strains of *E. histolytica.*

4. *C* *E. histolytica* is the cause of amebic dysentery.

5. *A* *Naegleria fowleri* causes primary amebic meningoencephalitis.

6. *B* *Acanthamoeba* causes granulomatous amebic encephalitis.

7. *D* *Entamoeba coli* is nonpathogenic.

8. *F* Chromatoidal bodies are found in young cysts of the genus *Entamoeba*. They are bundles of crystalline RNA.

9. *B* The cyst is the resistant infectious stage of amebae.

10. *A* The trophozoite is the motile, reproductive stage of amebae.

OTHER INTESTINAL PROTOZOAL INFECTIONS AND TRICHOMONIASIS

FLAGELLATES

Dientamoeba fragilis and *Giardia lamblia* are intestinal flagellates with pathogenic potential. Other flagellates of the intestinal tract that have not been associated with disease include *Chilomastix mesnili, Pentatrichomonas (Trichomonas) hominis,* and the less common organisms, *Retortomonas intestinalis* and *Enteromonas hominis.*

Trichomonas tenax is a commensal organism found in the mouth. *Trichomonas vaginalis* is a parasite of the urogenital tract that frequently causes disease.

DIENTAMOEBA INFECTION

Dientamoeba infection is caused by *D. fragilis.*

Transmission

The exact mode or modes of transmission are not definitively proven. Electron microscroscopic study of pinworm (*Enterobius vermicularis*) eggs have shown structures resembling *D. fragilis* within the eggshell. Experimental and epidemiologic data also support the possibility that infection with *D. fragilis* is acquired concommitantly with pinworm.

Geographic Distribution and Epidemiology

The organism is found worldwide and its prevalence varies widely. It is more common in children and may have higher prevalence rates in institutionalized individuals.

Habitat

The parasite is found in the crypts of the colonic mucosa.

Properties of the Organism

The organism only occurs in the trophozoite stage. Although the parasite has no flagella, and was thought for many years to be an ameba, electron microscopic studies show its relationship to the flagellates. It is now classified with the trichomonads. The trophozoite usually ranges from 7 to 12 μ in diameter. A high percentage of organisms seen in diagnostic smears are binucleate (Fig. 51.1). These nuclei are in an arrested telophase. The nuclei typically contain 4–8 large chromatin granules, and the cytoplasm is highly vacuolated.

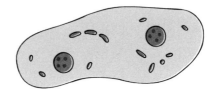

Figure 51.1

Trophozoite of *D. fragilis*.

Clinical Manifestations

Infections are often asymptomatic, but as many as 25% of infected individuals may have diarrhea, abdominal pain, flatulence, or other nonspecific GI complaints.

Laboratory Diagnosis

Identification of the parasite in permanent stained stool specimens is essential. It is important that the specimen be fresh, or it should be immediately preserved in PVA fixative.

Treatment

Iodoquinol, tetracycline, and paromomycin have been found to be effective in *D. fragilis* infections.

GIARDIASIS

Giardiasis is caused by *G. lamblia,* also called *Giardia intestinalis* by European authors.

Transmission

Infection results from the ingestion of cysts from feces. Contaminated water is a frequent source and a few food borne outbreaks have been reported. Transmission may also occur in association with certain sexual practices. Many animals have *Giardia* that have the ability to infect humans.

Geographic Distribution and Epidemiology

Infection with *G. lamblia* is found worldwide. Higher prevalence rates are associated with areas where conditions are crowded and sanitation is poor. High rates are seen in day care centers, in hikers who drink untreated mountain stream water, and in male homosexuals. Many water borne outbreaks have been attributed to municipal water supplies that have not been treated with flocculation and filtration. *Giardia* cysts are relatively resistant to chlorination. Many animals, including dogs and cats, harbor *Giardia.* However, the role of animal reservoirs in human infection is not known.

Habitat

Trophozoites attach to the mucosa of the proximal small intestine.

Properties of the Organism

The pear-shaped trophozoite is dorsoventrally flattened and has a large ''sucking disk'' on its ventral surface with which it attaches to the intestinal mucosa. It has two nuclei, eight flagella, and a pair of prominent curved bodies in the center of the organism called ''median bodies.'' The trophozoite is 9–21 μ in length, and reproduction is through binary fission (Fig. 51.2). The oval cyst is about 8–14 μ in length and contains four nuclei, the median bodies, and numerous linear structures that are the intracytoplasmic components of the flagella (Fig. 51.2).

Studies of *Giardia* by isoenzyme analysis and molecular techniques reveal wide diversity among different isolates. Whether different strains have varying capacities to produce disease is not yet known. There is evidence that the organisms have the ability to express a variety of surface antigens. This variability may assist in avoiding the host's immunologic defense mechanisms.

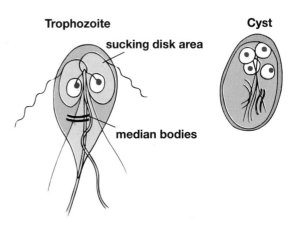

Figure 51.2
Trophozoite and cyst of *G. lamblia.*

Clinical Manifestations

Some infections may be asymptomatic. When symptoms occur, they may vary from severe acute diarrhea to chronic mild diarrhea associated with flatulence, abdominal discomfort, and fatigability. In some instances, significant intestinal malabsorption occurs. Lactose intolerance may develop and may persist after elimination of the parasites. Patients with immunoglobulin deficiencies are especially susceptible to symptomatic giardiasis.

Laboratory Diagnosis

Routine examinations of stool for ova and parasites will reveal parasites in most infections. Cysts are more likely to be seen in formed or semiformed stools. Trophozoites may be seen in diarrheic stools. For some patients who excrete very low numbers of organisms, it may be necessary to examine multiple fecal specimens to find parasites. Invasive techniques can also be used. The "string test" (Entero-Test™) allows sampling directly from the small intestine. A length of nylon yarn is introduced into the duodenum by means of a weighted gelatin capsule. The capsule is swallowed and the free end of the string is retained by taping it to the cheek or looping it over a tooth. After several hours, the string is retrieved and mucus removed from the distal end is examined for *Giardia* trophozoites. Intestinal biopsy and collection of specimens at gastroduodenoscopy are useful but expensive and uncomfortable procedures.

Monoclonal antibody can be used with an immunofluorescent method to detect organisms in fecal specimens. An ELISA can detect *Giardia* antigen in stool by using antibody to a specific *Giardia* protein. These tests have recently become commercially available.

Treatment

There are three major drugs used for the treatment of giardiasis in the United States. Metronidazole is often used, but is considered investigational in giardiasis. Furazolidone and quinacrine are approved by the FDA for use in this infection.

TRICHOMONIASIS

Trichomoniasis is an infection of the urogenital tract caused by *T. vaginalis.*

Transmission

Sexual intercourse is the mode of transmission for the majority of infections. Fomites, such as moist towels, are possible sources. There are rare instances of neonatal infections acquired during birth.

Geographic Distribution and Epidemiology

Trichomoniasis is found worldwide. It may occur in 5–10% of healthy women of child bearing age. Peak incidence occurs between 16 and 35 years. More than 50% of patients attending sexually transmitted disease clinics have been found to be infected. Risk factors for infection include multiple sex partners and poor personal hygiene. Trichomoniasis is commonly found associated with other sexually transmitted infections.

Habitat

The organisms are found in the vagina and urethra in females and in the urethra, seminal vesicles, and prostate in males.

Properties of the Organism

Trophozoites average about 13 μ in the longest dimension and have a single nucleus located at the anterior end. There are four anterior flagella. An **undulating membrane** extends from the anterior pole to about halfway down the body. Beneath the undulating membrane there is a supporting structure called the costa. There is a rigid rod, the axostyle, which runs the length of the body and protrudes from the posterior end (Fig. 51.3). Granules located along the costa and axostyle are organelles called hydrogenosomes, which participate in pyruvate metabolism and the generation of molecular hydrogen. *T. vaginalis* has no cyst form.

Clinical Manifestations

Asymptomatic infections are common, but as many as 50% of infected women will have vaginitis and cervicitis with large amounts of yellowish, frothy discharge. The vaginal mucosa is hyperemic. Concommitant infection with path-

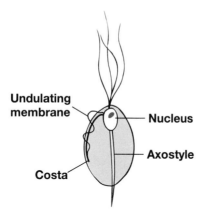

Figure 51.3
Trophozoite of *T. vaginalis*.

ogenic bacteria or yeasts is very common. When vaginitis is present, symptoms of burning, itching, dysuria, and frequency of urination are common. Males are usually asymptomatic, but occasionally develop urethritis or prostatitis.

Laboratory Diagnosis

Motile organisms can be demonstrated in wet mounts of vaginal secretions in about 80% of infections. Culture of vaginal discharge is the most sensitive method of diagnosis, but this technique requires several days of incubation. A rapid test using monoclonal antibody with direct immunofluorescence appears to be nearly as accurate and sensitive as culture techniques.

Treatment

Metronidazole is usually effective in a single dose. It is important to treat the patient's sexual partners even if they are asymptomatic. A few strains of *T. vaginalis* are relatively resistant to metronidazole.

APICOMPLEXA (SPOROZOA)

The Apicomplexa that infect the human intestinal tract are *Cryptosporidium parvum* and *Isospora belli*. *Sarcocystis* species are also parasites of humans but are rarely reported and will not be discussed here.

CRYPTOSPORIDIOSIS

Cryptosporidiosis is caused by *C. parvum.*

Transmission

The infection is acquired by the ingestion of **oocysts** from the feces of infected humans or animals.

Geographic Distribution and Epidemiology

The infection is worldwide with higher prevalence rates in areas of poor sanitation. Outbreaks have been reported from day care centers. There are probably many mammalian reservoir hosts. Cryptosporidiosis has been reported in veterinarians dealing with infected cattle.

Habitat

The organisms are seen in the brush border of the intestinal epithelium of both small and large bowel. Parasites have been seen in the gallbladder, tonsillar epithelium, and bronchi in patients with AIDS.

Properties of the Organism

The form of the organism excreted in the stool is called an oocyst. It contains four **sporozoites.** Following ingestion, the sporozoites escape from the oocyst and penetrate the intestinal epithelium, where they undergo asexual multiplication. The organisms appear to be attached to the cell's surface at the brush border, but are actually under the cell membrane external to the cytoplasm (Fig. 51.4A,B). Sexual stages develop and unite to form an oocyst that is shed in the feces. Some oocysts release sporozoites before they are excreted in the stool. These sporozoites enter intestinal epithelial cells and continue the cycle (internal autoinfection). The oocysts excreted in the stool are 4–5 μ in diameter (Fig. 51.4C).

The taxonomy of *Cryptosporidium* is still evolving. It is generally accepted that *C. parvum* is the species that infects humans and cattle.

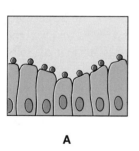 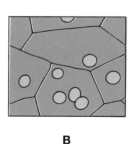 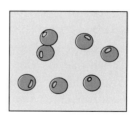

A   B   C

Figure 51.4

Cryptosporidium. (A) Organisms in brush border of intestinal epithelium. (B) Scanning electron micrograph of *Cryptosporidium* in intestinal epithelium. (C) Oocysts of *Cryptosporidium* in feces.

Clinical Manifestations

In immunocompetent individuals, the infection is associated with low-grade fever, nausea, occasional vomiting, and a self-limited watery diarrhea. The illness rarely lasts more than 2 weeks. In immunocompromised patients, the diarrhea is chronic, often severe, and may be fatal. It has been a major problem in patients with AIDS.

Laboratory Diagnosis

It is necessary to use a modified acid-fast stain to differentiate oocysts from yeasts in stool specimens. The oocysts stain red with the acid-fast technique. A sensitive direct immunofluorescent technique using monoclonal antibody is now commercially available.

Treatment

There is no effective treatment available. Immunocompetent patients do not require treatment and the infection resolves spontaneously. An analog of somatostatin, octreotide, has been helpful in relieving the chronic diarrhea in patients with AIDS. This drug affects only the symptoms, and has no effect on the causative organisms.

CYCLOSPORA INFECTION

Cyclospora **infection** is caused by an organism that was initially described as a cyanobacteriumlike or a cocidianlike body (CLB). It has been determined to be an apicomplexan of the genus *Cyclospora,* closely resembling *Cryptospori-*

dium. The oocysts of *Cyclospora,* measuring 8–10 μ in diameter, are larger than those of *Cryptosporidium.* The oocysts require 1–2 weeks to sporulate and become infectious. The diarrheal illness caused by *Cyclospora* is similar to that of cryptosporidiosis, but may be more chronic with average duration of about 6 weeks. It may also cause chronic infection in AIDS patients. The modified acid-fast stain is used for stool specimens but the affinity of the oocysts for the stain is highly variable within the same specimen. A recent report suggests that trimethroprim-sulfamethoxazole may be useful in treating this infection.

ISOSPORIASIS

Isosporiasis is caused by the parasite *I. belli.* The infection is uncommon in the United States but occurs more frequently in South America and Southeast Asia. It was noted in Haitian patients with AIDS who had immigrated to the United States. Subsequently, it has been reported as a cause of chronic diarrhea in AIDS patients. *I. belli* has a life cycle similar to that of *Cryptosporidium,* but it is located deep within the cytoplasm of the intestinal epithelial cell. The oocysts excreted in the stool measure about 30 μ in length. Two spherical **sporoblasts** are seen within the oocyst. The sporoblasts mature into **sporocysts,** each containing four sporozoites (Fig. 51.5). The acute infection is similar to cryptosporidiosis, but is often accompanied by eosinophilia. Patients with AIDS and other immunosuppressed individuals may develop chronic, debilitating diarrhea. The diagnosis is dependent on finding oocysts in fecal concentrates or in modified acid-fast stains of stool. Treatment is usually not needed in the self-limited illness seen in immunocompetent individuals, but the combination of trimethroprim and sulfamethoxazole appears effective. Patients with AIDS may require long-term suppressive treatment.

CILIATES

Balantidiasis is caused by *Balantidum coli,* the only ciliate found in humans. Infections have been reported from many countries, but balantidiasis is very rare in the United States. Although the infection is found in a variety of mammals, the pig is the major reservoir. Many patients give a history of contact with pigs. Human-human transmission is also common. The infection is acquired by the ingestion of cysts. The parasites are found in the colon. The trophozoites vary in size and can reach 150 μ in their largest dimension. Trophozoites are covered with cilia and have a funnellike **cytostome** at the anterior pole. The cytoplasm contains

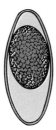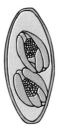

Figure 51.5

I. belli. (Left) Immature oocyst. (Right) Mature oocyst with sporozoites in sporocysts.

a very large, kidney-shaped macronucleus and an inconspicuous micronucleus (Fig. 51.6). Cysts measure about 60 μ in diameter. The majority of infections are asymptomatic but the parasite has the ability to produce colonic ulcerations similar to those found in amebiasis. Symptoms also resemble those seen in invasive amebiasis. Diagnosis is made by finding trophozoites or cysts in the stool. Treatment with tetracycline or metronidazole is effective.

MICROSPORIDIA

Microsporidia were rarely found in humans until recently when it was recognized that these infections are a complication of AIDS. The intestinal and systemic infections are probably acquired by the ingestion of spores, and disease usually develops only in the immunosuppressed. The source of human infections is unknown. The organisms are characterized by their small size (<5 μ), intracellular location, and the morphology of their spores (Fig. 51.7). The spore con-

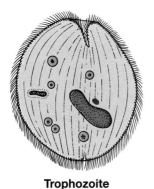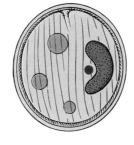

Trophozoite   **Cyst**

Figure 51.6

Trophozoite and cyst of *B. coli.*

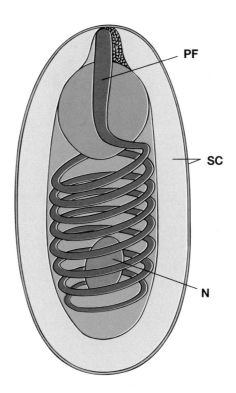

Figure 51.7

Internal structure of a microsporidian. PF, polar filament; SC, spore coats; N, nucleus.

tains a coiled polar tube or filament. When this polar tube is extruded, it penetrates a host cell and provides the means for transfer of infectious sporoplasm into the host cell. Several species have been involved in human infections. Most infections have been reported in AIDS patients as intestinal infections caused by *Enterocytozoon.* A new species of intestinal microsporidian, *Septata intestinalis,* has been described in AIDS patients. This organism may disseminate to many extraintestinal sites and may be excreted in urine as well as feces. Ocular infection, encephalitis, and generalized infections have been associated with other species. Diagnosis is usually made by demonstrating the organism in biopsies. Giemsa-stained touch preparations from intestinal biopsies often reveal the intracellular parasites. Fecal films stained with a concentrated trichrome stain may be diagnostic of intestinal microsporidiosis when prepared and examined by a skilled and experienced technologist. Electron microscopy is required to determine the species of microsporidia. Recent reports suggest that albendazole may produce symptomatic improvement in intestinal microsporidiosis, but the infection persists and relapse is common.

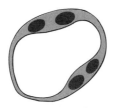

Figure 51.8
B. hominis.

UNCERTAIN CLASSIFICATION

The organism, *Blastocystis hominis,* was thought to be a yeast for many years. Evidence has been presented that it is a protozoan, but definitive classification requires more study. Infection with *Blastocystis* is very common. Although prevalence rates vary widely in different surveys, rates of 10–20% are often reported. It is presumed, but not proven, that the mode of transmission is fecal-oral. The form of the organism most commonly recognized varies widely in diameter from 5 to 30 µ. It contains a large, amorphous central body with a rim of cytoplasm containing small nuclei (Fig. 51.8). There are many anecdotal reports of diarrheal disease associated with this organism. Studies provide conflicting conclusions concerning the organism's pathogenicity. The issues of classification and pathogenicity are still unsettled.

SUMMARY

Table 51.1 summarizes the major characterestics of intestinal protozoa and *Trichomonas vaginalis*.

REFERENCES

Aucott JN, Ravdin JI (1993): Amebiasis and ''nonpathogenic'' intestinal protozoa. Infect Dis Clin North Am 7:467.

Boreham PFL, Stenzel DJ (1993): *Blastocystis* in humans and animals: morphology, biology and epizootiology. Adv Parsitol 32.1.

Cross JH (1990): Balantidiasis and other intestinal protozoa. In Warren KS, Mahmoud AAF (eds): Tropical and Geographical Medicine. 2nd ed. New York: McGraw-Hill Book Co.

Curry A, Canning EU (1993): Human microsporidiosis. J Infect Dis 27:229.

Dubey JP, Speer CA, Fayer R (1990): Cryptosporidiosis in Man and Animals. Boca Raton, FL: CRC Press.

Hill DR (1993): Giardiasis. Issues in diagnosis and management. Infect Dis Clin North Am 7:503.

Honigberg BM (ed) (1990): Trichomonads Parasitic in Humans. New York: Springer-Verlag.

TABLE 51.1. Summary of Intestinal Protozoal Infections and Trichomoniasis

Organism	Transmission	Location	Clinical manifestations	Laboratory diagnosis	Treatment
Entamoeba histolytica	Fecal–oral (ingestion of cysts)	Colon	Diarrhea, dysentery, hepatic abscess	Fecal exam, colon biopsy, serology	Metronidazole, iodoquinol, other drugs
Dientamoeba fragilis	Pinworm eggs?	Colon	Diarrhea, abdominal pain	Fecal exam	Tetracycline, iodoquinol
Giardia lamblia	Fecal–oral (ingestion of cysts)	Small intestine	Diarrhea, flatulence, bloating, malabsorption	Fecal exam, "string test," fecal antigen test	Metronidazole, quinacrine or furazolidone
Trichomonas vaginalis	Sexual intercourse	Vagina, urethra, prostate, seminal vesicles	Vaginal discharge, dysuria, frequency, burning, itching	Wet mount, culture, monoclonal fluorescent antibody test	Metronidazole
Cryptosporidium	Fecal–oral (ingestion of oocysts)	Small intestine and colon	Watery diarrhea. Chronic diarrhea in immunosuppressed	Fecal exam with acid-fast stain, monoclonal fluorescent antibody	Symptomatic treatment with octreotide
Cyclospora	Fecal–oral (ingestion of oocysts)	Small intestine	Watery diarrhea. Chronic diarrhea in immunosuppressed	Fecal exam with acid-fast stain	Possibly trimethoprim-sulfamethoxazole
Isospora belli	Fecal–oral (ingestion of oocysts)	Small intestine	Watery diarrhea, eosinophilia. Chronic diarrhea in immunosuppressed	Fecal exam	Trimethoprim-sulfamethoxazole
Balantidium coli	Fecal–oral (ingestion cysts)	Colon	Diarrhea, dysentery	Fecal exam	Tetracycline, metronidazole
Microsporidia (several species)	Probably ingestion of spores	Intestine, brain, eye, other sites	Diarrhea, encephalitis, conjunctivitis, keratitis	Biopsy and electron microscopy, special stain for feces	Possibly albendazole
Blastocystis hominis	Probably fecal–oral	Intestine	Possibly causes diarrhea	Fecal exam	Efficacy is unproven, but metronidazole and iodoquinol are often used

Meyer EA (ed) (1990): Giardiasis. In Ruitenberg EJ, MacInnis AJ (eds): Human Parasitic Diseases. Vol. 3. New York: Elsevier Science Publishing Co.

Ortega YR et al. (1993): *Cyclospora* species—A new protozoan infection of humans. N Engl J Med 328:1308.

Soave R, Johnson WD Jr (1988): *Cryptosporidium* and *Isospora belli* infections. J Infect Dis 157:225.

Thompson RC et al. (1993): *Giardia* and giardiasis. Adv Parasitol 32:71.

Wittner M et al. (1993): Parasitic infections in AIDS patients. Cryptosporidiosis, isosporiasis, microsporidiosis, cyclosporiasis. Infect Dis Clin North AM 7:569.

REVIEW QUESTIONS

> For questions 1 to 3, choose the ONE BEST answer or completion.

1. Giardiasis is found more frequently in the following *except*
   a) mountain hikers who drink untreated surface water
   b) male homosexuals
   c) pregnant women
   d) patients with immunoglobulin deficiencies
   e) children in day care centers

2. Which of the following parasites may be transmitted by pinworm eggs?
   a) *Dientamoeba fragilis*
   b) Microsporidia
   c) *Cryptosporidium*
   d) *Trichomonas vaginalis*
   e) *Isospora belli*

3. Which of the following parasites is commonly transmitted by sexual intercourse?

a) *Giardia lamblia*
b) *Cryptosporidium*
c) *Dientamoeba fragilis*
d) *Trichomonas vaginalis*
e) Microsporidia

> For questions 4 to 8, a list of lettered options is followed by several numbered items. For each numbered item, select the ONE lettered option that is most closely associated with it. Each lettered option may be selected once, more than once, or not at all.

A) *Giardia lamblia*
B) *Dientamoeba fragilis*
C) *Cryptosporidium*
D) *Trichomonas vaginalis*
E) *Balantidium coli*
F) *Blastocystis hominis*
G) *Isospora belli*
H) Microsporidia

For the characteristic features listed below, select the appropriate organism.

4. Attaches to small bowel mucosa with "sucking disk."

5. Develops within intestinal mucosal cells under host cell membrane but outside of host cytoplasm. May cause fatal diarrhea in AIDS patients. May infect cattle.

6. Spores contain a coiled polar tube. May cause intestinal infection in AIDS patients.

7. Usually causes no symptoms in infected males. May rarely be acquired by the baby during childbirth.

8. Unclassified organism. Controversy concerning its status as a pathogen.

ANSWERS TO REVIEW QUESTIONS

1. *c* Although pregnant women may have severe symptomatic giardiasis, there is no evidence of increased incidence in this group. Mountain hikers, male homosexuals, and children in day care centers have a greater likelihood than the general population of acquiring giardiasis. Patients with immunoglobulin deficiency are particularly susceptible to infection with *G. lamblia.*

2. *a Dientamoeba fragilis* is associated with pinworm infection and has been seen within pinworm eggs.

3. *d Trichomonas vaginalis* is commonly transmitted by sexual intercourse. The other parasites discussed in this chapter are acquired or thought to be acquired by ingestion of infectious stages.

4. *A Giardia lamblia* attaches with its "sucking disk."

5. *C Cryptosporidium* develops intracellularly outside of the host cell cytoplasm. *Isospora belli* and microsporidia develop within the host cell cytoplasm. All of the other parasites listed are extracellular organisms.

6. *H* Microsporidia spores have a coiled polar tube and the microsporidian, *Enterocytozoon,* infects the intestine of AIDS patients.

7. *D T. vaginalis* usually causes no symptoms in males and rarely may be acquired by female babies during birth.

8. *F Blastocystis hominis* is an unclassified organism. Investigators differ as to its potential for causing disease.

EOSINOPHILIA AND PARASITIC INFECTIONS

THE EOSINOPHIL

Three types of polymorphonuclear leukocytes are found in human blood and tissue: neutrophils, basophils, and **eosinophils.** Eosinophils are distinguished by their large intracytoplasmic granules that stain red with the dye eosin. The nuclei of eosinophils are usually bilobed compared with three or more lobes in neutrophils and basophils. Although eosinophils contain several different types of granules, the most prominent are the eosinophilic granules, which contain a crystalloid core surrounded by a less dense matrix. The core consists of a cationic protein called major basic protein. It is toxic for larval helminth parasites. Other toxic proteins, including a neurotoxin, are also found within the granule. Eosinophils are also very rich in a variety of enzymes. One enzyme, lysophospholipase, is found in the plasma membrane of the cell. When the eosinophil breaks down, the lysophopholipase forms Charcot-Leyden crystals. These slender, hexagonal, bipyramidal structures are frequently seen in exudates and granulomas containing eosinophils. The surface of the eosinophil has receptors for IgG, IgE, and complement.

Eosinophils originate in the bone marrow where they accumulate in a large reserve of mature cells. The eosinophils leave the bone marrow and briefly circulate in the blood before entering the tissues. Skin, GI tract, and lungs are major sites of eosinophil migration. It is estimated that there are about 100 eosinophils in the tissues for every one found in the blood. Several chemotactic factors are known to cause eosinophil migration. A cytokine named IL-5 appears to be an important mediator of the eosinophilia of parasitic infections.

The number of eosinophils in the circulation varies widely. Values for the normal ranges of eosinophils per cubic millimeter of are 125 ± 100 with slightly higher values for children. Eosinophils are also expressed as a percentage of the total WBC with a normal range of 2–4%, however, this method is not as accurate as a total eosinophil count. Elevation of the eosinophil count above the normal range is called **eosinophilia.** Clinicians frequently conclude that a significant eosinophilia is present when the eosinophils exceed 5% of the total WBCs.

EOSINOPHIL FUNCTION

Although the eosinophil is capable of ingesting a variety of microorganisms and antigen-antibody complexes, it is much less efficient at phagocytosis and intracellular killing than the neutrophil. It appears to function much more effectively in extracellular reactions. Eosinophils bind to certain parasites and other types of cells. Complement and IgG are commonly involved in attachment, but lectins and IgE may also serve in this process. Following adherence, the eosinophil degranulates, and the cytotoxic effects are observed. This cytotoxicity may be of benefit in the protection against some helminth infections, but it also has the potential to contribute to the pathology of certain conditions, such as allergic disorders.

EOSINOPHILIA

Eosinophilia occurs in association with a wide variety of infectious neoplastic and idiopathic diseases, but it is most commonly associated with allergic conditions and with invasive helminth infections. The presence of significant eosinophilia often alerts the clinician to consider parasitic disease in the differential diagnosis of the condition.

The highest levels of eosinophilia occur in helminth infections in which larvae migrate in the tissues, such as visceral larva migrans (toxocariasis) and trichinosis. Moderate to high levels of eosinophilia occur in the early stages of intestinal nematode infections that have an extraintestinal migration phase, filarial infections, and infections with blood stream or tissue dwelling trematodes. Higher levels of eosinophilia are seen in the early stages of infection. The number of eosinophils tends to fall toward normal over a period of weeks or months after the acute infection. Chronic infections may be associated with mildly elevated or normal eosinophil counts. Lumen dwelling parasites, such as *Enterobius vermicularis* and the large tapeworms, *Taenia solium, Taenia saginata,* and *Diphyllobothrium latum,* do not usually cause eosinophilia. *Trichuris trichiura,* even though it is partially imbedded in the superficial mucosa of the colon, does not produce eosinophilia. The only occurrence of significant eosinophilia with protozoan infections is seen with *Isospora belli.*

The Table 52.1 shows the usual responses in those helminth infections that are associated with eosinophilia.

TABLE 52.1. Responses in Helminth Infections associated with Eosinophilia

Disease	Eosinophilia
Schistosomiasis	Moderate, highest in the early stages
Liver fluke infection (clonorchiasis) (opisthorchiasis)	Moderate, highest in the early stages
Lung fluke infection (paragonimiasis)	Moderate, highest in the early stages
Dwarf tapeworm infection (hymenolepiasis nana)	Low
Cysticercosis (*Taenia solium* larvae)	Usually absent. Cerebrospinal fluid may show eosinophilia in some cases of CNS involvement
Hydatid disease (*Echinococcus granulosus*)	Rarely present in established infections unless there is leakage of hydatid cyst fluid
Ascariasis	Moderate during larval migration stage. Low to moderate in established infection
Hookworm infection (*Ancylostoma, Necator*)	Low to moderate. Higher levels during larval migration stage
Strongyloidiasis	Moderate. May be high during early stage of infection
Trichinosis	Very high
Visceral larva migrans (toxocariasis)	Very high
Lymphatic filariasis (*Wuchereria, Brugia*)	Low to moderate. High in the syndrome of tropical pulmonary eosinophilia
Onchocerciasis	Moderate

SUMMARY

1. The eosinophil is a type of leukocyte that is characterized by the presence of large intracytoplasmic granules that stain red with eosin.

2. Eosinophils circulate in the blood but most are found in the tissues.

3. An elevation in the numbers of eosinophils in the circulation above the normal range is called eosinophilia.

4. A major function of the eosinophil is the killing of certain parasites with toxic cationic proteins. Complement and antibody participate in the cytotoxicity.

5. *Isospora belli* is the only protozoan consistently associated with eosinophilia.

6. Helminths that invade tissues commonly cause significant eosinophilia (see Table 52.1).

REFERENCES

Gleich GJ (1988): Current understanding of eosinophil function. Hosp Pract 23:137.

Nutman TB, Cohen SG, Ottesen EA (1988): The eosinophil, eosinophilia, and eosinophil-related disorders. I. Structure and development. Allergy Proc 9:629.

Nutman TB, Cohen SG, Ottesen EA (1989): The eosinophil, eosinophilia, and eosinophil-related disorders. II. Eosinophil infiltration and function. Allergy Proc 9:641.

Nutman TB, Cohen SG, Ottesen EA (1989): The eosinophil, eosinophilia, and eosinophil-related disorders. III. Clinical assessments and eosinophil related disorders. Allergy Proc 10:33.

Nutman TB, Cohen SG, Ottesen EA (1989): The eosinophil, eosinophilia, and eosinophil-related disorders. IV. Eosinophil related disorders (continued). Allergy Proc 10:47.

REVIEW QUESTIONS

For questions 1 to 4, choose the ONE BEST answer or completion.

1. Eosinophil granules contain
   a) antibody
   b) eosin
   c) toxic cationic proteins
   d) lysophospholipase

2. The major effect of eosinophils on parasites is
   a) the extracellular killing of the organisms
   b) phagocytosis and intracellular digestion of the parasite
   c) the production of specific antibody by the eosinophil
   d) caused by the activation of mononuclear cells by the eosinophil

   e) caused by the activation of neutrophils by the eosinophil

3. In a normal individual, which of the following sites would be expected to contain large numbers of eosinophils?
   a) Brain
   b) Muscle
   c) Heart
   d) Liver
   e) Gastrointestinal tract

4. Of the following infections, which one is NOT associated with eosinophilia?
   a) Strongyloidiasis
   b) Enterobiasis
   c) Trichinosis
   d) Ascariasis
   e) Hookworm infection

ANSWERS TO REVIEW QUESTIONS

1. *c* The granules contain several toxic cationic proteins. The core of the large granule contains major basic protein. The granules stain with eosin but do not contain it. Lysophospholipase is an enzyme located in the cytoplasmic membrane.

2. *a* The eosinophil kills parasites by degranulating on the surface of the parasite, therefore, the killing is extracellular. Although eosinophils may function as phagocytic cells, this is not the principle mechanism used against parasites. Eosinophils are not antibody producing cells, nor do they activate mononuclear cells or neutrophils.

3. *e* The tissue eosinophils are concentrated in the GI tract, skin, and lung.

4. *b* The cause of enterobiasis, *Enterobius vermicularis,* lives in the lumen of the intestine and does not elicit an eosinophilia. In strongyloidiasis, hookworm infection, ascariasis and trichinosis, larvae migrate through the tissues or in the circulation causing an eosinophilic response.

INTESTINAL, LIVER, AND LUNG TREMATODE INFECTIONS

Although the schistosomes are trematodes, they differ widely from the other organisms in this group. The schistosomes will be discussed in Chapter 54. The trematodes that infect the intestinal tract, the liver, and the lung are discussed here. The key aspects of these infections are summarized in Table 53.1.

Trematodes or flukes are leaf-shaped, bilaterally symmetrical, and usually dorsoventrally flattened. These organisms have a muscular oral sucker and a ventral sucker. Both sexes are present within the same organism (hermaphroditic), and the sex organs are usually represented by two testes and one ovary. The intestinal tract begins at the oral sucker and branches to form two ceca that end blindly at the posterior of the worm (Fig. 53.1). The outer layer of the organism, the tegument, is coated with a glycocalyx that protects the trematode from the host's digestive enzymes. The eggshell has a lidlike structure, called an **operculum,** which covers the opening through which the larva hatches.

The life cycle of trematodes begins with the development of a ciliated larva (miracidium) inside the egg. The miracidium hatches from the egg and penetrates the tissues of the first intermediate host, a snail. Asexual multiplication takes place in the snail. A motile larva, the **cercaria,** escapes from the snail and encysts on aquatic vegetation or in the tissues of a second intermediate host depending on

TABLE 53.1. Key Points of the Three Major Examples of Trematode Infections

Organism	Transmission	Location	Clinical manifestations	Diagnosis
Fasciolopsis buski	Ingestion of aquatic plants	Intestine	Diarrhea, eosinophilia	Fecal examination
Clonorchis sinensis	Ingestion of raw, pickled, or undercooked fish	Bile ducts	Acute: Fever, abdominal pain, eosinophilia (may be asymptomatic) Chronic: Cholangitis	Fecal examination
Paragonimus westermani	Ingestion of raw, pickled, or undercooked freshwater crabs or crayfish	Lung	Cough, hemoptysis, increased sputum, chest pain. Eosinophilia in early infections	Sputum examination Fecal examination Serology

the species of trematode. The encysted larva is called a **metacercaria.** Infection is acquired when the metacercaria is ingested. The larval worm migrates to the preferred location within the body, develops to an adult and begins producing eggs. In liver and intestinal trematode infections the eggs are excreted in the feces and, in lung fluke infections are excreted in the sputum and feces.

INTESTINAL TREMATODE INFECTION

Many trematode species are capable of parasitizing the human intestine. *Fasciolopsis buski* is used as an example.

Organism

Fasciolopsiasis is caused by the intestinal fluke, *F. buski.*

Transmission

The infection is acquired by the ingestion of metacercariae on freshwater aquatic plants, such as water chestnuts, water caltrop, water bamboo, and watercress.

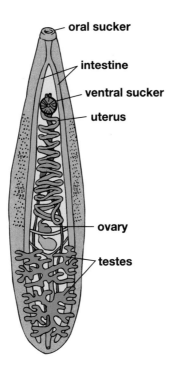

Figure 53.1.

C. sinensis adult as example of trematode morphology.

Geographic Distribution and Epidemiology

The infection is found in China, Taiwan, Indonesia, Malaysia, Southeast Asia, India, and Bangladesh. About 10 million individuals are infected. Pigs, dogs, and rabbits are reservoir hosts. Ponds used for growing aquatic plants are often contaminated with pig feces and the plants fed to the pigs, thus maintaining the cycle. Snail intermediate hosts have a wide distribution.

Habitat

Adult worms are adherent to the mucosa of the small intestine.

Properties of the Organism

Adult worms are 2–7.5 cm in length. Eggs are ellipsoidal and measure 130–140 µ in length. The eggshell is transparent and has a small operculum at the more pointed end (Fig. 53.2A).

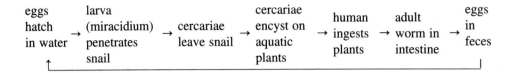

eggs hatch in water → larva (miracidium) penetrates snail → cercariae leave snail → cercariae encyst on aquatic plants → human ingests plants → adult worm in intestine → eggs in feces

Clinical Manifestations

The severity of symptoms is probably in proportion to the number of parasites. Heavier infections produce abdominal pain that may mimic peptic ulcer disease. Diarrhea is common. In severe infections, there is edema and ascites, which may reflect hypoalbuminemia caused by protein loss in the stool. Eosinophilia is usually present.

Laboratory Diagnosis

Routine stool examinations should reveal eggs.

Treatment

Praziquantel given in a single dose is highly effective.

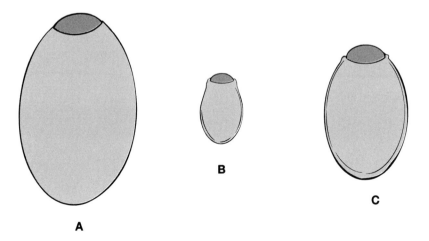

Figure 53.2.

Trematode ova. (A) *F. buski.* (B) *C. sinensis.* (C) *P. westermani.*

LIVER TREMATODE INFECTION

Organism

Clonorchiasis is caused by the Oriental liver fluke, *Clonorchis sinensis,* which is also called *Opisthorchis sinensis.*

Transmission

The infection is acquired by ingestion of raw, pickled, smoked, or dried freshwater fish containing metacercariae.

Geographic Distribution and Epidemiology

The infection is endemic in China, Taiwan, Vietnam, Korea, and Japan. Imported fish from China have caused high prevalence rates in Hong Kong. Liver flukes closely related to *C. sinensis* are found in Thailand, the Soviet Union, and parts of Europe. The infection occurs in areas where there is a cultural preference for raw or fish that has been inadequately treated to kill the metacercariae. Pigs, dogs, cats, and rats serve as reservoir hosts.

Habitat

The adult worms are found in the bile ducts. The most common location is in the intrahepatic bile ducts, but the parasites may also be seen in the extrahepatic ducts, the pancreatic duct, and gallbladder.

Properties of the Organism

The adult worms are slender and measure 1–2 cm in length (Fig. 53.2B). The eggs are small, brownish-yellow in color, and measure about 35 μ in length. These eggs are difficult to distinguish from the eggs of some other species of intestinal flukes.

eggs
ingested → cercariae → cercariae → human → adult worms → eggs in
by snail   leave snail   encyst in   ingests fish   in bile ducts   feces
                          fish

Clinical Manifestations

Most infections are asymptomatic. Heavy infection acquired at a single exposure may cause fever, diarrhea, abdominal pain, and eosinophilia. Chronic heavy infections may predispose to bile duct obstruction, intrahepatic stone formation, and cholangitis.

There is thickening and dilatation of bile ducts with biliary ductal hyperplasia. Metaplastic change may occur in the biliary epithelium. Infection has been associated with the occurrence of cholangiocarcinoma. Animal experiments show that a combination of carcinogen in the diet plus infection with liver flukes can produce cholangiocarcinoma.

Laboratory Diagnosis

Routine stool examinations, which include a concentration technique, are usually adequate for recovering eggs.

Treatment

Praziquantel is effective.

LUNG TREMATODE INFECTION

Organism

Paragonimiasis, or lung fluke infection, is caused by *Paragonimus westermani* and other species of *Paragonimus.*

Transmission

The infection is acquired by the ingestion of freshwater crabs or crayfish containing metacercariae.

Geographic Distribution and Epidemiology

The infection is found in China, Korea, Japan, eastern India, Papua New Guinea, Solomon islands, Samoa, Sri Lanka, and West Africa. Many different species of crab-eating mammals can serve as reservoir hosts.

Habitat

The adult worms are found in the lungs. Ectopic location of the worms in the brain, abdominal cavity, and subcutaneous tissue may occur.

Properties of the Organism

The adult flukes are about 1 cm in length and 0.5 cm in thickness. Worms are often found in pairs. Inflammatory reaction around adult worms in the lung progresses to fibrosis. Eggs are discharged from the fibrous capsule into the bronchi. The eggs are 80–120 μ in length and have pronounced ''shoulders'' at the junction of the operculum and the eggshell (Fig. 53.2C).

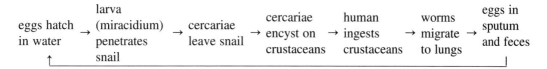

eggs hatch in water → larva (miracidium) penetrates snail → cercariae leave snail → cercariae encyst on crustaceans → human ingests crustaceans → worms migrate to lungs → eggs in sputum and feces

Clinical Manifestations

Cough, hemoptysis, increased sputum production, and chest pain may occur. Severity of symptoms may be relative to the numbers of worms. Chest X-rays may show patchy infiltrates, which may progress to nodular or cystic lesions. The lower and midlung fields are more commonly involved. The infection is often confused with pulmonary tuberculosis. Eosinophilia is more likely to be present in the early stages of infection.

Laboratory Diagnosis

Although the eggs appear in the sputum, both stool and sputum examinations should be done because sputum containing the eggs is frequently swallowed. A variety of serologic tests have been developed that appear to be sensitive and specific. These tests are not generally available in the United States; however, an immunoblot test is performed at the Centers for Disease Control and Prevention in Atlanta, Georgia.

Treatment

Praziquantel is the drug of choice in paragonimiasis.

OTHER COMMON TREMATODE INFECTIONS

Heterophyes heterophyes and *Metagonimus yokogawai* are very small intestinal trematodes that are acquired by the ingestion of metacercariae in raw or marinated freshwater fish. These infections are usually found in India, Japan, China, Taiwan, Korea, the Philippines, and Indonesia. Other endemic areas are the Middle East, the Balkans, the Soviet Union, and Spain. The parasites attach to the intestinal mucosa. Symptoms of diarrhea and abdominal discomfort may occur. The eggs, which are similar to those of *Clonorchis sinensis,* are detected by fecal examination.

The sheep liver fluke, *Fasciola hepatica,* causes facioliasis. Infection is acquired by the ingestion of raw aquatic vegetation, often watercress, contaminated with metacercariae. The infection is found worldwide in sheep-raising areas. The adult flukes are located in the large bile ducts and gallbladder. Sheep and other herbivores are reservoir hosts. The adult organisms are 2–3 cm in length. Ingested metacercariae excyst in the intestine. The larvae penetrate the bowel wall, migrate through the peritoneal cavity, and enter the liver. Adult worms deposit eggs in the bile ducts. The eggs, which resemble those of *F. buski,* are carried into the intestine with the bile and pass out of the body in the feces. Symptoms of fever, abdominal pain, hepatomegaly, and eosinophilia are common in the early stages of infection. Chronic infection may be associated with nonspecific GI complaints or with symptoms caused by bile duct obstruction. Eggs are recovered by routine fecal examination. Praziquantel is not an effective treatment for fascioliasis compared with other trematode infections. Bithionol is frequently used.

SUMMARY

1. Trematodes other than the schistosomes are hermaphroditic, dorsoventrally flattened organisms.

2. All trematodes have snail intermediate hosts.

3. Transmission occurs through the ingestion of infective larval stages.

4. The diagnosis of trematode infections is made by the demonstration of the eggs of the parasites.

5. Table 53.1 summarizes the key points of the three major examples of trematode infections.

6. Praziquantel is highly effective in the treatment of all of these infections with the exception of *Fasciola hepatica.*

REFERENCES

Harinasuta T, Bunnag D (1990): Liver, Lung and Intestinal Trematodiasis. In Warren KS, Mahmoud AAF (eds): Tropical and Geographical Medicine, 2nd ed. New York: McGraw-Hill Book Co.

Harinasuta T et al. (1993): Trematode infections. Opisthorchiasis, clonorchiasis, fascioliasis, and paragonimiasis. Infect Dis Clin North Am 7:699.

Hughes DL (1985): Trematodes excluding the schistosomes with special emphasis on *Fasciola.* Curr Top Microbiol Immunol 120:241.

Lin AC, Chapman SW, Turner HR, Wofford JD Jr (1987): Clonorchiasis: An update. South Med J 80:919.

Sun T (1984): Pathology and immunology of *Clonorchis sinensis* infection of the liver. Ann Clin Lab Sci 14:208.

REVIEW QUESTIONS

For questions 1 to 5, choose the ONE
BEST answer or completion.

1. The following characteristics are common to
   all intestinal, liver, and lung flukes, *except*
   a) the adult contains both sexes (hermaph-
      roditic)
   b) snails are intermediate hosts
   c) the infection is acquired by ingesting in-
      fectious stages
   d) eosinophilia is common in the early
      stages of infection
   e) there are no reservoir hosts

2. Paragonimiasis would most likely be associated with
   a) gastrointestinal bleeding
   b) hemoptysis (coughing up blood)
   c) jaundice
   d) skin rash
   e) enlargement of the liver

3. Fasciolopsiasis is acquired by

a) ingestion of raw or pickled freshwater
   crustaceans (crabs, crayfish)
b) ingestion of raw or undercooked freshwater fish
c) ingestion of raw or undercooked freshwater snails
d) ingestion of raw aquatic vegetation
e) penetration of the skin by infectious
   stages in fresh water

4. For optimal diagnosis of paragonimiasis, the
   following should be performed
   a) stool examination
   b) sputum examination
   c) stool and sputum examination
   d) examination of biliary drainage
   e) skin tests

5. Adults of *Clonorchis sinensis* are usually
   found in
   a) the lumen of the intestine
   b) the intrahepatic bile ducts
   c) the portal blood vessels in the liver
   d) the lung parenchyma
   e) the hepatic parenchyma

ANSWERS TO REVIEW QUESTIONS

1. *e* The intestinal, liver, and lung flukes all have several reservoir hosts that harbor the adult parasites.

2. *b* Paragonimiasis (lung fluke infection) is most likely to be associated with hemoptysis (coughing up blood). In some infections with species of *Paragonimus* the adult worms migrate to the brain, subcutaneous tissue or abdomen causing symptoms related to these sites.

3. *d* Fasciolopsiasis (intestinal fluke infection) is acquired by the ingestion of raw aquatic vegetation, such as water chestnuts, water bamboo, caltrop, and so on.

4. *c* Although eggs of *Paragonimus* are often found in the sputum, the best approach is to examine both stool and sputum. Bronchial mucus containing eggs is swallowed and the stool examination may be positive at times when the sputum is negative.

5. *b* The adult worms of *Clonorchis sinensis* are most frequently found in the intrahepatic bile ducts although they may be seen in the extrahepatic bile ducts, pancreatic duct, and gallbladder.

SCHISTOSOMIASIS

GENERAL CONSIDERATION

Organism

Schistosomiasis is caused by infection with one of several species of **schistosome** (blood fluke). Schistosomes are trematodes, but they differ considerably in morphology and life cycle from the trematodes discussed in Chapter 53. The major species that infect humans are *Schistosoma mansoni, Schistosoma japonicum,* and *Schistosoma haematobium.* Less common species, *Schistosoma mekongi* and *Schistosoma intercalatum* have similar life cycles and will not be discussed here. About 250 million people have schistosomiasis. Characteristics of the three major species are given in Table 54.1.

Transmission

Infection with any of the species of schistosome is acquired by exposure to fresh water containing infected snails. A larval stage, called a **cercaria,** which is shed from the snails, penetrates unbroken skin.

TABLE 54.1. Characteristics of the Three Major Species of Schistosome

Organism	Transmission	Distribution	Location	Clinical manifestations	Laboratory diagnosis
Schistosoma mansoni	Skin penetration by cercariae in fresh water	Africa, Middle East, South America, Caribbean	Veins of colon	Acute: Fever, abdominal pain, lymphadenopathy, tender liver, diarrhea, eosinophilia Chronic: Diarrhea, abdominal pain, hepatosplenomegaly, ascites	Fecal examination, rectal biopsy, serology
Schistosoma japonicum	Skin penetration by cercariae in fresh water	China, Japan, Philippines	Veins of small bowel	Acute: Fever, abdominal pain, lymphadenopathy, tender liver, diarrhea, eosinophilia Chronic: Diarrhea, abdominal pain, hepatosplenomegaly, ascites	Fecal examination, rectal biopsy, serology
Schistosoma haematobium	Skin penetration by cercariae in fresh water	Africa, Middle East	Veins of urinary bladder	Dysuria, frequency of urination, hematuria	Examination of urine, nucleopore filter, rectal biopsy, serology

Properties of the Organism

Unlike the other trematodes, the sexes are separate. The adult male worm appears cylindrical with a groove down the ventral surface (gynocophoral canal). The adult female is cylindrical and slender. The female lies in the canal of the male assuring continued fertilization (Fig. 54.1). The intestine of the female appears dark because of ingested blood. Both males and females have prominent anterior and ventral suckers.

The female deposits eggs in venules. The eggs do not possess an operculum as do the eggs of the other trematodes. A ciliated larva, the **miracidium,** develops within the egg. When the egg is excreted into fresh water, the larva hatches from the egg and penetrates a snail intermediate host. The larva undergoes asexual multiplication in the snail resulting in the production of thousands of infectious larvae called cercariae (Fig. 54.2). The cercariae escape from the snail and move

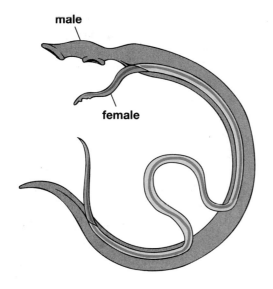

Figure 54.1.
Schistosoma adult male and female.

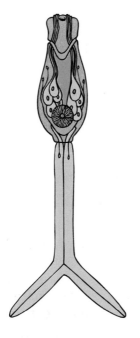

Figure 54.2
Schistosome cercaria.

about in the water using their forked tails. When they contact skin, they burrow through the epidermis into the blood vessels and are carried by the circulation to eventually locate in the liver. After development to adults in the vessels of the liver, the worms migrate to their final location in veins of the intestine or urinary bladder depending on the species of schistosome.

Eggs deposited in the venules of the bowel or bladder are able to penetrate the wall of the viscus and enter the lumen. Depending on the species, the eggs are excreted in the urine or the feces. Eggs that do not penetrate the tissues may be swept into the venous blood flow and embolize in the liver or lung. Cell mediated reactions to the eggs in the tissues produce granulomas that cause the serious complications of schistosomiasis. Adult schistosomes are able to survive for many years in the human host. During the first stage of infection, the invading schisto-somes are susceptible to destruction by the combined action of host IgE antibody, complement, and eosinophils. Macrophages also participate in killing the young schistosomes. Soon after infection, the parasites are able to incorporate or produce host antigens on their surface. This antigenic "camouflage" may protect the par-asites from the host's immune defense mechanisms.

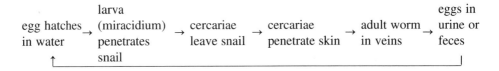

SCHISTOSOMIASIS MANSONI

Schistosomiasis mansoni is caused by *S. mansoni.*

Transmission

Cercariae from infected snails penetrate unbroken skin following exposure to freshwater.

Geographic Distribution and Epidemiology

The infection is found in tropical Africa, North Africa, the Arabian peninsula, the eastern part of South America, including Brazil, Venezuela and Surinam, and some Caribbean islands including Puerto Rico. Foci of infection are related to the fecal contamination of fresh water, which contains snail intermediate hosts. The prevalence in the population reflects the degree of exposure to infected water. There are no significant reservoir hosts for *S. mansoni.*

Habitat

Adult worms are found in the venules of the colon and rectum, but may occur in ectopic locations.

Properties of the Organism

The life cycle is outlined above. The adult worms are found in the veins of the colon and rectum. Eggs deposited in the venules, pass through the bowel wall, and are excreted in the feces. The eggs are about $150 \times 50 \mu$ and possess a prominent lateral spine (Fig. 54.3A). The adult male is about 1 cm in length and the female is about 1.5 cm long.

Clinical Manifestations

A transient rash may occur at the site of cercarial invasion. The early phase of infection is often asymptomatic. The signs and symptoms of acute schistosomiasis **(Katayama fever)** occur several weeks after infection. The symptoms usually coincide with the beginning of egg deposition, usually 1–3 months after infection. Fever, malaise, hives, abdominal pain, lymphadenopathy, and liver tenderness are common. Diarrhea, which may contain blood, may occur. The

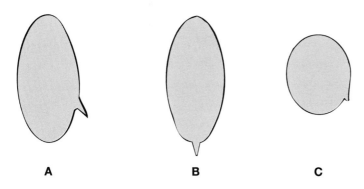

A   B   C

Figure 54.3

Diagnostic features of schistosome ova. (A) *S. mansoni.* (B) *S. haematobium.* (C) *S. japonicum.*

severity of symptoms is usually related to the number of worms. Chronic involvement of the colon produces symptoms of abdominal cramping and bloody diarrhea. Intestinal pseudopolyps may form. **Hepatosplenic schistosomiasis** develops when eggs deposited in the intestinal veins are carried into the portal system, and cause inflammatory reactions in the intrahepatic portal venules. The resulting presinusoidal cirrhosis causes obstruction of blood flow and increased pressure in the portal vein (portal hypertension). Advanced stages show intense fibrosis of the vein walls producing the so-called clay-pipestem appearance. The liver and spleen are enlarged. Increased collateral circulation around the obstructed intrahepatic portal vessels produces esophageal varices that are susceptible to rupture and hemorrhage. Ascites and abdominal distention may develop. Eggs deposited by the worms in the colonic veins may be carried by the dilated collateral vessels to embolize in the lung. In the lung, the eggs produce an endarteritis, which leads to pulmonary hypertension and right ventricular failure (cor pulmonale). Eggs carried to the spinal cord by venous anastomoses result in neurologic impairment.

Laboratory Diagnosis

Formalin-ethyl acetate concentrates of stool usually recover the characteristic eggs. Rectal biopsy is the most sensitive technique for detecting very light infections. Fresh biopsies of the rectal mucosa are compressed between two microscope slides and viewed under the low power of the microscope for the presence of the eggs. Serologic tests, such as ELISA are helpful in screening for light infections that are difficult to diagnose by stool examination. Newer tests, such as immunoblotting, appear highly sensitive and can discriminate between the species of schistosome.

Treatment

Praziquantel is the drug of choice. Oxamniquine is also effective, but geographic strains of *S. mansoni* vary in their sensitivity to this drug.

SCHISTOSOMIASIS JAPONICA

Schistosomiasis japonica is caused by *S. japonicum.*

Transmission

Cercaria from infected snails penetrate unbroken skin following exposure to freshwater.

Geographic Distribution and Epidemiology

The infection is found in China, Taiwan, Japan, the Philippines, and Sulawesi. Many species of mammals serve as reservoir hosts.

Habitat

Adult worms are more commonly found in the venules of the small intestine, but usually are also present in the veins of the colon and rectum.

Properties of the Organism

The life cycle is noted in general considerations above. Eggs pass through the bowel wall and are excreted in the feces. The eggs are about $75 \times 50 \mu$ and may possess a very small and inconspicuous knoblike spine (Fig. 54.3). The adult male is about 2 cm, and the female is about 2.5 cm in length.

Clinical Manifestations

The illness is similar to *S. mansoni* infection. Hepatosplenic complications occur more frequently than in infection with *S. mansoni*. Neurologic complications with cerebral involvement are not uncommon.

Laboratory Diagnosis

The same techniques are used as for *S. mansoni* infection.

Treatment

Praziquantel is an effective drug.

SCHISTOSOMIASIS HAEMATOBIA

Schistosomiasis haematobia is caused by *S. haematobium.*

Transmission

Cercariae from infected snails penetrate unbroken skin following exposure to freshwater.

Geographic Distribution and Epidemiology

The infection is wide spread in Africa and the Middle East. Foci of infection occur on Mediterranean islands, Portugal, and in one area of India. There are no significant reservoir hosts for *S. haematobium.*

Habitat

Adult worms are found in the venules of the urinary bladder (vesical plexus). These worms also commonly occur in rectal veins.

Properties of the Organism

The life cycle is outlined in General Considerations above. Eggs are deposited in venules of the urinary bladder. The eggs penetrate the bladder wall and are excreted in the urine. The eggs are about 150 x 50 μ and have a prominent terminal spine. The adult males are about 1.5 cm and the females are about 2 cm in length.

Clinical Manifestations

Involvement of the urinary bladder causes hematuria and urinary tract symptoms, such as dysuria and frequency of urination. The hematuria often is noted at the end of urination (terminal hematuria).

Deposition of eggs in the ureter may lead to obstruction and hydronephrosis. There is an association between infection with *S. haematobium* and the occurrence of squamous cell carcinoma of the bladder. Because the veins of the urinary bladder drain into the inferior vena cava, hepatosplenic involvement is rare. Pulmonary and cardiac disease secondary to the embolization of eggs in the lungs may occur but is not common. Neurologic complications related to spinal cord involvement have been reported.

Laboratory Diagnosis

Eggs may be found on examination of the urinary sediment. The urine specimen has a higher yield of eggs if it is collected between noon and 3 o'clock in the afternoon. Filtration of the urine through a nucleopore filter is a very efficient technique for recovering eggs for diagnosis. Bladder biopsy or rectal biopsy is infrequently needed for definitive diagnosis. Serologic tests may be helpful.

Treatment

Praziquantel is the drug of choice. Metrifonate, an anticholinesterase compound, is also effective. Because of its lower cost, it has been widely used in endemic areas.

CERCARIAL DERMATITIS

Cercarial dermatitis (swimmer's itch) is caused by a variety of schistosomes of birds. Snail intermediate hosts are found in both fresh or salt water. When humans are exposed to the water containing cercariae shed from the snails, the cercariae penetrate the skin but do not enter the circulation and are unable to develop. The cercariae cause a papular, erythematous, pruritic rash that may last for several days.

SUMMARY

1. Adult schistosomes live in veins and venules. The sexes are separate and the eggs are not operculated.

2. Snails are intermediate hosts, and the infection is acquired by contact

with fresh water containing cercariae shed from the snails. The cercariae penetrate the unbroken skin.

3. Table 54.1 summarizes the characteristics of infection with the three major species of schistosome.

4. The pathology of schistosomiasis develops in response to the local deposition of eggs in the bowel or urinary bladder and to the embolization of eggs in the portal system and pulmonary arterioles.

5. Hepatosplenic schistosomiasis develops from the reaction to eggs embolized in the portal venules of the liver. Presinusoidal cirrhosis and portal hypertension cause enlargement of the liver and spleen, ascites, and esophageal varices. Hepatosplenic complications are more common in infections with *Schistosoma mansoni* and *Schistosoma japonicum*.

6. Pulmonary schistosomiasis may occur in infections of all three schistosome species. Eggs lodging in the pulmonary arterioles cause pulmonary hypertension and right ventricular failure.

7. Praziquantel is an effective treatment of infections with all three species.

8. Cercarial dermatitis is a papular, pruritic skin condition caused by the penetration of cercariae from species of schistosomes found in birds.

REFERENCES

Boros DL (1989): Immunopathology of *Schistosoma mansoni* infection. Clin Microbiol Rev 2:250.

Davis A (1986): Recent advances in schistosomiasis. Q J Med 58:95.

Evengard B (1989): Schistosomiasis. Immunological, serological and clinical aspects. Scand J Infect Dis Suppl 63:1.

Gonzalez E (1989): Schistosomiasis, cercarial dermatitis, and marine dermatitis. Dermatol Clin 7:291.

Lusey DR, Maguire JH (1993): Schistosomiasis. Infect Dis Clin North Am 7:635.

Rollinson D, Simpson AJG (eds) (1987): The Biology of the Schistosomes: From Genes to Latrines. San Diego: Academic Press.

REVIEW QUESTIONS

For questions 1 to 2, choose the ONE BEST answer or completion.

1. Schistosomiasis (all species) is acquired by
   a) ingestion of raw or pickled freshwater fish
   b) penetration of the skin by larval stages in fresh water
   c) ingestion of raw or pickled freshwater crustaceans (crab or crayfish)
   d) ingestion of aquatic vegetation, such as water chestnuts
   e) ingestion of raw or pickled snails

2. Which of the following conditions has been attributed to *Schistosoma haematobium* infections?
   a) carcinoma of the colon
   b) cholangiocarcinoma (carcinoma of bile ducts)
   c) carcinoma of the ureter
   d) carcinoma of the urinary bladder
   e) carcinoma of the gall bladder

For questions 3 to 8, a list of lettered options is followed by several numbered items. For each numbered item, select the ONE lettered option that is most closely associated with it. Each lettered option may be selected once, more than once, or not at all.

A) *Schistosoma mansoni* only
B) *Schistosoma japonicum* only
C) *Schistosoma haematobium* only
D) Both *S. mansoni* and *S. haematobium*
E) Both *S. mansoni* and *S. japonicum*
F) All three species

For the following statements, select the appropriate parasite or parasites.

3. Infection is found in China

4. Infection is found in South America

5. Infection is found in Africa

6. Infection may cause hematuria (blood in the urine)

7. Diagnosis may be made by rectal biopsy

8. Diagnosis is made by fecal concentration techniques

ANSWERS TO REVIEW QUESTIONS

1. *b* All species of schistosomes infect humans by penetration of the skin by cercariae in fresh water.

2. *d* There is an epidemiologic association between infection with *Schistosoma haematobium* and carcinoma of the urinary bladder.

3. *B* *Schistosoma japonicum* is found in China.

4. *A* Only *Schistosoma mansoni* is found in South America.

5. *D* Both *S. mansoni* and *S. haematobium* are found in Africa.

6. *C* *S. haematobium* localizes in veins of the urinary bladder and causes hematuria.

7. *F* All three species may have eggs deposited in rectal mucosa even though the primary location may be the urinary bladder (*S. haematobium*) or small intestine (*S. japonicum*).

8. *D* Eggs of *S. mansoni* and *S. japonicum* are shed in the feces. *S. haematobium* eggs are found in the urine.

CESTODE INFECTIONS

Adult cestodes, or tapeworms, are ribbonlike. The worm possesses an attachment organ, called a **scolex,** at its anterior end. With the exception of *Diphyllobothrium latum*, the species discussed here have scoleces with four circular suckers that are used to grasp the host's intestinal mucosa Fig. 55.1A,B). Some species also have circular rows of hooks on the scolex that assist in attachment. The scolex of *D. latum* has two longitudinal grooves that serve the same purpose (Fig. 55.1C). Behind the scolex, is an undifferentiated region of rapid growth called the neck. Further down the length of the worm, transverse divisions separate the worm into a series of connected segments. The segments are called **proglottids.** Maturation of organs within the proglottids occurs as the proglottids grow more distal from the scolex. The mature proglottid contains both male and female sex organs. After fertilization takes place, the uterus fills with eggs. The gravid proglottids are found at the most distal portion of the worm (Fig. 55.2). Tapeworms have no intestinal tract but they are able to take up nutrients through their tegument. Glucose is the major source of energy in the metabolism of cestodes. All tapeworms require larval development in one or more intermediate hosts. The major types of larvae can be categorized by their morphology as follows:

Cysticercus: A cystic structure containing fluid and a single scolex (*Taenia solium* and *Taenia saginata*).

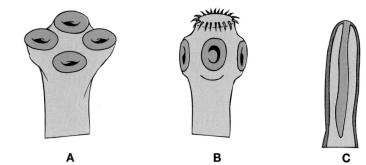

Figure 55.1.

Tapeworm scoleces. (A) *T. saginata*. (B) *T. solium*. (C) *D. latum*.

Hydatid cyst: A fluid-filled cystic structure that is lined with a germinal membrane with **brood capsules** and many **protoscolices** (*Echinococcus granulosus*).

Cysticercoid: A solid structure containing a single inverted scolex (*Hymenolepis nana*).

Plerocercoid: A ribbonlike worm with anterior grooves that become the grooved suckers of *D. latum*. Plerocercoid larvae of *Spirometra* species cause sparganosis.

Adult tapeworms are always found in the intestine. Eggs or proglottids containing eggs are excreted in the stool. Eggs are ingested by the intermediate host, and the embryos that hatch from the eggs develop into larvae. When the definitive host ingests the tissues of the intermediate host, the larvae develop into adult tapeworms in the intestine. Depending on the species of tapeworm, humans may serve as the definitive host or as an accidental intermediate host. A list of important tapeworms that have humans as definitive hosts follows:

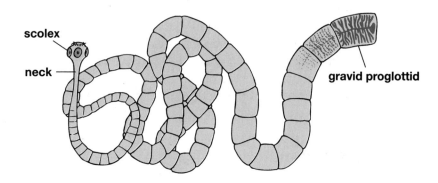

Figure 55.2.

T. solium adult. The scolex is smaller and the worm is much longer than shown.

Taenia saginata: beef tapeworm
Taenia solium: pork tapeworm
Diphyllobothrium latum: fish tapeworm
Hymenolepis nana: dwarf tapeworm

Humans are accidental intermediate hosts in infections with the following tapeworms:

Echinococcus granulosus: causing hydatid disease
Taenia solium: causing cysticercosis
Spirometra species: causing sparganosis

Infections with *Hymenolepis nana* are unique, because humans are both definitive and intermediate hosts.

The characteristics of the major cestode infections are summarized in Table 55.1.

TAENIASIS SAGINATA

Taeniasis saginata is caused by *T. saginata,* the beef tapeworm.

Transmission

The infection is acquired by the ingestion of raw or undercooked beef containing larvae of *T. saginata.*

Geographic Distribution and Epidemiology

The infection is found worldwide with high prevalence rates in countries where poor sanitation and the eating of raw or rare beef coincide. Infrequent infections occur in the United States.

Habitat

The adult worms attach in the small intestine.

TABLE 55.1. Characteristics of Cestode Infections

Organism	Transmission	Location	Clinical manifestations	Laboratory diagnosis	Treatment
Taenia saginata	Ingestion of cysticerci in raw or rare beef	Intestine	Nonspecific GI complaints. Migration of proglottids	Fecal exam for ova, examination of proglottids	Niclosamide, praziquantel
Taenia solium	Ingestion of cysticerci in raw or rare pork	Intestine	Nonspecific GI complaints. Passing proglottids	Fecal exam for ova, examination of proglottids	Niclosamide
Taenia solium (cysticercosis)	Ingestion of eggs from human feces	Central nervous system, muscle, subcutaneous tissue, eye and so on	Seizures, headache, meningismus, subcutaneous nodules, visual disturbance	Serologic tests or biopsy	Surgery, praziquantel, albendazole
Diphyllobothrium latum	Ingestion of larvae in undercooked or raw freshwater fish	Intestine	Nonspecific GI complaints. Passing proglottids	Fecal exam for ova, examination of proglottids	Niclosamide, praziquantel
Spirometra species (sparganosis)	Ingestion of water with infected copepod or ingestion of plerocercoid in frog, snake, etc.	Subcutaneous tissues	Migratory subcutaneous nodule	Examination of excised parasite	Surgical excision
Hymenolepis nana	Ingestion of eggs from human feces	Larva in intestinal wall, adult in intestinal lumen	Diarrhea, abdominal pain, eosinophilia	Fecal exam for ova	Praziquantel, niclosamide
Echinococcus granulosus (hydatid disease)	Ingestion of eggs from dog feces	Liver and lung are the most common sites	Hepatic cysts cause pain in the area of the cyst. Rupture of cysts causes allergic reactions and eosinophilia	Imaging techniques, serologic tests	Surgery, albendazole

Properties of the Organism

The scolex has four muscular suckers (Fig. 55.1A). The worm is usually about 15–20 ft in length. The motile, gravid proglottids often migrate from the anus. The morphology of the uterus in the gravid proglottid is characteristic for the species (Fig. 55.3A). Cattle acquire the infection by ingestion of eggs contaminating grass or feed. The eggs hatch in the intestine of the cattle, the embryos penetrate the mucosa and enter blood vessels. The embryos are disseminated by way of the circulation, lodge in various tissues, including muscle, and develop into cysticerci. The cysticercus larva is a cystic structure about 1–2 cm in diameter. Inside the cyst is a small, solid mass that contains the scolex. When beef muscle containing cysticerci is ingested, the cysticerci develop into adult tapeworms. Usually, only one adult tapeworm survives and develops to maturity. The eggs of *T. saginata* are spherical, have a striated layer surrounding the embryo, and have a brownish eggshell. The embryo, called an **onchosphere,** contains six hooks that are used to burrow through the intestinal wall. The eggs are morphologically identical to those of *T. solium* (Fig. 55.4A).

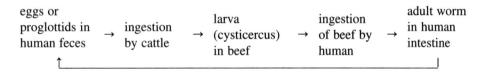

Clinical Manifestations

Although many GI complaints have been associated with *T. saginata* infection, a cause and effect relationship is difficult to prove. Patients who know that they have a tapeworm infection are much more likely to report symptoms than those who are unaware of their infection. The most distressing symptom is the migration of proglottids from the anus.

Laboratory Diagnosis

The differentiation of *T. saginata* from *T. solium* is based on the morphology of gravid proglottids. The uterus has a central stem with lateral branches. By counting the primary lateral branches on one side of the uterine stem, the species may be separated. The uterus of *T. solium* has 12 or less branches and *T. saginata* has more than 12 (Fig. 55.3A,B). The eggs of both species are morphologically

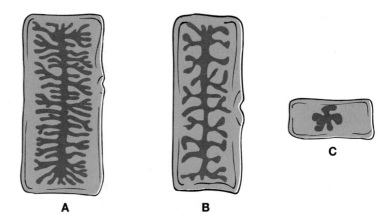

Figure 55.3.

Tapeworm gravid proglottids. (A) *T. saginata.* (B) *T. solium.* (C) *D. latum.*

identical (Fig. 55.4A). Recent successful use of DNA probes to differentiate the eggs may become practical in the future.

Treatment

Niclosamide and praziquantel are both highly effective.

TAENIASIS SOLIUM

Taeniasis solium is caused by *T. solium,* the pork tapeworm.

Transmission

The infection is acquired by the ingestion of raw, cured, or inadequately cooked pork containing cysticerci of *T. solium.*

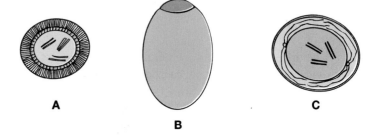

Figure 55.4.

Tapeworm ova. (A) *T. solium.* (B) *D. latum.* (C) *H. nana.*

Geographic Distribution and Epidemiology

The highest prevalence rates are seen in countries where pork is a major part of the diet, such as Mexico, Latin America, Spain, Portugal, Africa, India, Southeast Asia, and China. Infections with adult worms are infrequently seen in the United States.

Habitat

The adult worm attaches in the small intestine.

Properties of the Organism

The life cycle is identical to that of *T. saginata;* however, the intermediate host is the pig instead of the cow. *T. solium* differs from *T. saginata* also in that eggs of *T. solium* are infectious for humans and may produce a disease called cysticercosis.

Clinical Manifestations

Infected individuals are usually asymptomatic or have nonspecific GI complaints.

Laboratory Diagnosis

See Taeniasis saginata.

Treatment

Niclosamide and praziquantel are effective. Praziquantel must be used with caution in case the patient with adult *T. solium* infection has developed cysticercosis.

CYSTICERCOSIS

Cysticercosis is caused by infection with larval stages of *Taenia solium*.

Transmission

Infection is caused by the ingestion of eggs of *T. solium* from human feces. Eggs may contaminate food or beverages. The person infected with adult *T. solium* may disseminate eggs to others and/or cause infection in himself/herself. The source of infection (eggs of *T. solium*) is always human.

Geographic Distribution and Epidemiology

The distribution is the same as for *T. solium.* Nearly all cysticercosis in the United States is seen in immigrants from these areas. Occasionally, infection is acquired in the United States by contact with immigrants harboring adult *T. solium.*

Habitat

Cysticerci may be found in many different tissues, but sites that are clinically prominent are muscle, CNS, eye, and subcutaneous tissue.

Properties of the Organism

Humans are accidental intermediate hosts. Ingested eggs hatch in the intestine. The liberated embryos penetrate the mucosa and are carried by the circulation to sites of development (muscle, brain, etc.). The embryos grow into cysticerci. The cysticercus is about 1–2 cm in diameter, and is usually spherical or ovoid. This fluid-filled cystic structure contains a rounded, dense mass on one side that contains the scolex (Fig. 55.5).

Clinical Manifestations

The clinical picture is dependent on the location and numbers of cysticerci as well as the local host tissue response. Healthy cysticerci produce little inflammatory response, but dead or degenerating organisms cause a granulomatous re-

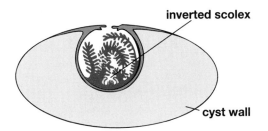

inverted scolex

cyst wall

Figure 55.5.
Cystircercus of *T. solium.*

action that contains eosinophils. Subcutaneous cysticercosis produces nodular lesions that resemble lipomas. Ocular involvement in the aqueous or vitreous humor causes visual impairment. Cerebral cysticercosis is divided into three types: (1) cysts in the brain parenchyma that produce seizures or a mass effect, (2) meningeal involvement may cause symptoms of meningitis or may obstruct cerebrospinal fluid flow with resulting hydrocephalus, (3) intraventricular cysts that also may cause hydrocephalus. Spinal cysticercosis causes a variety of neurological abnormalities related to the degree of spinal cord involvement.

Laboratory Diagnosis

Subcutaneous lesions are usually biopsied for a definitive diagnosis. The diagnosis of nervous system involvement is based on the clinical picture, the likelihood of exposure and characteristic findings on computed tomography or magnetic resonance imaging of the brain. Serologic tests on serum may be helpful. The combination of an enzyme linked immunosorbent assay and an immunoblot test appears very sensitive and specific, but false negatives are common when there are single lesions in the cerebral parenchyma.

Treatment

Asymptomatic cysts or cysts that cause seizures that are easily controlled probably do not require specific treatment. Medical treatment is possible using praziquantel or albendazole, but there is no universal agreement on the indications for the use of these drugs. Patients undergoing therapy with praziquantel or albendazole often have worsening of symptoms because of inflammatory reactions about the dead or dying parasites. Corticosteroids have been used to minimize these reactions. Hydrocephalus from intracranial hypertension may require cerebrospinal fluid shunting procedures.

DIPHYLLOBOTHRIASIS

Diphyllobothriasis is caused by *D. latum,* the fish tapeworm.

Transmission

Infection is acquired by the ingestion of raw, undercooked, pickled, or lightly smoked freshwater fish containing the larvae of the tapeworm.

Geographic Distribution and Epidemiology

The infection is reported from nearly all areas of the world, but higher prevalence rates occur in Finland, Russia, Scandinavia, and Canada, where freshwater fish is traditionally eaten raw, pickled, or lightly smoked. Efforts at preventing contamination of freshwater lakes with human feces have dramatically reduced the prevalence of this infection.

Habitat

The adult worm attaches in the small intestine.

Properties of the Organism

Eggs are operculated and measure about $70 \times 50 \mu$ (Fig. 55.4B). When the eggs are excreted and reach fresh water, a ciliated larva develops and hatches through the opened operculum. The larva is ingested by a freshwater crustacean (copepod). After a period of development in the copepod, the larva becomes infective for fish. When the infected copepod is eaten by a fish, the larva migrates to the muscle, and becomes an elongated and ribbonlike plerocercoid. The infected fish may be eaten by larger fish causing the larva to migrate into the muscle of the new host fish. Eventually, game fish containing the larvae are eaten by humans. The larva attaches to the mucosa of the small intestine and develops to an adult tapeworm. Eggs are excreted in the stool. It is not unusual for chains of proglottids to be passed in the stool. The adult worm has an elongate scolex with two parallel grooves that are used in attachment (Fig. 55.1C). The adult reaches lengths greater than 30 ft.

eggs hatch in water → larva eaten by copepod → copepod eaten by fish → fish eaten by bigger fish → fish eaten by human → adult worm in human intestine → eggs in feces

Clinical Manifestations

Most patients are asymptomatic, but a variety of nonspecific GI symptoms have been reported to be associated with the infection. A small percentage of infected individuals develop a megaloblastic anemia, which is indistinguishable from pernicious anemia. This complication is rarely reported outside of Finland. The tapeworm competes with the host for vitamin B_{12} and also interferes with the host's absorption of vitamin B_{12}.

Laboratory Diagnosis

Eggs are easily recovered from the stool. The gravid proglottid contains an egg-filled, "rosette" shaped uterus that is diagnostic (Fig. 55.3C).

Treatment

Niclosamide and praziquantel are effective drugs.

SPARGANOSIS

Species of the tapeworm genus *Spirometra* are morphologically similar to *Diphyllobothrium* and have a similar life cycle. The plerocercoid larva of this genus, also called a **sparganum,** may infect humans, producing the disease **sparganosis.** The infection is acquired by the ingestion of water containing copepods infected with the first-stage larva or by ingesting the second intermediate hosts such as tadpoles, frogs, or snakes that contain plerocercoid larva. Incidence of sparganosis has been reported in every continent. In the United States, most infections have originated in southern or southeastern states.

The plerocercoid larva recovered from humans is a whitish, ribbonlike worm that is a few millimeters in width and a variable length to a few centimeters. Its surface is wrinkled, and the anterior end may show the groovelike indentations that are the precursors to the sucking grooves of the scolex of the adult worm. Dogs and cats are definitive hosts.

Sparganosis may involve all tissues in the body excepting bone. The most common form is subcutaneous sparganosis, which appears as a migratory subcutaneous nodule. The treatment is sugical removal and the diagnosis is confirmed by examination of the excised parasite. Ocular sparganosis is relatively common in China and Vietnam. It results from the application of poultices of frog flesh to the eye for medicinal purposes. Plerocercoid larvae from the frog migrate into the periorbital and retroorbital tissues producing edema and inflammation.

HYMENOLEPIASIS

Hymenolepiasis is caused by *H. nana,* the dwarf tapeworm.

Transmission

The infection is acquired by ingesting the eggs of *H. nana* in food or beverages or from contaminated fingers. The eggs are excreted in the stools of infected humans.

Geographic Distribution and Epidemiology

The infection is found worldwide with greater prevalence rates in regions with poor sanitation. Prevalence is much higher among children, possibly because of lower levels of personal hygiene. In some areas of India and the Middle East, prevalence rates among children exceed 20%. High rates are also seen in Latin America and central Europe.

Habitat

Adult worms attach to the mucosa of the small intestine. Larvae develop in intestinal villi.

Properties of the Organism

The adult worm is usually less than 4 cm in length. The scolex has four suckers and a circular row of hooks. Proglottids disintegrate in the lumen of the intestine, and the infectious eggs are excreted in the stool. When an egg is ingested, the embryo hatches and burrows into the intestinal villus where it develops into a cysticercoid larva. A few days later, the larva breaks out into the intestinal lumen and matures to an adult worm. It is possible for one individual to harbor several thousand adult worms. The egg contains a six-hooked embryo within an envelope that has two polar knobs from which extend several filaments (Fig. 55.4C). Eggs liberated from proglottids in the intestinal lumen may hatch and cause internal autoinfection. Eggs from stool can be ingested from contaminated fingers causing external autoinfection.

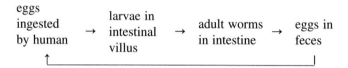

Eggs are infectious for several species of beetles and fleas. Larval stages develop in the insect. Accidental ingestion of the insect intermediate host can cause infection in humans. This indirect cycle is probably relatively unimportant in the epidemiology of human infections.

Clinical Manifestations

Infections with less than 1000 parasites may be asymptomatic or cause loose stools. Infections with more than 3000 worms are associated with diarrhea, abdominal pain, and other nonspecific complaints. Eosinophilia may be present.

Laboratory Diagnosis

The characteristic eggs are usually easy to recover in direct smears or concentrates of the stool.

Treatment

Praziquantel is preferred over niclosamide because it is effective in a single dose.

HYDATID DISEASE

Hydatid disease or echinococcosis is caused by *E. granulosus.*

Transmission

Humans are accidental intermediate hosts. Infection is acquired from ingesting eggs of the parasite from dogs or other definitive hosts, such as wolves or foxes. Eggs are present in dog feces and contaminate the dog's fur and the environment. Close contact with dogs or exposure to the contaminated environment fosters transmission.

Geographic Distribution and Epidemiology

The highest prevalence rates occur in sheep raising areas where the custom of feeding sheep viscera to the dogs is practiced. Endemic areas are found in South America, Africa, the Mediterranean area, the Middle East, Central Asia, and areas of Australia and New Zealand. Foci of infection are also present in California, Arizona, New Mexico, Utah, Alaska, and Canada. Although sheep are the most important intermediate hosts, cattle, pigs, goats, horses, buffalo, and camels can also serve in this role.

Habitat

Hydatid cysts develop most frequently in the liver. Other sites are lung, brain, kidney, spleen, bone, and the heart.

Properties of the Organism

The adult worm is very small and has only three proglottids. Dogs are often infected with thousands of adult worms. Eggs are excreted in dog feces and contaminate the grass. Sheep grazing on the grass ingest the eggs. The eggs hatch in the intestine, the embryos burrow into the mucosa, enter the blood vessels, and are carried to the liver. Usually, the embryos are trapped in the liver, but some may be disseminated in the general circulation to lodge in other organs. The embryo develops into the hydatid cyst. The cyst consists of an outer acellular, laminated membrane that is lined with a thin cellular layer called the germinal membrane. Spherical structures, called brood capsules, bud from the membrane. Protoscolices grow from the inner surface of the brood capsules (Fig. 55.6). Each protoscolex has the potential to become an adult worm when it is ingested by the definitive host. When sheep are slaughtered by sheepherders, it is common practice to feed the viscera to the sheep dogs. The dogs ingest the cyst material, and each protoscolex develops to an adult worm in the dog's intestine. Human infections occur when the eggs from dog feces are ingested and hydatid cysts develop in the human.

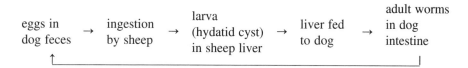

Clinical Manifestations

Hydatid cysts develop relatively slowly, usually about 1 cm/year. These cysts produce symptoms because of the space occupying mass or because of leakage, rupture, or secondary bacterial infection. Liver cysts usually cause pain when they

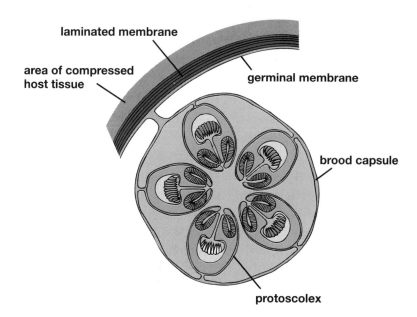

Figure 55.6.

Section of hydatid cyst (larva of *E. granulosus*).

reach a significant size. Cysts of diameters of 15–20 cm are not uncommon. Leakage or rupture may produce severe allergic reactions including anaphylaxis. Lung cysts are often asymptomatic and are discovered on routine chest X-ray. Older cysts may calcify. Cysts in other locations, such as the brain and heart, cause symptoms related to their mass effect. Cysts in bone may cause pathological fractures.

Laboratory Diagnosis

Cysts are best defined by the imaging techniques of ultrasound, computed tomography (CT), and magnetic resonance (MRI). A history of exposure in an endemic area is helpful. Serologic tests are useful when positive, however, negative tests occur in 10–15% of liver cysts and 50% of lung cysts. At operation, the finding of **hydatid sand** (protoscolices and hooks of protoscolices) in the fluid is diagnostic.

Treatment

Surgical removal of accessible cysts is the preferred approach. Surgical procedures risk the spillage of cyst contents with the potential complications of severe allergic reactions or the development of secondary cysts from the protoscolices. Medical therapy with albendazole has become standard in some countries but is considered investigational in the United States. Albendazole has been used with some success in an attempt to avoid surgery and in cases where surgery is not feasible. This drug appears most useful as an adjunct to surgery in the prevention of the development of secondary cysts.

ALVEOLAR HYDATID DISEASE

Alveolar hydatid disease is caused by *Echinococcus multilocularis,* which resembles *E. granulosus* in morphology and life cycle. The intermediate hosts are rodents, and the definitive hosts usually are foxes, but dogs may become infected by eating rodents. The disease is found only in the Northern Hemisphere. Although cases are reported in the northern United States, adjacent Canada, and parts of Europe, the greatest number of human infections are reported from Alaska, the Soviet Union, and northern Japan. The cysts in the intermediate hosts, including humans, bud externally producing an aggressively growing, tumorlike mass in the liver. The cysts may even spread hematogenously to the lungs and brain. Imaging techniques and a highly specific serologic test aid in the diagnosis. Surgery is curative if the masses can be removed early in the course of the disease. Chemotherapy with albendazole has been of benefit in some cases.

SUMMARY

1. The adult tapeworm has an attachment organ, called the scolex, at its anterior end.

2. The ribbonlike body of the adult tapeworm is made up of segments called proglottids.

3. Each proglottid contains both male and female sex organs. Gravid proglottids contain eggs.

4. All tapeworms require intermediate hosts for the development of larval stages.

5. Humans serve as definitive hosts for *Taenia saginata*, *Taenia solium*, and *Diphyllobothrium latum*.

6. Humans are accidental intermediate hosts for *T. solium* (cysticercosis), *Spirometra* species (sparganosis), *Echinococcus granulosus* (hydatid disease), and *Echinococcus multilocularis* (alveolar hydatid disease).

7. Humans are both intermediate and definitive hosts for *Hymenolepis nana*.

8. Characteristics of the common tapeworm infections are summarized in Table 55.1.

REFERENCES

Botero D, Tanowitz HB, Weiss LM, Wittner M (1993): Taeniasis and cysticercosis. Infect Dis Clin North Am 7:683.

Cook GC (1988): Neurocysterosis: parasitology, clinical presentation, diagnosis, and recent advances in management. Q J Med 68:575.

Jueco N (1982): *Hymenolepis nana* Infection. In Steele JH (ed): CRC Handbook Series in Zoonoses. Section C: Parasitic Zoonoses. Arambulo P (Section ed). Vol. I. Boca Raton, FL: CRC Press.

Kammerer WS, Shantz PM (1993): Echinoccocal disease. Infect Dis Clin North Am 7:605.

Pawlowski ZS (1982): Taeniasis and cysticercosis. In Steele JH (ed): CRC Handbook Series in Zoonoses. Section C: Parasitic Zoonoses. Arambulo P (Section ed). Vol. I. Boca Raton, FL: CRC Press.

Schantz PM, Okelo GB (1990): Echinococcosis (Hydatidosis). In Warren KS, Mahmoud AAF (eds): Tropical and Geographical Medicine. 2nd ed. New York: McGraw-Hill Book Co.

Thompson RCA (ed) (1986): The Biology of Echinococcus and Hydatid Disease. Boston: Allen & Unwin.

Von Bonsdorff B (1977): Diphyllobothriasis in Man. New York: Academic Press.

REVIEW QUESTIONS

For questions 1 to 7, a list of lettered options is followed by several numbered items. For each numbered item, select the ONE lettered option that is most closely associated with it. Each lettered option may be selected once, more than once, or not at all.

A) *Taenia solium*
B) *Taenia saginata*
C) *Echinococcus granulosus*
D) *Hymenolepis nana*
E) *Diphyllobothrium latum*

For the statements below, select the appropriate parasite.

1. The pig is the intermediate host.

2. Humans acquire the infection by ingesting eggs from dog feces.

3. Eggs are excreted in human feces. If these eggs are ingested by humans, cystic larval stages may develop in the CNS.

4. When humans ingest eggs of this parasite, larval stages develop in the intestinal villus.

5. Sheep serve as intermediate hosts.

6. Humans acquire the infection by eating raw, undercooked, or pickled freshwater fish.

7. When humans ingest the eggs of this parasite, large cystic structures may develop in the liver or lung.

ANSWERS TO REVIEW QUESTIONS

1. *A* The pig develops larval stages (cysticerci) in muscle.

2. *C* The adult stages of *Echinococcus granulosus* are in the dog intestine. Humans become accidental intermediate hosts when they ingest eggs shed in dog feces.

3. *A* Cysticercosis of the nervous system may develop following ingestion of eggs of *Taenia solium* from human feces. Hydatid cysts of the CNS may develop after ingestion of eggs from *dog* feces.

4. *D* Humans serve as both definitive and intermediate hosts of *Hymenolepis nana*. The larval stage develops in the intestinal villus.

5. *C* Sheep develop the larval stages of *E. granulosus* (hydatid cysts) in liver and other viscera.

6. *E* *Diphyllobothrium latum* larvae are found in freshwater fish.

7. *C* Hydatid cysts of *E. granulosus* develop most commonly in liver and lung when eggs from dog feces are ingested.

INTESTINAL NEMATODE INFECTIONS AND TRICHINOSIS

INTESTINAL NEMATODE INFECTIONS

Nematodes, or roundworms, are cylindrical in shape and have a complete intestinal tract, with the mouth located at the anterior end and the anus at the posterior end. The sexes are separate. The female worm is larger than the male. The male has a sharply curved posterior end or an expansion of the posterior, called a bursa, which is used in clasping the female. The male also possesses one or two copulatory spicules that aid in the mating process. The testes and ovaries are cylindrical. The ovaries are continuous with the uteri. Usually, the vulva is located near the midbody of the female. Larvae develop within the egg, and in some species, hatch from the egg to continue development in the soil. The first stage larva is noninfectious. This larva has a muscular esophagus with a prominent esophageal bulb. After additional development it becomes infectious, a larva with a slender esophagus without a bulb. The common intestinal nematodes, with the exception of *Enterobius vermicularis,* are often referred to as soil-borne nematodes because infection is acquired by the ingestion of eggs from soil or by the active penetration of the skin by larvae dwelling in the soil. The intestinal nematodes do not have intermediate hosts, but they require a period of maturation outside the human host. There are no significant reservoir hosts for the intestinal nematodes. Table 56.1 summarizes the major characteristics of the common intestinal nematode infections.

STRONGYLOIDIASIS

Strongyloidiasis is caused by *Strongyloides stercoralis.*

Transmission

Infection is acquired by direct contact with soil containing infective larvae. The larvae penetrate unbroken skin.

Geographic Distribution and Epidemiology

The infection is found worldwide, but the highest prevalence rates are concentrated in warm, humid environments where sanitation is poor and soil is contaminated with human feces, or fecal material is used as fertilizer. It is estimated that there are up to 100 million infections.

Habitat

The adult female worms are embedded in the mucosa of the duodenum and jejunum.

Properties of the Organism

Adult females are about 2–3 mm in length. These females produce eggs in the duodenal mucosa that hatch and release noninfective larvae (Fig. 56.1). The larvae, which are about 250 μ in length, are excreted in the stool. In the soil, the noninfectious larvae may develop by a direct cycle into infective larvae. (See Direct Cycle, p. 903.) The infective larvae can penetrate the unbroken skin. Noninfective larvae in the soil may develop into free-living adult worms, which may have one or more generations before producing infective larvae. (See Indirect Cycle, p. 904.) Infective larvae, which penetrate the skin, are carried by the blood-

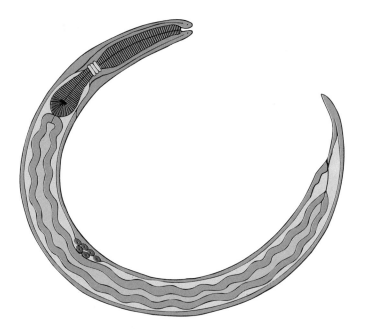

Figure 56.1.
Strongyloides stercoralis
noninfective larva.

stream to the alveolar capillaries where they rupture into the alveoli. These larvae undergo further development and are brought up in bronchial mucus and swallowed into the GI tract. The adult females are parthenogenetic and deposit eggs without the aid of fertilization by the male. In some circumstances, the noninfective larvae released into the intestinal lumen, may rapidly transform into infective larvae, penetrate the mucosa, and be carried to the lungs to initiate another cycle of development. This process is called internal autoinfection. External autoinfection can occur when noninfective larvae transform into infective larvae in fecal material contaminating the anal and perianal skin. Both types of autoinfection insure that the host will remain infected for many years, if not for life.

(A) Direct Cycle

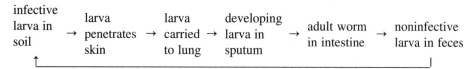

infective larva in soil → larva penetrates skin → larva carried to lung → developing larva in sputum → adult worm in intestine → noninfective larva in feces

(B) Indirect Cycle

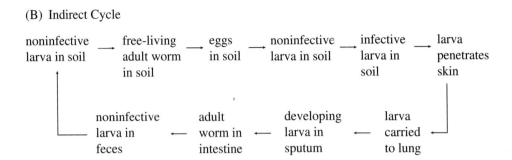

Clinical Manifestations

Skin penetration by the larvae may go unnoticed, or it may cause local erythema and pruritus. Migration of the larvae in the lung may cause symptoms of cough, wheezing, and transient pulmonary infiltrates. There is an eosinophilia that may be quite high. The combination of transient pulmonary infiltrates and eosinophilia is called **Loeffler's syndrome** and may occur in other conditions. When the female worms invade the intestinal wall, there may be symptoms of epigastric pain and diarrhea. An urticarial rash (hives) is common in chronic infection. When large numbers of larvae transform into infective stages and invade the intestine, severe diarrhea and bloody diarrhea may occur. This condition is called **hyperinfection.** Because of the large numbers of larvae migrating through the lungs, there may also be symptoms of cough, dyspnea, wheezing, and hemoptysis. When the migrating larvae produce symptoms in other organs, such as the liver, heart, kidneys, or CNS, the condition is called **disseminated strongyloidiasis.** Hyperinfection and dissemination occur in debilitated, malnourished or immunosuppressed patients. Dissemination has often been associated with the administration of high doses of corticosteroids. Fatalities are not uncommon as a result of hyperinfection or disseminated disease. Eosinophilia may be absent in severe infections.

Laboratory Diagnosis

Larvae may be demonstrated in fecal wet mounts and formalin-ethyl acetate fecal concentrates. The larvae also may be concentrated from fecal specimens by using a funnel (Baermann) or filter paper strips (Harada-Mori). Both techniques require the collection of fresh feces. In the **Baermann technique,** a large portion of feces is placed on supporting wire and gauze in contact with the surface of water in a large funnel. Larvae migrate from the feces into the water and fall to the bottom of the funnel. After about 12 h a small amount of water is drawn from the bottom of the funnel into a centifuge tube. The sediment is examined for larvae after centrifugation. In the **Harada-Mori technique,** a small amount of feces is smeared on the central portion of a strip of filter paper that is placed in a centrifuge tube containing a few milliliters of water. The water moistens the filter paper and the larvae migrate down into the water. After 10 days a small amount of water is removed and examined for larvae. The string test of duodenal contents (Entero-Test[R]) recovers larvae and occasionally eggs. Larvae of *Strongyloides* must be differentiated microscopically from larvae of the hookworms. Serologic tests, such as the ELISA test, will detect antibody to *S. stercoralis,* but cannot distinguish between current and past infections.

Treatment

Thiabendazole is effective in a 2-day course in immunocompetent patients, but it may be necessary to administer the drug for 7 days or more in immunosuppressed patients. Side effects are common with the use of thiabendazole. Careful follow-up is important to be sure that the infection has been eliminated.

HOOKWORM INFECTION

Hookworm infection is caused by *Ancylostoma duodenale* and *Necator americanus.*

Transmission

The infection is acquired by direct contact with soil containing infective larvae. *A. duodenale* infection may also be acquired by ingestion of larvae.

Geographic Distribution and Epidemiology

The infection is widely distributed throughout regions where sanitation is poor and the climate provides warmth and moisture. Approximately one-fourth of the world's population is thought to be infected. In some rural areas, prevalence rates reach 90%. Although there are differences in the distribution of the two species of hookworm, this is of little clinical significance, and the two species may be considered together.

Habitat

The adult worms attach to the mucosa of the duodenum and proximal small intestine.

Properties of the Organism

The adult parasites measure about 1 cm in length and have specialized buccal capsules for sucking on the intestinal mucosa. The anterior end of the worm is sharply curved, the "hook" of the name hookworm. The male worm has a characteristic copulatory bursa at its posterior end. The species of hookworm can be differentiated by their buccal cavities that either contain cutting plates (*N. americanus*) (Fig. 56.2A) or pairs of "teeth" (*A. duodenale*) (Fig. 56.2B). The eggs of the two species are identical (Fig. 56.3B). When the eggs are passed in the

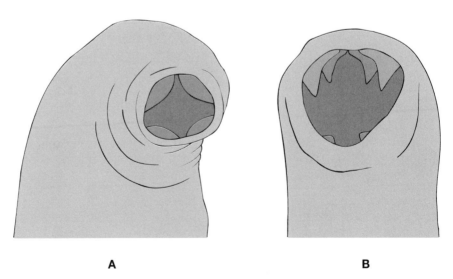

A   **B**

Figure 56.2.

Hookworm mouthparts. (A) *N. americanus.* (B) *A. duodenale.*

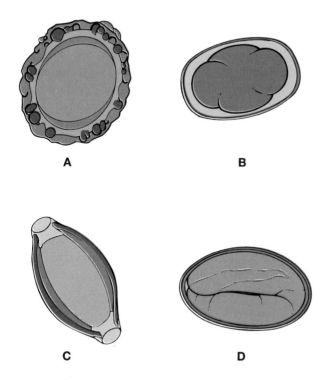

Figure 56.3.

Intestinal nematode ova.
(A) *A. lumbricoides.* (B)
Hookworm. (C) *T. trichiura.* (D) *E. vermicularis.*

stool, the embryo is in a very early stage of development. A first stage larva develops within the egg, hatches within 48 h, and begins feeding on organic material in the soil. It transforms into a nonfeeding, infective larva in about 1 week. When an infective larva comes in contact with human skin, it penetrates and is carried by the blood stream to the lungs where it breaks into an alveolus. It continues development and is brought up in bronchial mucus and swallowed into the intestinal tract. The maturing worm attaches to the mucosa and begins sucking blood. The worms mate in the lumen of the intestine, and the females begin laying eggs. The life span of the hookworms is usually 1–5 years.

eggs hatch in soil → noninfective larva in soil → infective larva in soil → larva penetrates skin → larva carried to lung → developing larva in sputum → adult worm in intestine → eggs in feces

Clinical Manifestations

Skin lesions may occur where larvae penetrate. These lesions are erythematous and pruritic. There may be transient pulmonary infiltrates and eosinophilia (Loeffler's syndrome) during the lung migration phase. Intestinal infection may be asymptomatic in light infections. Symptoms usually are proportional to the worm burden. Moderate infections tend to cause epigastric pain and diarrhea associated with a mild eosinophilia. Anemia secondary to blood loss will depend on the numbers of worms, the dietary iron intake, and iron stores of the patient.

Laboratory Diagnosis

Examination of fecal specimens by concentration techniques should discover nearly all significant infections. Larvae may hatch in fecal specimens that are not fresh. These larvae must be differentiated from *Strongyloides* larvae.

Treatment

Mebendazole and pyrantel pamoate are effective drugs.

CUTANEOUS LARVA MIGRANS

Cutaneous larva migrans (creeping eruption) is caused by hookworm parasites of dogs and cats. The infective larvae develop in soil contaminated with dog or cat feces. The larvae penetrate the skin causing erythematous, serpiginous, and pruritic lesions. The lesions may last weeks or months. The parasites are unable to complete their life cycle and wander about in the skin producing the linear skin lesions. The infection is treated with thiabendazole topically or orally. Recent reports indicate that albendazole is highly effective and less toxic.

ASCARIASIS

Ascariasis is caused by *Ascaris lumbricoides*.

Transmission

The infection is acquired by the ingestion of embryonated eggs from fecally contaminated food or beverages, or from fomites or dirty fingers.

Geographic Distribution and Epidemiology

The infection is found worldwide in association with poor sanitation. Highest prevalence rates occur in areas where human excreta is used to fertilize vegetable crops. Estimates of worldwide prevalence are as high as 1 billion infections.

Habitat

Adult worms are found in the lumen of the small intestine.

Properties of the Organism

Adult worms are 20–35 cm in length (Fig. 56.4). The eggs are 45–75 μ in length and have a "bumpy" outer coat that is usually brownish in color (Fig. 56.2A). The egg becomes infectious after 2–3 weeks of larval development inside the eggshell. Following ingestion of an embryonated egg, the larva hatches from the egg and penetrates the intestinal wall. The larva is carried to the lung where it ruptures into the alveolus. The maturing larva is transported in the bronchial mucus and swallowed into the GI tract where it becomes an adult. A female worm

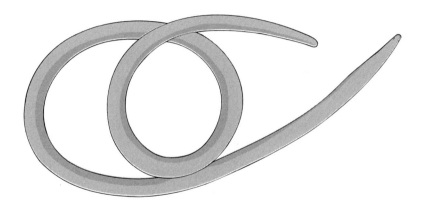

Figure 56.4.

Adult *A. lumbricoides* female.

may deposit more than 200,000 eggs per day. It is estimated that the parasites live about 1 year.

embryonated egg in soil → egg ingested → larva hatches and penetrates intestine → larva carried to lung → developing larva in sputum → adult worm in intestine → eggs in feces

Clinical Manifestations

Larval migration in the lung is usually asymptomatic but in heavy infections or in sensitized individuals, there may be a pneumonia or at least transient pulmonary infiltrates and eosinophilia (Loeffler's syndrome). The intestinal phase of the infection may produce abdominal pain, diarrhea, and other nonspecific GI complaints. In heavy infections in children, intestinal obstruction may occur. Invasion of the bile ducts may produce liver abscesses, cholangitis, bile duct obstruction, and pancreatitis. In some instances, the worms may be vomited or actively migrate up the esophagus and out through the nasopharynx. Mild-moderate eosinophilia is common.

Laboratory Diagnosis

Routine fecal examination should easily reveal eggs of *Ascaris*.

Treatment

Mebendazole and pyrantel are effective drugs.

VISCERAL LARVA MIGRANS

Visceral larva migrans (toxocariasis) is caused by roundworms of dogs and cats (*Toxocara canis,* and *Toxocara cati*). The infection is acquired by the ingestion of eggs from contaminated soil. Large numbers of eggs may be excreted into the environment in the feces of infected puppies. The infection is most commonly seen in children under the age of 4 who are known dirt eaters. After the embryonated eggs are ingested, the larvae hatch and penetrate the intestine, but cannot develop to adult worms in the human host. The larvae migrate in various organs producing an inflammatory response. Light infections may have eosinophilia without symptoms. Heavier infections may cause fever, tender hepatomegaly, cough, pulmonary infiltrates, and marked eosinophilia. **Ocular larva migrans** usually occurs without other symptoms and is caused by one or more larvae migrating in the retina. Diagnosis of visceral or ocular larva migrans is suggested by the clinical findings with support from serologic tests. The ELISA appears relatively sensitive and highly specific. Thiabendazole has been used in treatment with some success. Albendazole is less toxic, and a recent report suggests that it is at least as effective as thiabendazole.

ANISAKIASIS

Anisakiasis is caused by species of roundworms of the genus *Anisakis* and related genera. The definitive hosts for these worms are marine mammals, such as whales and seals. Humans acquire the infection by ingesting infective larvae in raw or marinated marine fish or squid. Larvae do not mature in the human host. The infection is endemic in Japan and sporadic cases occur throughout the world where raw fish is consumed. The illness may begin a few hours to a few days after the ingestion of the larvae. There is usually nausea, vomiting, and progressive abdominal pain. If endoscopy is performed soon after symptoms begin, larvae may be seen penetrating the gastric or duodenal mucosa. In some instances, symptoms are minor and the patient reports "coughing up" the larval worm. If parasites are not seen at endoscopy, serologic tests performed by specialized laboratories may be helpful in supporting the clinical diagnosis. There is no treatment for the infection other than removal of the worms at endoscopy.

TRICHURIASIS

Trichuriasis is caused by the whipworm, *Trichuris trichiura.*

Transmission

The infection is caused by the ingestion of embryonated eggs from an environment contaminated with human feces.

Geographic Distribution and Epidemiology

The infection is worldwide and closely parallels the distribution of ascariasis. Poor sanitation and the use of human feces as fertilizer contributes to a high prevalence. There may be as many as 800 million infections. Children tend to have the most clinically significant infections.

Habitat

The adult worms embed their anterior ends in the superficial mucosa of the colon and rectum.

Properties of the Organism

The adult worms are 3–5 cm in length. The anterior portion of the worm is very thin and threadlike (the lash of the ''whip''), and the posterior is thick and contains the reproductive organs. The males have curled posterior ends (Fig. 56.5). Following the ingestion of an embryonated egg, the larva hatches and develops to an adult in the intestinal epithelium. The slender anterior end of the adult worm

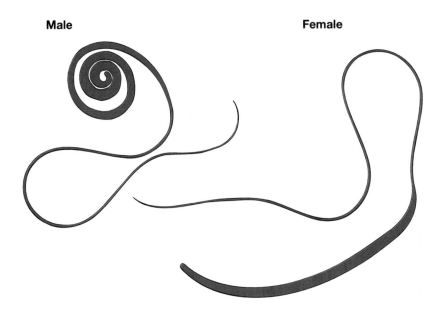

Male   **Female**

Figure 56.5.

Adult *T. trichiura*.

remains embedded in the superficial mucosa of the cecum, colon, and rectum. The barrel shaped eggs are shed in the feces. The eggs measure 50–54 μ in length and have clear polar plugs at each end (Fig. 56.3C). The life span of the worm is usually about 1 year but longer lived infections are common.

embryonated egg in soil → egg ingested → egg hatches in intestine → adult worm in colon → eggs in feces

Clinical Manifestations

Light infections may be asymptomatic. Heavy infections that frequently occur in children in endemic areas may produce severe bloody diarrhea and rectal prolapse. Chronic infection in children has been associated with growth retardation.

Laboratory Diagnosis

Routine stool examinations should reveal eggs in any clinically significant infection.

Treatment

Mebendazole and albendazole are effective.

ENTEROBIASIS

Enterobiasis is caused by infection with the pinworm, *Enterobius vermicularis.*

Transmission

Ingestion of eggs from the environment. A common autoinfection route in children is transfer of eggs from the perianal region to the mouth by contaminated fingers. Infection is also acquired from inhalation of eggs that adhere to mucus membranes and eventually are swallowed.

Geographic Distribution and Epidemiology

The infection is found worldwide with the highest prevalence in school children. It is the most common helminthic infection in the United States. Prevalence rates are variable but 20–60% of school age children are probably infected.

Habitat

The adult worms live in the proximal colon, cecum, and appendix.

Properties of the Organism

The adult females are about 1 cm in length. These females have a sharply pointed posterior end that gives them the name, "pinworm" (Fig. 56.6). Male and female pinworms inhabit the cecum, appendix, and adjacent colon. The gravid females migrate down the colon, through the anus, and lay their eggs on the perianal skin (Fig. 56.3D). The migration occurs at night while the host is sleeping. The eggs become infectious within a few hours and may be directly ingested on contaminated fingers or spread to the environment by air currents.

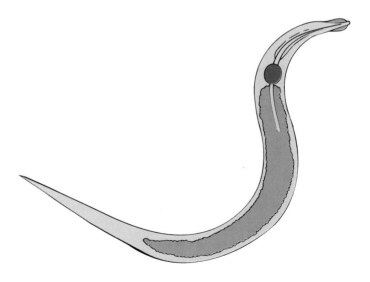

Figure 56.6.
Adult female *E. vermicularis*.

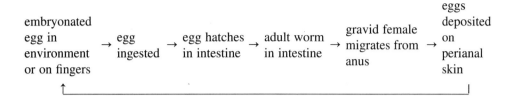

Clinical Manifestations

The vast majority of infections are asymptomatic. However, some individuals will develop anal pruritus. In some instances, vaginal pruritus develops, probably as a result of worms migrating into the vagina. There is no firm evidence that the parasite causes appendicitis.

Laboratory Diagnosis

Cellulose tape swabs (Scotch tape) are applied to the anal folds and perianal skin in the morning before the patient bathes or goes to the bathroom. The tape is examined microscopically for the presence of pinworm eggs. Although seven consecutive negative daily swabs are necessary to exclude the diagnosis of enterobiasis, three or four swabs will detect the majority of infections.

Treatment

Mebendazole and pyrantel pamoate are highly effective in a single dose. Patient education concerning the nature of the infection and the common occurrence of reinfection is most important. Extra efforts in hygienic measures are worthless. There rarely is justification for treating all family members. Reinfection can be expected and retreatment will be indicated for those who develop symptoms.

TRICHINOSIS

Trichinosis is caused by the nematode, *Trichinella spiralis.*

Transmission

Infection is acquired by the ingestion of undercooked or raw pork, bear meat, wild boar, and so on, containing larvae of *T. spiralis.*

Geographic Distribution and Epidemiology

The infection occurs worldwide. Subclinical infection is probably common, but the disease is most frequently recognized in outbreaks. Trichinosis was common in the United States before the 1950s when laws prohibiting the feeding of raw garbage to hogs sharply reduced the incidence. From 1983 to 1987, there were 33 outbreaks reported in the United States with 162 cases and 1 death. Outbreaks are sometimes associated with homemade sausage or the consumption of bear meat. In Alaska, the eating of walrus meat has caused human infection.

Habitat

The adult worms are found in the proximal small intestine. Larvae encyst in skeletal muscle.

Properties of the Organism

Encysted larvae ingested in infected meat are liberated by digestive juices and develop to adult worms in the mucosa of the small intestine within 48 h. The female adults deposit larvae in the intestinal wall. The larvae are carried by the blood stream throughout the body and encyst in skeletal muscle cells. When the larva is mature, it appears tightly coiled and surrounded by a capsule formed from the host skeletal muscle cell (Fig. 56.3). The domestic cycle of infection is maintained by feeding uncooked garbage containing pork scraps or infected rodents to hogs. Rats become infected by cannibalism or eating pork scraps. Many carnivorous or omniverous animals are infected with *Trichinella.* Bear meat, walrus, and wild pigs have been significant sources of infection in humans.

Clinical Manifestations

Symptoms from the GI phase of the infection, when present, may occur within 2 days of ingesting the infected meat. These early symptoms usually consist of diarrhea, nausea, vomiting, and resemble nonspecific gastroenteritis. The stage

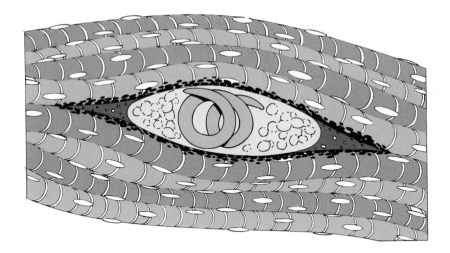

Figure 56.7.
T. spiralis larva in muscle.

of muscle invasion by the larvae usually begins about 1 week after infection and is marked by symptoms of fever, muscle pain, and swelling of the tissues around the eyes (periorbital edema). A very high eosinophilia is characteristic. Symptoms usually peak in the third or fourth week. Severe infections may develop myocarditis, meningitis, or encephalitis. Fatalities have been associated with these complications. Convalescence may take weeks or months.

Laboratory Diagnosis

The diagnosis is usually made based on epidemiologic factors and the clinical picture. It is difficult or impossible to demonstrate positive serologic tests or positive muscle biopsies until 2–3 weeks after ingesting the infected meat. When muscle biopsies are done to confirm the diagnosis, the biopsy should be taken from a muscle that is painful. Tests that detect antigens of *Trichinella* in the early stages of infection are under development.

Treatment

Mebendazole has an effect on both adult worms and the larvae. Corticosteroids are also used in severe infections to reduce the inflammatory reaction.

TABLE 56.1. Major Characteristics of Intestinal Nematode Infections and Trichinosis

Organism	Transmission	Location of adult worms	Larval migration in humans	Clinical manifestations	Laboratory diagnosis	Treatment
Strongyloides stercoralis	Skin penetration by larvae	Embedded in the mucosa of the proximal small intestine	Lungs (may cause Loeffler's syndrome)	Epigastric pain, diarrhea, eosinophilia. Superinfection or dissemination in immuno-suppressed	Fecal exam for larvae. Larval concentration methods (Baermann, Harada–Mori). Duodenal "string" test. Serology	Thiabendazole
Hookworms (*Ancylostoma duodenale* and *Necator americanus*)	Skin penetration by larvae	Attached to the mucosa of the proximal small intestine	Lungs (may cause Loeffler's syndrome)	Epigastric pain, diarrhea, eosinophilia	Fecal exam for ova	Mebendazole, pyrantel
Dog and cat hookworms (causing cutaneous larva migrans)	Skin penetration by larvae	Adult worms do not develop	Skin	Erythematous, serpiginous, pruritic skin lesions	Characteristic skin lesions	Thiabendazole orally or topically
Ascaris lumbricoides	Ingestion of embryonated eggs	Lumen of the small intestine	Lungs (may cause Loeffler's syndrome)	Abdominal pain, diarrhea, eosinophilia	Fecal exam for ova	Mebendazole, pyrantel

Organism	Transmission	Location	Migration	Symptoms	Diagnosis	Treatment
Dog and cat roundworms (*Toxocara canis* and *T. cati* causing visceral and ocular larva migrans)	Ingestion of embryonated eggs	Adult worms do not develop	Liver, lungs, CNS, eye, and so on	Fever, tender hepatomegaly, cough, lung infiltrates, high eosinophilia. Retinal lesions in ocular disease	Clinical picture and serologic tests	Thiabendazole, albendazole
Anisakis	Ingestion of raw marine fish or squid	Adult worms do not develop	Penetrates stomach or small intestine	Nausea, vomiting, abdominal pain	Endoscopy and serologic tests	Removal at endoscopy
Trichuris trichiura	Ingestion of embryonated eggs	Partially embedded in superficial mucosa of colon and rectum	None	Diarrhea or bloody diarrhea	Fecal exam for ova	Mebendazole
Enterobius vermicularis	Ingestion of embryonated eggs	Colon	None	Perianal and vaginal itching	Cellulose tape swabs	Mebendazole, pyrantel
Trichinella spiralis	Ingestion of larvae in raw or undercooked pork, bear meat, and so on	Proximal small intestine	Larvae encyst in skeletal muscle	Fever, periorbital edema, muscle pain, eosinophilia	Clinical picture, serologic tests, muscle biopsy	Mebendazole, corticosteroids

SUMMARY

1. Intestinal nematodes (roundworms) are cylindrical and possess a complete GI tract. The sexes are separate.

2. The eggs or larvae of intestinal nematodes require a period of maturation outside the host before they become infectious.

3. The common intestinal nematodes, *Strongyloides stercoralis*, the hookworms, *Ascaris lumbricoides*, *Trichuris trichiura*, and *Enterobius vermicularis* do not have intermediate hosts or significant reservoir hosts.

4. Adult worms of *Trichinella spiralis* develop in the intestine and larvae encyst in skeletal muscle cells. *T. spiralis* is infectious for a wide variety of hosts.

5. Table 56.1 summarizes the major characteristics of the infections discussed in this chapter.

REFERENCES

Bundy DA, Cooper ES (1989): Trichuris and trichuriasis in humans. Adv Parasitol 28:107.

Campbell WC (ed) (1983): Trichinella and Trichinosis. New York: Plenum Press.

Crompton DWT, Nesheim MC, Pawlowski AS (eds) (1985): Ascariasis and its Public Health Significance. Philadelphia: Taylor & Francis.

Gilman RH (1982): Hookworm disease: Host-pathogen biology. Rev Inf Dis 4:824.

Glickman LT, Magnaval J-F (1993): Zoonotic roundworm infections. Infect Dis Clin North Am, 7:717.

Grove DI (ed) (1989): Strongyloidiasis: A Major Roundworm Infection of Man. London: Taylor & Francis.

Hotez PJ (1989): Hookworm disease in children. Pediatr Infect Dis J 8:516.

Keystone JS (1989): Enterobiasis. In Goldsmith R, Heyneman D (eds): Tropical Medicine and Parasitology. Norwalk: Appleton & Lange.

Leicht SS, Youngberg GA (1987): Cutaneous larva migrans. Am Fam Physician 35:163.

Liu LX, Weller PF (1993): Strongyloidiasis and other nematode infections. Infect Dis Clin North Am 7:655.

Markell EK (1985): Intestinal nematode infections. Pediatr Clin North Am 32:971.

Schantz PM (1989): Toxocara larva migrans now. Am J Trop Med Hyg 41, No. 3:21.

REVIEW QUESTIONS

For questions 1 to 2, choose the ONE
BEST answer or completion:

1. Cutaneous larva migrans is caused by larvae
   of
   a) *Ascaris lumbricoides*
   b) *Enterobius vermicularis*
   c) dog roundworms
   d) dog hookworms
   e) *Trichinella spiralis*

2. Eosinophilia is common in these infections,
   except in
   a) trichuriasis
   b) strongyloidiasis
   c) ascariasis
   d) trichinosis
   e) visceral larva migrans

For questions 3 to 9, a list of lettered
options is followed by several numbered
items. For each numbered item, select the
ONE lettered option that is most closely
associated with it. Each lettered option
may be selected once, more than once, or
not at all.

   A) *Ascaris lumbricoides*
   B) *Trichuris trichiura*

C) *Strongyloides stercoralis*
D) Hookworms
E) *Enterobius vermicularis*
F) *Trichinella spiralis*

For the statements below, select the
appropriate parasite.

3. This parasite may cause a fatal, disseminated
   disease in immunosuppressed patients.

4. Definitive diagnosis may be made by muscle
   biopsy.

5. The infection is acquired by ingesting raw or
   inadequately cooked pork.

6. The infection is acquired by ingesting eggs
   from the soil or on raw vegetables. Larvae
   migrate from the intestine to the lung; adult
   worms develop in the intestine.

7. Heavy infections may cause an iron deficiency anemia.

8. Diagnosis is made using cellulose tape swabs
   on the perianal skin.

9. The anterior portion of the adult worm is embedded in the superficial mucosa of the colon
   and rectum.

ANSWERS TO REVIEW QUESTIONS

1. *d* Dog hookworms cause cutaneous larva migrans. Dog roundworms *(Toxocara canis)* cause visceral larva migrans.

2. *a* Trichuriasis is not associated with eosinophilia. The parasites do not have stages that migrate in the tissues.

3. *C* Strongyloidiasis may have fatal dissemination in the immunosuppressed patient.

4. *F* Muscle biopsy may reveal larvae of *T. spiralis* and is a technique for definitive diagnosis.

5. *A* Trichinosis is acquired from eating raw or undercooked pork.

6. *A* Ingestion of *Ascaris lumbricoides* eggs from soil or contaminated vegetables is followed by migration of larvae to the lung. Adult worms develop in the intestine.

7. *D* Hookworms cause significant blood loss and can produce an iron deficiency anemia.

8. *E* Enterobiasis is diagnosed by observing eggs on cellulose tape swabs of the perianal skin.

9. *B* *Trichuris trichiura* adults have their anterior ends embedded in the superficial mucosa of the colon and rectum.

FILARIAL INFECTIONS AND DRACUNCULIASIS

The filarial parasites are slender nematodes that have complex life cycles involving insect intermediate hosts. A definitive diagnosis is based on the recovery and identification of the embryonic worms called **microfilariae.** The diseases produced by these parasites are significant causes of morbidity in tropical areas. Table 57.1 summarizes the characteristics of the major filarial infections.

LYMPHATIC FILARIASIS

Lymphatic filariasis is caused by *Wuchereria bancrofti* and *Brugia malayi* (bancroftian and malayan filariasis). A third species, *Brugia timori,* is limited to two Indonesian islands and will not be discussed.

Transmission

Many species of mosquito serve as intermediate hosts and transmit the infection during biting.

TABLE 57.1. Characteristics of Major Filarial Infections and Dracunculiasis

Organism	Transmission	Location of adult worms	Location of larvae	Clinical manifestations	Laboratory diagnosis	Treatment
Wuchereria bancrofti Brugia malayi	Bite of mosquito	Lymphatics	Microfilarae in blood. Nocturnal periodicity except *W. bancrofti* in Pacific area	Lymphangitis, lymphadenitis, lymphedema, fever, eosinophilia. Elephantiasis	Blood films, concentration or filtration techniques for microfilariae	Diethyl-carbamazine
Onchocerca volvulus	Bite of black fly	Subcutaneous tissues in fixed nodules	Microfilariae in skin	Subcutaneous nodules, dermatitis, pruritus, eye lesions, eosinophilia	Skin snips or shavings for microfilariae. Mazzotti test	Ivermectin
Loa loa	Bite of mango fly	Migratory in subcutaneous tissues	Microfilariae in blood. Diurnal periodicity	Transient subcutaneous swellings, eosinophilia	Blood films, concentration or filtration techniques for microfilariae	Diethyl-carbamazine
Dracunculus medinensis	Ingestion of infected copepod in drinking water	Subcutaneous tissues	Discharged by adult worm through skin lesion	Palpable cord in skin. Blister that develops into painful ulcer	Presence of worm in ulcer. Discharge of larvae from worm	Mechanical removal

Geographic Distribution and Epidemiology

Bancroftian filariasis is widely distributed throughout the tropical zone, especially in humid areas. It is found in Africa, Asia, Southeast Asia, Pacific islands, Central and South America, and some Caribbean islands. There are no significant reservoir hosts for *W. bancrofti*. Malayan filariasis is found in Southeast Asia, Indonesia, India, Sri Lanka, China, Korea, and Japan. There is a variety of reservoir hosts including monkeys, cats, and pangolins. Worldwide prevalence of lymphatic filariasis is estimated to be 90 million infections.

Habitat

The adult worms are found in lymphatics and lymph nodes. Microfilariae are found in the blood.

Properties of the Organism

The adult worms are threadlike and measure 4–10 cm in length. These worms develop in the lymphatics and lymph nodes. The fertilized adult females produce embryonic worms called microfilariae. The microfilaria is about 250 μ in length and is surrounded by a flexible sheath (Fig. 57.1). The two species can be differentiated by the arrangement of nuclei in the tail of the microfilaria. Microfilariae circulate in the peripheral blood. They may be taken up by the mosquito during

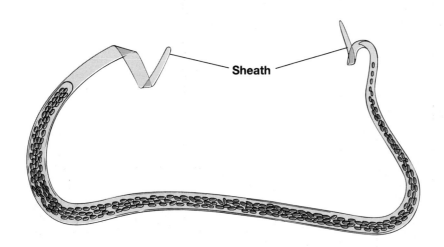

Sheath

Figure 57.1.

Microfilaria.

a blood meal. In the mosquito, the microfilariae develop to more advanced larval stages in the thoracic muscles. Eventually, they migrate to the mosquito's mouth parts. When the mosquito bites, the larvae gain access to the host's tissues, and the adult worms develop in the lymphatics. Most geographic strains of *Wuchereria* and all strains of *Brugia* have microfilaremias that are nocturnally periodic (i.e., the microfilariae appear in the peripheral blood in the greatest numbers at night). The strain of *Wuchereria* found in the Pacific area has the maximal microfilaremia in the daytime.

In most infections, there is a lack of protective immune responsiveness both humoral and cell mediated. There is active suppression of the immune response to filarial antigens. Although high IgE levels may develop, IgG blocking antibodies prevent allergic manifestations from occurring.

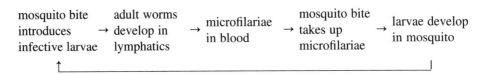

Clinical Manifestations

Early symptoms are lymphangitis, lymphadenitis, and in males, epididymitis, funiculitis, or orchitis. Often fever and malaise are associated with the lymphatic involvement. As the infection becomes chronic, there may be repeated bouts of lymphangitis with the development of lymphedema. Eventually, the tissue becomes infiltrated and fibrous with permanent enlargement of involved extremities **(elephantiasis)** (Fig. 57.2). Scrotal involvement is common. Hydrocoeles and scrotal elephantiasis may be seen. Extremities with lymphedema are very susceptible to bacterial infections. These additional insults may further damage the lymphatics. Other complications of lymphatic filariasis are hematuria or proteinuria or both. The appearance of chyle in the urine (chyluria) is caused by rupture of lymphatics in the renal pelvis. Abscesses of the lymphatics may also develop.

Eosinophilia is common in early lymphatic filariasis but may be absent in the chronic stages.

Many infections in the indigenous population of an endemic area are asymptomatic. Visitors to endemic areas who acquire the infection are much more likely to have significant symptoms.

Tropical pulmonary eosinophilia is associated with immune hyperresponsiveness, antibody to the microfilarial sheath, and the trapping of microfilariae in the lung. Microfilariae are not found in the peripheral blood. The syndrome is

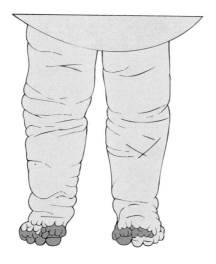

Figure 57.2.
Elephantiasis.

characterized by paroxysmal coughing and wheezing, which is frequently worse at night. Chest X-rays may show a fine mottling (miliary pattern). The disease is associated with very high eosinophil counts and marked elevation in IgE. A high titer of antifilarial antibody is present, and the condition responds well to treatment with the filaricide, diethylcarbamazine.

Laboratory Diagnosis

The definitive diagnosis of lymphatic filariasis is made by demonstrating microfilariae in blood smears, concentrations, or by the use of special filters. Blood specimens must be collected at the correct time of day to coordinate with the periodicity of the microfilaremia. Microfilariae may not appear in the blood for up to 1 year after exposure. The clinical signs of retrograde lymphangitis or inflammatory reactions in the male genitalia may lead to early suspicion of filarial infection. Serologic tests are available, but are specific only for the whole group of filarial infections. These tests are of limited value in endemic areas where the majority of the population is positive.

Treatment

The drug diethylcarbamazine is rapidly effective in killing the microfilariae and will also destroy the adult worms when given over a period of several weeks. Ivermectin is currently being tested as a possible alternative.

Several different surgical approaches have been used to attempt to reduce the burden of elephantiasis of the extremities or genitalia. A recently developed technique connects veins with the lymphatics to allow direct drainage of lymph into the venous system.

ONCHOCERCIASIS

Onchocerciasis is caused by *Onchocerca volvulus.*

Transmission

Infection is acquired through the bite of infected black flies (*Simulium*).

Geographic Distribution and Epidemiology

The infection is found in Central and West Africa, Yemen, Saudi Arabia, Mexico, Guatemala, Venezuela, Colombia, Ecuador, and Brazil. About 17 million infections occur worldwide. In West Africa, where the disease is called river blindness, up to 10% of the population in endemic areas has been blinded by the infection. Because the black flies breed in rapidly flowing water, disease transmission is most intense near rivers and streams.

Habitat

Adult worms are found in subcutaneous nodules. Microfilariae are found in the skin and eye.

Properties of the Organism

Adult male and female worms lie coiled in fibrous nodules in the subcutaneous tissues. The female worm is about 0.5 mm in diameter but may be 50 cm in length. The male is only about 5 cm in length. The females produce microfilariae that migrate in the dermis and eye. The microfilariae are taken up by the black fly when it takes a blood meal. The parasites undergo larval development in the fly and eventually migrate to the proboscis and are introduced when the infected fly bites.

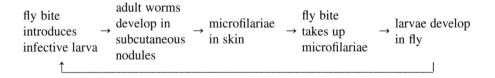

Clinical Manifestations

The subcutaneous nodules are usually found over bony prominences and are painless. The reactions to the microfilariae produce the signs and symptoms. A maculopapular, pruritic rash is common. Eventually, there is thickening of the skin and loss of elasticity. Patchy changes in pigmentation may occur. Lymph node enlargement may occur and is often prominent in African infections. Eye involvement often begins with small precipitates around microfilariae in the cornea. Sclerosing keratitis may cause visual impairment. More serious complications can occur in the iris and retina, which can produce blindness. Eosinophilia is usually present in all forms of onchocerciasis.

Laboratory Diagnosis

Microfilariae are demonstrable in skin snips or skin shavings that are incubated in saline. The microfilariae migrate out of the tissue into the saline and can be identified by specific morphologic features. In some cases of ocular involvement, slit lamp examination will reveal microfilariae in the cornea or anterior chamber. A provocative test is performed occasionally, using small doses of diethylcarbamazine **(Mazzotti test).** An exacerbation of the pruritic dermatitis within 24 h of the test dose indicates the presence of onchocerciasis. A careful ophthalmologic examination must be done before administering diethylcarbamazine to rule out ocular involvement. Serologic tests for filariasis are usually positive but are not specific for onchocerciasis.

Treatment

Microfilariae are easily killed by diethylcarbamazine, but this often causes severe allergic reactions to the dead and dying parasites. Diethylcarbamazine has no effect on adult worms. Suramin, a toxic drug that has to be given intravenously, was used until recently for killing the adult parasites. The introduction of a new drug (ivermectin) has changed the strategy for the treatment of onchocerciasis in endemic areas. Ivermectin can be given in a single oral dose. Although it does not kill the adult worms, it prevents the female worms from producing microfilariae for a period of at least 6 months. Because the pathology of onchocerciasis is caused by microfilariae, elimination of these forms prevents symptoms and ocular complications. Doses given to the entire population in an endemic area at 6 monthly intervals has the possibility of preventing disease and ending transmission of the infection and eventually eliminating it.

OTHER FILARIAL INFECTIONS

Loiasis, caused by *Loa loa* is transmitted by mango flies *(Chrysops).* The infection is found in West Africa, the Congo basin, and parts of the Sudan. Adult worms migrate in the subcutaneous tissues and occasionally cross the eye under the conjunctival membrane. Microfilariae are found in the blood and have a diurnal periodicity. The most common symptom is the development of transient, localized subcutaneous edema **(Calabar swellings).** Eosinophilia is common.

Three species of the genus *Mansonella* infect humans. These species are transmitted by the bite of midges *(Culicoides),* and *Mansonella ozzardi* is also transmitted by black flies.

Mansonella ozzardi is found in parts of South and Central America and in many Caribbean islands. Adult worms are found in the mesentery and visceral fat. The nonperiodic microfilariae are found in the blood and skin. Infections may be asymptomatic, but inguinal lymphadenopathy, pruritic skin lesions and fever have been reported. Eosinophilia is prominent.

Mansonella perstans infections occur in many parts of Africa as well as South and Central America and many Caribbean islands. Adult worms live in connective tissues and the nonperiodic microfilariae are found in the blood. Hives, pruritus, fever, and Calabar swellings have been reported.

Mansonella streptocerca is found in the Congo river basin of Africa. Adult worms probably live in the subcutaneous tissues. Microfilariae are found in the skin and blood. Symptoms and signs are similar to onchocerciasis but without subcutaneous nodules or ocular involvement.

DRACUNCULIASIS

Dracunculiasis (dracontiasis) is caused by the guinea worm, *Dracunculus medinensis.* Infection is acquired by drinking water containing infected copepods. The disease is found in West and Central Africa, the Arabian peninsula, India, and Pakistan. It occurs in rural areas where drinking water is obtained from shallow, unprotected wells, ponds, and water holes. After the host ingests the infected copepod, the larva migrates to deep connective tissues. About 1 year from initial infection, the adult female worm appears subcutaneously, usually in the legs, where it produces a painful blister in the skin overlying the worm's anterior end. The blister ruptures, and the worm discharges a fluid containing larvae. When larvae are discharged into a water source containing copepods, they are eaten by the copepods and develop to infective stages. The adult female worms reach 1 m in length and may be felt as a firm cord in the subcutaneous tissue.

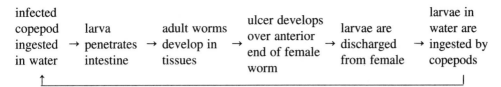

The painful ulcer caused by the parasite may be disabling, and often becomes secondarily infected. Gradual removal of the worm by gentle traction takes several days. Extraction may be facilitated by several drugs that reduce the inflammation around the worm.

Infected copepods can easily be filtered from drinking water, and this technique is being used in the current efforts to eradicate dracunculiasis worldwide.

SUMMARY

1. The features of the major filarial infections and dracunculiasis are outlined in Table 57.1.

2. Tropical pulmonary eosinophilia consists of pulmonary symptoms, elevated IgE, high eosinophilia, high titre of filarial antibody, and absence of microfilariae in the peripheral blood.

REFERENCES

Duke BO (1990): Onchocerciasis—an overview of the disease. Acta Leiden 59:9.
Wong MM (1989): Tropical eosinophilia. In Goldsmith R, Heyneman D (eds): Tropical Medicine and Parasitology. San Mateo, CA: Appleton & Lange.
Muller R (1971): Dracunculus and dracunculiasis. Adv Parasitol 9:73.
Nanduri J, Kazura JW (1989): Clinical and laboratory aspects of filariasis. Clin Microbiol Rev 2:39.
Ottesen EA (1993): Filarial infections. Infect Dis Clin North Am 7:619.
Sasa M (1976): Human Filariasis. Baltimore: University Park Press.

REVIEW QUESTIONS

For questions 1 to 8, a list of lettered options followed by several numbered items. For each numbered item, select the ONE lettered option that is most closely associated with it. Each lettered option may be selected once, more than once, or not at all.

A) *Wuchereria bancrofti* and *Brugia malayi*
B) *Onchocerca volvulus*
C) *Loa loa*
D) *Dracunculus medinensis*

For the statements below, select the appropriate parasite(s).

1. A painful skin ulceration develops.

2. Adult worms are found in lymphatics and lymph nodes.

3. Adult worms are found in subcutaneous nodules.

4. Eye involvement may progress to blindness.

5. Microfilariae appear in greatest numbers in peripheral blood during the daytime (diurnal periodicity).

6. Transmission is by mosquitos.

7. Elephantiasis may develop.

8. Diagnosis is made by finding microfilariae in skin shavings or skin snips.

ANSWERS TO REVIEW QUESTIONS

1. **D** A painful skin ulcer develops near the anterior end of the female *Dracunculus medinensis*. Larvae are discharged through the ulcer.

2. **A** Adults of *Wuchereria bancrofti* and *Brugia malayi* are found in lymphatics and lymph nodes.

3. **B** Adults of *Onchocerca volvulus* are found in fixed, painless, subcutaneous nodules.

4. **B** Onchocerciasis may cause lesions of the cornea, iris, and retina, which can produce blindness.

5. **C** The microfilariae of *Loa loa* appear in greatest numbers during the daytime. The mango fly vector bites during the daytime.

6. **A** Both *W. bancrofti* and *B. malayi* are transmitted by mosquitos.

7. **A** Elephantiasis is a complication of infection with *W. bancrofti* and *B. malayi*.

8. **B** Onchocerciasis is diagnosed by finding microfilariae in skin shavings or skin snips.

MALARIA AND BABESIOSIS

MALARIA

Malaria is caused by apicomplexan parasites of the genus *Plasmodium.* The four species that infect humans are *Plasmodium vivax, Plasmodium falciparum, Plasmodium malariae,* and *Plasmodium ovale.*

Transmission

The infection is acquired through mosquito bites by members of the genus *Anopheles.* Blood transfusion and the sharing of contaminated hypodermic needles are other modes of transmission. Congenital malaria may also occur.

Geographic Distribution and Epidemiology

Malaria is endemic throughout the major tropical areas of the world. Areas of high prevalence exist in Africa, parts of South America, Central America and Mexico, the subcontinent of India, Southeast Asia, and many of the South Pacific islands exclusive of Polynesia. Approximately 270 million people are infected with malaria, and one-half of the world's population lives in areas where malaria is transmitted. It is estimated that 1 million children die of malaria in Africa each year. Continued surveillance is required in temperate zones to prevent the reintroduction of malaria into areas where it has been eradicated. Worldwide, *P. vivax* and *P. falciparum* are the predominant species. *P. vivax* is widely distributed throughout all areas where malaria is transmitted. Its range extends into temperate regions. *P. falciparum* has a tropical and subtropical distribution while *P. malariae* is less commonly reported from temperate and subtropical areas. *P. ovale* is most frequently reported from West Africa, but it is also found sporadically in other parts of tropical Africa, South America, and Asia.

Habitat

The parasites are intracellular in hepatocytes (liver parenchymal cells) and erythrocytes.

Properties of the Organism

The mosquito introduces infective stages (sporozoites) into the human host in its saliva during biting. The sporozoites enter hepatocytes and multiply asexually until the parasites rupture from the cell. The released parasites infect erythrocytes and begin a cycle of asexual reproduction within the RBCs. This asexual cycle in the RBCs has the following stages:

1. The **ring stage** is the earliest form seen in the red cell. It consists of a ring of cytoplasm containing a dot of nuclear material (Fig. 58.1A). The central area of the ring is a vacuole containing hemoglobin.
2. The **trophozoite** is the ameboid growing form of the organism before there is any division of nuclear material (Fig. 58.1B). As the trophozoite develops, brownish or black granular material appears within the cytoplasm. This malaria pigment is the iron-containing, end product of hemoglobin metabolized by the parasite.
3. The **early schizont** stage begins with the first nuclear division. The cytoplasm of the parasite has not yet undergone division.
4. The **mature schizont** (segmenter) has undergone complete division of the nuclear material and the cytoplasm to form individual organisms called **merozoites** (Fig. 58.1C). When the erythrocyte containing the mature schizont ruptures, the merozoites are released and penetrate other RBCs to continue the cycle.

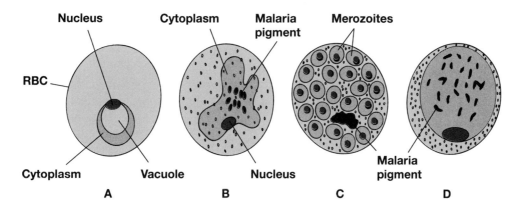

Figure 58.1.

P. vivax in RBCs. (A) Ring stage. (B) Motile trophozoite in enlarged RBC with Schüffner's dots. (C) Mature schizont with merozoites, clumped malaria pigment. Enlarged RBC shows Schüffner's dots. (D) Female gametocyte.

P. vivax, P. falciparum, and *P. ovale* have asexual cycles that take 48 h from ring stage to mature schizont and *P.* malariae takes 72 h to complete the cycle. After several asexual cycles, some merozoites do not progress through asexual development, but remain compact organisms that enlarge and differentiate into either male (**microgametocyte**) or female (**macrogametocyte**) forms (Fig. 58.1D). These **gametocytes** circulate in the blood and are unable to develop further unless taken up by an anopheline mosquito during a blood meal. Completion of sexual development occurs within the mosquito and results in the appearance of sporozoites in the mosquito's salivary gland.

In infections caused by *P. vivax* and *P. ovale,* some of the sporozoites that penetrate the hepatocytes do not immediately undergo division, but remain dormant as **"hypnozoites."** It is the delayed activation of the hypnozoite that is responsible for relapses of clinical disease. *P. falciparum* and *P. malariae* do not have stages that persist in the liver cells. **Relapse** and **recrudescence** are terms applied to the recurrence of clinical malaria after a period without symptoms. True relapses occur when a patient who has had all RBCs cleared of parasites develops a new infection of the erythrocytes from hypnozoites in the liver. *P. vivax* and *P. ovale* cause relapsing malaria, while *P. falciparum* and *P. malariae* infect the liver cells during the initial phase of infection, but do not persist in the liver. However, parasitemias that are too low to cause illness may occur with these species. These low parasitemias may persist for varying periods and then increase to a level that produces symptoms. This process is called recrudescence. *P. falciparum* infections usually have recrudescences within days or weeks. Recrudescence may occur in *P. malariae* infections up to 50 years or more after the initial infection.

Characteristics of the different species follow:

P. vivax infects young RBCs. The parasites cause enlargement of the infected cell and produce stainable alterations of the red cell membrane called Schüffner's dots. The trophozoites are very ameboid and the mature schizont contains 12–24 merozoites (Fig. 58.1).

P. falciparum is able to infect RBCs of any age. The ring stage is small and delicate and may have two chromatin (nuclear) dots (Fig. 58.2C). Gametocytes are cresent shaped (Fig. 58.2D). Only rings and gametocytes are seen in the peripheral blood. The more advanced stages of asexual development take place in venules where the infected red cells adhere to the vascular endothelium.

P. malariae infects mature RBCs and these cells do not enlarge as the parasites develop. The trophozoites tend to extend from one side of the red cell to the other in a band (Fig. 58.2A). Mature schizonts contain 6–12 merozoites.

P. ovale infects young RBCs causes them to enlarge and produces Schüffner's dots. The infected cells are often ovoid and have ragged margins (Fig. 58.2B). The trophozoite remains relatively compact, and the mature schizont usually has 4–12 merozoites.

Synchronous rupture of the red cells containing merozoites produces chills and fever. Anemia develops, not only from the destruction of infected cells, but

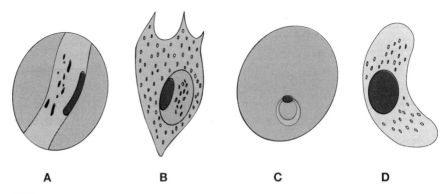

A   B   C   D

Figure 58.2.

Other *Plasmodium* species. (A) Trophozoite (band form) of *P. malariae* in normal size RBC. (B) Trophozoite of *P. ovale* in enlarged, oval RBC with ragged edges and prominent Schüffner's dots. (C) Ring stage of *P. falciparum*. (D) *P. falciparum* female gametocyte.

from hemolysis and phagocytosis of uninfected red cells. The latter effect is thought to be caused by immunologic mechanisms. Hyperplasia of the mononuclear phagocyte system occurs with resulting hepatosplenomegaly. Uptake of malaria pigment by phagocytes darkens the tissues of the liver, spleen, and bone marrow. Stimulation of the immune system results in high levels of polyclonal gamma globulin. Thrombocytopenia may be caused by sequestration of platelets in the spleen and damage to platelets by immune mechanisms. In falciparum malaria, the membranes of infected RBCs develop electron-dense knobs that adhere to the endothelium of the small venules and capillaries. This phenomenon causes plugging of the vasculature with subsequent ischemia of the involved tissues.

The cytokine, TNF, is thought to play a significant role in malaria. The release of TNF may produce some of the symptoms associated with the rupture of infected RBCs. Some severe effects of malaria in experimental animals appear to be caused by TNF, and TNF levels in humans have been correlated with the severity of infection with *P. falciparum.*

Clinical Manifestations

After a variable incubation period that is determined by the species, strain and previous prophylaxis, there may be a prodrome resembling a ''flulike'' illness with low-grade fever, headache, and malaise. This condition may last a few days before the onset of the true malaria **paroxysms.** The paroxysm consists of shaking chills and high fever followed by a fall in temperature and profuse sweating. In the nonimmune person, paroxysms may initially occur irregularly or daily, but may begin or rapidly evolve into the cyclic pattern typical for the particular species of malaria. Splenomegaly and mild hepatomegaly develop. Peripheral blood usually shows a normal or reduced leukocyte count. Thrombocytopenia is common and anemia of a varying degree develops. Malaria may be complicated by intercurrent infection, especially pneumonia.

Falciparum malaria is potentially fatal and may present with several clinical syndromes. A list of these syndromes follow:

Cerebral malaria may have variable neurologic manifestations, but often presents with confusion, which progresses to stupor, coma, and death.

Pulmonary edema commonly is difficult to manage and often leads to a fatal outcome.

Renal failure is usually caused by acute tubular necrosis, but cases of glomerulonephritis also have been reported.

Bilious remittent fever results from liver involvement with marked jaundice.

Algid malaria refers to the condition of vascular collapse and shock that is associated with a fall in temperature. Adrenal insufficiency may be a component of this syndrome.

Dysentery and other GI symptoms may occur.

Blackwater fever describes the hemoglobinuria seen in association with massive hemolysis and acute renal failure.

Malaria is also implicated as a cause of two other syndromes that appear to involve immunologic processes:

Tropical splenomegaly is a syndrome consisting of significant splenomegaly associated with a severe hemolytic anemia and lymphocytic infiltrates in the hepatic portal triads. Both the IgM and antimalarial antibody levels are elevated. Patients respond to treatment with antimalarial drugs.

Endemic nephrosis represents renal immune complex disease associated with *P. malariae* antigens. The clinical manifestations are similar to nephrotic syndrome of other etiologies. Response to treatment is often poor.

Immunology

Acquired immunity is usually strain specific and not completely protective. Many individuals will continue to have low parasitemias, with minimal or no symptoms. Transplacental immunity is important in areas of high prevalence. It protects infants from fatal falciparum malaria. Genetic resistance also occurs. *P. vivax* merozoites require the presence of the Duffy blood group antigen on the surface of the RBC in order to penetrate and infect the cell. A very high percentage of West African Blacks are Duffy blood group negative and are protected from infection with *P. vivax*. There are many genetic abnormalities of hemoglobin formation and of red cell enzymes. The geographic distribution of these abnormalities in the population is similar to that of *P. falciparum* infection. It is thought that these genetic polymorphisms provide a selective advantage in evasion of the lethal effects of falciparum malaria. The protective effect of hemoglobin S has been demonstrated. Hemoglobin S homozygotes have potentially fatal sickle cell disease because the abnormal hemoglobin deforms the red cell at low oxygen tensions, and the misshapen cells (sickle cells) cause obstruction of blood vessels. Hemoglobin S heterozygotes, however, do not develop sickle cell disease and are protected from high parasitemias and severe effects of falciparum malaria. In an infected red cell that contains hemoglobin S, reduced oxygen tension causes a loss of intracellular potassium, which results in the death of the parasite. Glucose-6-phosphate dehydrogenase deficiency and thalassemia may also confer some degree of protection. A common genetic defect in a RBC transmembrane protein causes Southeast Asian ovalocytosis. The abnormally rigid, oval-shaped erythrocytes are resistant to infection with *P. falciparum.*

Laboratory Diagnosis

Currently, the definitive diagnosis of malaria is made by identifying the parasites in blood films. The optimal stain for malaria parasites is Giemsa; however, parasites should be easily recognized in films stained with Wright's stain. Both thick and thin films should be made. The thick film concentrates the organisms and is useful for screening. The thin film allows better morphologic examination for the determination of the species. Blood films should be made frequently (every 4–6 h) in situations where the diagnosis is not immediately apparent. Because falciparum malaria may be rapidly fatal, a diagnosis of infection with this species constitutes a medical emergency and must be reported immediately. Rapid screening for malaria parasites may be performed using a commercially available centrifugation technique called Quantitative Buffy Coat (QBC) for analysis. Infected RBCs are separated by centrifugation in a glass capillary tube. The organisms, stained with acridine-orange, can be detected in the capillary tube using fluorescent microscopy.

Serologic tests may be useful in unusual clinical circumstances and in epidemiologic studies. Molecular techniques utilizing the PCR and DNA probing may someday be generally available for the diagnosis of malaria. Probes that recognize malarial ribosomal RNA are under development.

Treatment and Prevention

Chloroquine is used for prophylaxis of all species of *Plasmodium,* except for chloroquine-resistant strains of *P. falciparum* (CRPF). The CRPF strains are now widespread in South America, India, and Southeast Asia and Africa. Currently, mefloquine or doxycycline are the drugs most commonly recommended for prophylaxis of CRPF. Treatment of the clinical attack of malaria for all species of malaria except CRPF is with chloroquine. The relapsing malarias (vivax and ovale malaria) require primaquine, in addition to chloroquine, to eliminate persisting liver stages (hypnozoites). Treatment of CRPF is with mefloquine or a combination of quinine, pyrimethamine and sulfa, or a combination of quinine and tetracycline. Halofantrine is being used outside the United States for the treatment CRPF.

In patients infected with *P. falciparum,* exchange transfusion is considered as an adjunct to drug treatment when the parasitemia is very high.

The use of insect repellents, protective clothing, and insecticide-impregnated bed nets are highly effective in reducing malaria transmission.

Vaccines

There is a vigorous effort to develop effective vaccines for malaria. Progress is difficult because of the antigenic variability of the parasites and because the vaccine must be highly effective to protect against a parasite that reproduces so rapidly. Although vaccines are being developed for all stages of the parasite, including merozoites and gametes, the most advanced efforts target the sporozoite. Recombinant DNA techniques have been used to produce antigens identified in the protein coat of the sporozoites (circumsporozoite protein). Unfortunately, these antigens have not been highly immunogenic. Currently, there are attempts to enhance the immune response by the use of various adjuvants. A synthetic peptide vaccine for falciparum malaria has shown a significant degree of protection in trials in South America and Africa.

BABESIOSIS

Babesiosis is caused by apicomplexan parasites of the genus *Babesia.* The organisms are transmitted by tick bites and infect RBCs. Sporadic cases of babesiosis are reported from various parts of the world, usually in individuals who have been splenectomized. *Babesia microti* is endemic in southern New England and infects people with intact spleens. Rodents serve as reservoir hosts. The parasites develop in the RBCs where they resemble malaria organisms. Patients develop fever, chills, sweats, myalgia, and fatigue. Unlike malaria, the fever is not periodic. Hemolytic anemia develops. *B. microti* infections are rarely fatal. The diagnosis is made by identifying the parasites in stained blood films. The organisms do not produce pigment. An immunofluorescent antibody test may be useful. A combination of quinine and clindamycin appears to be an effective treatment.

SUMMARY

1. Malaria is caused by *Plasmodium vivax*, *Plasmodium falciparum*, *Plasmodium malariae*, and *Plasmodium ovale*.

2. All species of malaria parasites are transmitted by anopheline mosquitos. Other modes of transmission are blood transfusion, contaminated hypodermic needles, and congenital infection.

3. Malaria parasites develop initially in hepatic parenchymal cells, and then penetrate RBCs to continue cycles of asexual reproduction. These cycles result in the synchronous destruction of RBCs. *P. vivax*, *P. ovale*, and *P. falciparum* have cycles of approximately 48 h and *P. malariae* has a 72-h cycle.

4. Some parasites in the RBCs develop into sexual stages that are infectious for the mosquito host.

5. The rupture of the RBCs by asexual parasites causes the onset of the malaria paroxysm that consists of chills and fever followed by profuse sweating. The periodicity of the paroxysms is dependent on the species of *Plasmodium*. There is hyperplasia of the mononuclear phagocyte system resulting in splenomegaly.

6. *P. falciparum* infections are often fatal because of the potential of this species for infecting high numbers of RBCs and the adherence of infected cells to the vascular endothelium. Cerebral malaria is a common, serious complication caused by obstruction of cerebral capillaries.

7. *P. vivax* and *P. ovale* may cause relapses because of persisting stages in the hepatic parenchymal cells (hypnozoites).

8. *P. falciparum* and *P. malariae* may cause recrudescences because of organisms persisting in low numbers in the RBCs.

9. Sickle cell hemoglobin, other hemoglobinopathies, and RBC enzyme deficiencies may be protective against the lethal effects of falciparum malaria. Individuals lacking Duffy blood group antigen are protected from infection with *P. vivax*.

10. Diagnosis of malaria is made by demonstrating the parasites in blood films.

11. Chloroquine is used for treatment and prophylaxis of *P. vivax*, *P. ovale*, *P. malariae*, and susceptible strains of *P. falciparum*, *P. vivax* and *P.*

ovale infections also require treatment with primaquine to eliminate the hypnozoites in the liver. Mefloquine is used for the prophylaxis and treatment of chloroquine resistant strains of *P. falciparum*.

12. Babesiosis is transmitted by tick bites and rodents are reservoir hosts.

13. *Babesia microti* is the species reported most frequently from humans in the United States.

14. Parasites develop in the RBCs and cause fever, chills, and myalgia. These manifestations are not cyclic or periodic as is seen in malaria.

15. Babesiosis is diagnosed by demonstrating parasites in blood films and differentiating them from malaria organisms.

REFERENCES

Bruce-Chwatt LJ (1985): Essential Malariology. 2nd ed. New York: Wiley.

Holder AA (1993): Developments with anti-malarial vaccines. Ann NY Acad Sci 700:7.

Gordon DM (1990): Malaria vaccines. Infect Dis Clin North Am 4:299.

Ristic M (1988): Babesiosis of Domestic Animals and Man. Boca Raton, FL: CRC Press.

Wernsdorfer WH, McGregor I (eds) (1988): Malaria. Principles and Practice of Malariology. Vols. 1 and 2. New York: Churchill Livingstone.

Zucker JR, Campbell CC (1993): Malaria. Principles of prevention and treatment. Infect Dis Clin North Am 7:547.

REVIEW QUESTIONS

For questions 1 to 4, choose the ONE BEST answer or completion.

1. Sporozoites of *Plasmodium* species penetrate and develop in
   a) mononuclear phagocyte cells of the spleen
   b) mononuclear phagocyte cells of the liver
   c) endothelial cells of small blood vessels
   d) hepatocytes (hepatic parenchymal cells)
   e) red blood cells

2. The stage of malaria parasites that is found in red blood cells and undergoes further development in the mosquito is the
   a) gametocyte
   b) ring
   c) hypnozoite
   d) merozoite
   e) schizont

3. The major cause of the complications of *Plasmodium falciparum* infections, such as cerebral malaria, is
   a) phagocytosis of uninfected red blood cells
   b) hyperplasia of the mononuclear phagocyte system
   c) nonspecific immunosuppression caused by the infection
   d) adherence of infected red blood cells to the endothelium of small blood vessels

   e) marked elevation of body temperature caused by rupture of infected red blood cells

4. Babesiosis has the following characteristics, *except*
   a) transmission by tick bite
   b) organisms initially develop in liver
   c) asexual reproduction occurs in red blood cells
   d) episodes of fever are not periodic
   e) anemia commonly develops

For questions 5 to 9, a list of lettered options is followed by several numbered items. For each numbered item, select the ONE lettered option that is most closely associated with it. Each lettered option may be selected once, more than once, or not at all.

A) *Plasmodium malariae*
B) *Plasmodium vivax*
C) *Plasmodium falciparum*
D) *Plasmodium ovale*
E) *Plasmodium malariae* and *Plasmodium falciparum*
F) *Plasmodium vivax* and *Plasmodium ovale*
G) All *Plasmodium* species

For the statements below, select the appropriate parasite(s).

5. Malarial pigment is produced in infected red blood cells.

6. Endemic nephrosis is associated with chronic infection.

7. Paroxysms of chills, fever, and sweats occur every 72 h.

8. Relapse of clinical illness is caused by the red blood cell infection developing from persisting hypnozoites in the liver.

9. Recrudescence of clinical illness is caused by an increase in the numbers of parasites persisting in red blood cells.

ANSWERS TO REVIEW QUESTIONS

1. *d* Sporozoites from mosquito saliva penetrate and develop asexually in hepatocytes (hepatic parenchymal cells).

2. *a* Gametocytes are the sexual stages circulating in the blood. These parasites complete the sexual cycle in the mosquito, eventually producing infective sporozoites in the mosquito's salivary glands.

3. *d* Adherence of infected RBCs to the vascular endothelium causes plugging of the vessels with subsequent ischemia of tissues supplied by the affected vessels.

4. *b* Babesia organisms directly infect RBCs. There is no initial development within liver cells as is the case with *Plasmodium* species.

5. *G* All species of *Plasmodium* produce malaria pigment.

6. *A* Endemic nephrosis results from renal damage caused by immune complexes containing *Plasmodium malariae* antigen.

7. *A* *P. malariae* causes paroxysms every 72 h. The other species have 48-h cycles.

8. *F* *Plasmodium vivax* and *Plasmodium ovale* are relapsing malarias. These parasites have dormant stages in liver cells (hypnozoites) which, when activated cause infection of RBCs and recurrence of clinical symptoms.

9. *E* *P. malariae* and *Plasmodium falciparum* infections can persist with low levels of infected RBCs. The patient is without symptoms until the number of infected RBCs increases to a certain level. The recurrence of symptoms in this instance is called recrudescence.

LEISHMANIASIS AND TRYPANOSOMIASIS

The flagellate parasites of blood and tissue, the hemoflagellates, consist of two genera, *Leishmania* and *Trypanosoma*. These parasites are transmitted by insect vectors and have characteristic morphologic features. The following parasitic forms are important in human disease:

Amastigote: This form is round or oval and measures 2–5 μ in diameter. It is found intracellularly and has a prominent nucleus and a dark staining, bar-shaped structure called a **kinetoplast** (Fig. 59.1A). The kinetoplast is a modified mitochondrion, which contains DNA arranged in circular ''minicircles'' and ''maxicircles.'' Electron microscopy reveals a flagellar pocket containing a short flagellum that does not extend beyond the surface of the organism. Intracytoplasmic vesicles, called glycosomes, contain the enzymes of glycolysis.

Promastigote: This form of *Leishmania* develops in the insect vector and in diagnostic cultures. The promastigote is elongated, measuring about 1.5–3.5 μ in width by 15–20 μ in length. A single flagellum projects from the anterior end. The kinetoplast appears as a dark, short bar at the base of the flagellum. The nucleus of the promastigote is located in the mid-region of the parasite (Fig. 59.1B).

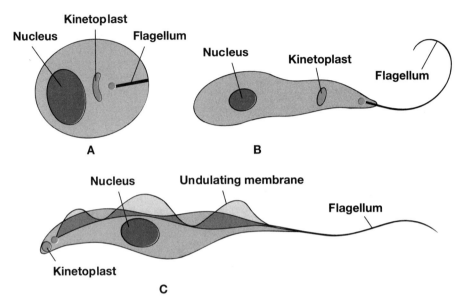

Figure 59.1.
Morphologic stages of hemoflagellates. (A) Amastigote. (B) Promastigote. (C) Trypomastigote.

Trypomastigote: This form has a flagellum that originates at the posterior end of the organism, runs the length of the body as an undulating membrane, and may extend beyond the anterior end as a free flagellum. The kinetoplast is also located at the posterior end near the origin of the flagellum (Fig. 59.1C). A single, large mitochondrion extends from the posterior to near the anterior end of the organism. Trypomastigotes also contain glycosomes. A summary of the major characteristics of leishmaniasis and trypanosomiasis is found in Table 59.1.

LEISHMANIASIS

The taxonomy of the *Leishmania* is complex and is frequently revised. A simplified classification is used here. Isoenzyme analysis has been used to differentiate subspecies of *Leishmania*. The recent use of DNA probes to detect specific sequences in the minicircles of kinetoplast DNA should make a major contribution to clarifying the classification problem.

Infectious promastigotes of *Leishmania* are transmitted by the bite of the sandfly (genera *Phlebotomus* and *Lutzomyia*). The promastigotes are phagocytized by mononuclear phagocytes. Complement, specifically C3, adhering to the parasite facilitates phagocytosis by binding to receptor sites on the macrophage. Two parasite surface proteins (lipophosphoglucan and glycoprotein 63) are important in C3 binding and may also be involved in binding to macrophage receptors independent of complement. Phagocytized parasites are able to inhibit the production of toxic metabolites by the macrophage, and they are able to survive and reproduce in a vacuole that contains the macrophage's digestive enzymes.

fly bite takes up amastigotes → amastigotes develop to promastigotes in gut of fly → promastigotes in proboscis of fly → fly bite introduces promastigotes → amastigotes in mononuclear phagocytic cells

VISCERAL LEISHMANIASIS

Visceral leishmaniasis (kala-azar) is caused by *Leishmania donovani* (several subspecies).

Transmission

Many species of sandfly serve as vectors for leishmaniasis. The promastigotes are introduced when the fly bites.

Geographic Distribution and Epidemiology

The infection is found in the Mediterranean basin, tropical Africa, Indian subcontinent, Southeast Asia, China, South, and Central America. In China, West Africa, and South America, dogs are reservoir hosts. Humans are the only significant hosts in India and some parts of Africa. The vector sandfly usually requires moist soil or ground debris for breeding.

Habitat

The amastigotes are found in the mononuclear-phagocyte system of the liver, spleen, and bone marrow. In cutaneous complications of visceral leishmaniasis, the parasites can be found in macrophages in the skin.

Properties of the Organism

The amastigotes multiply in the macrophages and may occasionally be found in cells in the circulation. The sandfly ingests amastigotes when taking a blood meal. The amastigotes transform into promastigotes in the gut of the sandfly, migrate to the proboscis, and are introduced when the sandfly bites. Promastigotes that are injected by the fly are phagocytized by macrophages and undergo transformation into amastigotes.

Clinical Manifestations

The incubation period varies from 2 weeks to more than 1 year. Onset may be insidious or abrupt. Fever, with double diurnal spikes, is common. Progressive hepatosplenomegaly occurs as a result of hyperplasia of the parasitized mononuclear phagocytes. There may also be lymphadenopathy. Weight loss, nose bleeds, diarrhea, and cough are common. There is pancytopenia (reduction in all formed elements of the blood) and a dramatic increase in gamma globulin (polyclonal hyperglobulinemia) with IgG predominating. During active infection, cell mediated responses to leishmanial antigens are absent, but develop following successful treatment. Untreated patients frequently die from concomitant bacterial infections, such as pneumonia or tuberculosis.

Some patients who have recovered from visceral leishmaniasis develop skin lesions called post kala-azar dermal leishmaniasis. The lesions frequently appear as papules or nodules on the face or ears. Flat, hypopigmented lesions also occur. The papular or nodular lesions contain many parasites.

Laboratory Diagnosis

Amastigotes may be found on smears made of white cells or bone marrow aspirates. Diagnostic spleen punctures are performed in some parts of the world. Cultures of blood and bone marrow can be done using blood agar slants of Nicolle, Novy, MacNeal (NNN medium) or liquid medium (Schneider's). Promastigotes develop in culture at room temperature within 4 weeks. Sensitive strain-specific DNA probes and PCR techniques are being developed.

Treatment

Pentavalent antimonial drugs (sodium stibogluconate and meglumine antimoniate) are the drugs of choice in treatment. Pentamidine has been used in resistant cases, and amphotericin B is a treatment of last resort because of its toxicity. Allopurinol, a structural analog of the purine base hypoxanthine, has been used experimentally. Because the parasites cannot synthesize purines, they incorporate the allopurinol into their RNA causing inhibition of RNA function.

CUTANEOUS LEISHMANIASIS

Cutaneous leishmaniasis is caused by several species and subspecies of *Leishmania.* The important organisms are categorized as follows:

Old World   *Leishmania tropica*
              Leishmania major
              Leishmania aethiopica

New World   *Leishmania mexicana* (several subspecies)
              Leishmania braziliensis (several subspecies)

Transmission

As with all *Leishmania,* the infection is transmitted through the bite of the sandfly.

Geographic Distribution and Epidemiology

L. tropica infections occur in urban areas of the Mediterranean basin, Middle East, Pakistan, and parts of India. Reservoir hosts are not important. *L. major* occurs in rural areas, usually dry desert regions of central Asia, southern Russia, Middle East, and Africa, where rodents serve as reservoir hosts. *Leishmania aethiopica* is found in northeast Africa. *L. mexicana* and *L. braziliensis* occur in Mexico, Central, and South America. A few cases have been reported from central Texas. A wide variety of reservoir hosts have been reported in the Western Hemisphere.

Habitat

The amastigotes are found in the mononuclear phagocytes of the skin.

Properties of the Organism

The parasites are morphologically identical to those causing visceral leishmaniasis. The life cycle is similar to that described for *L. donovani,* but infection is limited to the skin.

Clinical Manifestations

Cutaneous leishmaniasis presents as nodular and ulcerated skin lesions. The clinical picture varies depending on the subspecies of parasite. In some areas, single lesions are the rule, and in others, satellite lesions may be common. In Mexico and Central America, chronic, progressive lesions of the pinna of the ear are common among forest workers. Most cutaneous leishmaniasis will heal spontaneously in a few months to 1 year with residual scarring. Healed cutaneous leishmaniasis caused by *L. tropica, L. major,* or *L. mexicana* is associated with lifelong immunity to the infecting strain. Diffuse cutaneous leishmaniasis, with multiple nodular skin lesions, develops rarely, except in *L. aethiopica* infection, and is probably related to impaired immune response of the host.

Laboratory Diagnosis

Biopsy of the tissue for histopathology and for culture may reveal organisms. Culture of aspirates from the active edge of the skin lesion using NNN or liquid Schneider's media is often diagnostic. A delayed hypersensitivity skin test (Montenegro test) is used in some endemic areas. Serologic tests are not generally available, but could become useful with the development of simple tests employing specific antigens. Tests are being developed for the detection of specific parasite DNA in biopsy specimens.

Treatment

Often, no treatment is given because the lesions will heal spontaneously. Treatment may be indicated because of the location of the lesion or the numbers of lesions. The threat of later development of mucocutaneous disease in infections acquired in the Western Hemisphere may warrant preventive treatment. Drugs listed for visceral leishmaniasis are used. Some strains of *Leishmania* are sensitive to heat, and local heat treatments may hasten healing.

MUCOCUTANEOUS LEISHMANIASIS

Mucocutaneous leishmaniasis is usually caused by subspecies of *L. braziliensis,* but there have been reports of mucocutaneous disease associated with *L. mexicana* infection. Usually there is an initial skin lesion that heals spontaneously. Months to years later, progressively destructive lesions develop in the buccal cavity or nasopharynx. Severe destruction of the tissues of the midface lead to death by starvation or aspiration pneumonia. Diagnosis from biopsies and cultures may be difficult because organisms are few even though the lesions are extensive. Serologic tests, where available, may be helpful. Molecular techniques for detecting parasite DNA could be the most sensitive. Treatment is the same as for visceral leishmaniasis.

TRYPANOSOMIASIS

AFRICAN TRYPANOSOMIASIS

African trypanosomiasis (sleeping sickness) is caused by two species of parasites: *Trypanosoma brucei gambiense* causes West African or Gambian trypanosomiasis and *Trypanosoma brucei rhodesiense* causes East African or Rhodesian trypanosomiasis.

Transmission

The organisms are inoculated into the human host during the bite of the tsetse fly (*Glossina* species).

Geographic Distribution and Epidemiology

The distribution of the disease is confined to areas infested by the vector tsetse fly. *T. b. gambiense* infections are found in West and Central Africa near rivers and streams. Animal reservoirs are considered to be relatively insignificant.

T. b. rhodesiense infections occur in East and Central Africa in the savanna environment where wild game animals are major reservoir hosts. About 25,000 new cases of African trypanosomiasis occur annually.

Habitat

After initial development in the skin, the trypomastigotes are found in blood, lymph nodes, and cerebrospinal fluid.

Properties of the Organism

The form found in humans is called a **trypomastigote** (or **trypanosome**). It varies greatly in length from 17 to 30 μ. It has an undulating membrane that runs the length of the organism. In the long, slender forms, the undulating membrane terminates in a free flagellum at the anterior end (Fig. 59.2A). There is a prominent nucleus in the midbody region. The kinetoplast is found near the origin of the flagellum and undulating membrane at the posterior of the organism. The infective stage is introduced into the skin during the bite of the tsetse fly. There is local multiplication of the parasites in the skin followed by dissemination into the blood. Eventually, infection of the lymphatics and then the CNS occurs. When a tsetse fly bites infected humans or animals, it takes up trypomastigotes with the blood

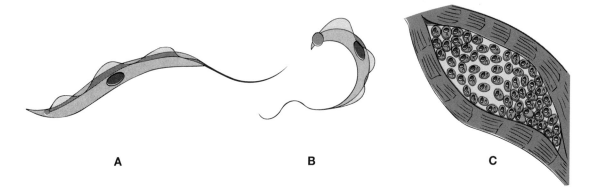

A   B   C

Figure 59.2.

Trypanosoma species. (A) Trypomastigote of *T. b. gambiense*. (B) Trypomastigote of *T. cruzi*. (C) *T. cruzi* amastigotes in heart muscle.

meal. The organisms develop in the fly, and eventually migrate to the salivary glands. When the fly bites, infective organisms are injected with the saliva.

The trypomastigotes possess a coat of glycoprotein molecules called the variant surface glycoprotein (VSG). As the population of trypomastigotes increases in the blood stream, the host develops humoral antibody to the VSG and the trypomastigotes are destroyed by antibody mediated mechanisms. A few parasites that express a different VSG survive and multiply causing a new wave of parasitemia. The organisms have the potential for the expression of many different VSGs. These antigenic variations allow the parasite to evade the humoral immune response of the host. Because of its variability, VSG cannot be used as antigen in vaccine development.

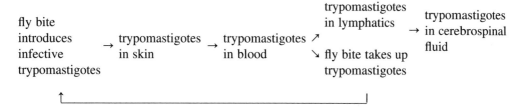

Clinical Manifestations

A primary lesion, the trypanosomal chancre, may develop at the site of the fly bite. The chancre is a circular, raised, erythematous, painful lesion which may be several centimeters in diameter. Fever is one of the earliest signs of generalized infection. It usually begins within a few days to weeks in the Rhodesian form, but may be delayed months to years in the Gambian form. The fever may be cyclic with the peaks related to increased parasitemia representing a new population of parasites expressing different VSG molecules. Infection with *T. b. rhodesiense* is associated with a rapidly progressive illness with invasion of the CNS occurring within a few weeks. Patients with the Rhodesian form may die of myocarditis before the nervous system is invaded. The Gambian form is much more insidious, with fever, malaise, and lymphadenopathy and hepatosplenomegaly progressing slowly over a period of months. Prominent posterior cervical lymphadenopathy is called **Winterbottom's sign.** The onset of CNS disease may also be subtle, with personality changes, insomnia, or irritability as early signs. Nervous system involvement may not occur until 1 year or more after infection. The encephalopathy leads to apathy, somnolence and coma (sleeping sickness). Death is usually caused by intercurrent infection, such as pneumonia. There is polyclonal elevation of serum gamma globulin with IgM predominating.

Laboratory Diagnosis

In the early stages, trypomastigotes can be seen in blood smears. Higher parasitemias are seen with Rhodesian trypanosomiasis. When lymphadenopathy is present, aspiration of lymph nodes can reveal organisms. When the nervous system is involved, parasites can be recovered from centrifuged cerebrospinal fluid. Detection of IgM in the cerebrospinal fluid of a patient with trypanosomiasis is diagnostic of nervous system invasion. Serologic tests are not highly sensitive or specific. Both PCR and DNA hybridization techniques are promising.

Treatment

Suramin and pentamidine are used in early cases without evidence of CNS involvement. Pentamidine is useful only in the Gambian infections. When there is nervous system invasion, an arsenical drug, melarsoprol, has been used. Recent use of a polyamine synthesis inhibitor, eflornithine (diflouromethylornithine, DFMO) has led to dramatic recovery in Gambian trypanosomiasis.

AMERICAN TRYPANOSOMIASIS

American trypanosomiasis (Chagas' disease) is caused by *Trypanosoma cruzi.*

Transmission

Infective organisms appear in the feces of blood-sucking reduviid bugs, also called kissing bugs or cone-nosed bugs (genera *Triatoma, Rhodnius,* and *Pan-strongylus*). The infection is acquired when the bug's feces contact the site of the bug bite or contact mucus membranes. The infection is also transmitted by blood transfusion and congenital infections have been reported.

Geographic Distribution and Epidemiology

The infection is found in Mexico, Central, and South America, with prevalence rates of about 17 million. Infections usually occur in rural areas where houses made of mud, sticks, and thatch provide ideal conditions for harboring the insect vectors. Dogs, cats, opposums, rodents, and armadillos are important reservoir hosts. Isolated human infections have been reported from Texas and California.

Properties of the Organism

Organisms excreted in the bug's feces enter the skin at the bite site or through contaminated mucus membranes. There is local multiplication in the tissues in the form of intracellular amastigotes, these transform into trypomastigotes as they are released from the ruptured host cell. The trypomastigote is about 20 μ in length and has a very prominent kinetoplast at the posterior end (Fig. 59.2B). Trypomastigotes circulate in the blood stream, but do not reproduce. These organisms are able to penetrate many different types of host cells where they transform into amastigotes (Fig. 59.2C). Bugs become infected by ingesting trypomastigotes during a blood meal. The organisms multiply in the hindgut of the bug and infective forms are deposited in the bug's feces.

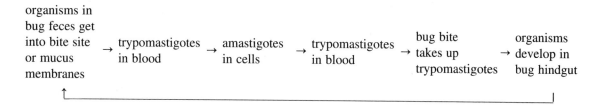

Clinical Manifestations

Initial infection is often asymptomatic, but may become evident many years later as the chronic form of the disease. Acute disease associated with the initial infection is more common in children. Unilateral periorbital edema (Romaña's sign) represents the reaction to the local multiplication of organisms that have been inoculated in the conjunctiva. Introduction of parasites at other locations often produce localized swelling and discoloration of the skin called a chagoma. The local lesion is followed by fever, lymphadenopathy, subcutaneous edema, and hepato-splenomegaly. Myocarditis is common and meningoencephalitis is a serious complication. Trypomastigotes are demonstrable in the blood. Chronic Chagas' disease may develop many years after the initial infection. Cardiomyopathy with congestive heart failure or arrhythmias may be seen. Impaired function and dilatation of the esophagus or colon is another complication of chronic infection

TABLE 59.1. A Summary of Leishmaniases and Trypanosomiases

Disease	Organism	Transmission	Location	Clinical manifestations	Laboratory diagnosis	Treatment
Visceral leishmaniasis (kala-azar)	*Leishmania donovani* (several subspecies)	Bite of sandfly	Amastigotes in macrophages of liver, spleen, bone marrow, and lymph nodes	Fever, hepatosplenomegaly, lymphadenopathy, pancytopenia, and hyperglobulinemia (IgG)	Smears and culture of blood, bone marrow, or splenic aspirate	Antimony compounds
Cutaneous leishmaniasis						
Old World	*Leishmania tropica* *Leishmania major*	Bite of sandfly	Amastigotes in macrophages of skin	Ulcerative skin lesions	Smears and cultures of aspirates or scrapings. Biopsy for staining and culture.	Antimony compounds
	Leishmania aethiopica			May also cause diffuse cutaneous leishmaniasis		
New World	*Leishmania mexicana* (several subspecies) *Leishmania braziliensis* (several subspecies)					

Disease	Organism	Transmission	Location/Forms	Symptoms	Diagnosis	Treatment
Mucocutaneous leishmaniasis	Usually *Leishmania braziliensis* (several subspecies)	Bite of sandfly	Amastigotes in macrophages of skin, and mucus membranes	Ulcerative skin lesion followed by metastatic spread to the tissues of nose and oropharynx	Smears and cultures of aspirates or scrapings. Biopsy for staining and culture. Organisms often difficult to find or culture.	Antimony compounds amphotericin B
African trypanosomiasis West African (Gambian)	*Trypanosoma brucei gambiense*	Bite of tsetse fly	Trypomastigotes in blood, lymphatics, brain, and cerebrospinal fluid	Early: fever, lymphadenopathy, increased IgM Late: CNS symptoms, coma and death	Examination of blood, lymph, and cerebrospinal fluid for trypomastigotes	Suramin, pentamidine, eflornithine
East African (Rhodesian)	*Trypanosoma brucei rhodesiense*	Bite of tsetse fly	Trypomastigotes in blood, brain, and cerebrospinal fluid	Fever, myocarditis, encephalitis	Examination of blood and cerebrospinal fluid for trypomastigotes	Suramin, pentamidine
American trypanosomiasis (Chagas' disease)	*Trypanosoma cruzi*	Feces of reduviid bug in bite or in mucus membranes	Trypomastigotes in blood. Amastigotes in heart, skeletal muscle, GI tract, and so on	Acute: chagoma, fever, hepatosplenomegaly, meningoencephalitis. Chronic: cardiomyopathy, megasyndromes of colon, or esophagus.	Examination of blood for trypomastigotes in acute stage. Serology and xenodiagnosis in chronic stage	Nifurtimox, benznidizole

that is seen more frequently in Brazil. This complication has been referred to as the **"megasyndrome"** referring to megaesophagus or megacolon. The pathogenesis of chronic disease is not clear, but antibodies have been detected in the serum of infected individuals that cross-react with substances in cardiac and nervous tissues.

Laboratory Diagnosis

Examination of stained blood smears or smears made from the white cell layer during the acute disease usually show trypomastigotes. In chronic infection, serologic tests are most useful. Parasites may be detected using **xenodiagnosis.** Xenodiagnosis is performed by having laboratory-reared, uninfected bugs bite the patient. The intestinal contents of the bugs are examined for organisms 1 and 2 months later. Xenodiagnosis may be replaced with PCR and DNA hybridization techniques directed to the kinetoplast DNA minicircles.

Treatment

There is no completely effective treatment for Chagas' disease. Nifurtimox and benznidazole may eliminate the parasitemia in the acute phase of the disease, but long-term follow-up of treated patients often reveals positive xenodiagnostic tests. Recently, allopurinol has been found to be at least as effective as nifurtimox and benznidazole. It also is much less toxic than the latter two drugs. Treatment of chronic complications, such as cardiomyopathy and the megasyndrome, is symptomatic.

SUMMARY

1. A summary of leishmaniases and trypanosomiases can be found in Table 59.1.

REFERENCES

Englund PT, Smith DH (1990): African Trypanosomiasis. In Warren KS, Mahmoud AAF (eds): Tropical and Geographical Medicine. 2nd ed. New York: McGraw-Hill Book Co.
Evans TG (1993): Leishmaniasis. Infect Dis Clin North Am 7:527.

Kirchhoff LV (1993): Chagas disease. American trypanosomiasis. Infect Dis Clin North Am 7:487.

Nogueira N, Rodrigues Coura J: American Trypanosomiasis (Chagas' Disease). In Warren KS, Mahmoud AAF (eds): Tropical and Geographical Medicine. 2nd ed. New York: McGraw-Hill Book Co.

Peters W, Killick-Kendrick R (eds) (1987): The Leishmaniases in Biology and Medicine. Vols. I and II. New York: Academic Press.

Russell DG, Talamas-Rohana P (1989): Leishmania and the macrophage: a marriage of inconvenience. Immunol Today 10:328.

REVIEW QUESTIONS

For questions 1 to 2, choose the ONE BEST answer or completion.

1. Amastigotes of *Leishmania* are found in
   a) human mononuclear phagocytes
   b) human hepatocytes (liver parenchymal cells)
   c) the proboscis of sand flies
   d) the salivary glands of tsetse flies
   e) human heart muscle (myocardial) cells

2. The following statements about *Trypanosoma brucei rhodesiense* are true, *except*
   a) game animals are reservoir hosts
   b) trypomastigotes can be found in the cerebrospinal fluid when the central nervous system is involved
   c) a skin lesion may develop at the site of the bite of the vector
   d) the disease progresses relatively rapidly compared to *Trypanosoma brucei gambiense* infection
   e) eosinophilia is common in acute infections

For questions 3 to 10, a list of lettered options is followed by several numbered items. For each numbered item, select the ONE lettered option that is most closely associated with it. Each lettered option may be selected once, more than once, or not at all.

A) Sand fly
B) Tsetse fly
C) Reduviid bugs
D) *Leishmania tropica*
E) *Leishmania mexicana*
F) *Leishmania braziliensis*
G) *Leishmania donovani*
H) *Trypanosoma b. gambiense*
I) *Trypanosoma b. rhodesiense*
J) *Trypanosoma cruzi*

For the statements below, select the appropriate organism.

3. Amastigotes may be found in myocardial (heart muscle) cells.

4. The organism that transmits *Leishmania*.

5. This organism causes ulcerative skin lesions in humans in the Middle East area.

6. Transmission of disease occurs through contamination of mucus membranes or bite site with the feces of this organism.

7. The organism that is the most common cause of mucocutaneous leishmaniasis.

8. Chronic infections with the organism may be associated with megaesophagus or megacolon.

9. Infections cause fever, hepatosplenomegaly, and a marked increase in gamma globulin, especially IgG, and organisms are found in mononuclear phagocytes.

10. The organism that is transmitted by tsetse flies in West Africa.

ANSWERS TO REVIEW QUESTIONS

1. **a** *Leishmania* amastigotes are found in mononuclear phagocytes. Promastigotes develop in sand flies and are the infective stages introduced when the fly bites.

2. **e** Eosinophilia is not a feature of any of the diseases caused by either *Leishmania* or *Trypanosoma*.

3. **J** Amastigote forms of *Trypanosoma cruzi* may be found intracellularly in many tissues including myocardial cells.

4. **A** Sand flies are vectors for *Leishmania*.

5. **D** *Leishmania tropica* causes cutaneous leishmaniasis in the Middle East area. Subspecies of *Leishmania mexicana* and *Leishmania braziliensis* cause cutaneous leishmaniasis in the Western Hemisphere.

6. **C** Reduviid bugs transmit *T. cruzi* in their feces.

7. **F** *L. braziliensis* is the most common cause of mucocutaneous leishmaniasis.

8. **J** Chronic infection with *T. cruzi* may cause megaesophagus or megacolon.

9. **G** Fever, hepatosplenomegaly, and markedly increased IgG are features of visceral leishmaniasis caused by *L. donovani*. The organisms are found in the mononuclear phagocytes of the liver, spleen, and bone marrow.

10. **H** *Trypanosoma brucei gambiense* is transmitted by tsetse flies in West Africa.

TOXOPLASMOSIS AND *PNEUMOCYSTIS* INFECTION

TOXOPLASMOSIS

Toxoplasmosis is caused by the apicomplexan parasite, *Toxoplasma gondii.*

Transmission

The infection is acquired by the ingestion of oocysts from cat feces or by ingestion of cysts in inadequately cooked or raw meat, including pork, lamb, or beef. Transplacental transmission causes congenital toxoplasmosis.

Geographic Distribution and Epidemiology

The infection is found worldwide in a wide variety of mammals and birds and has been reported with varying prevalence rates in all human populations tested. Prevalence rates are dependent on the degree of exposure to cats and upon the frequency of eating rare or raw meat. Prevalence rates increase with age. In some areas of the United States, 25% of the population is infected by age 25. In France, almost all women who eat rare or raw meat are infected. In the United States, between 1 and 6 pregnant women per 1000 acquire toxoplasmosis with the associated risk of congenital disease.

Habitat

Toxoplasma is an intracellular parasite that has the ability to infect any nucleated cell. Major target organs are the lymph nodes, the brain, skeletal muscle, and the retina.

Properties of the Organism

The definitive host for *Toxoplasma* is the domestic cat and other felids. The cat acquires the infection by eating infected rodents or birds that contain tissue cysts or by ingesting oocysts from the feces of other cats. In the cat, the parasite undergoes reproduction in the intestinal epithelium. Sexual stages in the intestine result in the production of oocysts that are excreted in the cat's feces. The oocysts are infectious for a wide variety of birds and mammals including humans and other cats. When animals or humans ingest oocysts from cat feces, organisms escape from the oocyst and develop into trophozoites called tachyzoites. Tachyzoites are elongated, crescent-shaped organisms about 4–7 μ in length (Fig. 60.1A). The posterior end of the organism is more rounded than the anterior end that contains the apical complex. There is a single nucleus. Tachyzoites actively penetrate host cells, multiply intracellularly, and cause the rupture and death of the host cell. While the tachyzoite is transiently free in the extracellular environment, it is susceptible to lysis by antibody and complement. Once it has entered a cell, it is protected from the lethal effects of humoral antibody. In macrophages, the tachyzoites survive by inhibiting the fusion of lysosomes with the phagosome containing the parasite. Eventually, some tachyzoites form cysts, most frequently in brain, skeletal muscle, and heart (Fig. 60.1B). The organisms that develop within the cysts are called bradyzoites. Cysts measure up to 200 μ in diameter and may contain as many as 3000 organisms. The formation of cysts may be in response to growing immunity of the host. When ingested, tissue cysts are infectious to humans and animals including cats. Many infections are acquired by adults from the ingestion of rare or raw meat containing tissue cysts. Pork and lamb are more commonly infected than beef.

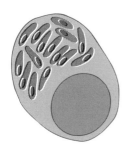
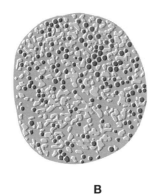

A   **B**

Figure 60.1.

Stages of *Toxoplasma* found in humans. (A) *Toxoplasma* tachyzoites in a macrophage. (B) *Toxoplasma* tissue cyst containing bradyzoites.

THE COMMON MODE OF INFECTION IN CATS

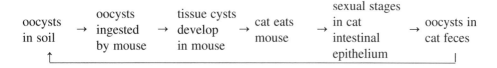

oocysts in soil → oocysts ingested by mouse → tissue cysts develop in mouse → cat eats mouse → sexual stages in cat intestinal epithelium → oocysts in cat feces

TWO MODES OF INFECTION IN HUMANS

oocysts from cat feces → ingestion of oocysts → tachyzoites in tissues → cysts containing bradyzoites in tissues

tissue cysts containing bradyzoites in meat → ingestion of cysts in raw or rare meat → tachyzoites in tissues → cysts containing bradyzoites in tissues

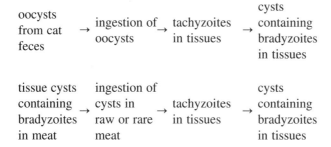

Clinical Manifestations

The two major categories of infection are acquired and congenital. Most acquired infections are asymptomatic. When clinical evidence of infection is present, the most common presentation of acquired infection is lymphadenopathy, usually cervical, without associated symptoms. Some acquired infections may have systemic manifestations, such as fever, headache, myalgia, lymphadenopathy, rash, and splenomegaly. The complex of symptoms may mimic infectious mononucleosis or a ''flu-like'' illness. There are rare case reports of acquired toxoplasmosis causing hepatitis, encephalitis, myocarditis, and pneumonia. Although eye involvement (retinochoroiditis) may occasionally occur in acute acquired infections, this condition usually represents activation of a congenital infection.

Congenital infections occur only when the mother acquires the infection immediately prior to or during pregnancy. Women who have antibody to *Toxoplasma* prior to becoming pregnant are not at risk for having an infected fetus or infant. Although congenital toxoplasmosis may be asymptomatic, it can cause mild-to-severe disease. Infants with inapparent infection at birth may develop significant ocular and neurologic sequelae in later childhood. Infections acquired by the fetus early in the gestational period are more likely to result in serious complications recognized at birth.

Severe, generalized congenital infections cause fever, jaundice, splenomegaly, hepatomegaly, pneumonia and rash, and also may have ocular and neurologic involvement. Infants with predominant neurologic findings usually have bilateral retinochoroiditis, and may have seizures, intracerebral calcifications, and hydrocephalus or microcephaly. Asymptomatic congenital infections may become clinically evident in older children and adults as unilateral retinochoroiditis unassociated with other symptoms.

Symptomatic toxoplasmosis may develop in AIDS patients and in other immunosuppressed individuals from activation of a congenital infection, from activation of previously asymptomatic acquired infection, or from a newly acquired infection. In these immunocompromised patients, the disease often presents as encephalitis, commonly as localized lesions resembling abscesses. About one third of AIDS patients that are seropositive for toxoplasmosis will eventually develop encephalitis.

Laboratory Diagnosis

Although the presence of antibodies to *T. gondii* is common in the general population, serologic tests are the principal means of diagnosis. Differentiation between IgM antibody, which occurs early in infection and IgG antibody, which develops later, is very helpful. The finding of IgM antibody in a newborn is presumptive evidence of congenital infection. One of the most specific and sensitive techniques for IgM antibody is called the double sandwich IgM enzyme-linked immunosorbent test. Recent studies show that IgA antibody specific for a *Toxo-*

plasma surface protein may be a more sensitive indicator of both acquired and congenital infections than IgM antibody. Both IgM and IgA antibodies should be measured when possible. An ELISA technique has also been used to detect antigens of *Toxoplasma* in serum of acute acquired infections and in blood, CSF, and urine of congenitally infected infants. Serum antibody tests are not as useful in ocular toxoplasmosis. It may be necessary to measure antibody in ocular fluids. In immunocompromised patients with cerebral involvement, brain biopsy with immunofluorescent or peroxidase-antiperoxidase staining may be necessary. Lymph node biopsy may show characteristic histologic features. Because asymptomatic infection is widespread, the demonstration of organisms in tissue or by animal inoculation is not proof of acute infection with the exception of congenital disease.

Treatment

Most infections are asymptomatic and do not require treatment. When treatment is indicated, a combination of pyrimethamine and sulfa drugs is used. Folinic acid is added to the regimen to prevent the development of megaloblastic anemia. Spiramycin, a macrolide antibiotic, has been used for many years in countries other than the United States to treat toxoplasmosis, especially in pregnant women. It is available as an investigational drug in the United States. Other drugs that have significant antitoxoplasma activity and are undergoing clinical evaluation are clindamycin, azithromycin, clarithromycin, and atovaquone. Prevention of congenital disease requires reducing the exposure to infection of antibody-negative pregnant women. These women should avoid cleaning cat litter boxes and children's sand boxes, as well as gardening in soil that may be contaminated with cat feces. Meat should be thoroughly cooked.

Vaccine development may be possible using mutant strains of *Toxoplasma* that do not cause persistent infections.

PNEUMOCYSTIS INFECTION

***Pneumocystis* infection** is caused by the unclassified organism *Pneumocystis carinii.* Although *Pneumocystis* usually is described as a protozoan parasite, analysis of the organism's ribosomal RNA shows a closer relationship to fungi than to protozoa.

Transmission

The mode of transmission is presumed to be by inhalation of droplets containing organisms. The organism is widespread and exposure must be extremely common. Overt infections in older children and adults may represent reactivation of infection, which was initially asymptomatic. *Pneumocystis* is an opportunistic organism that does not produce symptomatic infection in normal, healthy individuals.

Geographic Distribution and Epidemiology

The organism is found worldwide and probably occurs as an asymptomatic infection early in life in most populations. Serologic studies show that 75% of children have antibody by the age of 4. Overt disease occurred in the past in outbreaks among malnourished, premature infants. *Pneumocystis* pneumonia still is associated with prematurity, but immunocompromised individuals are at greatest risk. In the United States, over 60% of patients with AIDS develop pnemocystis pneumonia. Although *Pneumocystis* organisms are found in a wide variety of domestic and wild animals, they are different immunologically from *P. carinii* found in humans. It is unlikely that animals are a significant source of human infection.

Habitat

The organisms are found in the pulmonary alveoli.

Properties of the Organism

The organism develops and reproduces extracellularly. Organisms that are phagocytized by macrophages are destroyed. The forms of the organism seen in the lung are the cyst and the trophozoite. The thick-walled cyst is about 5–12 μ in diameter (Fig. 60.2A,B). It contains up to eight intracystic bodies, each with a stainable nucleus (Fig. 60.2A). The trophozoite is ovoid, measures about 2–4 μ in diameter, and has a simple nucleus. *P. carinii* is able to attach tightly to type 1 pneumocytes. The alveoli become filled with a foamy material containing many organisms. In premature infants, there is thickening of the alveolar septae and an infiltrate of plasma cells. In older children and adults, there is interstitial edema

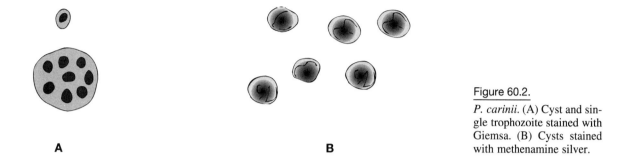

A   **B**

Figure 60.2.
P. carinii. (A) Cyst and single trophozoite stained with Giemsa. (B) Cysts stained with methenamine silver.

and infiltration with neutrophils and lymphocytes, but there is no plasma cell infiltrate.

Clinical Manifestations

Those at risk for *Pneumocystis* pneumonia are premature infants, congenital immunodeficiencies, malnourished children, AIDS patients, and individuals receiving immunosuppressive treatment for cancer, tissue transplants, or other conditions.

Symptoms in older children and adults tends to be abrupt with fever, tachypnea, dry cough, and cyanosis with progressive respiratory failure. The onset of the illness in infants and AIDS patients may be more insidious without fever. Chest X-rays usually show a diffuse alveolar infiltrate, but atypical presentations are frequent in AIDS patients.

Laboratory Diagnosis

Specimens may be obtained by a variety of techniques for examination for the organisms. Sputum induced by a saline mist gives a fairly high yield in AIDS patients, but may be inadequate in other situations. A more invasive technique may be necessary, such as bronchoscopy with brochoalveolar lavage or transbronchial needle biopsy. Open lung biopsy may be necessary in a few patients. Material obtained by these methods should be stained with Gomori methenamine silver stain. This stain makes cysts stand out as black structures. Giemsa stain will demonstrate trophozoites and intracystic bodies, but is much more difficult to interpret. Serologic tests may be useful in epidemiologic studies, but they are not yet sufficiently refined to be helpful in the clinical illness.

Treatment

Infections are usually treated initially with a combination of trimethoprim and sulfamethoxazole. Several other dihydrofolate reductase inhibitors are also being used alone or in combination with sulfas or sulfone. Pentamidine and eflornithine are also useful. Inhalation of aerosolized pentamidine has been found to be an effective treatment and prophylaxis in AIDS patients. Prophylactic regimens are recommended in HIV infected patients with low CD4+ lymphocyte counts even before their first episode of *Pneumocystis* pneumonia. Another treatment regimen includes a combination of the antimalarial primaquine and the antibiotic clindamycin. The new antiprotozoal drug atovaquone also shows promise.

SUMMARY

1. Toxoplasmosis is caused by *Toxoplasma gondii*. Infection is acquired by ingestion of oocysts from cat feces or by ingestion of tissue cysts in rare or raw meat.

2. In humans, the organisms occur in two forms, the tachyzoite and the cyst. The organisms may infect any nucleated cell and are commonly found in skeletal muscle, lymph nodes, brain, and retina.

3. Cats are definitive hosts for *T. gondii*. Stages develop in the intestinal epithelium that result in the production of infectious oocysts in the cat's feces. A wide variety of mammals and birds are susceptible to infection.

4. Acquired toxoplasmosis is usually asymptomatic. The most common clinical manifestations are (1) localized lymphadenopathy, (2) an infectious mononucleosis-like syndrome, (3) cerebral involvement in immunosuppressed individuals. Retinochoroiditis infrequently occurs in acute acquired infection, but is usually a late manifestation of congenital infection.

5. Congenital toxoplasmosis may develop when a woman acquires an acute infection during pregnancy.

6. Clinical features of congenital disease may include retinochoroiditis, encephalomyelitis, hydrocephalus or microcephaly, and intracerebral calcifications and seizures.

7. Diagnosis of toxoplasmosis usually relies on serologic tests. The detection of IgM or IgA antibody indicates an acute infection.

8. Toxoplasmosis is treated with a combination of pyrimethamine and sulfa compounds.

9. *Pneumocystis carinii* causes pneumonia in immunocompromised individuals, such as AIDS patients, premature infants, malnourished children, patients undergoing immunosuppressive therapy, and in children with congenital immunodeficiencies.

10. *P. carinii* is seen in the pulmonary alveoli as thick-walled cysts with intracystic bodies and as trophozoites.

11. The illness may be abrupt or insidious in onset. Fever and difficulty breathing are common symptoms. Death from progressive pulmonary failure usually occurs in untreated patients.

12. Diagnosis is made by Gomori methenamine silver stain of sputum, bronchoalveolar lavage fluid, needle biopsy material, or open lung biopsy for the characteristic cysts. Giemsa stain is necessary to detect intracystic bodies or trophozoites.

13. Treatment of *Pneumocystis* infection is usually with a combination of trimethoprim and sulfamethoxazole or with pentamidine. Prophylaxis is used in AIDS patients and in HIV infected patients with low CD4 ± lymphocyte counts.

REFERENCES

Cook GC (1990): *Toxoplasma gondii* infection: a potential danger to the unborn fetus and AIDS sufferer. Q J Med 74:3.

Davey RT Jr, Masur H (1990): Recent advances in the diagnosis, treatment, and prevention of *Pneumocystis carinii* pneumonia. Antimicrob Agents Chemother 34:499.

Dubey JP, Beattie CP (1988): Toxoplasmosis of Animals and Man. Boca Raton, FL: CRC Press.

Frenkel JK (1990): Toxoplasmosis in human beings. J Am Vet Med Assoc 196:240.

Glatt AE, Chirgwin K (1990): *Pneumocystis carinii* pneumonia in human immunodeficiency virus-infected patients. Arch Int Med 150:271.

Gutierrez Y (1989): The biology of *Pneumocystis carinii*. Semin Diagn Pathol 6:203.

Hopkin JM, Wakefield AE (1993): Molecular and cell biology of opportunistic infections in AIDS. *Pneumocystis carinii*. Mol Cell Biol Hum Dis Ser 2:187.

McCabe R, Chirurgi V (1993): Issues in toxoplasmosis. Infect Dis Clin North Am 7:587.

Walzer PD, Cushion MT (1989): Immunobiology of *Pneumocystis carinii*. Pathol Immunopathol Res 8:127.

REVIEW QUESTIONS

> For questions 1 to 5, choose the ONE
> BEST answer or completion.

1. The diagnosis of acute toxoplasmosis may be based on the following, *except*
   a) the demonstration of IgM or IgA antibody to *Toxoplasma* in an adult
   b) the demonstration of IgM or IgA antibody to *Toxoplasma* in a newborn
   c) the demonstration of positive immunofluorescent test on brain biopsy from AIDS patients
   d) the demonstration of organisms by animal inoculation from lymph node biopsy of an adult
   e) the demonstration of organisms by animal inoculation from lymph node biopsy of newborn

2. A 30-year-old pregnant woman with a history of enlarged lymph nodes caused by toxoplasmosis 5 years previously is found to have IgG antibody to *Toxoplasma* during the first trimester of her pregnancy. She should
   a) be counseled that the fetus is at high risk of severe infection and termination of the pregnancy should be considered
   b) be started on treatment to protect the fetus from infection
   c) undergo sampling of the amniotic fluid to determine if the fetus is infected

d) be counseled to continue with the pregnancy because there is no risk to the fetus
   e) be counseled to continue with the pregnancy but have the newborn tested immediately for congenital toxoplasmosis

3. The following groups are at high risk of acquiring *Pneumocystis* pneumonia, *except*
   a) the fetuses of pregnant women exposed to *Pneumocystis* during pregnancy
   b) children with congenital immunodeficiencies
   c) premature infants
   d) AIDS patients
   e) individuals receiving immunosuppressive treatment

4. The following statements about *Pneumocystis carinii* are true, *except*
   a) the organism is probably a fungus
   b) the cysts stain with Gomori methenamine silver stain
   c) the intracystic bodies and trophozoites stain with Giemsa stain
   d) lymphadenopathy is common in the acute disease
   e) prophylactic treatment is used in many AIDS patients

5. The most common manifestation of reactivation toxoplasmosis in AIDS patients is
   a) pulmonary infection

b) generalized lymph node infection
c) central nervous system infection

d) cardiac infection
e) retinal infection

ANSWERS TO REVIEW QUESTIONS

---

1. *d* Many adults have chronic, asymptomatic toxoplasmosis. Recovering parasites from lymph nodes does not indicate that the illness is acute toxoplasmosis. Demonstration of organisms in the newborn is evidence of congenital infection as is the finding of IgM or IgA antibody. High levels of IgM or IgA antibody in an adult are diagnostic of acute infection. Demonstration of organisms on brain biopsy in an AIDS patient is evidence of *Toxoplasma* as the cause of CNS abnormalities.

2. *d* The patient has protective antibody from her previous infection. The fetus is not at risk of congenital infection.

3. *a* There is no risk to the fetus. If the pregnant woman is healthy, there is no risk for her even though she is exposed to individuals with *Pneumocystis* pneumonia.

4. *d* *Pneumocystis* infection is a pulmonary infection. Lymphadenopathy is not a feature of the disease.

5. *c* Patients receiving immunosuppressive therapy and AIDS patients are at high risk for reactivation of toxoplasmosis in the CNS. Pulmonary, cardiac, retinal, and generalized infections may occur but are not as common as CNS involvement.

ARTHROPODS

Some species of arthropods act as pests by biting or stinging; some may also serve as vectors for certain viral, bacterial, rickettsial, and parasitic infections. Other species may be true parasites that spend part of their life cycle developing in human tissues. The following text is a synopsis of some commonly seen conditions caused by arthropods. The text is summarized in tabular form in Table 61.1. The role of arthropods as vectors will not be discussed.

MITES

Scabies is caused by the itch mite, *Sarcoptes scabiei.*

Transmission

The infestation is acquired by direct contact with infested skin or with contaminated clothing or bedding.

Geographic Distribution and Epidemiology

Scabies is found worldwide with higher prevalence rates associated with crowded conditions and poor hygiene. Animals also have species of scabies mites that may cause transient rashes in humans, but they do not establish chronic infestations.

Location

In burrows in the upper layers of the epidermis.

Properties of the Organism

Adult mites burrow in the superficial layers of the epidermis. The females measure about 0.5 mm in diameter (Fig. 61.1) and the males are considerably smaller. The female deposits eggs in the burrows. The eggs hatch in about 3–4 days, and the newly hatched larvae also burrow in the skin and mature to adults within 4 days.

Clinical Manifestations

The areas most commonly affected are interdigital webs, the genitalia, the umbilicus, the areolae, the axillary folds, the extensor areas over the elbows and knees, and the flexor area of the wrists. The initial lesions are small, erythematous papules or vesicles that represent an allergic reaction to the mite's secretions. The lesions are intensely pruritic, and excoriation and secondary bacterial infection of excoriations is common. Many infestations will resolve spontaneously over a period of months, but some become chronic and may persist for years. In immunosuppressed individuals, a generalized scaling and crusting dermatitis called **Norwegian scabies** may develop.

Laboratory Diagnosis

Close observation of the skin with a hand lens may reveal the characteristic burrows. The diagnosis is made by scraping the skin lesions and demonstrating the mites or eggs in the scrapings.

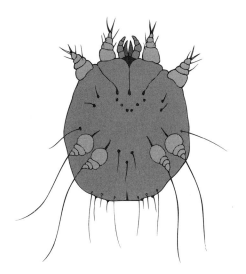

Figure 61.1.
Adult female *S. scabiei*.

Treatment

Lindane, crotamiton, and benzyl benzoate have been widely used, but the effectiveness of these compounds appears to be diminishing. Permethrin cream (5%) is highly effective.

Mite Dermatitis Caused by Species Other Than *Sarcoples scabiei*

Chigger bites are caused by species of trombiculid mites. The six-legged larvae of these mites attach to the skin and suck tissue fluids. The saliva from these mites causes an intensely pruritic inflammatory reaction that appears as a maculopapular lesion. The lesions tend to be located in areas where the clothing is tight, such as ankles, groin, waistline, and armpits. The eight-legged adult mites are not parasitic. Treatment is symptomatic.

Several species of mites may cause dermatitis in humans. Mites of rats, mice, and chickens have this potential as do mites that contaminate cheese, straw, and a variety of substances.

Mites Causing Allergy

The common allergy to house dust is, in fact, sensitivity to mites that feed on organic debris in the dust. The most common manifestation is asthma.

LICE

Pediculosis is caused by three species of louse: *Pediculus humanus humanus* (also called *Pediculus humanus corporis*), the body louse; *Pediculus humanus capitis,* the head louse; and *Pthirus pubis,* the crab louse or pubic louse.

Transmission

Louse infestations are usually acquired by direct contact. The sharing of clothing can transmit the body louse. The head louse may also be transmitted by the sharing of contaminated combs. Sexual contact is the common mode of transmission for the pubic louse.

Geographic Distribution

Infestation with the body louse is found worldwide in populations where crowding and poor personal hygiene are common. These conditions apply particularly to refugee populations. Louse infestations and louse-borne diseases have always been associated with wars and the populations displaced by the wars. Head louse infestations are common in children aged 3–10 years, regardless of good hygiene. Prevalence rates in schools in the United States range from 10 to 40%.

Habitat

P. h. humanus lives in clothing and intermittently feeds on the skin; *P. h. capitis* lives in the hair of the scalp; and *P. pubis* lives in the hair about the genitalia, but may also infest the hair of the axilla and the eyelashes.

Properties of the Organism

Lice are insects. The body louse and the head louse are about 2–3 mm in length (Fig. 61.2A). The pubic louse is about 2 mm in diameter and is oval in shape (Fig. 61.2B). With its clawlike legs and rounded body, it resembles a miniature crab. The body louse lives in clothing of the host and lays eggs (nits) along the seams of the material. The head louse and the pubic louse glue their nits to

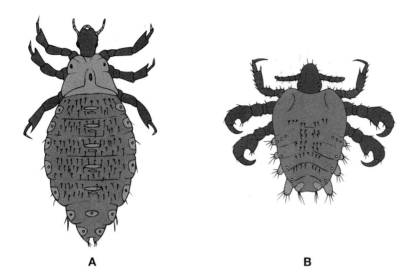

Figure 61.2.
Lice. (A) *P. humanus*. (B) *P. pubis*.

A   B

the hair shafts. Nymphs hatch from the eggs and mature to adults. The cycle takes about 1 month. Both nymphs and adults feed on blood.

Clinical Manifestations

Hemorrhagic macules or papules develop at the site of the bites. Pruritus and excoriation are common.

Laboratory Diagnosis

Adult lice or nits are seen in the hair or on clothing.

Treatment

Head lice are effectively treated with lindane, natural pyrethrins synergized with piperonyl butoxide, or permethrin. Body louse infestations require treatment of clothing with insecticide or drycleaning. The patient must also be treated with lindane or pyrethroids. Pubic lice infestations respond to the compounds noted above, but require retreatment after 10 days to eliminate the organisms.

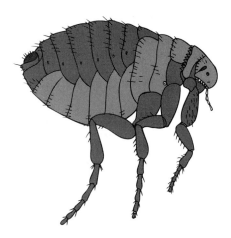

Figure 61.3.
Adult flea.

FLEAS

Fleas serve as vectors of several diseases and as pests because of their irritating bites (Fig. 61.3). The chigoe flea, *Tunga penetrans,* is a true parasite of humans and other mammals during a phase of its life cycle. Chigoe flea infestation is found in tropical Africa, South, and Central America. The infestation is acquired by contact with soil containing the adult fleas. The adult female flea burrows into the skin, usually beneath the toenail or elsewhere in the skin of the feet. The gravid female enlarges to the size of a pea and begins discharging eggs from her swollen abdomen. Eggs that reach the soil, develop into larvae, pupae and, eventually adults. The lesions contain a characteristic black spot, which is in the center of the posterior end of the female flea. Surgical removal of the gravid flea is the appropriate treatment. Secondary bacterial infection of the lesions is a common complication.

MYIASIS (FLY LARVA INFESTATION)

There are many species of fly that may infest human tissues in the larval stage causing **myiasis.** Some species require a mammalian host for larval development, others may deposit eggs in open sores or wounds as an alternative to decaying animal or vegetable material. The human bot fly, *Dermatobia hominis,* provides an example of cutaneous myiasis. The fertilized adult female fly attaches her eggs to the abdomen of a blood sucking fly or mosquito. When the fly or mosquito bites, the eggs hatch and larvae drop onto the skin. The larvae penetrate the skin and develop. A furuncle forms about each larva. This is a painful, red, nodular, boil-like lesion with a small central opening through which the larva obtains oxygen. After about 40 days, the larva emerges, falls to the ground, and pupates. The adult fly emerges from the pupa. The treatment for this condition is the application of an occlusive material, such as cellulose tape, to the opening. Later, the dead or dying larva may be extracted easily from the lesion with forceps.

Other common infestations with fly larvae occur with the Tumbu fly *(Cordylobia anthropophaga)* in Africa and the sheep nasal bot fly *(Oestrus ovis)* in rural sheep-raising areas throughout the world. The Tumbu fly larvae produce cutaneous lesions similar to those of the human bot fly noted above. The sheep nasal bot fly deposits larvae in the nose or conjunctiva where local irritation and inflammation develop. Human infections are usually conjunctival and this condition is called **ophthalmomyiasis.**

BITES AND STINGS

Many different arthropods cause disease in humans because of reactions to bites or stings. The substances introduced into the human body by the bite or sting may be directly toxic (e.g., black widow spider venom), or it may cause problems because of local allergy (flea and mosquito bites) or systemic allergy (bee stings or kissing bug bites). A few of these reactions are listed below.

1. Bee, wasp, and fire ant stings produce local reactions to the venom. Large numbers of stings may produce systemic reactions. Systemic allergic reactions are the usual cause of fatalities attributed to these stings.

2. Centipede bites, spider bites, and scorpion stings produce illness by the toxic effects of their venom. The severity of the reaction is variable depending on the species, the location of the bite, and the amount of venom injected. Children and debilitated individuals are at risk for the most severe reactions. Specific and polyvalent antivenins are available for use in treatment for many forms of envenomization. The bite of the black widow spider, *Latrodectus mactans,* is painless but may be followed by painful muscle cramping and rigidity and other systemic symptoms. Analgesics, calcium gluconate, and muscle relaxants are used in treatment. The violin spiders or brown spiders (*Loxosceles* spp.) may cause severe, progressive, necrotizing skin lesions (**necrotic arachnidism),** and in some instances, severe and even fatal systemic reactions. Antivenin is not availble to treat this condition. Local and systemic corticosteroids have been used in treatment, but their value is uncertain. Large lesions may require skin grafting procedures.

3. Tick paralysis is caused by toxin in the saliva of species of hard ticks

TABLE 61.1. Arthropods

Disease	Organism	Transmission	Location of organism	Clinical manifestations	Laboratory diagnosis	Treatment
Scabies	*Sarcoptes scabiei*	Direct contact with infested skin	Superficial epidermis	Pruritus, papules and vesicles	Examination of skin scrapings for mites and eggs	Topical permethrin, lindane, or crotamiton
Pediculosis	*Pediculus humanus humanus* (body louse)	Contaminated clothing, close contact	Clothing	Pruritic, hemorrhagic macules, or papules	Examination of clothing for lice and nits	Lindane, permethrin, treatment of clothing
Pediculosis	*Pediculus humanus capitis* (head louse)	Close contact, sharing combs	Scalp hair	Pruritic, hemorrhagic macules, or papules	Examination of hair for lice and nits	Lindane, permethrin, shampoos or rinses
Pubic pediculosis	*Pthirus pubis* (pubic or crab louse)	Sexual intercourse	Pubic hair	Pruritic, hemorrhagic macules, or papules	Examination of pubic hair for lice and nits	Lindane, permethrin
Chigoe flea infestation	*Tunga penetrans* (chigoe flea)	Skin contact with soil containing adult fleas	Beneath the toenail, skin of the feet	Irritating swellings surrounded by inflammation	Black spot in center of the lesion	Surgical removal
Cutaneous myiasis	*Dermatobia hominis* (human bot fly)	Larvae hatch from eggs attached to biting flies or mosquitoes	Skin	Painful, erythematous, nodular lesion with central opening	Appearance of lesion, identification of removed larva	Extraction after occlusive dressing

Condition	Organism	Source/Transmission	Location	Clinical features	Diagnosis	Treatment
Cutaneous myiasis	*Cordylobia anthropophaga* (tumbu fly)	Larvae in soil or clothing penetrate unbroken skin	Skin	Pruritic, erythematous, nodular lesion with central opening	Appearance of lesion, identification of removed larva	Extraction after occlusive dressing
Ophthalmomyiasis	*Oestrus ovis* (sheep nasal bot fly)	Fly deposits larvae in conjunctivae	Conjunctival sac	Conjunctivitis	Examination of the conjunctivae for larvae	Removal of larvae
Black widow arachnidism	*Latrodectus mactans* (black widow spider)	Bite	Bites are usually on exposed skin	Painful muscle cramps and rigidity	Examination of spider	Analgesic, muscle relaxant
Necrotic arachnidism	*Loxoceles* spp. (brown or violin spider)	Bite	Bites are usually on exposed skin	Enlarging necrotic ulcer at bite site	Examination of spider	Local and systemic steroids, surgical removal of lesion
Tick paralysis	Hard tick	Attachment of tick	Ticks may attach to skin in any location	Progressive paralysis	Recognition of tick	Removal of tick
Nasopharyngeal pentastomiasis	*Linguatula serrata*	Ingestion of nymphs in raw lymph nodes or liver of sheep, goats or cattle	Nasopharynx	Pain, coughing, sneezing, vomiting, nasal discharge	Examination of naso-pharynx for nymphs	Removal of nymphs
Visceral pentastomiasis	*Armillifer* species	Ingestion of eggs in water, vegetation or raw snake	Liver, spleen, peritoneal cavity, pleura, or lung	Inadequate information, often an incidental finding	Surgical removal, C-shaped calcification on x-ray	Treatment not usually required

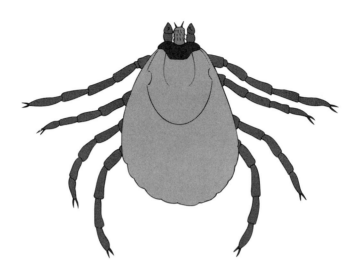

Figure 61.4.
Adult hard tick.

(Fig. 61.4). Progressive paralysis usually begins in the lower extremities, ascends to involve the upper extremities, and may compromise respiration. Removal of the tick results in recovery.

4. Mosquitos, fleas, mites, lice, and many blood-sucking arthropods cause an irritating dermatitis, which is a local allergic reaction to the bites. The kissing bugs (reduviid or cone-nosed bugs) may produce systemic allergic reactions.

PENTASTOMES

Pentastomes are placed in a separate phylum. These organisms share features of arthropods and annelids and are referred to as "tongue worms" because of their tonguelike shape. Infection with any species of pentostome is referred to as pentastomiasis. Nasopharyngeal infections, caused by *Linguatula serrata,* occur in North Africa, the Middle East, and the Sudan. The disease is acquired from the ingestion of raw lymph nodes or liver of sheep, goats, or cattle that contain the nymphal stage. The nymphs migrate to the tissues of the nasopharynx where their attachment causes local pain, coughing, sneezing, vomiting, and nasal discharge. There may be swelling of the face. Mechanical removal of the attached parasites is necessary.

Visceral infections are caused by species of *Armillifer.* Infections are reported from the Middle East, Africa, and Southeast Asia. It is believed that infection is acquired from the ingestion of water or aquatic plants that are contaminated with eggs of the parasite. Ingestion of raw snake also may cause infection. Snakes harbor the adult organisms and eggs in their respiratory tracts. Ingestion of the eggs by a human leads to the development of nymphs that migrate and encyst in the viscera. Encysted nymphs may be found in the liver, spleen, peritoneal cavity, pleura, or lung. There is little information on the clinical manifestations of infection. Most cases are diagnosed by the accidental finding of the nymphs at surgery, or the presence of the characteristic C-shaped calcification on X-ray.

SUMMARY

1. **The major features of arthropods are summarized in Table 61.1.**

2. **Arthropod bites and stings cause disease by toxic reactions to venom or by allergy to venom or secretions.**

REFERENCES

Blankenship ML (1990): Mite dermatitis other than scabies. Dermatol Clin 8:265.

Drabick JJ (1987): Pentastomiasis. Rev Infect Dis 9:1087.

Elgart GW (1990): Ant, bee, and wasp stings. Dermatol Clin 8:229.

Elgart ML (1990): Flies and myiasis. Dermatol Clin 8:237.

Goddard J (1993): Physician's Guide to Anthropods of Medical Importance. Boca Raton, FL: CRC Press.

Meinking TL, Taplin D (1990): Advances in pediculosis, scabies, and other mite infestations. Adv Dermatol 5:131.

Orkin M, Maibach HI (eds) (1985): Cutaneous Infestations and Insect Bites. New York: Marcel Dekker.

Wilson DC, King LE Jr (1990): Spiders and spider bites. Dermatol Clin 8:277.

REVIEW QUESTIONS

For questions 1 to 8, a list of lettered options is followed by several numbered items. For each numbered item, select the ONE lettered option that is most closely associated with it. Each lettered option may be selected once, more than once, or not at all.

A) *Sarcoptes scabiei*
B) Body louse
C) Head louse
D) Crab louse
E) Pentastomes
F) *Dermatobia hominis*
G) Black widow spider
H) Violin spider
I) Chigoe flea
J) Tick

For the statements or definitions below, select the appropriate term or organism.

1. Its bite causes necrotic ulcerations of the skin.

2. It deposits eggs in the seams of clothing.

3. Gravid females often found under the toenail.

4. Some species are associated with a paralytic condition.

5. It lives in the pubic hair.

6. Its bite causes painful muscle spasms.

7. It is transmitted by direct contact with infested skin, and it burrows in the epidermis causing pruritic lesions.

8. The organism causes cutaneous myiasis.

ANSWERS TO REVIEW QUESTIONS

1. **H** The violin spider or brown spider causes ulceration of skin at the site of the spider bite. The condition is called necrotic arachnidism.

2. **B** The body louse, *Pediculus humanus humanus,* deposits eggs on the seams of clothing.

3. **I** The chigoe flea, *Tunga penetrans,* usually enters the skin of the feet, often under the toenails.

4. **J** The secretions of certain hard ticks may cause tick paralysis.

5. **D** The crab louse or pubic louse, *Pthirus pubis,* lives in the pubic hair.

6. **G** Black widow spider bite may cause painful muscle spasms.

7. **A** *Sarcoptes scabiei* is transmitted by direct contact. The adult mites burrow in the epidermis causing the pruritic skin lesions of scabies.

8. **F** *Dermatobia hominis,* causes cutaneous myiasis (fly larva infestation of the skin).

GLOSSARY

Acid-fast stain: A differential staining procedure that identifies bacteria as members of the genera *Mycobacterium* and *Nocardia*. The procedure is a valuable aid in the diagnosis of mycobacterial diseases and nocardiosis.

Acidophile: A bacterium that requires very low pH conditions for growth.

Acrodermatitis chronica atrophicans (ACA): A sclerotic or atrophic skin lesion that may occur during the development of chronic disseminated Lyme borreliosis. It occurs more commonly in Europe than in the United States.

Active immunoprophylaxis: See **Immunoprophylaxis.**

Acute urethral syndrome: Symptomatic infection of the genitourinary tract of sexually active females characterized by pyuria and very low colony counts of bacteria.

Adhesin: Host cellular or microbial external structure (often an antigenic substance such as a protein) that mediates attachment to a substrate surface or another cell.

Aerobes: Cells that are able to utilize oxygen as a terminal electron acceptor; practically, those that can grow in room air.

Agent of spongiform encephalitis: As **Prion.**

A⁻H⁻U⁻ auxotrophs: Strains of gonococci that require arginine, hypoxanthine, and uracil for growth. Most of these strains are associated with gonococcal dissemination.

Ail (adherence invasion locus) gene: A chromosomal gene that encodes for a small molecular weight outer membrane protein present on the surface of *Yersinia enterocolitica* that contributes to adherence and cell entry.

Alcohol fermentation: Fermentation that results in ethanol formation from glucose.

Algid malaria: A complication of falciparum malaria consisting of vascular collapse and shock associated with a fall in body temperature.

Alginate: Extracellular polysaccharide mucoid "slime" produced by *Pseudomonas aeruginosa;* most closely associated with those strains that colonize cystic fibrosis patients.

Alkalophile: A bacterium that requires very high pH conditions for growth.

Alopecia: Loss of hair.

Alpha hemolysis: A partial lysis of erythrocytes by bacteria on blood agar plates. The reaction manifests as a green zone around the colonies.

Amastigote: The intracellular form of *Leishmania* species and *Trypanosoma cruzi* found in the human and reservoir hosts. The flagellum does not extend beyond the margin of the parasite and is inconspicuous.

Ameboma: A localized mass lesion or colonic wall thickening caused by *Entamoeba histolytica*.

Aminoglycoside: Class of antibiotics bactericidal to numerous aerobic bacteria by multiple mechanisms that require careful dosing and monitoring because of small differences between effective and toxic doses.

Anaerobes: Cells that do not require oxygen as a terminal electron acceptor for energy metabolism.

Anamorph: The somatic or reproductive structures of the asexual form of fungal growth.

Annellide: A conidiogenous fungal cell that produces conidia successively and bears multiple scars around the tip left by the released conidia. The tip of the annellide lengthens as more conidia are produced.

Annelloconidium: An enteroblastic conidium produced by a conidiogenous fungal cell called an annellide.

Antagonism: The effectiveness of one chemotherapeutic agent diminishes that of another agent when both are administered together.

Anthropophilic: To grow preferentially on humans rather than other animals.

Anti-DNase B (ADB) assay: An assay that measures the presence of antibody directed against DNase B as a measure of recent group A streptococcal infection. Sensitivity is greater than the ASO test in the diagnosis of group A streptococcal skin diseases. The test is a valuable adjunct in the diagnosis of the late sequelae of group A streptococci, namely, rheumatic fever and acute hemorrhagic glomerulonephritis.

Antibiotic: Substance produced by a fungus or bacterium that inhibits growth of other microorganisms. See **Antimicrobial** and **Chemotherapeutic agents.**

Antigenic drift: A point mutation that results in a change in the configuration of a specific epitope on the surface of a specific virion. Antibodies reactive against the epitope before the change are now less reactive against the changed epitope.

Antigenic shift: The replacement of a gene by an allele that results in a complete change in the configuration of a specific epitope on the surface of a virion. Antibodies reactive against the epitope before the change are now totally unreactive against the changed epitope.

Antimicrobial agent: Substance that either kills, inhibits, or prevents damage due to an infectious microorganism. See **Antibiotic** and **Chemotherapeutic agent.**

Antisepsis: The destruction or prevention of growth of pathogenic or potentially pathogenic microorganisms by chemical means. Usually refers to the external application of a chemical to tissues.

Anti-Streptolysin O (ASO) assay: An assay that measures the presence of antibody directed against Streptolysin O as a measure of recent group A streptococcal infection. The test serves as a valuable adjunct in the diagnosis of the late sequelae of group A streptococci, namely, rheumatic fever and acute hemorrhagic glomerulonephritis.

Apicomplexa: Intracellular protozoan parasites, characterized by organelles organized into an apical complex. The organelles are used in penetrating host cells.

Arthroconidium: A thallic conidium released by the fungus at maturity by fragmentation. (Also referred to as an arthrospore by some.)

Asaccharolytic: Cells that are unable to utilize sugars (glucose, sucrose) for energy metabolism.

Ascomycete: A fungus belonging to the phylum Ascomycota.

Ascospore: Sexual spores produced in an ascus. Characteristic of the Ascomycetes.

Attachment sites: Specific epitopes on the surface of a virion that can bind onto configuratively complementary epitopes on the cell surface. This binding initiates the virus replication cycle.

Attenuated vaccine: A vaccine composed of microorganisms treated in such a manner that they are no longer capable of producing disease, yet are still vaccinogenic and capable of growth and multiplication.

"Atypical" mycobacteria: Opportunistic or frank pathogens comprising four groups of *Mycobacteria* with characteristics different from *Mycobacterium tuberculosis* and *M. bovis.* They are thought to be transmissible from the environment, are not transmissible from human to human, and are difficult to treat effectively. Disseminated disease due to group III organisms (*M. avium-intracellulare* complex or MAC) in AIDS patients is of considerable concern.

Autoclave: An apparatus considered to be the most effective, practical, and common method of sterilization. The principle of operation is based upon the creation of high temperatures under steam pressure.

Autointerference: Progeny virions released from an infected cell are frequently a mixture of defective and nondefective virions. When another cell is infected simultaneously by both the defective and nondefective virions, the defective one interferes with replication of the nondefective one. See **Defective interfering particles.**

Bacillus of Calmette and Guerin (BCG) vaccine: A vaccine against tuberculosis consisting of a live, attenuated strain of *Mycobacterium bovis.* It has been used with variable degrees of success in countries where the prevalence of tuberculosis is high.

Bacteremia: Presence of bacteria in the bloodstream.

Bactericidal agent: Agent that kills microorganisms.

Bacteriocin: Substance produced by a strain or species of bacteria that inhibits growth of or destroys another strain.

Bacteriostatic agent: Agent that prevents the growth and multiplication of microorganisms.

Bacteriuria: Presence of bacteria in the urine. May or may not be associated with pyuria or symptomatic disease.

Baermann technique: A method of concentrating larvae of *Strongyloides stercoralis* from feces using a funnel filled with water.

Basidiomycete: A fungus belonging to the phylum Basidiomycota.

Basidiospore: A sexual spore produced on a basidium characteristic of the Basidiomycetes.

Benign gummas: Destructive, granulomatous lesions of the skin, bone, and viscera during the tertiary stage of syphilis. Spirochetes are rarely, if ever, found in the lesions.

Beta hemolysis: Complete lysis of erythrocytes by bacteria on blood agar plates. The reaction manifests as a clear zone around the colonies.

β-lactam: Antibiotic class that kills bacteria by interfering with cell wall synthesis. Based on a core structure similar to that of penicillin.

Bilious remittent fever: A complication of falciparum malaria consisting of impairment of liver function and the presence of marked jaundice.

Biologic vector: Infectious organisms require development or multiplication within the vector before they can be transmitted.

Blackwater fever: A complication of falciparum malaria consisting of massive hemolysis resulting in hemoglobinuria.

Blastic: Conidium formation by the blowing out of the fertile hyphae.

Blastoconidium: An asexual reproductive element formed by budding (called a blastospore by some).

Bradyzoite: The form of *Toxoplasma gondii* that develops within tissue cysts.

Brood capsule: The cystlike structures that originate from the germinal membrane of hydatid cysts. The brood capsule contains protoscoleces.

Bubo: Inflamed and swollen lymph gland (adnexal or inguinal), adjacent to site of bacterial infection.

"C" carbohydrate: Streptococcal wall polysaccharides whose antigenic diversity forms the basis for the classification of streptococci into 20 groups.

C5a peptidase: A surface-bound endopeptidase of most group A streptococci thought to contribute to the virulence of the organism by cleaving the C5a component of complement, resulting in the inability of the molecule to act as a chemoattractant of polymorphonuclear leukocytes to areas of inflammation.

Calabar swellings: Transient, localized subcutaneous edema associated with loiasis.

Capnophilic: Cells that require carbon dioxide concentrations greater than those in room air for optimal growth.

Capsid: The protein shell of a virus.

Capsid symmetry: The arrangement of capsomeres around the viral genome. Icosahedral symmetry refers to the arrangement that results in an icosahedron. Helical symmetry is the arrangement that results in a slender tube.

Capsomeres: Morphologic units that comprise the capsid of a virus.

Capsule: Mucoid structures, usually polysaccharide in nature, that closely surround the cell wall of some microorganisms. They may be antiphagocytic and/or vaccinogenic. Anticapsular antibody may be useful in the rapid identification of some encapsulated bacterial pathogens.

Carbuncle: A lesion resulting from the lateral and deeper extension of *Staphylococcus aureus* from the skin. It is characterized by multiple openings to the surface with pus discharge.

Carrier: A healthy person who is carrying and usually excreting an infectious agent.

Cell-associated virus: Virus that cannot be released from the infected cell.

Cell doubling time: Same as **Cell generation time.**

Cell generation time: The time needed by a cell to form two daughter cells from the mother cell.

Cell-mediated immunity: In tuberculosis, the mechanism in which alveolar macrophages, activated by the lymphokine macrophage activating factor (MAF) released from antigen-sensitized T lymphocytes, phagocytize and digest the organism.

Cell wall: A structure of unique chemical composition that lies in close apposition to the cytoplasmic membrane. It confers rigidity and shape to bacteria by virtue of its peptidoglycan content.

Cercaria: The larval stage of trematodes that leaves the snail intermediate host.

Cerebral malaria: A complication of falciparum malaria associated with cerebral capillary obstruction, brain congestion, and swelling.

Cestode: See **Tapeworm.**

CFU: Colony forming units; refers to numbers of bacterial colonies on agar cultures, each of which started as a single bacterium in the original specimen.

Chancre: A painless, indurated, well-circumscribed ulcer that develops during the primary stage of acquired syphilis.

Chemoprophylaxis: Attempt to prevent a disease or to reduce the severity of a disease by the administration of a specific drug. Preexposure chemoprophylaxis is the administration of the drug before exposure to the infectious agent (e.g., taking amantadine during an influenza epidemic). Taking a drug during incubation of a disease is postexposure chemoprophylaxis (e.g., taking acyclovir after exposure to chicken pox).

Chemotherapeutic agent: Substance, biologically or synthetically derived, used to treat disease (including noninfectious diseases). See **Antibiotic** and **Antimicrobial agent.**

Chlamydoconidium: A thallic conidium often formed internally but may occur terminally or laterally. (Also referred to as a chlamydospore by some.)

Chromatoidal body: Deeply staining bundles of crystalline RNA found in young cysts of the genus *Entamoeba*.

Chronic infection: The persistence of a replicating infectious agent in the host.

Ciliate: A protozoan that moves by the use of cilia which cover the organism's surface. The cilia resemble short flagella in structure and function.

Coagulase: An enzyme of *Staphylococcus aureus* that catalyzes the conversion of plasma fibrinogen to a fibrin clot in the presence of a co-reacting factor.

Co-cultivation: The cultivation of tissues from two sources. It is a sensitive laboratory procedure for detecting virus in latency.

Coenocytic: A cytoplasm containing many nuclei and uninterrupted by septa.

Coinfection: Simultaneous infection of the host by two infectious agents.

Commensalism: In a close association, one organism benefits without harming the host organism.

Common pili: Numerous hairlike, rigid, surface protein appendages originating in the cytoplasmic membrane of predominantly gram-negative bacteria. They may mediate adherence to host cell surfaces and/or exhibit antiphagocytic activity.

Complement: Series of serum proteins involved in mediation of immune reactions.

Complementation: See **Nongenetic interaction.**

Complete medium: A medium that contains each nutrient required for cell growth.

Composite transposon: A type of transposon that consists of a host gene, such as an antibiotic-resistant gene, flanked by insertion sequences.

Conidiogenous cell: The fertile fungal cell from which a conidium develops.

Conidiophore: A hyphal branch that bears conidia.

Conidium: An asexual reproductive propagule.

Conjugation: The exchange of genetic material between two cells through cell-to-cell contact.

Cross-neutralization: A method for determining immunogenic relatedness between two isolates of a virus. Antisera against each of the two isolates are prepared; neutralization titers of each serum against homologous and heterologous isolates are determined and compared.

Cyst: The infectious stage of parasitic protozoa that has a protective cyst wall and is resistant to environmental conditions.

Cysticercoid: The larval stage of *Hymenolepis nana* that consists of a solid structure containing a single inverted scolex.

Cysticercus: The larval stage of *Taenia solium* and *Taenia saginata* consisting of a cystic structure containing fluid and a single scolex.

Cytotoxin: Substance elaborated by microorganisms that damages structure or function of somatic cells of the host organism. An example is leukotoxins, which destroy white blood cells.

Cytokine: Soluble substance secreted by immunologically active cells that affects function of other cells.

Cytostome: A fixed area in the surface of a protozoan that serves as a "cell mouth" where nutrients are ingested.

Dark field microscopy: A form of microscopy in which organisms appear white against a dark background. Spirochetes that do stain poorly or not at all with the usual dyes are best observed in the living state by this method.

Death phase: Phase of cell's life where nutrients are exhausted and the cell dies.

Defective interfering particles: Defective virions that interfere with the replication of homologous virus through competition for a specific functional component which the defective virus lacks.

Defective virus: A virus that lacks one or more functioning genes required for replication.

Definitive host: A host that harbors the adult or sexual form of the parasite.

Deletion mutant: A type of mutation characterized by the loss of a portion of its genome.

Dematiaceous: Dark-colored.

Denticle: Projection upon which conidia or spores are borne.

Dermatophytes: A special group of fungi involved in the dermatophytoses, i.e., ringworm or tinea.

Deuteromycete: A fungus belonging to the phylum Deuteromycota (also known as Fungi Imperfecti).

Diarrhea: Syndrome in which patient suffers from bowel movements of greater frequency or greater volume than is normal for that patient. See **Dysentery.**

Dimorphic: Having two morphological forms, one displayed in the tissue of a host, the other in nature and commonly in cultures in the laboratory.

Diphtheria exotoxin: An extracellular, heat-labile protein of *Corynebacterium diphtheriae* consisting of two polypeptide fragments held together by a disulfide bond. The exotoxin acts by inhibiting protein synthesis at the ribosome level. Fragment B is required for transport into the mammalian cell of enzymatically active fragment A, which catalyzes ADP ribosylation and resultant inactivation of elongation factor (EF)-2.

Diphtheritic pseudomembrane: A well defined, extensive fibrinous exudate that manifests during the pathogenesis of diphtheria as a thick, closely adherent, dirty gray structure covering the pharynx, larynx, tonsils, or skin lesion.

Diphtheroids: Nontoxigenic corynebacteria that occupy the skin, nose, throat, nasopharynx, urinary tract, and conjunctiva of normal individuals. In rare instances, they may produce septicemia in immunosuppressed hospitalized patients resulting in a high case fatality rate due to multiple antibiotic resistance.

Diploid: Containing the double (2n) number of chromosomes (cf. haploid).

Diplopia: Double vision.

Disinfection: The destruction of pathogenic or potentially pathogenic microorganisms by chemical means. Usually refers to the treatment of inanimate objects (fomites).

Disseminated gonococcal infection (DGI) strains: Gonococcal strains mostly of the $A^-H^-U^-$ auxotype and associated with serum resistance and a high degree of penicillin susceptibility.

Dysentery: Gastrointestinal disease characterized by frequent small bowel movements accompanied by cramps, tenesmus (straining), and the presence of blood, mucus, and inflammatory cells in the feces. See **Diarrhea.**

Dysphagia: Difficulty in swallowing.

Dysphonia: Thickness of speech.

Early genes: Genes of DNA viruses are transcribed in blocks. Those that are transcribed right after the uncoating of virus genes are the early genes. Those that are transcribed after early gene products have reached sufficiently high concentrations are the late genes.

Ecthyma gangrenosum: Large (up to 5 cm across) round or oval cutaneous lesions with necrotic centers and erythematous or indurated edges seen in patients with *Pseudomonas aeruginosa* septicemia.

Ectoparasite: A parasite that lives on the surface of the host.

Ectothrix: A sheath of arthroconidia on the outside of a hair shaft.

Electron transport chain: Enzymes and electron carrier components that comprise the respiratory chain.

Electron-transport phosphorylation: Formation of ATP by the ATP synthase that is coupled to the electron transport chain derived electrochemical gradient.

Elementary body: A specialized form of *Chlamydia.*

Elephantiasis: Enlargement of the extremities or scrotum in chronic lymphatic filariasis.

Endemic nephrosis: Nephrosis associated with immune complex disease in *Plasmodium malariae* infections.

Endogenous: Microorganisms that are part of the indigenous microbiota of the intact host.

Endogenous virus: A virus that originates from within a cell. Generally refers to the oncornaviruses that are transmitted from generation to generation through the germ cell as provirus.

Endoparasite: A parasite that lives within the host.

Endosome: See **Karyosome.**

Endospores: Refractile bodies produced by the vegetative cells of *Bacillus* and *Clostridium* species under adverse conditions. They are metabolically inactive, highly resistant to heat and chemicals, and are able to survive many years in the environment.

Endothrix: A cluster of arthroconidia within a hair shaft.

Endotoxin (LPS): Lipopolysaccharide (LPS) component of gram-negative bacterial outer membranes that is released at cell destruction or during normal growth cycles.

Enteroblastic: A blastic conidium in which only the inner wall of the cell becomes the conidial cell wall. The other cell wall layers come to compose the lips of the conidiogenous cell. See **Phialide.**

Enterotoxin: Substance elaborated into the environment by a microorganism that causes damage to structure or function of intestinal epithelial cells involved in fluid and electrolyte transport; action of enterotoxin usually results in diarrhea.

Envelope: The membranous outermost layer of some viruses.

Episomal DNA: Viral DNA that exists as independent molecules rather than integrated with host DNA. See also **Provirus.**

Erysipelas: A group A streptococcal disease usually of the face and lower extremities. Primary disease is characterized by a fiery red, advancing erythema. Dissemination may occur.

Erythema migrans: The initial distinctive characteristic lesion(s) that forms at or near the infected *Ixodes* tick bite site during the pathogenesis of Lyme borreliosis. The macular, then papular lesion(s) gradually expands to form an annular, erythematous lesion that ranges from 5 cm to 70 cm in diameter.

Essential nutrient: A specific compound or nutrient that the cell must be provided.

Eukaryote: A cell with a membrane-bound nucleus (containing several chromosomes) and organelles such as mitochondria.

Exfoliative (epidermolytic) exotoxin: An extracellular product of some strains of *Staphylococcus aureus* responsible for the intraepidermal splitting of tissues and necrosis observed in scalded skin syndrome (SSS).

Exogenous: Infectious agents that are acquired from the environment; not normally found among the indigenous microbiota.

Exotoxin: Substance elaborated into the environment by a microorganism that causes damage to structure or function of affected target organisms or cells.

Exponential phase: Phase of rapid cell growth and division.

F-1 antigen: An "envelope" protein and protein-polysaccharide complex antigen of *Yersinia pestis* that exerts antiphagocytic activity.

Facultative anaerobe: The cell can grow either with or without oxygen present.

Facultative intracellular parasite: Intracellular organisms capable of multiplying in an in vitro acellular environment.

Fastidious nutrition: Need by the cell for numerous essential nutrients.

Fc receptors: Surface bacterial proteins that bind to the Fc domain of mammalian immunoglobulin. A group A streptococcal Fc receptor for human IgG may exhibit antiphagocytic activity during the pathogenesis of primary skin infections.

Fermentation: Anaerobic ATP generating process in which organic substrates are oxidized incompletely to form acids or alcohols.

Fibrinolysin: An extracellular enzyme capable of dissolving fibrin clots.

Fibronectin: Circulating and cell surface-associated glycoprotein that mediates nonspecific adherence of some bacteria (staphylococci), clearance of some circulating host components (fibrin), but may also inhibit attachment of other microorganisms to host cells.

Flagella: Long, slender protein appendages responsible for bacterial motility. They originate from a basal body and hooklike structure within the cytoplasmic membrane of several bacterial and protozoal species.

Flagellate: A protozoan that moves by the use of whiplike structures called flagella.

Flagellum: A whiplike structure used by flagellates for motility.

Flatworm: The term includes flukes (trematodes) and tapeworms (cestodes).

Fluke: Flukes (trematodes), with the exception of the schistosomes, are dorsoventrally flattened, leaf-shaped, hermaphroditic helminths with oral and ventral suckers. Snails are always first intermediate hosts. Eggs are operculated. Schistosomes are cylindrical; the sexes are separate and eggs are not operculated.

Fragment length polymorphism: Digestion of DNA genomes of different virus strains by restriction endonucleases may generate DNA fragments of different lengths; each strain may have a characteristic pattern for fragments. This fragment length polymorphism of a species of virus or bacterium is useful in tracing the source of a virus.

Fungus: A heterotrophic, eukaryotic organism that reproduces asexually or sexually. Possesses a well-defined cell wall typically chitinized and membranes comprised of sterols (e.g., ergosterol).

Furuncle: A painful, indurated, erythematous, single or multiple skin abscess caused by *Staphylococcus aureus*. It is further characterized by a central area of necrosis walled off from surrounding subcutaneous tissue.

Gametocyte: Either the male or female form of the malaria parasite within the RBC.

Gamma hemolysis: No lysis of erythrocytes by bacteria on blood agar plates. The erythrocytes remain intact and there is no change around the colonies.

General recombination: A process that involves the breakage and reunion of two homologous DNA molecules.

Generalized transduction: A type of transduction in which any one host gene has an equal chance of being transduced.

Geophilic: Soil inhabiting.

Germ tube: The initial tubular filament produced by a germinating spore or conidium.

Germicidal: As **Disinfection.**

Ghon complex: Calcified tuberculous lesions, including those in the hilar lymph nodes, at the primary pulmonary sites of infection.

Globi: The numerous packets of *Mycobacterium leprae* found within phagocytic foam cells in lepromatous leprosy.

Gluconeogenesis: Ability of the cell to synthesize glucose from pyruvate.

Glycolysis: Oxidation of glucose to pyruvate by the EMP pathway.

Gonococcal outer membrane protein (OMP) I: Protein I is the major OMP, which is antigenically diverse among strains and functions as a porin in complex with Protein III.

Gonococcal outer membrane protein (OMP) II: Protein II is an ''opacity'' protein that mediates attachment to host cells. Antigenic variation may contribute to the ability of the gonococcus to evade the immune response and cause repeated infection.

Gonococcal outer membrane protein (OMP) III: In addition to its function as a porin with Protein I, Protein III also appears to be the binding site for IgG blocking antibody that prevents complement-mediated bactericidal antibody function and thus may contribute to dissemination.

Gram stain: A differential staining procedure that permits the separation of bacteria into two broad groups, namely, gram-positive and gram-negative. It is useful as a diagnostic aid in the identification of pathogens. The organisms may exhibit differences in virulence factors, disease pathogenesis, and antimicrobial susceptibility.

Half-life: The amount of time required after administration of a chemotherapeutic agent for the serum concentration to fall to one-half of the peak concentration. Agents with short half-lives require more frequent dosing.

Haploid: Containing a single set (n) of chromosomes.

Harada-Mori technique: A method of concentrating larvae of *Strongyloides stercoralis* from feces using strip of filter paper and a small amount of water in a test tube.

Helper virus: A virus that enables a defective virus to replicate by providing the defective one with its missing functional component. See also **Defective virus.**

Hemorrhagic glomerulonephritis: A late sequela of group A streptococci occurring mostly in children one to five weeks after the onset of group A streptococcal pharyngeal or skin disease caused by any of 12 different serotypes. Renal damage is the result of immune complex deposition on the glomerular basement membrane.

Holoblastic: Blastic conidium formation in which all of the wall layers are involved in formation of the conidium wall.

Hyaluronidase: An extracellular enzyme capable of hydrolyzing the hyaluronic acid constituent of connective tissue ground substance and thereby facilitating the spread of organisms through tissue.

Hydatid cyst: The larval stage of *Echinococcus granulosus* consisting of a fluid-filled cystic structure lined with a germinal membrane. Brood capsules containing protoscoleces develop from the germinal membrane.

Hydatid sand: The gritty material from hydatid cysts containing protoscoleces and hooks of protoscoleces.

Hypha: The filament of a fungus that represents a vegetative unit.

Hypnozoite: The form of *Plasmodium vivax* and *P. ovale* that is dormant in liver cells, but when activated, divides and eventually causes relapses of clinical malaria.

Iatrogenic: Unintended byproduct of medical intervention. Example: iatrogenic urinary tract infection occurs after catheterization introduces fecal organisms into the previously sterile bladder.

IgA1 protease: An enzyme produced by the meningococcus and gonococcus that inactivates local secretory IgA and thus may play a role in facilitating adherence to mucosal surfaces.

Immortalization: The acquisition by a mammalian cell of the ability to multiply rapidly and persistently in vitro, usually due to infection by a virus. For example, the immortalization of human B lymphocytes by the EB virus.

Immunoprophylaxis: A procedure for enhancing the host's immunity against a specific infectious agent. Preexposure immunoprophylaxis implies that the procedure is administered to the host before exposure to the infectious agent (e.g., feeding polio vaccine to young infants). In postexposure immunoprophylaxis, the procedure is administered to the host after the host has been exposed to the infectious agent (e.g., the inoculation of rabies vaccine after a bite by a rabid animal). The administration of vaccine or preformed antibodies are referred to, respectively, as active and passive immunoprophylaxis.

Immunotype: The typing of virus isolates by cross-neutralization or equivalent test. Generally, the difference between neutralization titers against homologous and heterologous isolates must be at least 16-fold in order to designate the two isolates as different immunotypes.

Impetigo: A disease syndrome caused by *Staphylococcus aureus* and group A streptococci, alone or in combination, and usually seen in newborns and children. Lesions initiate on the face and are characterized as vesicular, crusting and/or pustular. Dissemination may occur.

Infectious nucleic acid: See **Transfection.**

Insertion mutation: In medical virology, this term usually refers to the integration of viral DNA into a host gene, thereby inactivating the host gene.

Insertion sequence: A type of transposon that consists of a transposase gene flanked by special DNA sequences necessary for its movement.

Interferons: Glycoproteins coded for by host cells. Have antiviral, antiproliferative, and immunologic functions. See also **Virus inhibitory proteins.**

Intermediate host: A host that harbors larval or asexual stages of the parasite.

Inv (invasin) **gene:** A chromosomal gene that encodes for a large molecular weight rare outer membrane protein present on the surface of *Yersinia enterocolitica* and *Y. pseudotuberculosis* that mediates adherence and cell entry.

Inversion: A mechanism that allows a specialized segment of DNA to invert its orientation in the genome.

K antigen: A heat-labile protein, located at the surface of the cell wall of *Corynebacterium diphtheriae*, that exhibits antiphagocytic activity and allows the organism to colonize prior to multiplication and exotoxin production.

Katayama fever: The acute stage of schistosomiasis characterized by fever, malaise, hives, lymphadenopathy, and liver tenderness.

Kinetoplast: An organelle found in *Leishmania* and *Trypanosoma*. It is a modified mitrochondrion containing DNA arranged in minicircles and maxicircles. It is located near the origin of the flagellum.

Lactic acid fermentation: Fermentation that results in lactate formation from glucose.

Lactoferrin: Iron-chelating compound present in neutrophil granules; aids in destruction of bacteria.

Lag phase: Phase of cell metabolism in which cells are preparing for cell biosynthesis and growth.

Laminar flow: A filtration system used to ventilate operating rooms, laboratories, and areas housing immunosuppressed and burn patients. A continual pistonlike displacement of regular circulating air in the area with filtered air is highly effective in reducing the numbers of airborne organisms.

Larva: The immature stages of helminths and arthropods.

Late genes: See **Early genes.**

Latency: A state in which an individual is infected with a microorganism, but exhibits no evidence of disease. In virology, latency usually implies the persistence of a virus in nonreplicating phase.

Latent infection: The persistence of a nonreplicating infectious agent in the host.

Lepromatous leprosy: The type of leprosy in which the organisms proliferate within macrophages (foam cells) at the site of entry and in epithelial tissues. Suppressor T lymphocytes are numerous, epithelioid and giant cells are rare or absent, CMI is impaired, and *Mycobacterium leprae* are numerous in macrophages.

Lepromin: An extract of *Mycobacterium leprae* utilized to determine the delayed type hypersensitivity (DTH) response in patients with leprosy. The method of inoculation and interpretation is the same as that for the tuberculin test (see **Tuberculin test**).

Leucocidin: An exotoxin of *Staphylococcus aureus* that contributes to the survival of the organism during host-parasite confrontation by destroying polymorphonuclear leukocytes.

Lichen: A symbiotic combination of a fungus and an alga; contained in a phylum called Mycophycophyta.

Lipooligosaccharide (LOS): An outer membrane component of meningococci and gonococci. It differs from LPS in that it has shorter, nonrepeat, O-antigenic side chains and thus a lower molecular weight. LOS is responsible for many of the toxic manifestations of disseminated meningococcal disease, attracts polymorphonuclear leukocytes to the primary site of gonococcal infection, and has been implicated as a potential cause of fallopian tube damage in patients with gonococcal salpingitis.

Lipoteichoic acid: A surface component of gram-positive bacteria covalently linked to the cytoplasmic membrane that participates in the adherence of group A streptococci to buccal cell epithelium.

Loeffler's syndrome: Transient pulmonary infiltrates on x-ray associated with peripheral eosinophilia.

Log phase: Same as **Exponential phase.**

LPS: See **Endotoxin.**

Lysogeny: A state in which the bacterial and viral genomes replicate synchronously in a virus-infected bacterium. The virus genome is integrated into the bacterial genome and is not expressed.

M proteins: Surface-exposed molecules of group A streptococci anchored to the cytoplasmic membrane and extending through the cell wall and capsule. It is the major virulence factor of the organism, exhibiting antiphagocytic activity and mediating adherence in concert with lipoteichoic acid. Its antigenic diversity is the basis for the recognition of more than 80 serotypes.

Macroconidium: The larger of two sorts of conidia produced by a single species of fungus.

Macrogametocyte: The female form of the malaria parasite within the RBC.

Matrix protein: Virus-coded protein on the inner surface of the virus envelope.

Mazzotti test: A provocative test for onchocerciasis using a low dose of diethylcarbamazine that causes a rash in infected persons.

Mechanical vector: Transmission of disease by transfer of organisms on body parts or in feces of vector.

Meningococcal outer membrane proteins (OMPs): Antigenically diverse proteins that form the basis for serotyping of meningococci. They also act as porins.

Merozoite: The form of the malaria parasite that results from asexual multiplication within the RBC. It is the form that is released from the mature schizont to infect other RBCs.

Mesosomes: Cytoplasmic membrane invaginations containing circular or tubular structures attached to DNA chromatin. They are thought to be associated with bacterial cell division.

Metacercaria: The larval stage of trematodes that is encysted in second intermediate hosts or on aquatic vegetation. It is infectious for the definitive host.

Microaerophile: The cell requires low oxygen levels for growth.

Microconidium: The smaller of two sorts of conidia produced by a single species of fungus.

Microfilaria: The embryonic worm produced by adult female filarial parasites including *Onchocerca volvulus.*

Microgametocyte: The male form of the malaria parasite within the RBC.

Microsporidia: Protozoa that are characterized by the production of spores containing coiled polar tubes.

Miracidium: The ciliated larva that hatches from the schistosome egg and then enters the snail intermediate host.

Mitogen: A substance that stimulates nonspecifically the proliferation of T lymphocytes.

Mixed-acid fermentation: Fermentation that results in formation of several types of organic acids from glucose.

Monokine: Soluble substance secreted by immunologically active monocytes that affects function of other cells.

Mould (mold): A multicellular fungus whose vegetative growth unit is a hypha. See **Hypha.**

Mycelium: A mass of hyphae constituting the thallus or colony of a fungus.

Necrotic arachnidism: The necrotizing skin lesion caused by the venom of violin spiders.

Necrotizing fasciitis: A rapidly spreading infectious process in which microbes multiply in the subcutaneous soft tissues, usually in the space between muscle sheaths, producing extensive tissue damage.

Negative staining: A procedure that stains the background of microorganisms or viruses, thereby leaving the microorganism contrastingly colorless or the virus components electron-translucent.

Neurotoxin: Substance that interferes with nerve functions, including those in the brain.

Nongenetic interaction: Interaction of virus gene products in a cell infected by two viruses. Genomes of progeny viruses remain unchanged. One example is complementation, where one virus produces a defective gene product and is incapable of replication; another virus provides the defective virus with a nondefective gene product and thereby enables the defective virus to replicate. Another example is phenotypic mixing, where one virus acquires in its virion the capsid protein or the envelope of another virion. When one virus acquires the envelope of another virus, the phenotypically mixed virion is known as a pseudotype.

Nonproductive infection: The failure of a virus-infected mammalian cell to release progeny virions, usually due to the suppression of late gene expression.

Norwegian scabies: The generalized scaling and crusting skin lesions seen in scabies in immunocompromised patients.

Nosocomial: Disease that is acquired by the patient during hospitalization or as a result of hospitalization.

Nosocomial infections: Infections acquired in the hospital.

Nucleocapsid: The nucleic acid of a virus enclosed in the capsid.

Obligate aerobe: Cell that requires oxygen for growth.

Obligate anaerobe: Cell that requires the absence of oxygen for growth.

Onchosphere: The embryo in the eggs of tapeworms. It possesses six hooks.

Oncogene: A regulatory gene of a mammalian cell that has been integrated into the genome of a retrovirus.

Oocyst: A stage of development in the life cycle of apicomplexans. The mature oocyst contains infectious sporozoites. It is the diagnostic form found in feces in infections with *Cryptosporidium*, *Cyclospora*, and *Isospora*.

Operculum: The lidlike portion of the eggshell of most trematodes and *Diphyllobothrium latum*. The larva hatches from the egg through the opening made by detachment of the operculum.

Ophthalmomyiasis: The involvement of the conjunctiva or other parts of the eye with fly larvae.

Opisthotonus: Spasmic contractions of the back muscles during the pathogenesis of tetanus.

Opportunistic infection: Infectious disease caused by microorganism(s) without major intrinsic virulence factors that takes advantage of a host's immunosuppression or a fortuitous environmental niche.

Osp A and B: Abundant subsurface lipoproteins of *Borrelia burgdorferi*.

Outer membrane: The convoluted, wrinkled, bilayer surface structure of gram-negative bacteria separated from the peptidoglycan layer by a periplasmic space. It is composed essentially of lipoproteins, phospholipids, porins, nonporins, and lipopolysaccharide (LPS).

Parasitism: One organism (the parasite) benefits at the expense of the host.

Paresis: Destruction of the brain parenchyma as the result of *Treponema pallidum* subsp. *pallidum* invasion during the tertiary stage of syphilis.

Passive immunoprophylaxis: See **Immunoprophylaxis.**

Pasteurization: The process whereby milk or milk products are exposed to temperatures for a time that destroys pathogenic and potentially pathogenic nonspore-forming bacteria transmissible by these products without affecting flavor.

Peplomers: Virus-coded glycoproteins inserted onto the virus envelope. Usually appear as projections from the envelope.

Peptidoglycan: A three-dimensional latticework layer of the bacterial cell wall that lies closest to the cytoplasmic membrane and is responsible for bacterial rigidity and shape.

Permissive infection: Opposite of nonproductive infection. See **Nonproductive infection.**

Persistent infection: The persistence of a replicating or nonreplicating infectious agent in the host.

Pharmacokinetics: The study of the concentrations achieved and activities of chemotherapeutic agents in the infected host.

Phenotypic mixing: See **Nongenetic interaction.**

Phialide: A conidiogenous fungal cell that produces enteroblastic conidia.

Phialoconidium: An enteroblastic conidium produced by a conidiogenous fungal cell called a phialide.

Plasmids: Autonomously replicating DNA molecules found in bacteria. They may be transferred from cell to cell.

Platyhelminth: See **Flatworm.**

Plerocercoid: The larval stage of *Diphyllobothrium latum* that is ribbonlike and possesses anterior grooves which become the grooves of the scolex of the adult worm. Plerocercoid larvae of *Spirometra* species cause sparganosis.

Polysaccharide A: A ribitol phosphate teichoic acid cell wall component of *Staphylococcus aureus* that possesses antiphagocytic activity.

Porin: Protein in bacterial cell outer membranes that forms channels that allow passage of substances through the cell wall and acts as attachment site for other substances.

Poroconidium: A holoblastic conidium produced through a pore by a conidiogenous fungal cell.

Postexposure chemoprophylaxis: See **Chemoprophylaxis.**

Postexposure immunoprophylaxis: See **Immunoprophylaxis.**

Postprimary pulmonary (reactivation) tuberculosis: Acquired by endogenous activation of *Mycobacterium tuberculosis* due to a waning acquired CMI resistance and reactivation of quiescent primary foci. The disease is severe and usually limited to the pulmonary tract.

Preexposure chemoprophylaxis: See **Chemoprophylaxis.**

Preexposure immunoprophylaxis: See **Immunoprophylaxis.**

Primary pulmonary (first-infection) tuberculosis: Acquired by children and adults by droplet nuclei mostly from patients infected with *Mycobacterium tuberculo-*

sis. The great majority of patients heal due to the development of an effective CMI response but may still retain organisms. Failure to mount an adequate CMI response results in unrestricted multiplication of the organisms in the lung and dissemination to most tissues resulting in miliary tuberculosis.

Prion: Acronym of "proteinaceous infectious agent."

Prion protein: A glycoprotein with molecular weight of 27 to 30 kd from which infectivity of prions cannot be separated.

Proglottid: The individual segment of a tapeworm. The mature proglottid contains both male and female sex organs. A gravid proglottid contains eggs.

Prokaryote: A cell lacking a membrane-bound nucleus and membrane-bound organelles.

Promastigote: The form of *Leishmania* species found in the sandfly vector and in culture. It is elongate and has a prominent anterior flagellum.

Prophylactic: Activities carried out to prevent development of a disease process.

Protein A: A cell wall component of *Staphylococcus aureus* covalently linked to peptidoglycan and consisting of a single polypeptide chain capable of binding to the Fc portion of IgG and to extracellular matrix glycoprotein. It may contribute to the adherence and antiphagocytic activity.

Protists: Eukaryotic microorganisms.

Proton motive force: Form of energy consisting of a difference in protons and electrical charge across the cytoplasmic membrane.

Protoplast: A shapeless gram-positive bacterium whose cell wall has been removed by lysozyme hydrolysis or inhibition of cell wall synthesis with an antimicrobial agent.

Protoscolex: The precursor to the scolex of an adult *Echinococcus granulosus*. The protoscoleces are found in the brood capsules and possess suckers and hooks.

Provirus: DNA intermediate of retroviral RNA genome that has integrated into host DNA.

Pseudohypha: A string of yeast cells produced by budding.

Pseudopod: The protrusion of cytoplasm (a "false foot") in protozoa is a mechanism for motility.

Pseudotype: See **Nongenetic interaction.**

Ptosis: Droopy eyelids.

Puerperal sepsis: A group A streptococcal disease of the uterine endometrium initiated in a susceptible host during or after delivery of the newborn by droplet nuclei from a case or carrier. Primary disease is characterized by a serosanguinous discharge. Direct extension and/or dissemination may occur.

Purpura: The purple splotchy rash that sometimes develops during meningococcemia.

Pyosin: Toxin produced by some strains or species of bacteria that can lyse cells of other strains or species of bacteria; used in epidemiologic typing schemes.

Pyrogenic (erythrogenic) exotoxins: Three antigenically distinct proteins one or more of which are produced by 95% of the strains of group A streptococci. Each can produce the rash of scarlet fever and exotoxin A is associated with a systemic toxic shocklike syndrome with a high case fatality rate.

Pyuria: Presence of inflammatory cells (polymorphonuclear leukocytes) in the urine; usually indicates presence of a urinary tract infection.

Quinolones: Class of antibiotics bactericidal to aerobic bacteria by inhibiting DNA gyrase activity.

Replicative intermediate: Double-stranded RNA formed during the synthetic phase of the virus replication cycle and serving as a template for the synthesis of RNA virus genome.

Reservoir host: A nonhuman host that can maintain the infection in nature in the absence of human hosts.

Rheumatic fever: A late sequela of group A streptococci occurring mostly among young children one to five weeks after the onset of group A streptococcal pharyngitis caused by any of the serotypes. The mechanism of pathogenesis is thought to be the result of the binding of anti-M protein antibody to cross-reactive epitopes on target tissues such as cardiac tissue.

Ring stage: The first stage of development of malaria parasites in the RBC. It consists of a ring of cytoplasm and a dot of nuclear material surrounding a vacuole.

Risus sardonicus: Sustained contraction of the facial muscles during the pathogenesis of tetanus.

Sabre shins: Damage to the long bones in early congenital syphilis.

Scalded skin syndrome: A disease syndrome caused by *Staphylococcus aureus* that usually occurs in infants and children four years of age or younger, and in the immunocompromised adult. Exfoliative exotoxin release by the organism causes intraepidermal splitting and bullous necrosis of tissue. Dissemination may occur.

Scarlet fever: A group A streptococcal disease characterized by a septic sore throat and a diffuse reddening of the skin with the rash most prominent on the trunk, neck, and extremities. Direct extension and/or dissemination may occur.

Schick test: The intradermal injection of a small amount of diphtheria exotoxin into one forearm and a heated toxin control into the other in order to determine susceptibility vs. immunity to diphtheria as measured by the development or absence of redness and induration. This procedure is used during outbreaks of diphtheria to determine which case contacts are susceptible to the disease and thus in need of immunization.

Schistosome: See **Fluke.**

Schizont: The form of asexual malaria parasite undergoing division in the RBC. The first division of nuclear material is called the early schizont. The mature schizont contains individual merozoites.

Scolex: The attachment organ at the anterior end of tapeworms. It possesses circular suckers or a sucking groove (*Diphyllobothrium*). Some species of tapeworm with circular suckers also have a crown of hooks.

Segmented genome: Viruses whose genomes consist of two or more molecules of nucleic acid.

Self assemblage: The automatic condensation of individual capsid protein molecules into a capsid.

Septic thrombophlebitis: Organisms growing in clot material within a blood vessel are seeded into the bloodstream, resulting in bacteremia. Intravenous catheters may induce endothelial cell damage that predisposes to clot formation.

Septicemia: Adverse host response to presence of bacteria or their products in the bloodstream; usually involves fever and other systemic symptoms.

Seroconversion: The appearance of specific antibodies in the serum against a specific infectious agent during or after infection by the agent.

Serologic marker: Antigens or antibodies in the serum that indicate infection by a specific agent.

Serotype: Same as **Immunotype.**

Sex pili: Hairlike, rigid, protein structures, one to four in number at random sites, originating in the cytoplasmic membrane of predominately gram-negative bacteria. They mediate the conjugation of donor and recipient cells and may participate in DNA transfer.

Slow virus infection: A virus infection characterized by long incubation (in years), insidious onset, relentless progression, and terminating in death.

Sparganum: A synonym for a **Plerocercoid** larva.

Specialized transduction: A type of transduction in which only the host gene adjacent to the phage DNA attachment site is transduced.

Spheroplast: A gram-negative bacterium that has retained some or all of its outer membrane components following lysozyme hydrolysis or inhibition of cell wall synthesis by antimicrobial agents.

Spirochetes: Unicellular, slender, helical-shaped or corkscrewlike, flexible organisms actively motile by virtue of periplasmic flagella that lie in the periplasmic space.

Sporangiophore: A hyphal branch bearing one or more sporangia.

Sporangiospore: A spore borne within a sporangium.

Sporangium: A saclike structure in which spores are produced endogenously.

Sporoblast: A stage of development seen in oocysts of *Isospora.* The spherical sporoblast matures into a sporocyst that contains infectious sporozoites.

Sporocyst: See **Sporoblast.**

Sporozoites: Forms of apicomplexan parasites that penetrate host cells and initiate infection.

Staphylococcal necrotizing colitis: A disease of patients whose normal bowel is altered by antibiotics that permit overgrowth by antibiotic-resistant, enterotoxin-producing strains of *Staphylococcus aureus.* Enterotoxin B damages the intestinal epithelium and produces fever, diarrhea, and abdominal cramps.

Staphylokinase: A fibrinolysin secreted by *Staphylococcus aureus.*

. . . static: A suffix denoting that the action of an antimicrobial agent will inhibit growth but not kill the targeted microbe, such as ''bacteriostatic.''

Stationary phase: Phase following cessation of log phase when cell growth stops.

Sterilization: The destruction or elimination of all microorganisms by physical means.

Streptokinases: Fibrinolysins produced by most strains of group A streptococci. See **Fibrinolysin.**

Streptolysin O: An extracellular, oxygen labile, antigenic protein produced by group A streptococci. The molecule lyses human erythrocytes and can damage or destroy polymorphonuclear leukocytes. Its ability to destroy adjacent cells and tissues contributes to the spread of the organism from local sites.

Streptolysin S: A largely cell membrane-bound, oxygen stable, nonantigenic protein of group A streptococci that lyses human erythrocytes and phagocytic cells by cell-cell contact, and exerts a leukotoxic effect upon polymorphonuclear leukocytes after phagocytosis.

Substrate-level phosphorylation: Formation of ATP from ADP by a kinase linked reaction involving a phosphorylated intermediate of catabolism.

Subvirion: Components of a virion. For example, a subvirion vaccine is a vaccine that contains the immunogenic component of a virus.

Sulfatides: Cell wall glycolipids of *Mycobacterium tuberculosis* and *M. bovis* that interact with polymorphonuclear leukocytes and macrophage lysosomal membranes to prevent their fusion with phagosomes.

Sulfur granules: Lobulated bodies in pus, sputum, or tissue biopsy material of patients with actinomycosis. They are composed of delicate tangled masses of gram-positive filaments of *Actinomyces israelii,* the ends of which are club-shaped.

Superantigen: Substance (protein) elaborated by microorganisms (including viruses) that acts independently as T-cell immune system modulator, stimulating release of cytokines and other immune system effectors.

Superinfection: An infection superimposed on a host that is already having an active infection by another infectious agent.

Symbiosis: In a close association between two organisms, both benefit.

Synergistic nonclostridial anaerobic myonecrosis: Also called "synergistic necrotizing cellulitis," is a destructive infection of the skin and subcutaneous tissues that usually involves mixtures of bacteria including anaerobic bacteria other than clostridia. Gas production in tissue may occur and bacteremia is even more likely.

Tabes: Destruction of the dorsal roots of the spinal cord by *Treponema pallidum* subsp. *pallidum* during the tertiary stage of syphilis.

Taboparesis: Destruction of the brain parenchyma and dorsal roots of the spinal cord by *Treponema pallidum* subsp. *pallidum* during the tertiary stage of syphilis.

Tachyzoite: The rapidly dividing, crescent-shaped form of *Toxoplasma gondii.*

Tapeworm: A ribbonlike helminth (cestode) that has an attachment organ called a scolex and developing segments called proglottids. The adult worm is found in the intestinal tract and larval stages occur in intermediate hosts.

Target organ: An organ in which a virus multiplies preferentially. Primary target refers to the organ in which a virus first multiplies after entry into the host. After multiplication in the primary target, the virus may reach distant organs via the blood lymph or peripheral nerve and multiplies in these distant organs. These distant organs are called secondary target organs.

Teichoic acids: Surface-exposed polymers of ribitol or glycerol phosphate covalently linked to the peptidoglycan of several gram-positive bacteria. They may exhibit antiphagocytic activity as, for example, during the pathogenesis of *Staphylococcus aureus* disease.

Teleomorph: The sexual or perfect state of a fungus.

Temperate phage: A type of bacterial virus that can, alternately, multiply rapidly in the host cell, thereby killing the host cell; or, integrate its genome into the host genome, thereby replicating harmoniously with the host genome.

Thallic: Conidium formation by the transformation of an entire preexistent hyphal element.

Tinea: The medical term for the ringworms. A defining adjective is added to indicate location, e.g., tinea capitis—ringworm of the scalp.

Toxic shock syndrome (TSS): A disease mostly, but not exclusively, of menstruating women that results from the enhancement of growth of TSST-1-producing endogenous *Staphylococcus aureus.* Elaboration of TSST-1 results in chills, fever, hypotension, shock, a sunburnlike macular rash, and subsequent exfoliation of skin on the feet and palms. Dissemination may occur.

Toxoid: An exotoxin whose toxicity but not antigenicity is inactivated by formalin.

Transduction: A process for the introduction of foreign genes into a cell through the use of viruses as vectors.

Transfection: The introduction of nucleic acid molecules into mammalian cells under rigidly controlled experimental conditions. The nucleic acid molecules used in transfection are usually virus genomes. If the transfection results in the release of progeny virions, the nucleic acid is said to be infectious.

Transformation: The acquisition of new heritable characteristic by a cell through the insertion of foreign DNA. In describing heritable change of a mammalian cell, transformation and immortalization are used interchangeably.

Translocation: A change in the location of a gene.

Transposons: Short segments of DNA that can move around within a cell to many positions on the host chromosome or the plasmid.

Trematode: See **Fluke.**

Treponematoses: Chronic inflammatory diseases, primarily of the skin and mucous membrane surfaces, caused by four human pathogens belonging to the genus *Treponema.*

Trismus: Stiffness of the jaw due to the spasmic contraction of the masseter muscle during the pathogenesis of tetanus.

Trophozoite: The motile, feeding form of protozoa.

Tropical splenomegaly: Splenomegaly, hemolytic anemia and lymphocytic infiltrates in hepatic portal triads associated with increased IgM and antimalarial antibodies.

Tropism: Affinity for a cell tissue or organ.

Trypanosome: See **Trypomastigote.**

Trypomastigote: Also called trypanosome. This form of the genus *Trypanosoma* is found in the human host. The organism is elongate. An undulating membrane runs the length of the body and extends as a flagellum from the anterior end.

TSST-1 (toxic shock syndrome toxin-1): An extracellular protein, produced by several strains of *Staphylococcus aureus,* responsible for the clinical manifestations of toxic shock syndrome.

Tubercles: Microscopic granulomas formed during the pathogenesis of tuberculosis. They are composed of central organized aggregations of enlarged macrophages resembling epithelial (''epithelioid'') cells, multinucleated Langhans giant cells (fused macrophage cytoplasm) containing tubercle bacilli, and peripheral lymphocytes, macrophages, and fibroblasts.

Tuberculin skin test: A measure of delayed type hypersensitivity (DTH) as determined by the intradermal injection of a tuberculoprotein of *Mycobacterium tuberculosis* referred to as purified protein derivative (PPD).

Induration of $\geq$ 10 mm after 48 to 72 hours is considered positive and indicates infection with *M. tuberculosis* or *M. bovis* as a result of first exposure and not necessarily disease.

Tuberculoid leprosy: The type of leprosy in which the organisms multiply at the site of entry and invade and colonize Schwann cells. *Mycobacterium leprae* induces helper T lymphocyte, epithelioid cell, and giant cell infiltration of the skin. DTH reactivity and CMI develop and remain vigorous during the course of the disease, accounting for the scarcity or absence of organisms within lesions.

Unconventional virus: As **Prion.**

Undulating membrane: A membrane that is found on the surface of some species of protozoan flagellates. Undulations of the membrane produce movement of the organism.

Variable outer membrane protein (VMP): An immunodominant protein of relapsing fever borreliae thought to account for the several antigenic variations observed within a given host during a single infection. The molecule undergoes changes in molecular weight and protein sequences with each episode of antigenic variation that occurs during the pathogenesis of the disease.

Vector: An arthropod that is responsible for the transmission of infection.

Vertical transmission: Transmission of a virus from one generation to another through the germ cell. Transplacental transmission is not vertical transmission.

Virion: A virus particle that has all its structural components. Also refers to virus in its extracellular phase.

Viroid: A class of infectious agents consisting of small molecules of naked RNA.

Virus inhibitory proteins: Specific proteins formed by host cells upon induction with interferons. The best studied ones are the elF kinase and oligoadenylate synthetase. Both proteins interfere with translation of virus mRNA. See **Interferons.**

Virus receptors: Specific epitopes on cell surface protein that permits the binding of a specific species of virus.

Virusoid: Same as viroid except that, in its extracellular phase, it is encapsidated in the nucleocapsid of a helper virus.

V-W antigens: Plasmid-mediated gene products of *Yersinia pestis, Y. enterocolitica,* and *Y. pseudotuberculosis* coordinately expressed with *Yersinia* outer membrane proteins (YOPs) only at 37°C in the presence of low Ca^{2+} concentration. They contribute to extracellular survival through antiphagocytic activity and to intracellular survival and multiplication within macrophages.

Waterhouse-Friderichsen syndrome: The massive hemorrhage and necrosis of the adrenals sometimes observed in infants during the pathogenesis of meningococcemia.

Winterbottom's sign: Prominent posterior cervical lymphadenopathy in West Africa trypanosomiasis.

Xenodiagnosis: Laboratory-reared, uninfected kissing bugs are used to bite the patient suspected of having Chagas' disease. The bugs are examined one to two months later for the development of *Trypanosoma cruzi* in their intestines.

Yeast: A unicellular fungus that reproduces by budding or by fission.

***Yersinia* outer membrane proteins (YOPs):** Plasmid-mediated gene products of *Yersinia pestis, Y. enterocolitica,* and *Y. pseudotuberculosis* coordinately expressed with F-1 antigen only at 37°C in the presence of low Ca^{2+} concentration. They contribute to extracellular survival through antiphagocytic activity and to intracellular survival and multiplication within macrophages.

Zoopathogenic: A pathogen of animals (including humans) as contrasted to phytopathogenic, a pathogen of plants.

Zoophilic: To grow preferentially on animals other than humans.

Zygomycete: A fungus belonging to the phylum Zygomycota.

Zygospore: A sexual spore produced by the Zygomycetes.

INDEX